The Paleo Approach

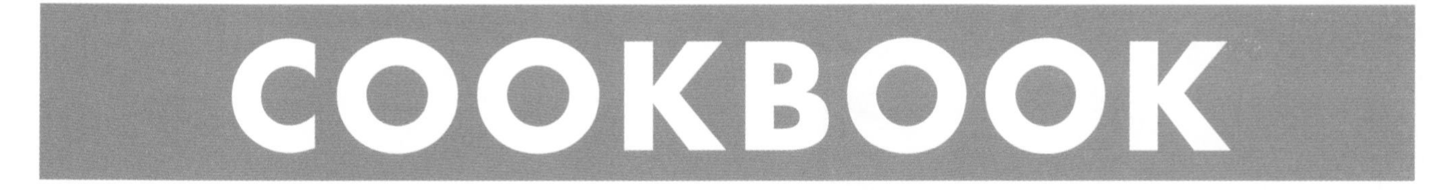

A Detailed Guide to Heal Your Body and Nourish Your Soul

Sarah Ballantyne, PhD
of ThePaleoMom.com

VICTORY BELT PUBLISHING INC.
Las Vegas

First Published in 2014 by Victory Belt Publishing Inc.

ISBN-13: 978-1-628600-08-7

The information included in this book is for educational purposes only. It is not intended nor implied to be a substitute for professional medical advice. The reader should always consult his or her healthcare provider to determine the appropriateness of the information for their own situation or if they have any questions regarding a medical condition or treatment plan. Reading the information in this book does not create a physician-patient relationship.

Printed in the U.S.A.

RRD 0214

Illustrations by Rob Foster

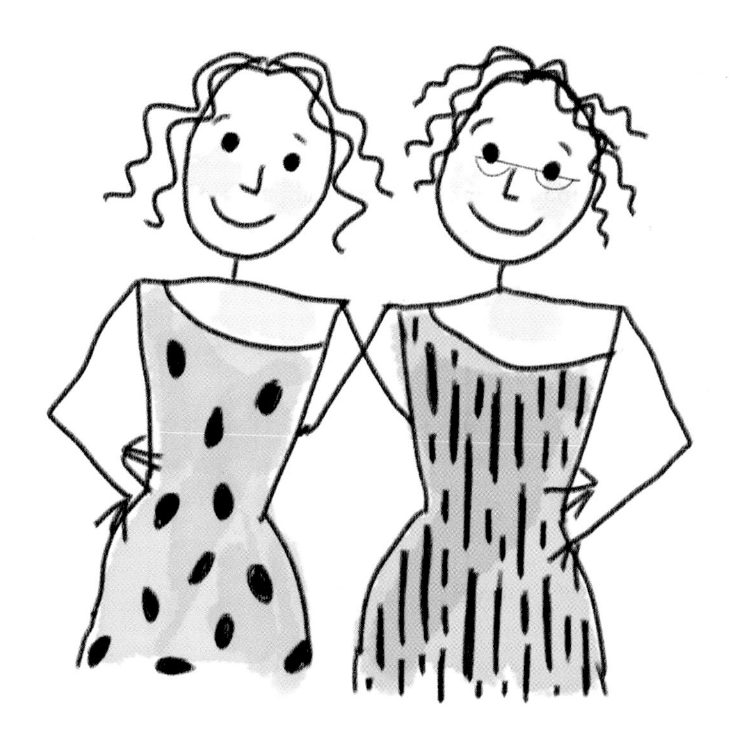

For my mom…

…who taught me how to cook and

nurtured my sense of adventure.

Thanks, Mom.

Table of Contents

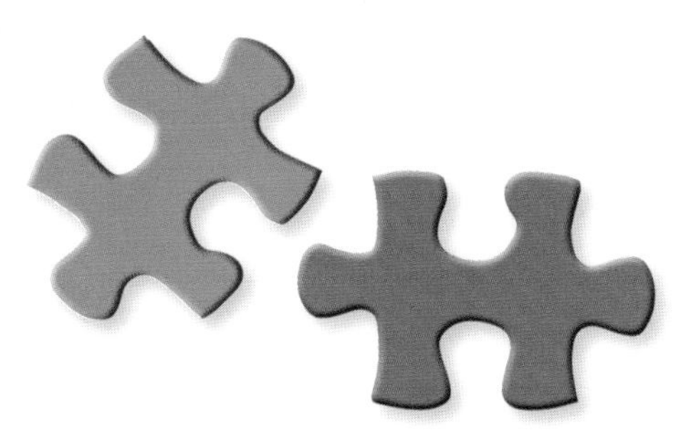

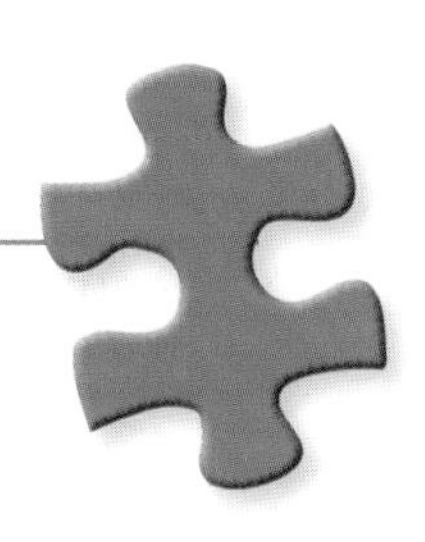

Part 1: The Basics

Chapter 1: The Paleo Approach Basics

Chapter 2: In the Kitchen

Chapter 3: Meal Plans and Shopping Lists

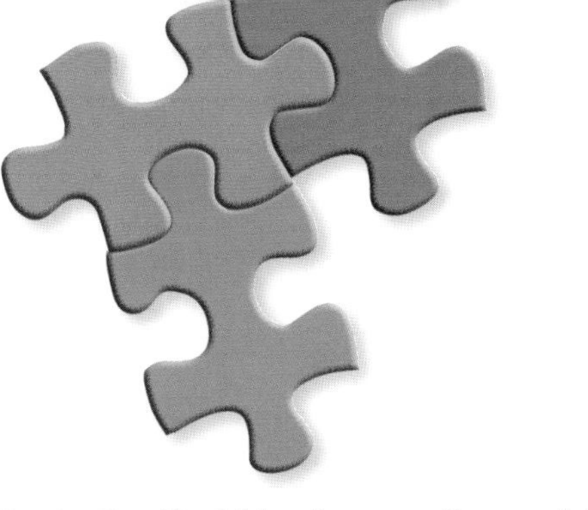
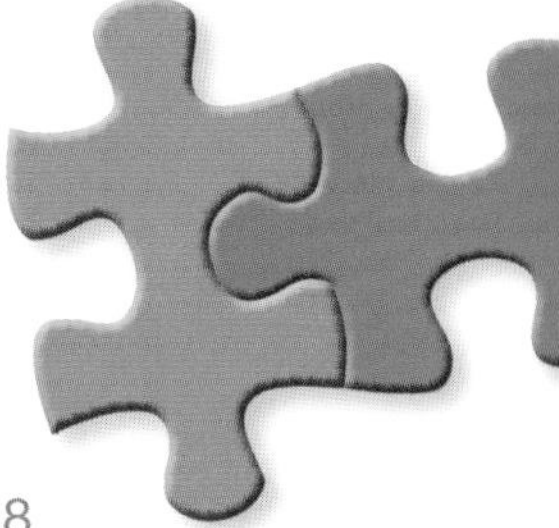

Part 2: The Recipes

Chapter 4: Kitchen Staples

Chapter 5: Breakfast Foods

Chapter 6: Appetizers, Salads, and Snacks

Chapter 7: Soups and Stews

Chapter 8: Meat and Poultry

Chapter 9: Fish and Shellfish

Chapter 10: Offal

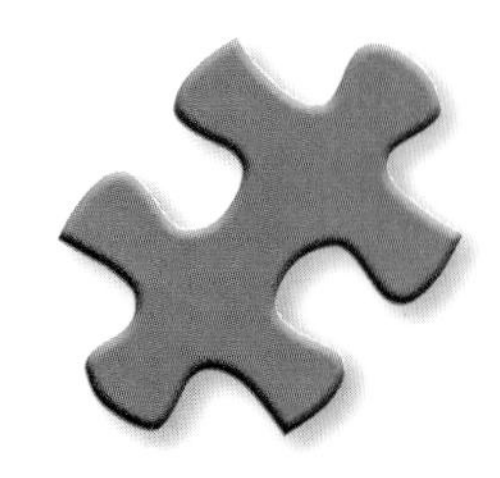

Chapter 11: Side Dishes

Chapter 12: Sweet Treats and Beverages

Resources

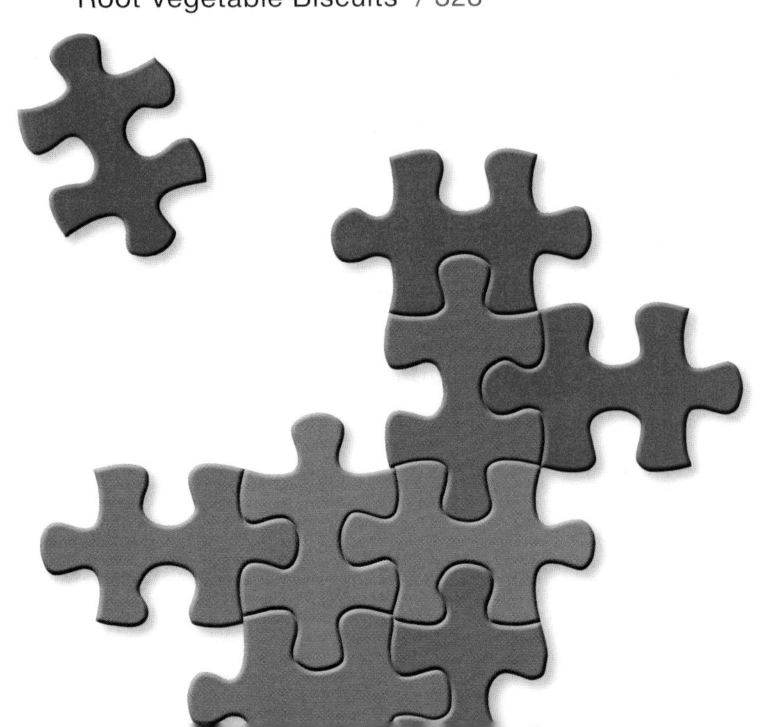

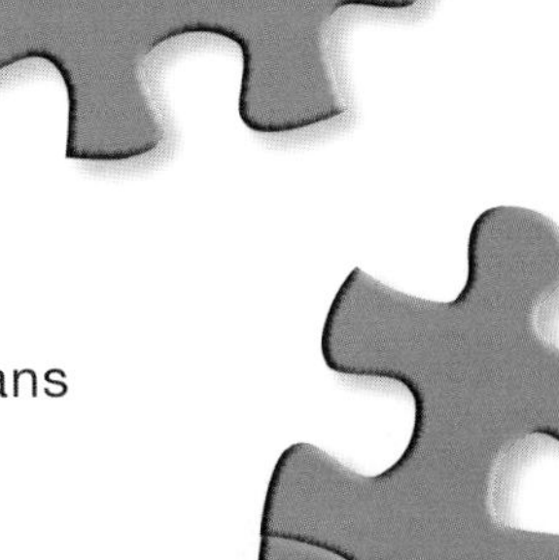

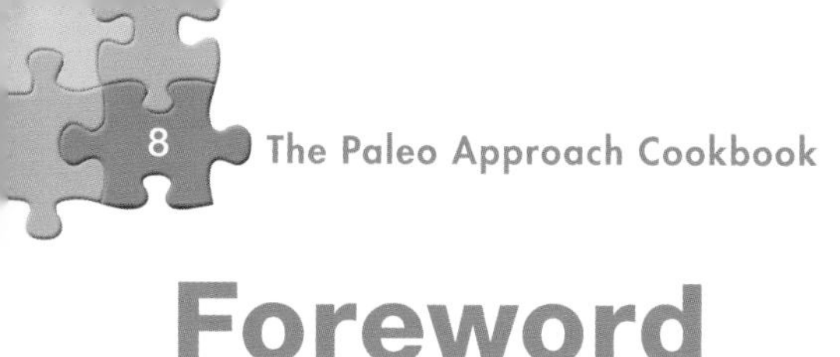

Foreword

Every day we choose what we will eat, and those choices can profoundly affect the course of health, energy, and vitality. Yet many Americans never learned that their choices at the table (or at the fast food counter) impact their very cells, even turning on and off genes that could determine future catastrophic health issues, from autoimmune disease and cancer to heart disease and diabetes. Furthermore, as the food industry has manipulated us to choose foods designed to induce overconsumption at the expense of health, we have surrendered our choices to corporate America. Very few Americans cook most of their meals anymore, and the result has been disastrous for our families and our country, as we shift our own genes toward more disease susceptibility, and pass those genes along to our children and our grandchildren.

I have learned this firsthand. In 2000, I was diagnosed with relapsing-remitting multiple sclerosis (MS). I went to the Cleveland Clinic and dutifully took the latest drugs. I was a doctor, so I believed I should do what the doctors told me to do. Still, within three years, my disease had transitioned to secondary progressive MS, the stage at which there are no more remissions or improvements. I took the recommended chemotherapy, got the tilt/recline wheelchair, and even took the "miracle drug" Tysabri, but continued to slowly decline. That is when I began reading the science myself, searching for what I could do to slow what looked like an inevitable slide into a bedridden life. I switched to the Paleo diet and began adding vitamins and supplements. Then I discovered Functional Medicine in 2007 and made additional refinements to my diet and supplement regimen. That is when the magic began to happen. Within three months of starting the new program, my fatigue was gone. At six months, I could walk without a cane, and at one year, I completed an 18-mile bicycle tour with my family.

Now I know how important it is that every bite sustain and nourish me rather than tear my system down. Cooking real whole food the human body is designed to eat is the only really effective and long-term strategy for reversing the trend of declining health. We need to take back our food supply and start cooking again.

Sarah Ballantyne and I have a lot in common. We are both research scientists, and we both suffered for years from autoimmune conditions. She and I also share a deep respect for one another's work and contributions teaching the public and our medical communities about addressing the environmental factors that can turn genes on or off—genes that can trigger disease or support health. We both responded to our illnesses by delving deeply into science for answers in order to recover, and we both eventually discovered Functional Medicine and the Paleo community. We were also both successfully able to restore our own health and vitality.

Our messages are remarkably similar, and it boils down to this: Food is absolutely critical. Instead of eating 150 pounds of sugar per person per year, instead of eating processed inflammatory fats and diets heavy in wheat, corn, soy, and dairy (and their many by-products—the primary ingredients in most processed foods), we need to eat real food—food that is filled with the vitamins, minerals, essential fats, and antioxidants that our cells need to do the chemistry of life properly. We need to eat food our bodies recognize, food that our bodies are designed to understand and utilize. Another thing Sarah and I have in common is our enthusiastic emphasis on micronutrient density. Too many people read a few lines about the Paleo diet and just eat a lot of meat, but true health goes far beyond meat. It involves eating a lot more vegetables in a wide variety and choosing more foods frequently off the menu, like organ meats and seaweed.

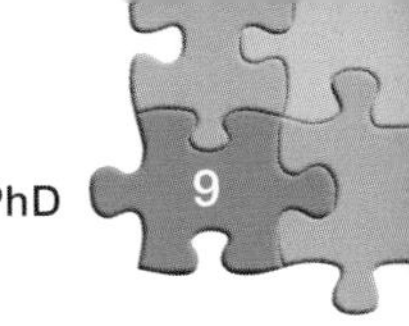

It all starts with cooking, and in this book, Sarah shows you exactly how to start, even if you've never attempted anything complicated in the kitchen. One of the things I love about this book is the long lists of foodstuffs for people to consider—foods that many of us never thought about eating, because the American diet is so limited in its range and variety. She stresses diversity, and also tells you how to use all those "strange" new foods. The book is encyclopedic in its explanation of cooking techniques, with step-by-step guidance for those who have forgotten or never were trained in cooking. Some of the dishes are quite simple, others more complex and time-consuming. People can choose the level of complexity and challenge they desire. The point is that they will be cooking again. For those who need help with ideas and how to begin, this is a very good start.

As you work through this book and transform your choices and your lifestyle, you will discover that your energy and moods will go up and your pain and fatigue will go down. You will learn how to engage your children in both cooking and eating for health. You will get your life back, and the lives of everyone you cook for, too. This is the power of the Paleo Approach, and this is a book to guide you.

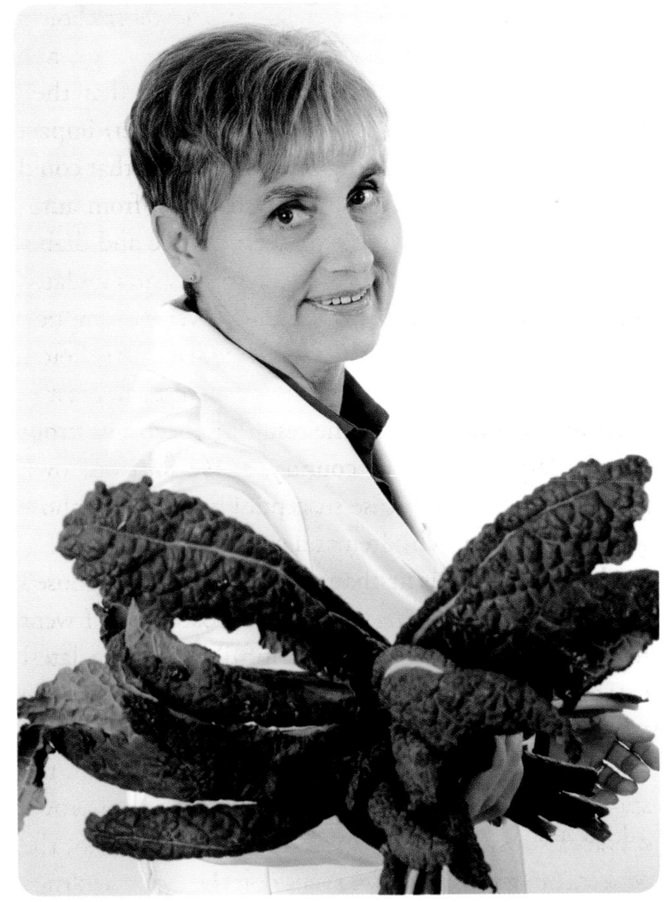

Photo credit: Jonathan D. Sabin

Terry Wahls, MD
Clinical Professor of Medicine, University of Iowa
Author of *The Wahls Protocol: How I Beat Progressive Multiple Sclerosis Using Paleo Principles and Functional Medicine*

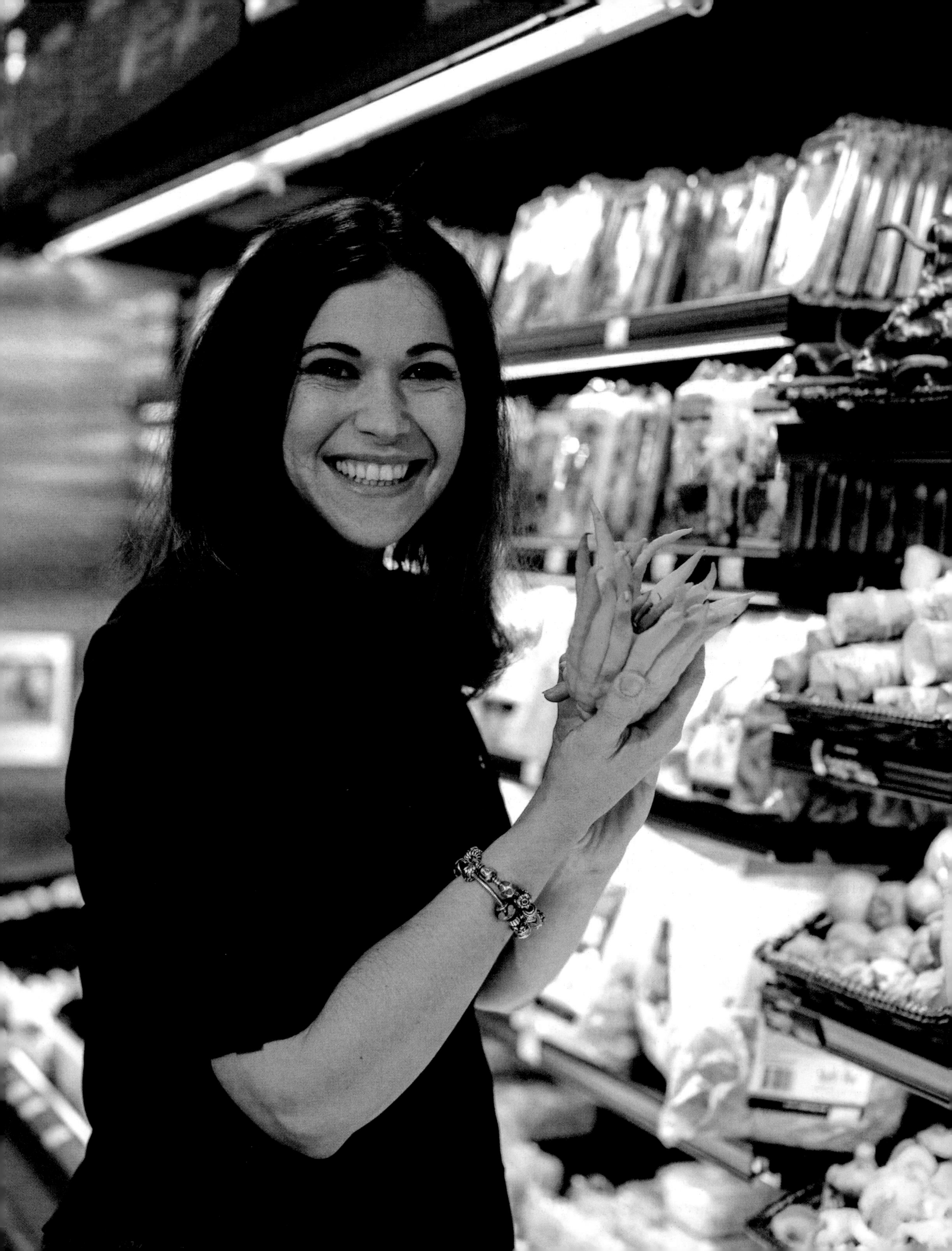

Preface: My Love of "Weird Stuff"

I love food. I have always loved food, and I will always love food. I also love to cook. I enjoy preparing food—whether it is an involved gourmet dish or a simple comfort food—and I use delicious meals as a way to show my love for my family and friends.

I used to be morbidly obese and extremely unhealthy, suffering not only from metabolic syndrome but also from more than a dozen immune- and autoimmune-related health conditions. Learning how to heal my body through healthful food choices was just as much about learning how to cook new foods in new ways as it was about learning what to eat and why.

I am naturally adventurous in both the foods I eat and the foods I prepare at home. When I was a kid, my grandparents would treat us to meals at ethnic restaurants for family gatherings. From a very early age, I associated fun, laughter, and the novelty of restaurants (which we never went to otherwise) with new and unique foods. Being adventurous with food earned you a badge of honor in my family. My uncles would dare my brothers, cousins, and me to eat the strangest foods on the menu. We would fight over who would get to eat the eyeballs from the whole fish at a Chinese restaurant, not because anyone particularly enjoyed them (although I thought they were tasty enough) but because of the status associated with being the kid who wasn't afraid to pop a whole eyeball into her mouth.

That doesn't mean I always enjoyed novel foods. I remember my first introduction to sushi. I just couldn't get over the texture and decided I didn't like it. When we had a second family gathering at a sushi restaurant a couple of months later, I reluctantly tried it again. This time, I knew what to expect from a textural standpoint, so I was able to notice the flavor—and I discovered that I loved it. Sushi became one of my favorite foods, and I vowed always to try something new twice, a philosophy that I continue to live by today in every aspect of my life.

Now, I geek out over unusual vegetables and new cuts of pasture-raised meat at my local farmer's market. I love it when my local Whole Foods imports exotic fruits, vegetables, herbs, and seafood. I have a rule: if I've never seen it before, I buy it. Being unafraid of new foods (or trying them even if I am a little afraid!) has enabled me not only to discover new favorites but also to provide my body with such a diversity of nutrition that I now feel and look better than I ever have in my adult life.

Just because some (okay, many) foods are excluded from the Paleo Approach doesn't mean that what you do eat needs to be bland, boring, or repetitive. You can make so many delicious, fulfilling meals with healthful foods that promote healing and help regulate your immune system. You don't need to feel deprived. You can still get joy out of food.

The recipes included in this book involve a broad spectrum of different ingredients, flavors, price points, and time commitments. Some meals are designed to provide you with several days' worth of leftovers. Other meals are designed to be quick to prepare on busy weeknights. Others are designed to deliver sophisticated flavor or make organ meat more palatable to you. These recipes will get you started in the kitchen and help make eating in this new way simpler and more approachable. And they'll show you just how delicious this way of eating can be! As you become more comfortable with new ingredients, new flavors, and new cooking methods, you may want to branch out and experiment—and that's great! Most of the recipes in this book include suggestions for variations so that you can be inspired to launch into new culinary directions in your kitchen every time you cook.

My journey toward health involved redefining what healthful food is, but it did not involve sacrificing flavor or enjoyment from food. And that is what this cookbook is all about: how to heal your body and love every bite.

> *The discovery of a new dish does more for human happiness than the discovery of a new star.*
>
> —Jean Anthelme Brillat-Savarin
> French lawyer and politician, 1755–1826

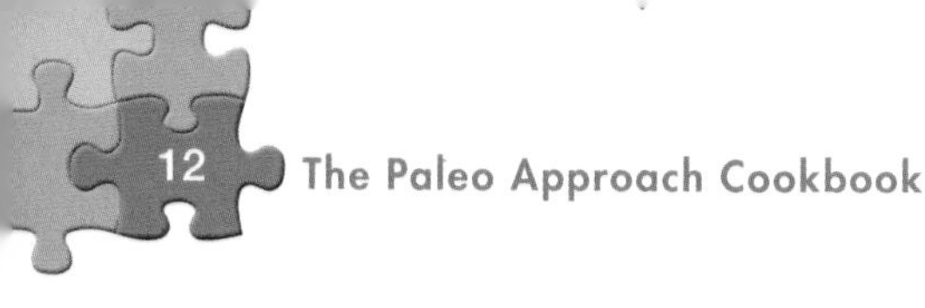

Acknowledgments

One of my earliest memories is of sitting on the floor under the kitchen table and watching my mom cook dinner while dancing and singing aloud to the radio. It's a memory I think of often because it is the heart of how I approach cooking. My mom taught me to cook by recruiting me to be her "helper" from a very young age; I always enjoyed cooking with her. Not only did she lay the foundation of kitchen skills that eventually matured into the ability to write this book, but she also taught me to have fun in the kitchen. And I would argue that fun is even more important than proficiency with a knife or good instincts with spices. Thanks, Mom.

This book would not exist without the support, encouragement, unconditional love, and commitment from my amazing husband, David. In early summer 2013, while buried in the massive undertaking that was *The Paleo Approach,* I turned to David and said, "I think I'm writing two books." When the decision was made to divide my originally overly ambitious project into a guidebook and a companion cookbook, the person most impacted was David, who found himself doing double duty for nearly a year longer than he had originally signed up for. He rose to the challenge of not only being the breadwinner with his own career, but also doing the lion's share of the housework and being responsible for remembering which days were school pajama days and getting the kids to swimming lessons on time.

My two beautiful and precocious daughters, Adele and Mira, provide me with so much inspiration, both personally and professionally. They also give honest feedback on the meals I create, and their enthusiasm (or lack thereof) greatly influenced the recipes in this cookbook (and the ones left out). And, of course, their antics make being in the kitchen fun.

I owe a debt of gratitude to my two assistants, Tamar England and Christina Feindel, not only for taking on various tasks associated with writing this book, but also for generally keeping ThePaleoMom.com and the associated social media active and flourishing. Their dedicated support is the reason I had any time at all to focus on writing this book.

I also want to thank Anne Angelone, Angie Alt, Amy Kubal, and Mickey Trescott for supporting me throughout this project. Beyond being core members of the Paleo autoimmune community, these talented professionals are the heart of ThePaleoMom Consulting, giving my readers and followers a means for getting expert one-on-one support for their health journeys, a service that is desperately needed but that I cannot provide myself.

The skills of some very talented people are on display in this book. I often say, "Everyone should have a Dawn," because Dawn Brewer (DawnBrewerPhotography.com) is one of the most brilliant photographers I've ever met. Beyond just plain ol' making me look good, Dawn has been a wonderful companion during so many fun days of shopping, visiting local farms, and cooking. Everyone should have someone in her life who both makes her look good and is just fun to be with. I was also fortunate to be introduced to Brian Grayson of Ink & Iron Garage. Brian has an amazing eye for design and beautiful wood, and his tables are on display in many of this book's photos.

I am passionate about supporting local farmers and sourcing high-quality, nutrient-dense foods. What's amazing is just how supportive my local farmers have been in return. Thank you to Bray Family Farm, Fry Farm, Owl Pine Farm, and TaylOrganic Farm, whose vegetables, fruits, meats, and faces are littered throughout this book. I also want to thank the Sandy Springs Farmer's Market for supporting our local farmers and other producers of high-quality foods (and for introducing me to them!). The high-quality products from Bos Creek Meats, GrassFed Traditions, Tendergrass Farms, Tropical Traditions, and US Wellness Meats are likewise heavily featured throughout this book. I also want to thank Whole Foods Merchants Walk, who truly have become like family to me and whose foods and faces can also be found throughout this book. Everyone should be so lucky as to be able to walk into her local grocery store and hug the fishmonger, butcher, produce manager, and store manager. It may slow down my shopping, but it makes food shopping one of the social highlights of my week!

My journey into the Paleo sphere, from amateur blogger to author and expert, was supported and guided by some pretty spectacular people. Thank you to George Bryant for showing me how to use a camera. Thank you to Stacy Toth and Matt McCarry for, well, everything and more! Thank you to Mira and Jayson Calton, Loren Cordain, Melissa Hartwig, Paul Jaminet, Chris Kresser, Diane Sanfilippo, Terry Wahls, Robb Wolf, and Liz Wolfe for welcoming me into the fold and providing so much support and advice and just generally geeking out with me.

Once again, it astounds me how much goes into a book beyond my ideas, words, and photographs. I can't begin to properly thank Erich Krauss, Michele Farrington, and all the amazing and talented people at Victory Belt Publishing for taking my efforts and turning them into a book!

I am also thankful for my supportive family, friends, and community. So many people contributed to this book in small ways, whether by testing recipes, watching my kids, or just offering words of encouragement. Special thanks to Noreen Ballantyne, Sandy and Cheryl Groulx, the McCarter clan, the Andrews family, Andrew Ballantyne, Jamie Anthony, René Groulx, Donny and Rachelle Groulx, Rachael Blaske, Kelly Posada, Rebecca Blaske, the Cochrans, the Kipps, the Goldberg family, the Kiesel family, the East Cobb YMCA, CrossFit Dwala, Red Door Playhouse, Rhythm Dance Centre, Mrs. Adams, Mrs. Baker, Mrs. Amsterdam, Mrs. Smart, the England family, the Brewer family, Kathryn and Michael Althauser, the Marraccini family, Dr. Flowers, Shelley Jordan, Misty Croft, Katherine Morrison, Dr. Hurt, Jason Sirotin, Debbie Bethea, Pam Chanin, Paula Coplon, Randi Dymkowski, Juan Esparza, Debbie Isbitts, Esti Klienman, Eileen Laird, Katherine Morrison, Elizabeth Ogletree, Erica Stein, Karen Stevenson, Jolaine Wiens, and all the other amazing people in my life and my children's lives.

Finally, I want to acknowledge the tremendous support and enthusiasm I've received from so many devoted blog readers and podcast listeners. Connecting with you through social media, the blog, e-mail, and the podcast has been an amazing and rewarding experience. Many of your questions and comments guided the structure and content of this book. And helping you has motivated me throughout the last two intense years of writing two essential resources for the autoimmune disease community.

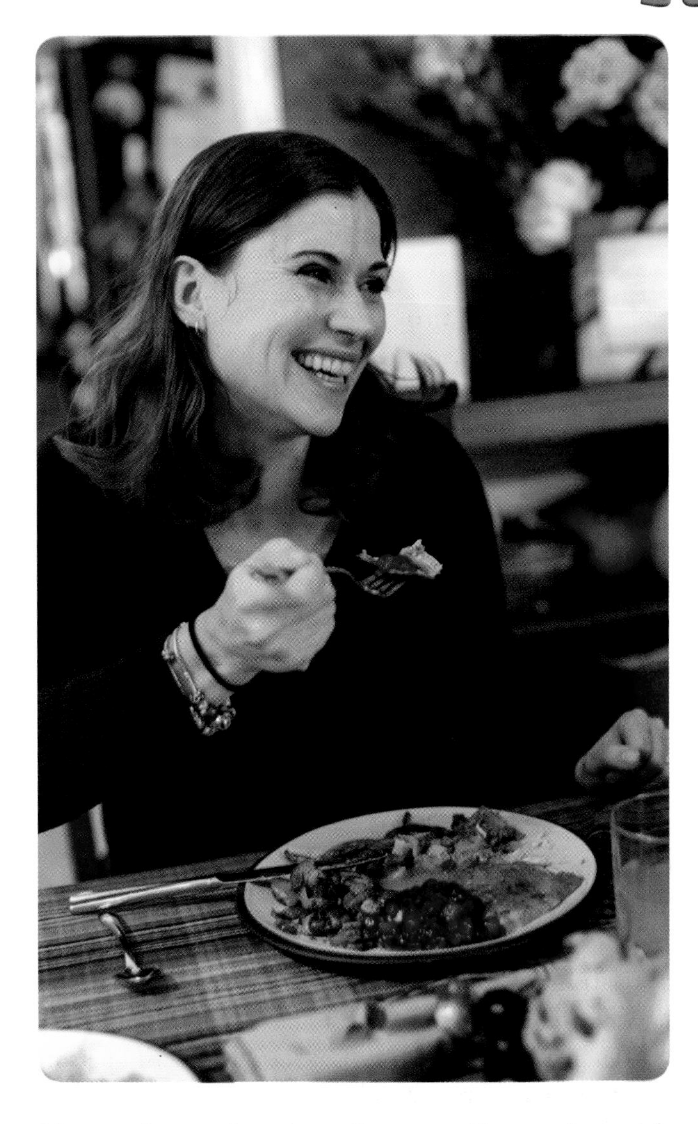

> *Dining with one's friends and beloved family is certainly one of life's primal and most innocent delights, one that is both soul-satisfying and eternal.*
>
> —Julia Child

Introduction

Autoimmune disease is an epidemic in our society, affecting an estimated 50 million Americans. But it doesn't have to be. Although genetic predisposition accounts for approximately one-third of your risk of developing an autoimmune disease, the other two-thirds comes from your environment, your diet, and your lifestyle. In fact, experts are increasingly recognizing that certain dietary factors are key contributors to autoimmune disease, placing these autoimmune conditions in the same class of diet- and lifestyle-related diseases as type 2 diabetes, cardiovascular disease, and obesity. This means that autoimmune disease is directly linked to your food choices and how you decide to live your life. It also means that you can manage and reverse autoimmune disease simply by changing how you eat and making more informed choices about sleep, activity, and stress . . . and that's some pretty darned good news!

There are more than 100 confirmed autoimmune diseases and many more diseases that are suspected of having autoimmune origins. The root cause of all autoimmune diseases is the same: our immune system, which is supposed to protect us from invading microorganisms, turns against us and attacks our proteins, cells, and tissues instead. Which proteins, cells, and tissues are attacked determines the autoimmune disease and its symptoms. The Paleo Approach is a powerful strategy that uses diet and lifestyle to regulate the immune system, putting an end to these attacks and giving the body the opportunity to heal.

The Paleo Approach works by addressing four key areas known to be important contributors to immune and autoimmune diseases. Drawing on insights gleaned from more than 1,200 scientific studies, these diet and lifestyle recommendations specifically target:

1. **Nutrient density.** The immune system (and indeed every system in the body) requires an array of vitamins, minerals, antioxidants, essential fatty acids, and amino acids to function normally. Micronutrient deficiencies and imbalances are key players in the development and progression of autoimmune disease. Focusing on consuming the most nutrient-dense foods available enables a synergistic surplus of micronutrients to correct both deficiencies and imbalances, thus supporting regulation of the immune system, hormone systems, detoxification systems, and neurotransmitter production. A nutrient-dense diet further provides the building blocks that the body needs to heal damaged tissues.
2. **Gut health.** Gut dysbiosis and leaky gut are key facilitators in the development of autoimmune disease. The foods recommended on the Paleo Approach support the growth of healthy levels and a healthy variety of gut microorganisms. Foods that irritate or damage the lining of the gut are avoided, while foods that help restore gut barrier function and promote healing are endorsed.

How Many People Suffer from Autoimmune Diseases?

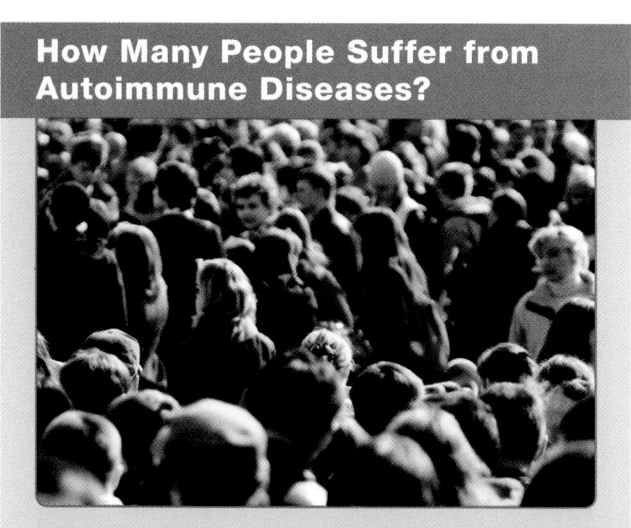

The National Institutes of Health used epidemiological studies pertaining to only 24 of the 100-plus autoimmune diseases to estimate that 23.5 million Americans have an autoimmune disease.

The American Autoimmune Related Diseases Association (AARDA) estimates that autoimmune disease has been diagnosed in 50 million Americans. AARDA used epidemiological studies, combined with individual patient group data, to show that approximately 20 percent of Americans are affected by autoimmune disease—that's about 63 million people!

Whether the true number of Americans who have an autoimmune disease is 23.5 million or 63 million, it's still way too many of us.

3. **Hormone regulation.** What we eat, when we eat, and how much we eat affect a variety of hormones that interact with the immune system. When dietary factors (like eating too much sugar or grazing rather than eating larger meals spaced farther apart) dysregulate these hormones, the immune system is directly affected (typically stimulated). The Paleo Approach diet is designed to promote regulation of these hormones, thereby regulating the immune system by proxy. These and other essential hormones that impact the immune system are also profoundly affected by how much sleep we get, how much time we spend outside, how much and what kinds of activity we get, and how well we reduce and manage stress.

4. **Immune system regulation.** Immune regulation is achieved by restoring a healthy diversity and healthy amounts of gut microorganisms, restoring the barrier function of the gut, providing sufficient amounts of the micronutrients required for the immune system to function normally, and regulating the key hormones that in turn regulate the immune system.

As you adopt the Paleo Approach, your food choices become focused on consuming the nutrients to support this healing—foods that provide everything your body needs to stop attacking itself, repair damaged tissues, and get healthy again: proteins, carbohydrates, and fats to sustain a normal metabolism, build new tissue, and produce hormones, important proteins, and signaling molecules; and the full range of fat-soluble vitamins, water-soluble vitamins, minerals, and antioxidants to get rid of inflammation, regulate the immune system, and support the normal functioning of all the body's systems.

This book is a companion cookbook to my first book, *The Paleo Approach. The Paleo Approach* explains in detail the scientific rationale behind each facet of the Paleo Approach diet and lifestyle. If you want to understand why it's important to avoid certain foods and eat more of others, you will not find that information here. Likewise, if you want to understand why changing your diet works or what to prioritize; if you need help with additional food sensitivities or troubleshooting; if you need guidance on which medical tests to have done, which medications to take or discontinue, how to navigate the complex world of supplements, or how to work with your doctor; or if you are keen to understand which foods you can reintroduce when, *The Paleo Approach* has the answers.

This cookbook assumes that you're sold on the Paleo Approach diet and you just need some help with the day-to-day implementation; some inspiration in the kitchen; and some quick reference guides to keep you organized. If you aren't interested in (or have already read about) *The Whys*, this book still sets forth *The Rules*. Summary guides and food lists are included here so that you don't need to run to your bedside table (or wherever you keep your copy of *The Paleo Approach*) every time you have a question about whether a food is okay to eat. Meal plans and shopping lists take the guesswork out of what to eat and help you prepare for the week ahead. Most important, this cookbook shows you how to put together delicious meals that comply with the Paleo Approach diet so that you can enjoy your food while you heal your body.

> *Leave your drugs in the chemist pot if you can heal the patient with food.*
> —Hippocrates

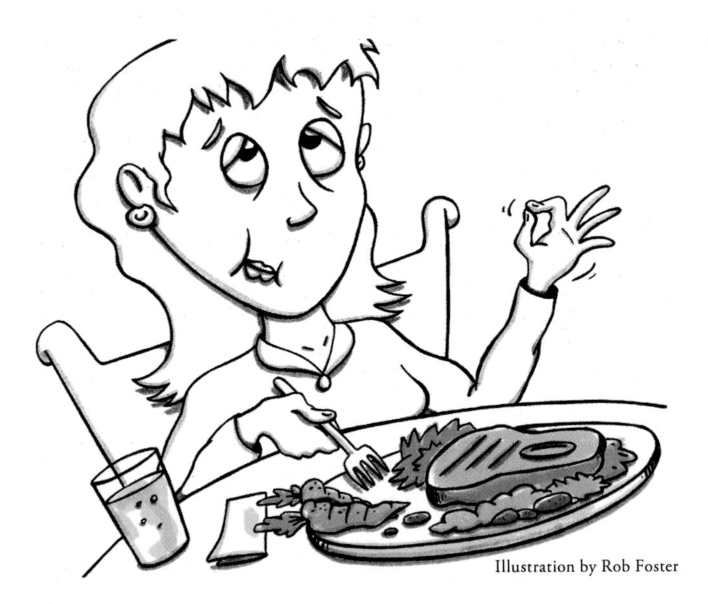

Illustration by Rob Foster

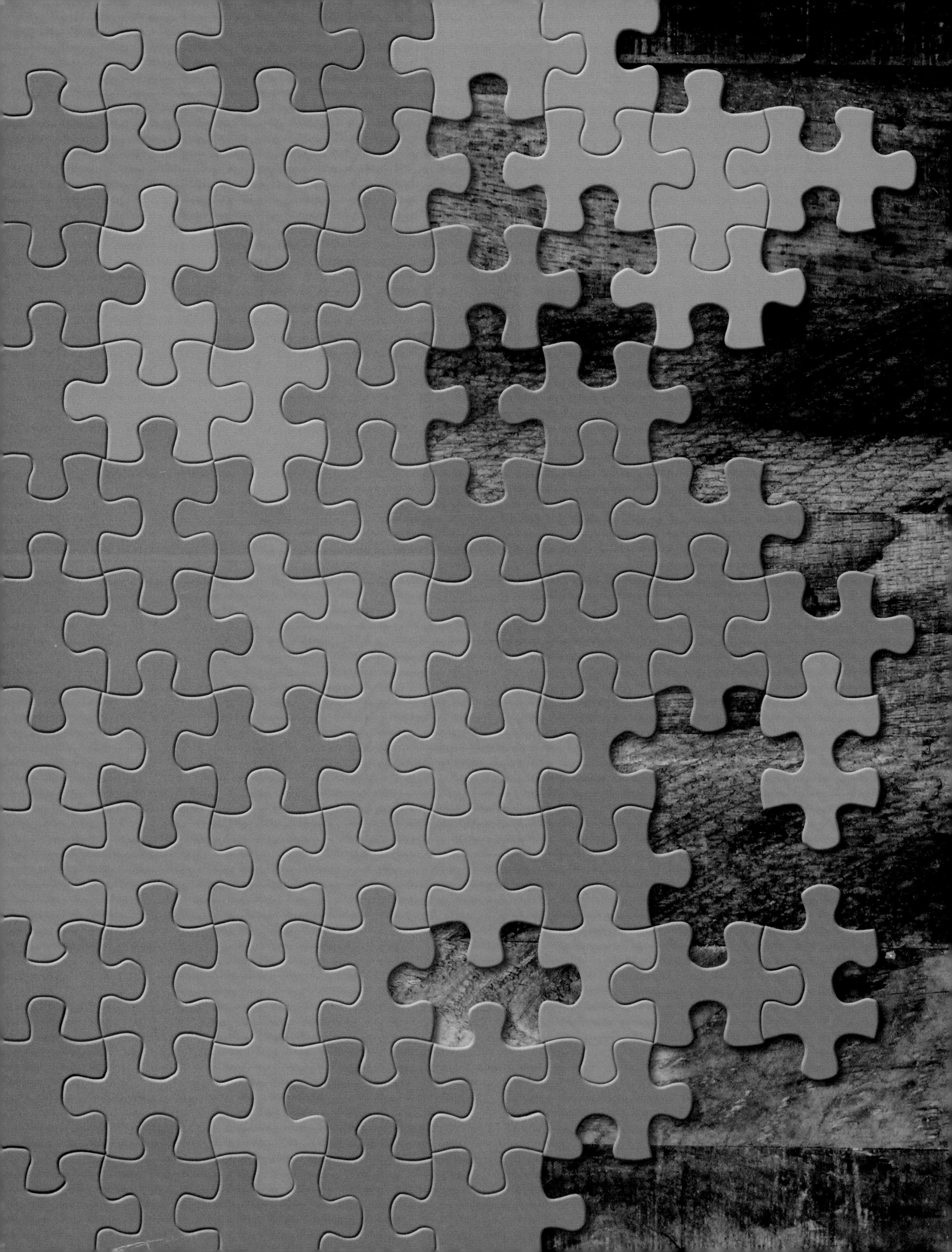

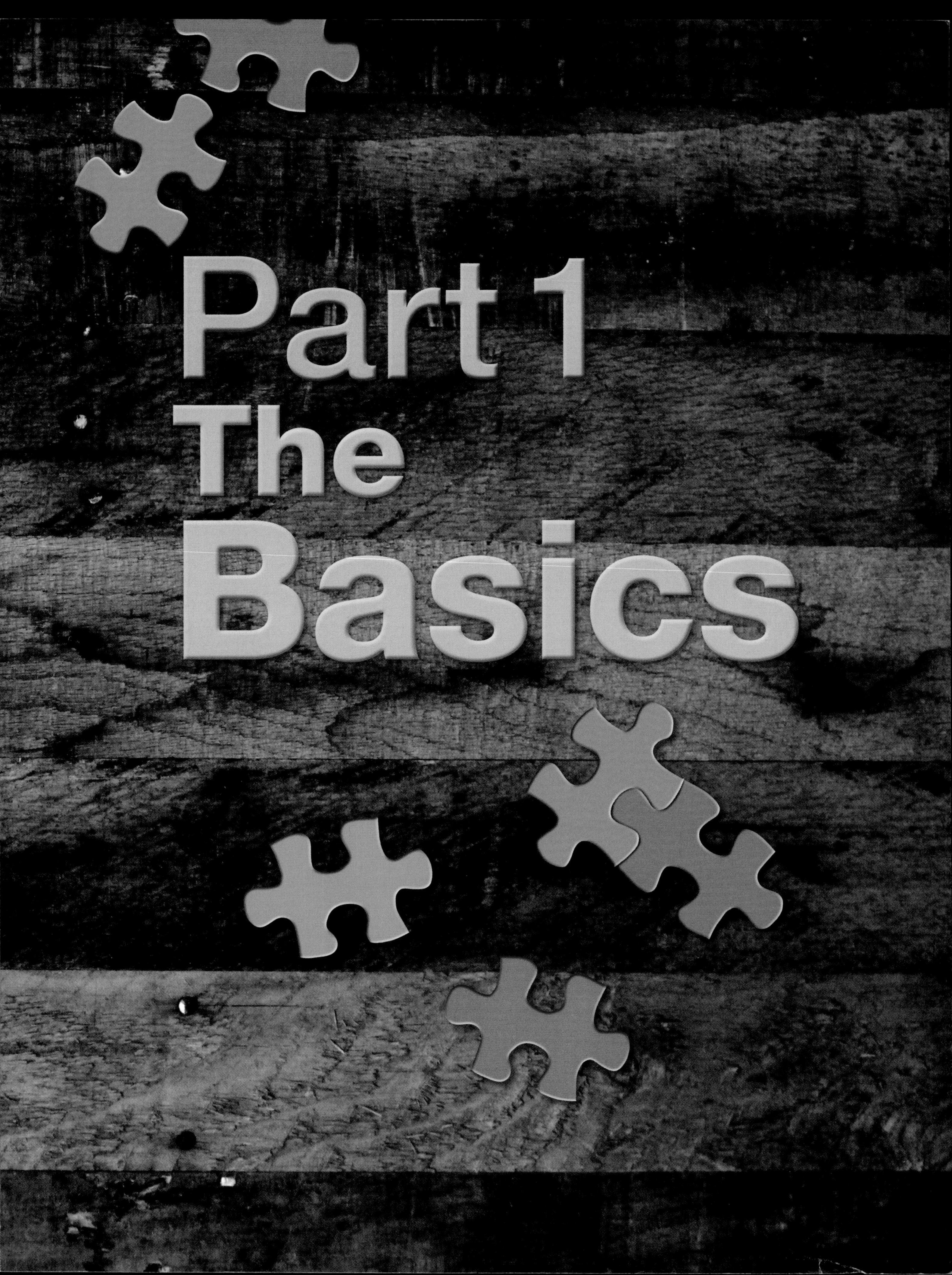

Part 1 The Basics

Chapter 1

The Paleo Approach Basics

Following the Paleo Approach diet involves increasing your intake of nutrient-dense, health-promoting foods while avoiding foods that may be triggers for your disease. In summary, the rules of what to eat are:

- ☑ Eat meat (including offal), poultry, fish, and shellfish.
- ☑ Eat plenty of vegetables and some fruit.
- ☑ Use quality fats for cooking and dressing your food.
- ☑ Source the best-quality ingredients you can.
- ☑ Eat as much variety as possible.

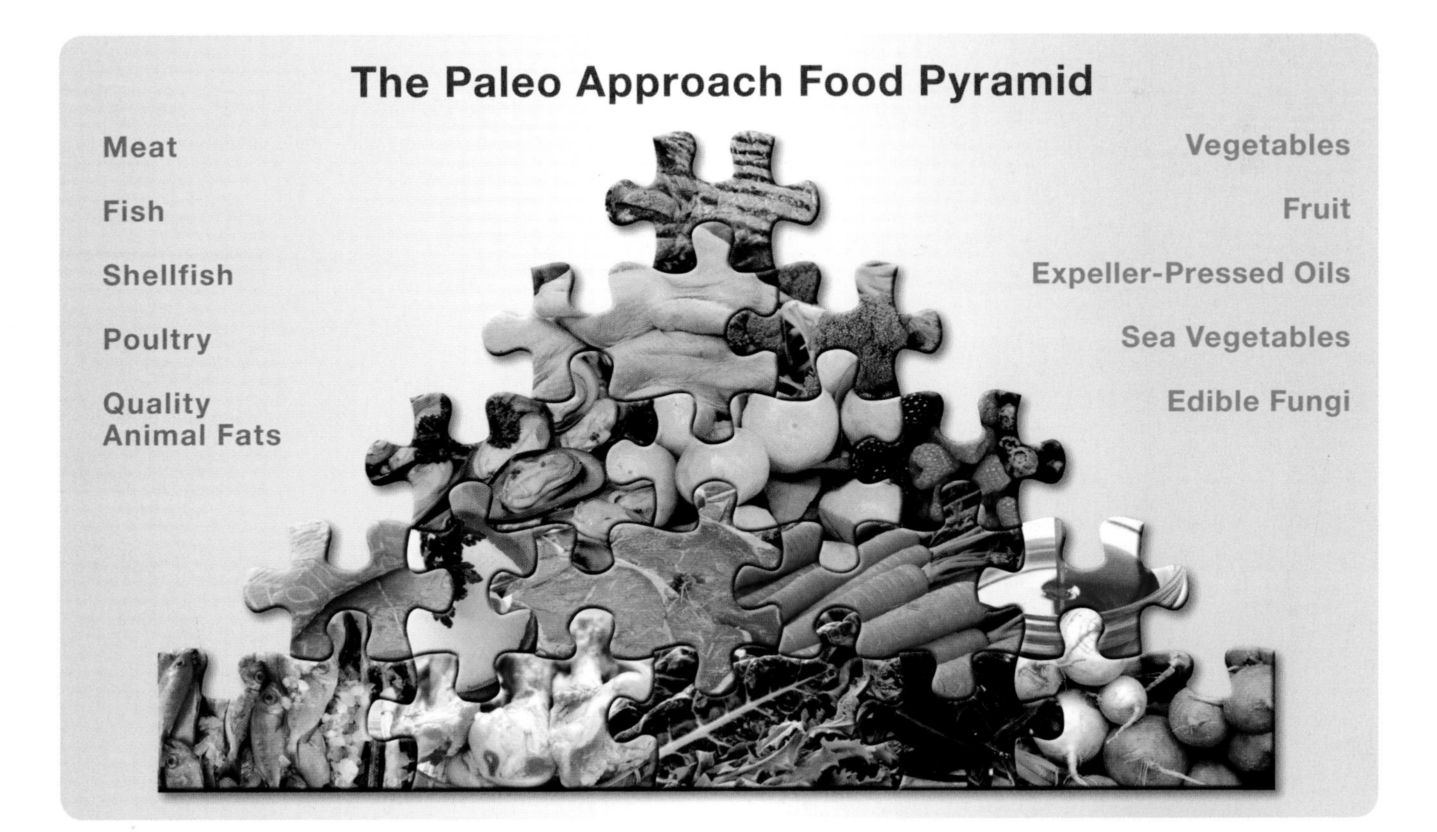

☒ Remove the following from your diet:

- Grains
- Legumes
- Dairy
- Refined and processed sugars and oils
- Nuts and seeds (including pseudograins, chocolate, and coffee)
- Nightshades
- Eggs
- Alcohol

! Moderate your intake of the following:

- Fructose (from fruits and starchy vegetables, aiming for between 10 and 20 grams per day)
- Salt (using only unrefined salt such as Himalayan pink salt or Celtic gray salt)
- Moderate- and high-glycemic-load fruits and vegetables (such as dried fruit, plantain, and taro root)
- Omega-6 polyunsaturated fatty acid–rich foods (such as poultry and fatty cuts of industrially produced meat)
- Black and green tea, and yerba mate
- Coconut

You may have noticed that I highlighted the simplicity of the *What to Eat* guidelines, while I tried to deemphasize the "no" foods and the "a little bit is okay" foods. Even after reading those short lists of what not to eat and what to moderate, you still might feel overwhelmed by the number of foods omitted from the Paleo Approach diet. But I don't want you to focus on what you can't eat. This book isn't about that. This book is about what you *can* eat—those delicious, nutrient-dense, comforting, and satisfying foods that will make you healthier.

You can enjoy an enormous wealth of meats, seafood, vegetables, fruits, quality fats, herbs, and spices that will provide the nutrition your body needs to regulate your immune system and heal itself. When you see the diversity of foods you get to eat—foods that foster health—you will quickly see that you don't need to be bored with your meals or feel limited by your choices. Mouthwatering, scrumptious meals that will make your taste buds dance with joy can be made with these foods. You won't be limited to bland, repetitive flavors (unless, of course, you like it that way).

If you need a more detailed list of what to avoid (and, in the case of certain ingredients, like gluten, dairy, soy, and corn, how to avoid them), you can find that information on page 29 and pages 368 to 371. Also, for quick reference, foods are listed in alphabetical order and labeled as to whether or not they are included in the Paleo Approach plan in the Resources section, starting on page 376. But let's not perseverate on the don'ts. Instead, I want to talk about the rich assortment of foods that will find their way onto your plate.

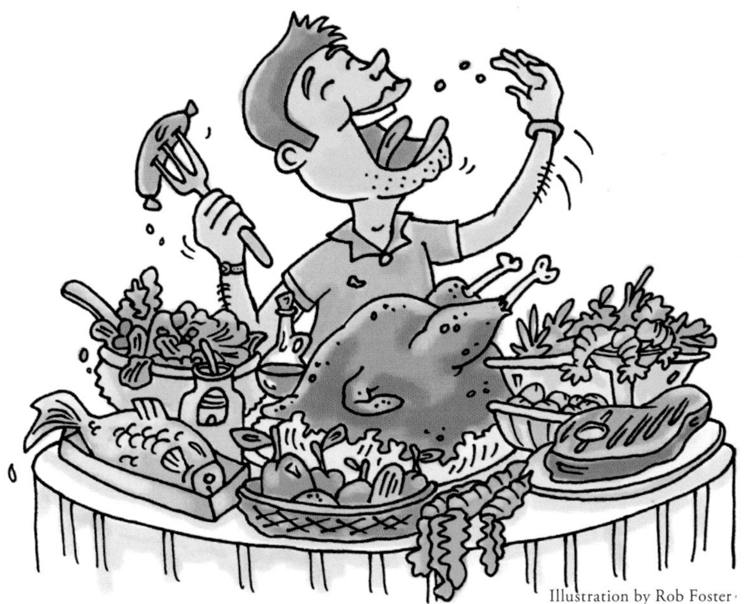

Illustration by Rob Foster

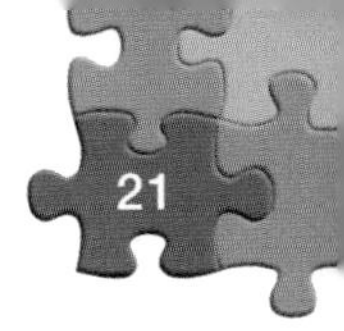

What to Eat

All the foods listed here are great to include in your diet. They are beneficial foods containing vital nutrients that will help regulate your immune system and your hormones and provide the building blocks that your body needs to heal. You don't need to eat all of these foods (it's okay if snails, frog legs, and crickets aren't your thing, and it's okay if you just can't get kangaroo meat or mizuna), but the idea is both to give you a definitive "yes list" and to introduce you to some innovative ways to increase variety and nutrient density by exploring new foods.

> *It's time to create an epidemic of health. And it starts with learning how to eat more nutrient-dense food.*
> —Dr. Terry Wahls

Red Meat

- antelope
- bear
- beaver
- beef
- bison/buffalo
- boar
- camel
- caribou
- deer
- elk
- goat
- hare
- horse
- kangaroo
- lamb
- moose
- mutton
- pork
- rabbit
- sea lion
- seal
- whale

(essentially, any mammal)

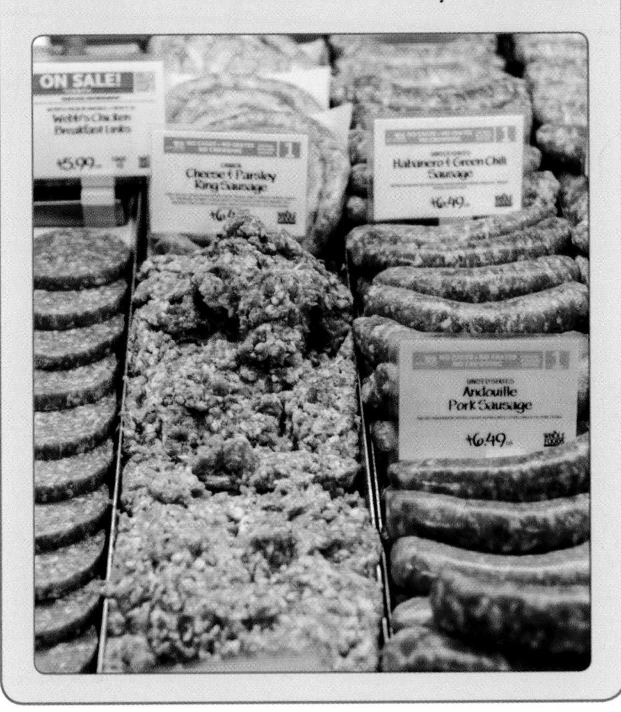

Poultry

- chicken
- dove
- duck
- emu
- goose
- grouse
- guinea hen
- ostrich
- partridge
- pheasant
- pigeon
- quail
- turkey

(essentially, any bird)

Amphibians and Reptiles

- crocodile
- frog
- snake
- turtle

Fish*

- anchovy
- Arctic char
- Atlantic croaker
- barcheek goby
- bass
- bonito
- bream
- brill
- brisling
- carp
- catfish
- cod
- common dab
- conger
- crappie
- croaker
- drum
- eel
- fera
- filefish
- gar
- haddock
- hake
- halibut
- herring
- John Dory
- king mackerel
- lamprey
- ling
- loach
- mackerel
- mahi mahi
- marlin
- milkfish
- minnow
- monkfish
- mullet
- pandora
- perch
- plaice
- pollock
- sailfish
- salmon
- sardine
- shad
- shark
- sheepshead
- silverside
- smelt
- snakehead
- snapper
- sole
- swordfish
- tarpon
- tilapia
- tilefish
- trout
- tub gurnard
- tuna
- turbot
- walleye
- whiting

*See page 387 for Selenium Health Benefit Values.

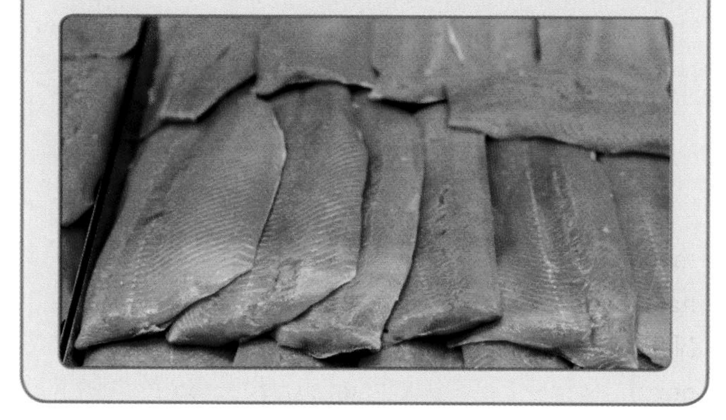

Shellfish

- abalone
- clam
- cockle
- conch
- crab
- crawfish
- cuttlefish
- limpet
- lobster
- mussel
- octopus
- oyster
- periwinkle
- prawn
- scallop
- shrimp
- snail
- squid
- whelk

Other Seafood

- anemone
- caviar/roe
- jellyfish
- sea cucumber
- sea squirt
- sea urchin
- starfish

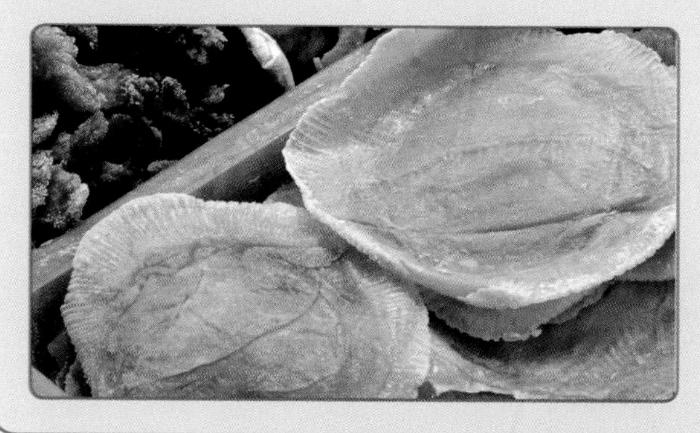

Offal

- blood
- bone broth
- bone marrow
- brain
- chitterlings and natural casings (intestines)
- fats and other trimmings (tallow and lard)
- fries (testicles)
- head meat (cheek and jowl)
- heart
- kidney
- lips
- liver
- melt (spleen)
- rinds (skin)
- sweetbreads (thymus gland or pancreas)
- tail
- tongue
- tripe (stomach)

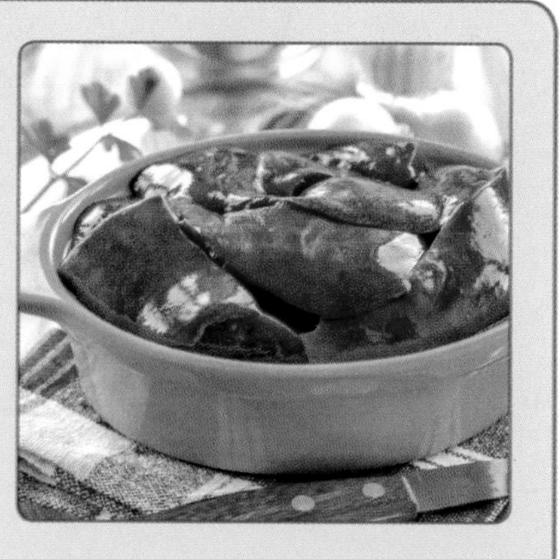

Glycine-Rich Foods

- most offal
- most seafood
- bone broth
- cheek and jowl
- chuck roast
- collagen supplements
- gelatin
- joint tissue and meat off the bone (trotters, duck feet, chicken wings)
- rinds (skin)

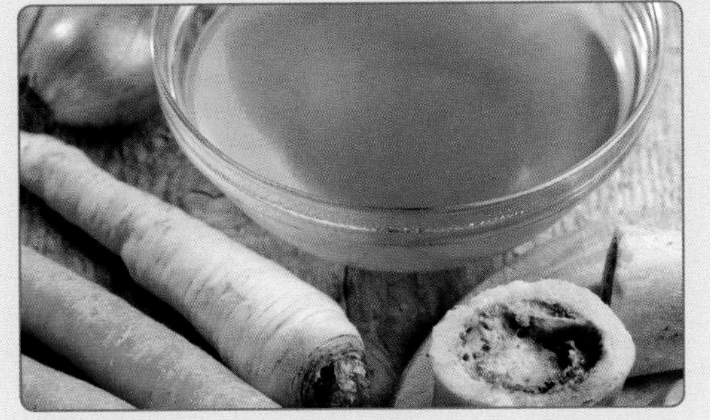

Edible Insects**

- agave worm
- ant
- bamboo worm
- bee larva
- centipede
- cicada
- cockroach
- cricket
- dragonfly
- dung beetle
- earthworm
- fly pupa
- grasshopper
- hornworm
- june bug
- locust
- mealworm
- sago worm
- silkworm

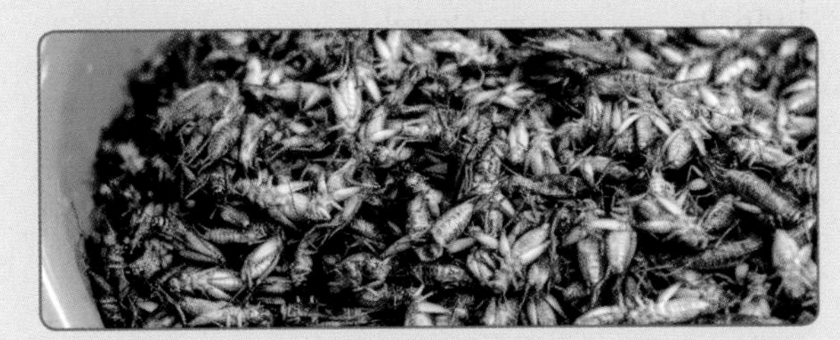

**Insects are eaten in cultural dishes around the world. They aren't all easy to get a hold of in Western countries, but cricket flour/powder is becoming easier to source.

Leafy Greens and Salad Veggies

- amaranth greens
- artichoke
- arugula
- asparagus
- beet greens
- bok choy
- borage greens
- broccoli
- broccoli rabe
- Brussels sprouts
- cabbage
- canola leaves
- capers
- cardoon
- carrot greens
- cat's-ear
- cauliflower
- celery
- celtuce
- Ceylon spinach
- chickweed
- chicory
- Chinese mallow
- chrysanthemum leaves
- collard greens
- cress
- dandelion
- endive
- fat hen
- fiddlehead
- Florence fennel
- fluted pumpkin leaves
- Good King Henry
- greater plantain
- kai-lan (Chinese broccoli)
- kale
- kohlrabi greens
- komatsuna
- Lagos bologi
- lamb's lettuce
- land cress
- lettuce
- lizard's tail
- melokhia
- mizuna
- mustard greens
- napa cabbage
- New Zealand spinach
- nopal
- orache
- pea leaves
- poke
- Prussian asparagus
- pumpkin sprouts
- radicchio
- radish sprouts
- samphire
- sculpit (stridolo)
- sea beet
- sea kale
- sorrel
- spinach
- squash blossoms
- summer purslane
- sunflower sprouts
- sweet potato greens
- Swiss chard
- tatsoi
- turnip greens
- water spinach
- watercress
- winter purslane

Stems, Flowers, and Flower Bud Vegetables

- asparagus
- broccoli
- capers
- cardoon
- cauliflower
- celery
- fennel
- nopal
- Prussian asparagus
- rhubarb (only the stems are edible)
- squash blossoms
- edible flowers (e.g. calendula, carnation, clover, dandelion, gladiolas, hibiscus, honeysuckle, lavender, marigold, nasturtium, pansy, primrose, scented geranium)

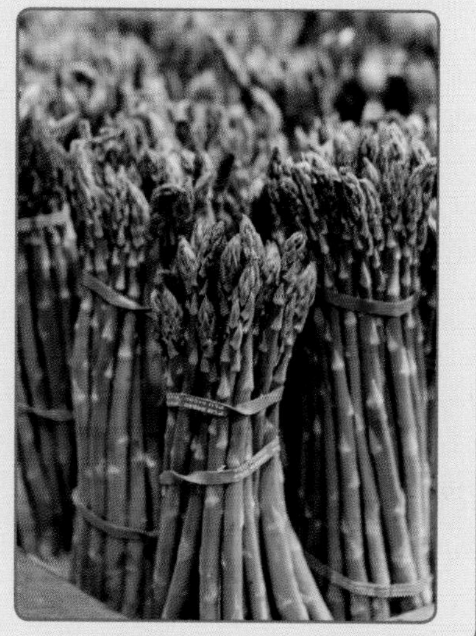

Alliums

- abusgata
- chives
- elephant garlic
- garlic
- kurrat
- leek
- onion
- pearl onion
- potato onion
- scallion
- spring onion
- shallot
- tree onion
- wild leek (aka ramp)

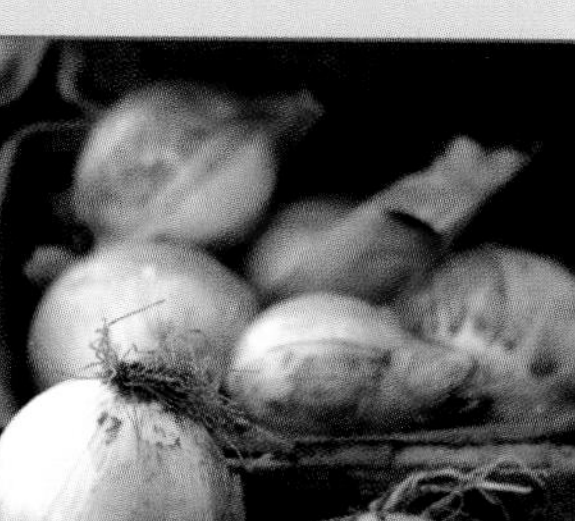

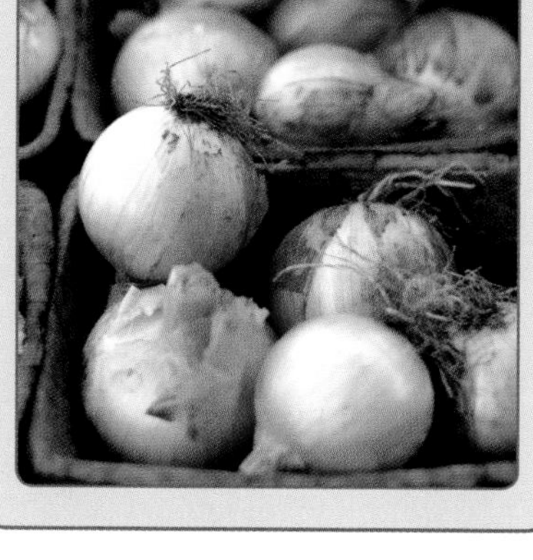

Roots, Tubers, and Bulb Vegetables

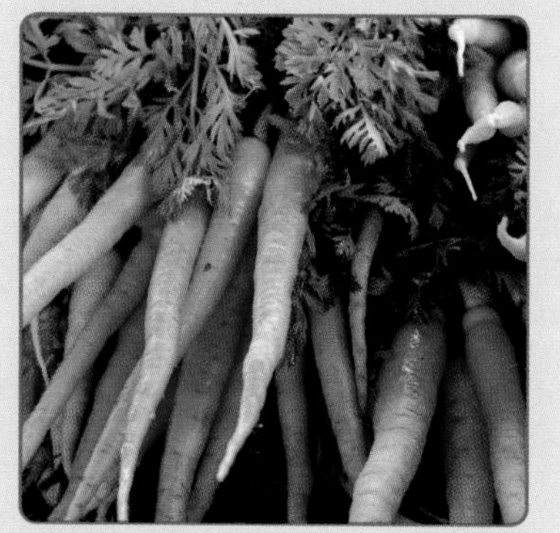

- arracacha
- arrowroot
- bamboo shoot
- beet root
- broadleaf arrowhead
- burdock
- camas
- canna
- carrot
- cassava (aka manioc, tapioca, yuca)
- celery root (aka celeriac)
- Chinese artichoke
- daikon
- earthnut pea
- elephant foot yam
- Ensete
- ginger
- Hamburg parsley
- horseradish
- Jerusalem artichoke
- jicama
- kohlrabi
- konjac
- kudzu
- lotus root
- maca
- mashua
- parsnip
- pignut
- prairie turnip
- radish
- rutabaga
- salsify
- scorzonera
- skirret
- swede
- sweet potato
- taro
- ti
- tigernut
- turnip
- ulluco
- wasabi
- water caltrop
- water chestnut
- yacón
- yam

Vegetables That Are Actually Fruits

- avocado
- bitter melon (aka bitter gourd)
- chayote
- cucumber
- ivy gourd
- loofa
- okra
- olive
- plantain
- pumpkin
- squash (see page 55)
- tinda
- West Indian gherkin
- winter melon
- zucchini

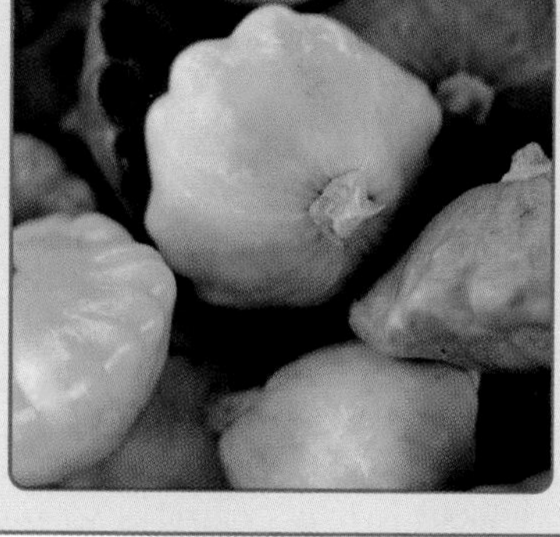

Sea Vegetables

- aonori
- arame
- carola
- dabberlocks
- dulse
- hijiki
- kombu
- laver
- mozuku
- nori
- ogonori
- sea grape
- sea kale
- sea lettuce
- wakame

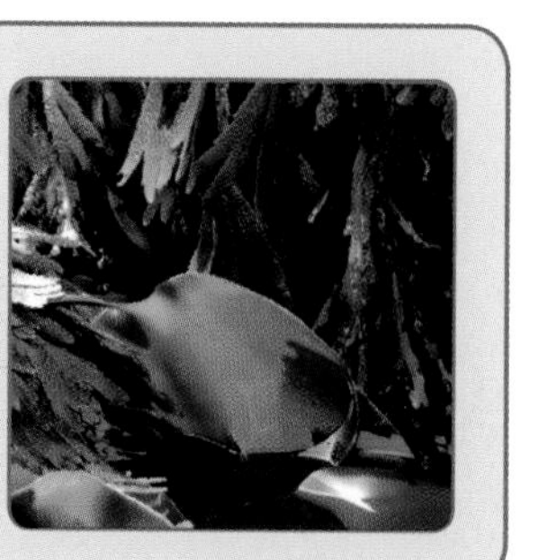

Edible Fungi

- beech mushroom (aka shimeji)
- boletus, many varieties
- button mushroom, many varieties (includes portobello and crimini)
- chanterelle, many varieties
- field blewit
- gypsy mushroom
- kefir (includes both yeast and probiotic bacteria)
- king trumpet mushroom
- kombucha (includes both yeast and probiotic bacteria)
- lion's mane mushroom
- maitake
- matsutake
- morel, many varieties
- oyster mushroom, many varieties
- saffron milk cap
- shiitake (aka oak mushroom)
- snow fungus
- *Sparassis crispa*
- straw mushroom
- sweet tooth fungus (aka hedgehog mushroom)
- tree ear fungus
- truffle, many varieties
- winter mushroom (aka enokitake)
- yeast (baker's, brewer's, nutritional)

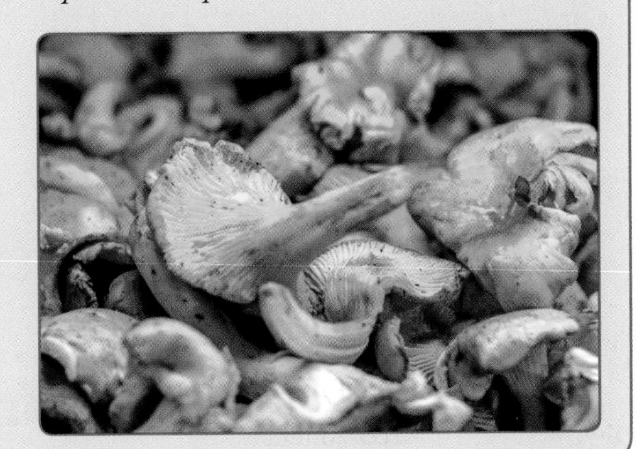

Berries

- açaí
- bearberry
- bilberry
- blackberry
- blueberry
- cloudberry
- cranberry
- crowberry
- currant
- elderberry
- falberry
- gooseberry
- grape
- hackberry
- huckleberry
- lingonberry
- loganberry
- mulberry
- muscadine
- nannyberry
- Oregon grape
- raspberry
- salmonberry
- sea buckthorn
- strawberry
- strawberry tree
- thimbleberry
- wineberry

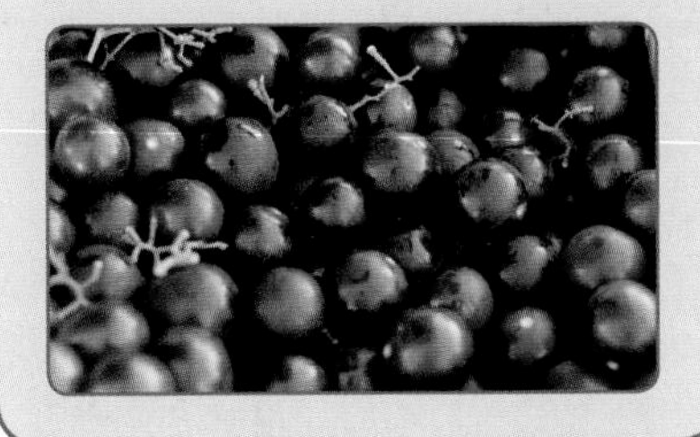

Rosaceae Family (Apple Family and Stone Fruits)

- apple
- apricot
- cherry
- chokeberry
- chokecherry
- crabapple
- greengage
- hawthorn
- loquat
- medlar
- nectarine
- peach
- pear
- plum
- quince
- rose hip
- rowan
- service tree
- serviceberry
- shipova

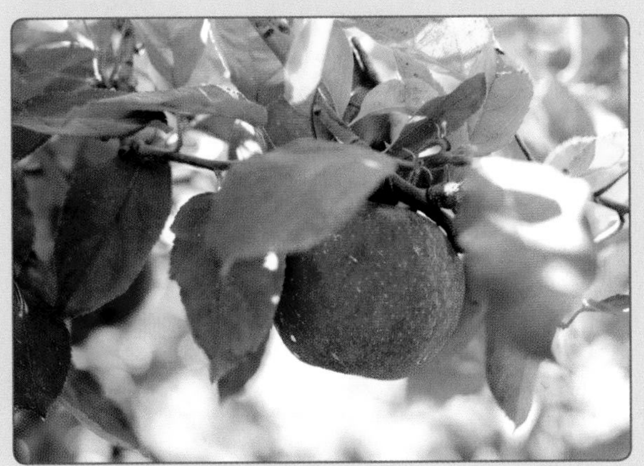

Melons

- canary melon
- cantaloupe
- casaba
- Charentais
- Christmas melon
- Crenshaw melon
- derishi
- Galia
- honeydew
- horned melon
- melon pear
- muskmelon
- net melon
- ogen melon
- pepino melon
- Persian melon
- Russian melon (aka Uzbek melon)
- sharlyn
- sweet melon
- watermelon
- winter melon

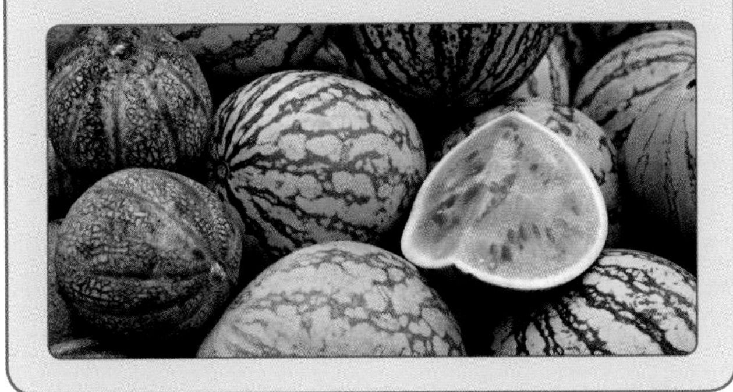

Citrus*

- amanatsu
- blood orange
- Buddha's hand
- cam sành
- citron
- clementine
- fernandina
- grapefruit, many varieties
- kaffir lime
- key lime
- kinnow
- kiyomi
- kumquat
- lemon, many varieties
- lime, many varieties
- limetta
- mandarin
- Meyer lemon
- orange, many varieties
- orangelo
- oroblanco
- pomelo
- pompia
- ponkan
- rangpur
- shonan gold
- sudachi
- tangelo
- tangerine
- tangor
- ugli
- yuzu

Tropical and Subtropical Fruits*

- abiu
- acerola
- ackee
- African moringa
- ambarella
- babaco
- banana
- biriba
- camucamu
- canistel
- ceriman
- chayote
- cherimoya
- coco plum
- coconut
- custard apple
- date
- dragonfruit
- durian
- fig, many varieties
- gambooge
- granadilla
- guanabana
- guava, many varieties
- guavaberry
- ilama
- jackfruit
- jujube
- karonda
- kiwi
- korlan
- kumquat
- longan
- loquat
- lychee
- mamey sapote
- mango
- mangosteen
- maypop
- medlar
- nance
- papaya
- passion fruit
- pawpaw
- peanut butter fruit
- persimmon
- pineapple
- plantain
- pomegranate
- pulasan
- quince
- rambutan
- riberry
- rose apple
- safou
- salak
- santol
- soursop
- star apple
- starfruit (carambola)
- sugar apple
- tamarind
- ugni
- vanilla bean
- wampee

*There are many more varieties of citrus and tropical fruits; these lists represent those that you are most likely to come across.

Good Fats

- avocado oil (cold-pressed)
- bacon fat (ideally from pasture-raised pigs)
- coconut oil (typically extra-virgin and expeller-pressed, but also naturally refined)
- lard (rendered fat from the backs of pigs, ideally pasture-raised)
- leaf lard (rendered fat from around pigs' kidneys and other internal organs, ideally pasture-raised)
- olive oil, extra-virgin and virgin
- palm oil (not to be confused with palm kernel oil; look for ethically and sustainably sourced)
- palm shortening (look for ethically and sustainably sourced)
- pan drippings
- poultry fat (typically duck, goose, or emu)
- red palm oil (look for ethically and sustainably sourced)
- salo (rendered fat from cured slabs of pork fatback, ideally pasture-raised)
- schmaltz (chicken or goose fat, ideally pasture-raised)
- strutto (clarified pork fat, ideally pasture-raised)
- tallow (rendered fat from beef, lamb, or mutton, ideally grass-fed)

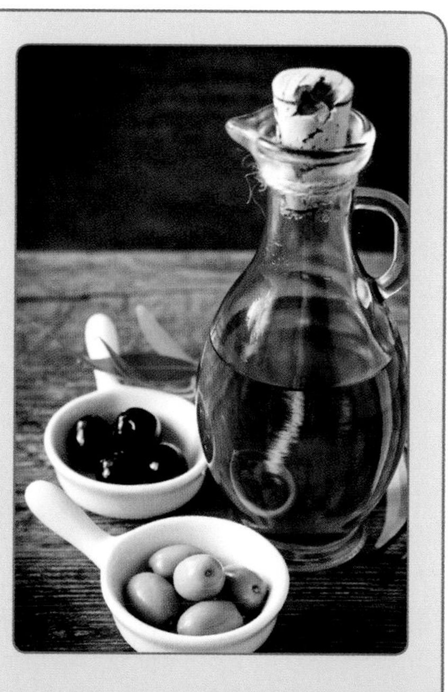

Probiotic Foods**

- beet and other vegetable kvasses
- kombucha
- coconut milk kefir or yogurt
- raw, unpasteurized, lacto- or wild-fermented vegetables (kimchi, beets, carrots, pickles)
- raw, unpasteurized, lacto- or wild-fermented fruits (green papaya, chutneys)
- raw, unpasteurized, lacto- or wild-fermented condiments (relishes, salsas)
- raw, unpasteurized sauerkraut
- water kefir

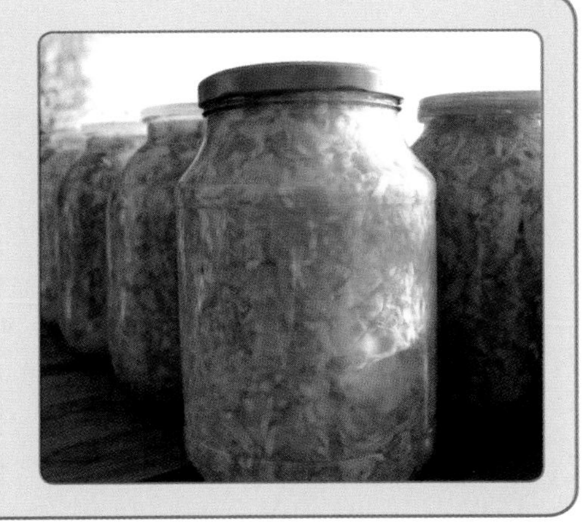

**Check ingredients to avoid nightshades, emulsifiers, and dairy.

Herbs and Spices

- asafetida (check ingredients)
- balm
- basil leaf (sweet, Thai, etc.)
- bay leaf
- chamomile
- chervil
- chives
- cilantro (aka coriander leaf)
- cinnamon
- cloves
- curry leaves
- dill weed
- fennel leaf
- fenugreek leaves
- galangal
- garlic
- garlic powder
- ginger
- horseradish (check ingredients for horseradish sauce)
- kaffir lime leaves
- lavender
- lemon balm
- lemongrass
- mace
- marjoram leaf
- mint (peppermint, spearmint, etc.)
- onion powder
- oregano leaf
- parsley
- perilla leaves (aka beefsteak leaves)
- rosemary
- saffron
- sage
- salt (Himalayan pink salt or Celtic sea salt)
- savory leaf
- sea vegetables
- tarragon
- thyme
- turmeric

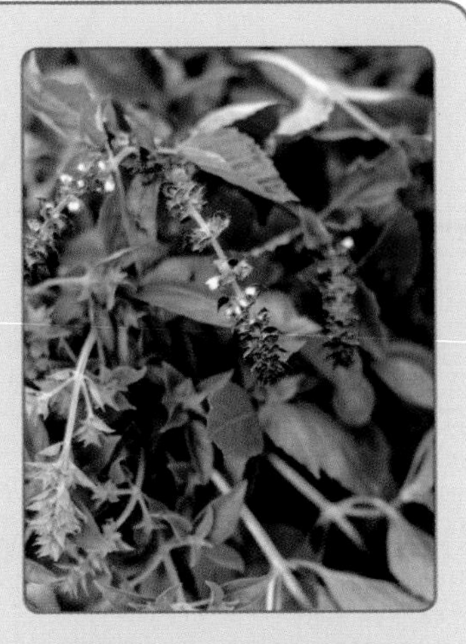

- truffle (whole truffles, truffle oil, or truffle salt)
- vanilla extract (if alcohol will be cooked off)
- vanilla powder (check ingredients)

Beverages

- beet and other vegetable kvasses
- carbonated or sparkling water
- coconut milk (emulsifier-free)
- coconut milk kefir
- coconut water
- homemade spa water (page 334)
- kombucha
- lemon or lime juice
- mineral water
- soda water
- tea, green or black
- tea, herbal (including chamomile, chicory, cinnamon, citrus rind, clove, dandelion root, dried fruit, ginger, hibiscus, honeybush, lavender, lemon balm, marshmallow root, milk thistle, mint, rose hip, rooibos, turmeric, and yerba mate)
- vegetable (green) juices and smoothies (in moderation)
- water
- water kefir

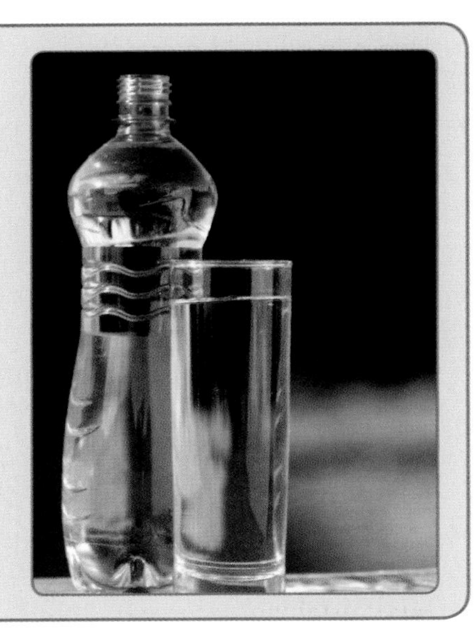

Pantry Items and Flavoring Ingredients

- agar agar
- anchovies or anchovy paste (check ingredients)
- apple cider vinegar
- arrowroot powder
- baking soda
- balsamic vinegar
- bonito flakes
- capers
- carob powder (in moderation)
- chutneys (in moderation; check ingredients)
- coconut aminos (a great soy sauce substitute)
- coconut butter (aka creamed coconut, coconut cream concentrate)
- coconut cream
- coconut flour
- coconut milk
- coconut water vinegar
- cream of tartar
- dried fruit (in moderation)
- fish sauce (check ingredients)
- gelatin
- green banana flour
- honey (in moderation)
- jams and jellies (in moderation; check ingredients)
- kuzu starch
- maple syrup (in moderation)
- molasses (in moderation)
- nutritional yeast (caution: common sensitivity)
- plantain flour (check ingredients: may be mixed with potato starch)
- pomegranate molasses (in moderation)
- red wine vinegar
- sea vegetable powder (or salt)
- shrimp paste (check ingredients)
- sweet potato flour or starch
- tamarind paste
- tapioca starch (caution: common sensitivity)
- truffle
- truffle oil (made with extra-virgin olive oil; check ingredients)
- truffle salt (check ingredients)
- umeboshi paste
- unrefined cane sugars
- vegetable powders (pumpkin, sweet potato, spinach, etc.)
- water chestnut flour
- white wine vinegar

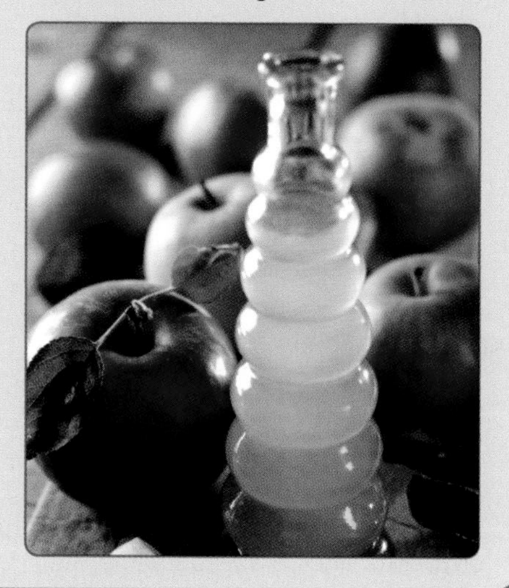

Do you feel better now? Do you see that there are tons of options of foods to eat? Do you see that eating a wide variety of foods won't really be that hard? Don't let any of the "weird stuff" intimidate you. You don't have to eat it—although any foods that give you the heebie-jeebies are probably the ones that are the most nutrient dense and will help support healing in your body the fastest. That sounds ironic, but it's really just a symptom of how much our food supply has changed in the last few decades. Not that long ago, what you may think of as "weird stuff" was considered "normal stuff," and some of our "normal stuff" was actually "weird stuff." For example, in my grandparents' generation, liver was part of the weekly rotation, steak and kidney pie was a treat, and lobster was a considered a food for "poor people." I ask you to let go of your preconceived notions about whether a food is yummy or normal, whether a food is a "breakfast food" or a "lunch food," and whether you can live without chocolate. Instead, I ask you to choose nutrient-dense foods from the above lists that will support your healing and to be open to the very real possibility that you will love them (or grow to love them as your taste buds adapt to the changes in your diet).

Regardless of whether you are intimidated, excited, or a mixture of both, this cookbook isn't about making you eat foods you don't like. It's about cooking with nutritious ingredients—yes, some that may be unfamiliar—in a way that doesn't cause stress in the kitchen and still puts delicious meals on your table. I promise that liver doesn't have to be yucky.

Foods to Consume in Moderation

Green tea, black tea, and yerba mate

Fructose: Aim for between 10 and 20 grams of fructose per day.

Salt: Use pink or gray salt because it is rich in trace minerals.

Omega-6 polyunsaturated fat–rich foods: Chicken, turkey, and other poultry; industrially produced fatty cuts of meat.

Moderate-glycemic-load vegetables and fruits: Such as some dried fruit, plantain, and taro root.

Coconut: See page 44 for guidelines.

☒ Foods to Avoid

Yes, we're focusing on the positives and the amazing foods you can eat. But, just so there's no miscommunication, here is a detailed list of foods to avoid while following the Paleo Approach. The reasons these foods are problematic for people with autoimmune disease are explained in great detail in *The Paleo Approach.*

☒ **Grains:** Barley, corn, durum, fonio, Job's tears, kamut, millet, oats, rice, rye, sorghum, spelt, teff, triticale, wheat (all varieties, including einkorn and semolina), and wild rice. See page 368 for hidden sources of wheat and page 369 for hidden sources of corn.

☒ **Gluten:** Barley, rye, wheat, and foods derived from these ingredients. See page 368 for hidden sources of gluten and gluten cross-reactors and commonly contaminated foods.

☒ **Pseudograins and grainlike substances:** Amaranth, buckwheat, chia, and quinoa.

☒ **Dairy:** Butter, butter oil, buttermilk, cheese, cottage cheese, cream, curds, dairy protein isolates, ghee, heavy cream, ice cream, kefir, milk, sour cream, whey, whey protein isolate, whipping cream, and yogurt. (Cultured grass-fed ghee might be tolerated.) See page 371 for hidden sources of dairy.

☒ **Legumes:** Adzuki beans, black beans, black-eyed peas, butter beans, calico beans, cannellini beans, chickpeas (aka garbanzo beans), fava beans (aka broad beans), Great Northern beans, green beans, Italian beans, kidney beans, lentils, lima beans, mung beans, navy beans, peanuts, peas, pinto beans, runner beans, split peas, and soybeans (including edamame, tofu, tempeh, other soy products, and soy isolates, such as soy lecithin). See page 370 for hidden sources of soy.

☒ **Processed vegetable oils:** Canola oil (aka rapeseed oil), corn oil, cottonseed oil, palm kernel oil, peanut oil, safflower oil, soybean oil, and sunflower oil.

☒ **Processed food chemicals and ingredients:** Acrylamides, artificial food color, artificial and natural flavors, autolyzed protein, brominated vegetable oil, emulsifiers (carrageenan, cellulose gum, guar gum, lecithin, xanthan gum), hydrolyzed vegetable protein, monosodium glutamate, nitrates or nitrites (naturally occurring are OK), olestra, phosphoric acid, propylene glycol, textured vegetable protein, trans fats (partially hydrogenated vegetable oil, hydrogenated oil), yeast extract, and any ingredient with a chemical name that you don't recognize.

☒ **Added sugars:** Agave, agave nectar, barley malt, barley malt syrup, beet sugar, brown rice syrup, brown sugar, cane crystals, cane juice, cane sugar, caramel, coconut sugar, corn sweetener, corn syrup, corn syrup solids, crystalline fructose, date sugar, dehydrated cane juice, demerara sugar, dextrin, dextrose, diastatic malt, evaporated cane juice, fructose, fruit juice, fruit juice concentrate, galactose, glucose, glucose solids, golden syrup, high-fructose corn syrup, honey, inulin, invert sugar, jaggery, lactose, malt syrup, maltodextrin, maltose, maple syrup, molasses, monk fruit (luo han guo), muscovado sugar, palm sugar, panela, panocha, rapadura, raw cane sugar, raw sugar, refined sugar, rice bran syrup, rice syrup, saccharose, sorghum syrup, sucanat, sucrose, syrup, treacle, turbinado sugar, and yacon syrup. See page 370 for hidden sources of added sugars. See page 56 for a list of the best sweeteners to use for occasional Paleo Approach–friendly treats.

☒ **Sugar alcohols:** Erythritol, mannitol, sorbitol, and xylitol. (Naturally occurring sugar alcohols found in whole foods like fruit are OK.)

☒ **Nonnutritive sweeteners:** Acesulfame potassium, aspartame, neotame, saccharin, stevia, and sucralose.

☒ **Nuts and nut oils:** Almonds, Brazil nuts, cashews, chestnuts, hazelnuts, macadamia nuts, pecans, pine nuts, pistachios, and walnuts, and any butters, flours, oils, or other products derived from these nuts. (Coconut is an exception and may be consumed in moderation, as discussed on page 44; macadamia nut oil and walnut oil might be tolerated.)

☒ **Seeds and seed oils:** Chia, flax, hemp, poppy, pumpkin, sesame, and sunflower seeds, and any butters, flours, oils, and other products derived from these seeds.

☒ **Nightshades or spices derived from nightshades:** Ashwagandha, bell peppers (aka sweet peppers), cape gooseberries (ground cherries, not to be confused with regular cherries, which are OK), cayenne pepper, eggplant, garden huckleberries (not to be confused with regular huckleberries, which are OK), goji berries (aka wolfberries), hot peppers (chili peppers and chili-based spices), naranjillas, paprika, pepinos, pimentos, potatoes (sweet potatoes are OK), red pepper, tamarillos, tomatillos, and tomatoes. (Note: Some curry powders contain nightshade ingredients.)

☒ **Spices derived from seeds (small amounts might be tolerated):** Anise, annatto, black caraway (aka Russian caraway, black cumin), celery seed, coriander, cumin, dill, fennel, fenugreek, mustard, and nutmeg.

☒ **Spices derived from berries and fruits (small amounts might be tolerated):** Allspice, star anise, caraway, cardamom, juniper, pepper (derived from black, green, pink, or white peppercorns; note that red pepper is a nightshade), sumac, and vanilla bean.

☒ **Eggs:** Although egg yolks might be tolerated.

☒ **Alcohol:** Although an occasional drink after remission might be tolerated.

☒ **Coffee:** Although an occasional cup might be tolerated.

☒ **Algae:** Spirulina and chlorella (might be tolerated).

☒ **High-glycemic-load foods:** Generally these foods are already avoided (examples include bread, pasta, grains, juice, sweetened beverages, cakes, cookies, and candy). Dried fruit that is high glycemic load might be used to flavor a dish.

The Quality of Your Food Matters

It's probably obvious to say that the higher the quality of your food, the better off you are. Higher-quality food provides more nutrition while containing fewer potentially problematic substances.

For red meat and poultry, high quality means grass-fed if the animal is an herbivore (like a cow, buffalo, or lamb), pasture-raised if the animal is an omnivore (like a pig, turkey, or chicken), or wild if the animal is a game animal, regardless of natural diet (like deer and boar). The meat from these animals tends to be leaner and more vitamin and mineral rich, with healthier fats (most notably a better ratio of omega-6 to omega-3 polyunsaturated fats, but also some other health-promoting fats, like conjugated linoleic acid), while never being treated with antibiotics or hormones.

For seafood, high-quality ideally means wild, caught from the ocean or from unpolluted lakes, rivers, and streams. However, farmed fish is still a great option (and far better than not eating fish); it provides high levels of beneficial long-chain omega-3 polyunsaturated fatty acids, highly digestible protein, and a plethora of vitamins and minerals that are essential for thyroid and immune function.

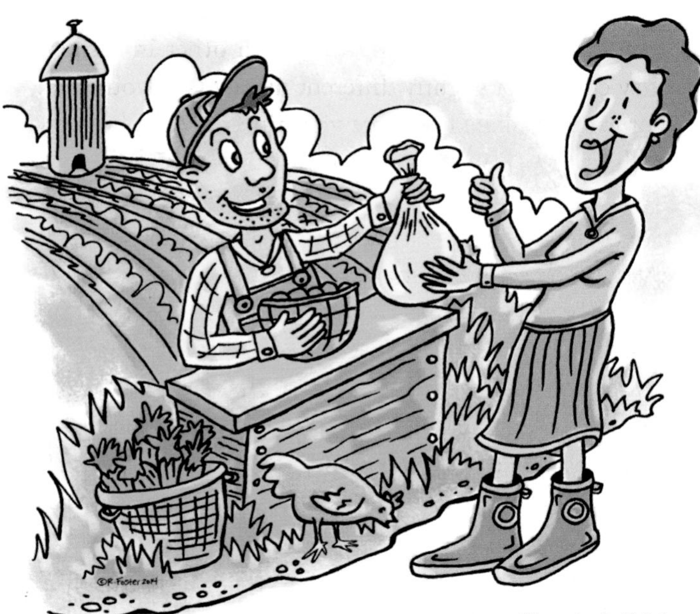

Illustration by Rob Foster

For produce, the ideal is to consume fresh, locally grown, organic, and in-season vegetables, fruits, and herbs. This may not be practical where you live, but whatever produce you can source from local farmers or grow in your backyard will be more nutrient dense than even organic produce purchased from a grocery store. Frozen organic vegetables and fruits are the next best thing to fresh, since they are frozen very soon after being harvested and are harvested ripe at the peak of the season. For mushrooms, the ideal is to consume wild mushrooms. For dried herbs and spices, the best choice is organic.

Animal fats should come from grass-fed and pasture-raised animals or wild game. Plant fats like coconut oil and olive oil should be cold pressed and ideally completely unrefined and as fresh as possible. If you are going to splurge on one high-quality ingredient, make it your cooking fats. If you're going to splurge on two high-quality ingredients, make the second one your salad dressing fats.

In general, you want to consume whole foods, which means unprocessed, unmanipulated ingredients or foods in their most natural state. Processing foods depletes nutrients. This doesn't mean you can't take advantage of prepackaged sweet potato chips or add tamarind paste or fish sauce to your meals. But it does mean that the vast majority of the foods you cook with should be recognizable and as close as possible to how they look while growing or roaming in the wild.

Eating the best-quality foods you can source is very important, but if you can't afford these high-quality ingredients or you just don't have access to them where you live, it's not a nonstarter. Even buying all your food from your regular neighborhood grocery store will have you feeling better when you know how to choose the best options available to you.

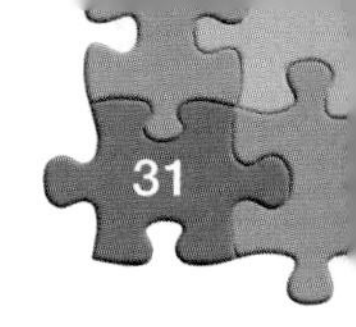

Variety Matters

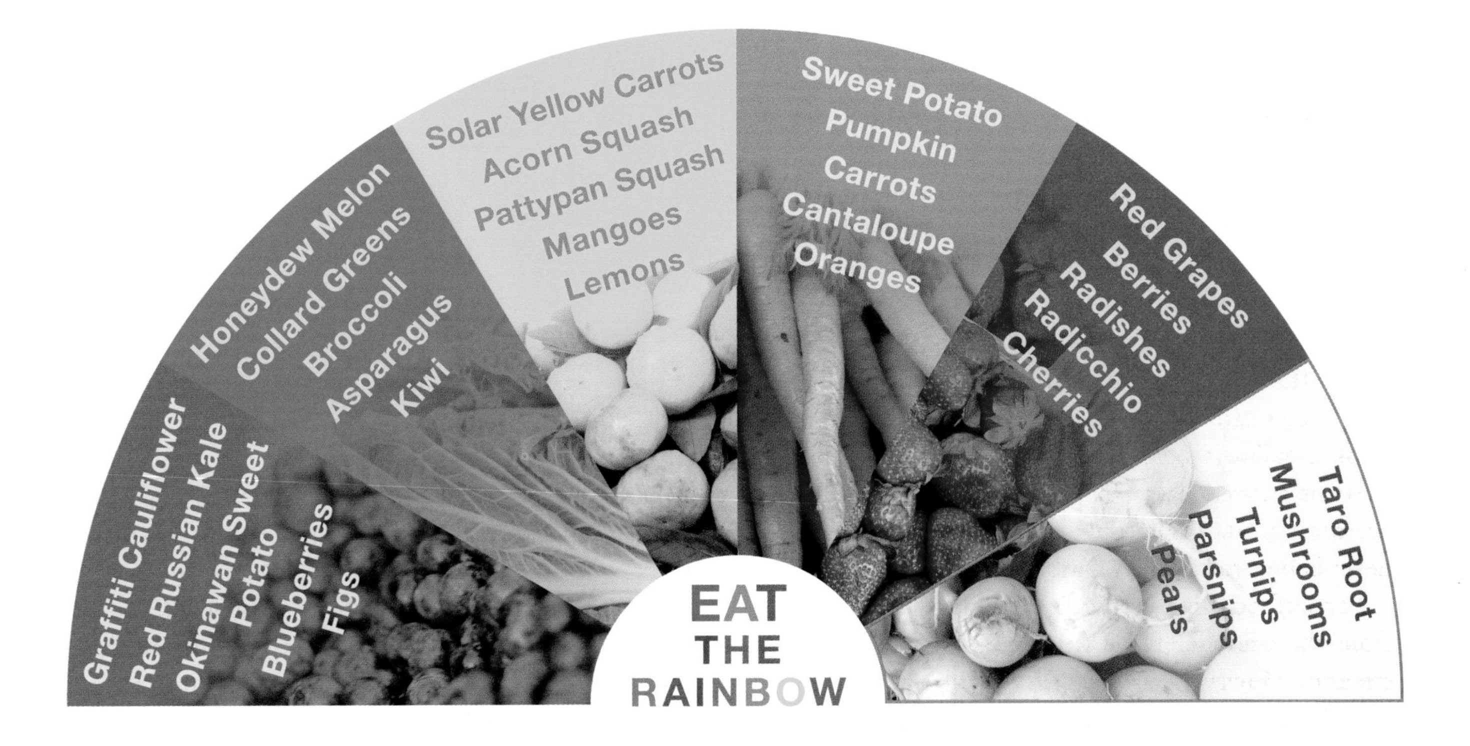

The single best way to ensure that you are getting the nutrition your body needs to heal is to eat as much variety as possible. This means both variety in the plant foods you are eating and variety in the animal foods you are eating.

It should come as no surprise that different foods contain different nutrients. When it comes to eating plants, it's important to "eat the rainbow." The same compounds that act as pigments in plants are also nutrients. For example, carotenoids, powerful antioxidants that are converted into vitamin A in the human body, impart yellow, orange, and red pigments to fruits and vegetables. Chlorophyll, known to prevent cancer, imparts green pigments to fruits and vegetables. Aim to eat at least two different-colored vegetables with every meal.

Just as it's important to eat a diversity of colors when choosing plant foods, it's also important to switch up foods within a particular color category. Even within one color of the rainbow, the nutrients you get from different plants can be very different. In fact, it may surprise you to know just how different highly related foods can be when it comes to their nutritional features. Kale and collard greens are both dense, slightly bitter leafy greens from the cruciferous family of vegetables. They are often prepared in similar ways, and you might see them as interchangeable in your cooking. But, while they might substitute nicely for each other in recipes, they contribute slightly different nutrients to your diet. For example, kale has more vitamin C and K, but collards contain more vitamin B_5 and B_9.

It is so important to eat large portions of a variety of vegetables. Studies consistently show that vegetable intake is associated with reduced risk of every chronic illness in which dietary risk factors have been evaluated. And studies that link other foods to cancer—for example, smoked foods, cured meats, and red meat—show no increase in cancer risk when people simultaneously include plenty of veggies, especially green ones, in their diets. When it comes to autoimmune disease, vegetables provide a huge assortment of essential antioxidants, vitamins, minerals, other phytonutrients, and fiber to support a healthy diversity of gut bacteria.

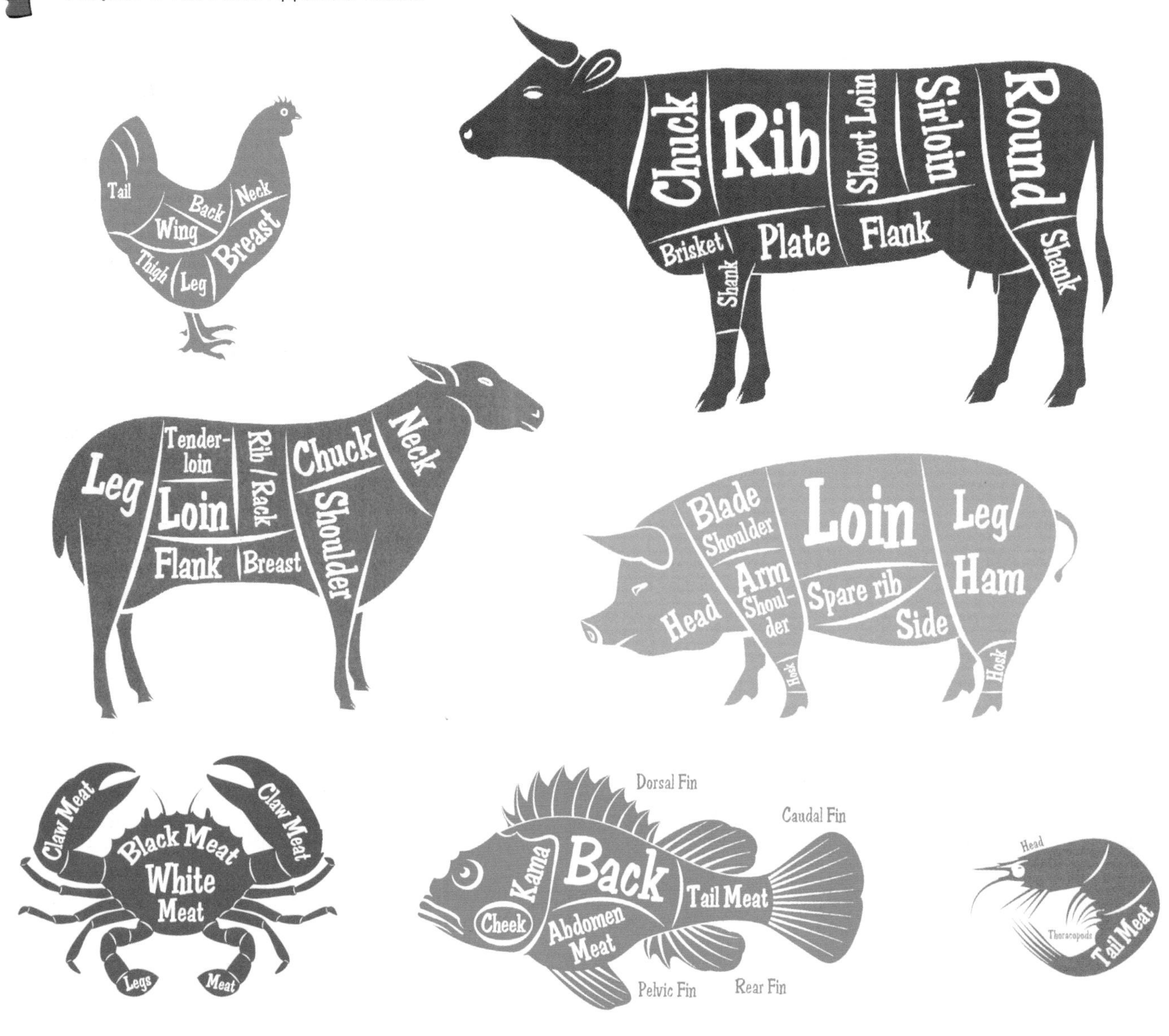

The same rule holds true for animal foods: variety ensures a greater breadth of nutrition. You might look at ground beef and ground lamb as being interchangeable. Both are red meat, after all, and you can easily substitute one for the other when making meatloaf, burgers, and pasta sauces. But whereas beef has more potassium and zinc, lamb contains more vitamin B_3 and selenium. And nutrition doesn't just vary by the animal; it also varies by the cut of meat! A beef rib-eye steak has more than double the vitamin B_{12} of a beef sirloin steak. And absolutely no muscle meat can compare with the nutrient density of any organ meat. Organs are powerhouses of nutrients and should find their way onto your plate at least four times per week.

The animal food version of eating the rainbow is to eat "snout to tail." This means eating every edible part of the animal. You can achieve this in one of two ways: you can make a concerted effort to buy different cuts of meat and source organ meat whenever you go shopping, or you can buy meat by the whole or substantial fraction of an animal (such as buying a whole pig or half a cow) and get everything that the meat processor or butcher will give you.

Just as it's super-important to eat every part of the animal, it's also important to eat a variety of different animals, including red meat, poultry, fish, shellfish, and some of those other options if you're feeling adventurous (you know, the ones I said you didn't have to eat if you didn't want to). The differences in nutrition between different types of animals can be substantial, not just in terms of vitamins and minerals offered but also in the relative quantities of various amino acids and essential fatty acids. Being too limited in your food choices can lead to nutrient deficiencies and excesses, neither of which are helpful when you're trying to heal your body!

Incorporating seafood into your diet is especially important, in part because of the extremely complementary nutrition that fish and shellfish have to meat from land animals. Seafood is your best source of a variety of essential vitamins and minerals (like vitamins A and D, zinc, and selenium), is your best source of essential long-chain omega-3 polyunsaturated fatty acids (well, unless you're eating brain), and provides the most digestible protein available. And don't forget sea vegetables; they're some of the most nutrient-dense plants and the only plant sources of long-chain omega-3 polyunsaturated fatty acids. (Sea vegetables contain DHA, whereas other plants provide the shorter-chain ALA, which is very inefficiently converted into DHA or EPA by the body.)

It's also important to vary how and whether you cook your foods. Cooking depletes some nutrients and causes others to form. Cooking improves the digestibility and bioavailability of many nutrients but inactivates some beneficial enzymes, kills probiotic organisms, and changes the quality of the fiber in foods. And different cooking techniques have different effects. For example, high-heat cooking can cause the formation of undesirable compounds (let me clarify: undesirable from a health standpoint because they are potential carcinogens, but typically very desirable from a taste standpoint). Boiling vegetables can cause nutrients to leach into the water. (Of course, if you're making soup, that's not an issue because you're going to drink that water!) Fermentation also changes the nutritional value of foods, typically increasing it. The way to get the best of all worlds is to vary your cooking techniques as much as you vary the types of foods you eat: sometimes steam your broccoli, sometimes eat it raw, sometimes ferment your vegetables, sometimes roast your meat, sometimes slow-cook it, sometimes eat sashimi.

When it comes to food choices, the more different ones you make within the food lists given here, the better. Variety is the key to getting all the nutrients you need in synergistic quantities for optimal health.

It's Fun Because It's Purple

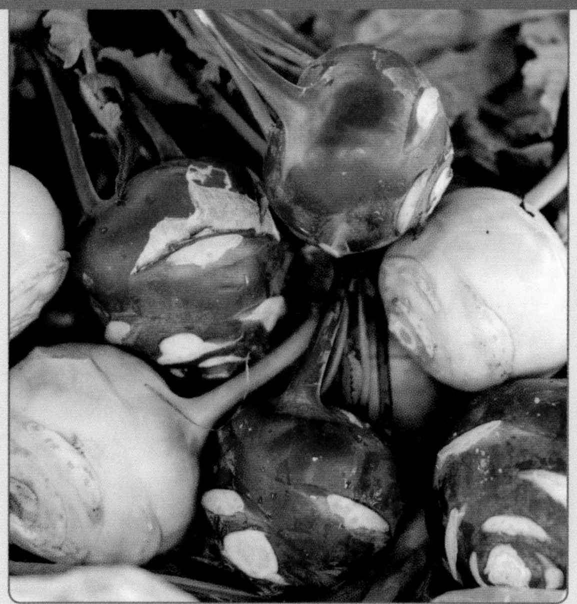

Many of the vegetables and fruits we think of as individual foods actually come in dozens, if not hundreds, of varieties. There are dozens of varieties of vegetables like carrots, sweet potatoes, beets, lettuce, kale, cauliflower, and squash. We're used to thinking of apples as coming in many different varieties, but other fruits do as well. For example, there are approximately 500 cultivars of peach! While grocery stores are stocking less-common varieties of some vegetables and fruits more regularly, the best place to find new varieties is your local farm or farmer's market. As you make an effort to eat a wide range of different vegetables, also try to source alternate varieties of each vegetable. Try purple carrots, white sweet potatoes, yellow beets, orange cauliflower, and purple kohlrabi. Try different varieties of radish, turnip, squash, cucumbers, and kale. The options are endless!

A Note on Salt

Himalayan pink and Celtic gray unrefined sea salt are always preferred over other choices because they are an important source of essential minerals, typically containing in excess of eighty different trace minerals. The recipes in this cookbook assume that you are using finely ground salt (table salt). If using coarsely ground salt instead, you may want to adjust the seasoning, since 1 teaspoon finely ground salt is equivalent to approximately 1¼ teaspoons coarsely ground salt. If you purchase pink or gray salt in rock form, you can easily grind it yourself in a spice grinder, mortar and pestle, food processor, or blender. Truffle salt can always be used as a substitute in savory dishes; look for a truffle salt with unrefined sea salt as its base.

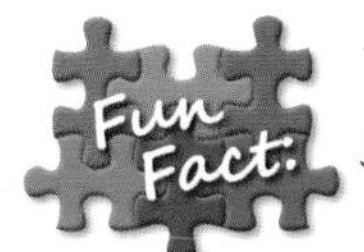

The most nutritious greens are actually the red, purple, and reddish-brown ones. This color indicates the presence of anthocyanins, which are powerful antioxidants.

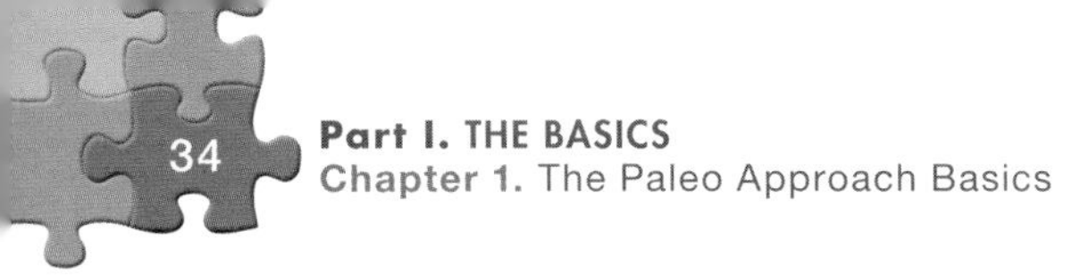

"Where Do I Buy These Foods?"

Okay, so you've perused the "foods to eat" lists, you've gotten over the initial panic when you read the words *earthworm* and *testicles,* and you're sold on the need to source the best-quality foods you can within your budget and to eat a variety of different foods (even if you're putting your foot down on sardines). Now you're trying to figure out where you are going to find all these foods. Actually, many of the foods listed are likely to be available at your local grocery store, but some will require a little more effort to source.

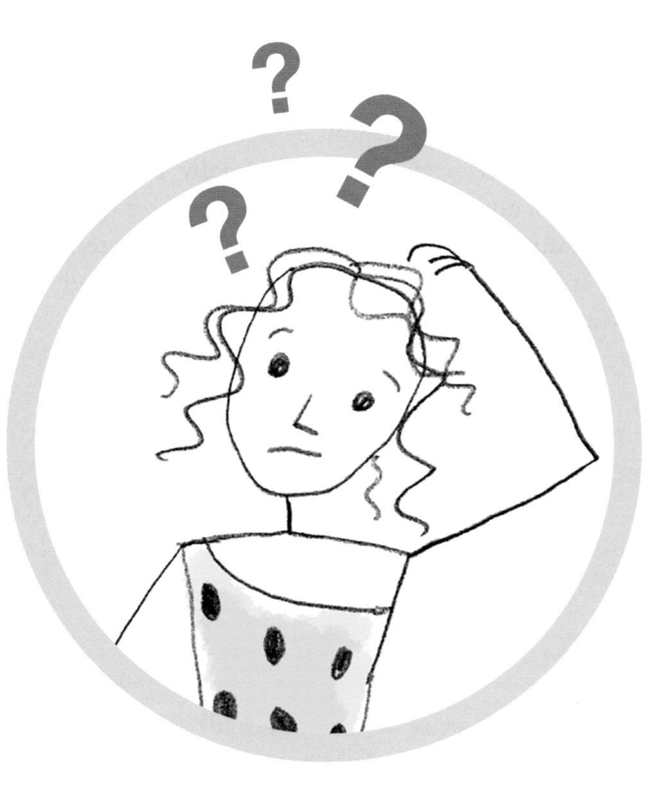

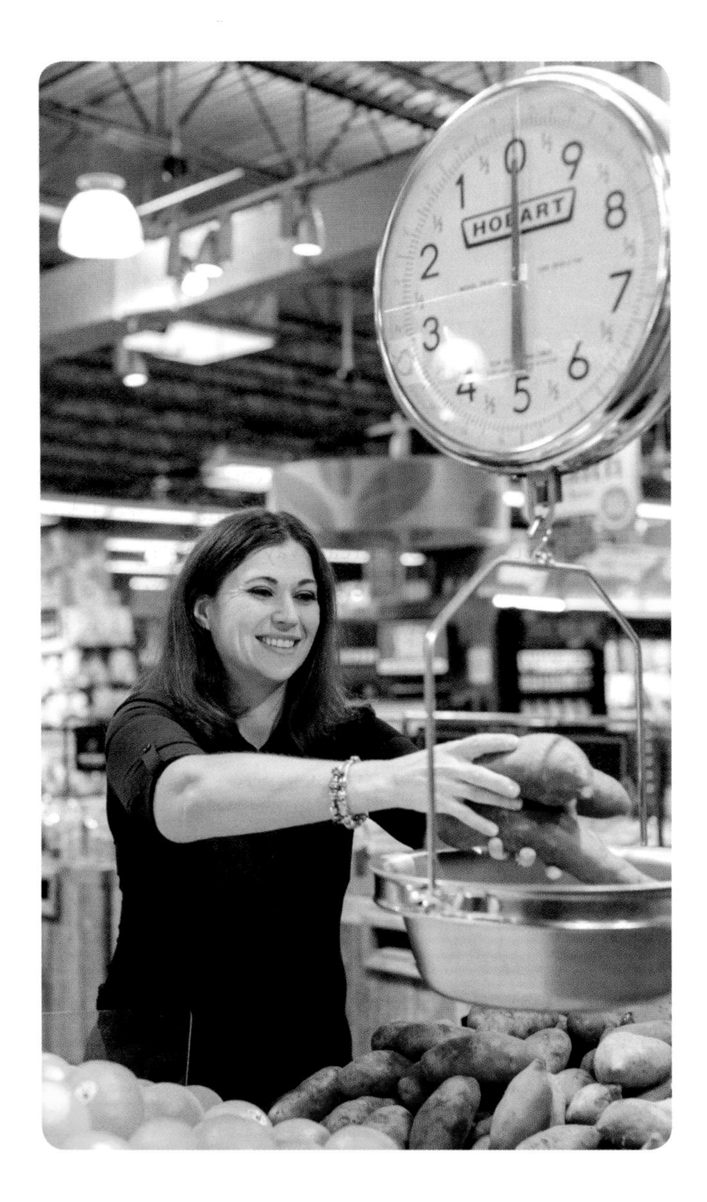

Standard grocery stores: More and more grocery stores are stocking grass-fed meat, free-range chicken, wild-caught fish and shellfish, and organic vegetables and fruits. If you don't see grass-fed meat or wild-caught fish, you can ask the butcher or fishmonger at the meat or fish counter. Some stores get limited quantities of grass-fed meat once a week, so they may carry it but are sold out by the time you do your shopping. Some stores stock only frozen wild-caught fish, and it's kept in a different aisle from the fresh fish. Many of the flavoring and pantry ingredients that will become staples in your kitchen can be found in the organic food aisles, gluten-free aisles, vegan/vegetarian food aisles (these are often combined into one space in a store), and cultural/international foods aisles. When in doubt, ask someone. Not all grocery stores are willing to special-order foods for you, but if a store perceives a market for an ingredient it doesn't usually carry, it may hop on the bandwagon.

Specialty stores (health food stores, natural food stores, supplement stores, cultural food markets, and co-ops): From big-chain natural food stores to mom-and-pop cultural food markets, these stores can be a boon to seekers of unusual ingredients and high-quality foods. When searching for a nonperishable item, it's helpful to know if it has an alternative name (for example, if you're looking for sweet potato noodles in a Korean market, it's helpful to know that they also go by the names *glass noodles* and *dangmyeon* and are traditionally used to make Japchae) and the cultural background of that food (for example, it's easiest to find pomegranate molasses in a Lebanese market, but you might find it in other Middle Eastern markets). Cultural markets are a great place to find unusual fruits and vegetables, too, typically imported, though sometimes locally grown if there's a large ethnic community to cater to. Even supplement stores and small health food stores often stock local produce. When in doubt, ask a store clerk or manager about a specific ingredient or about where the store sources the foods it carries.

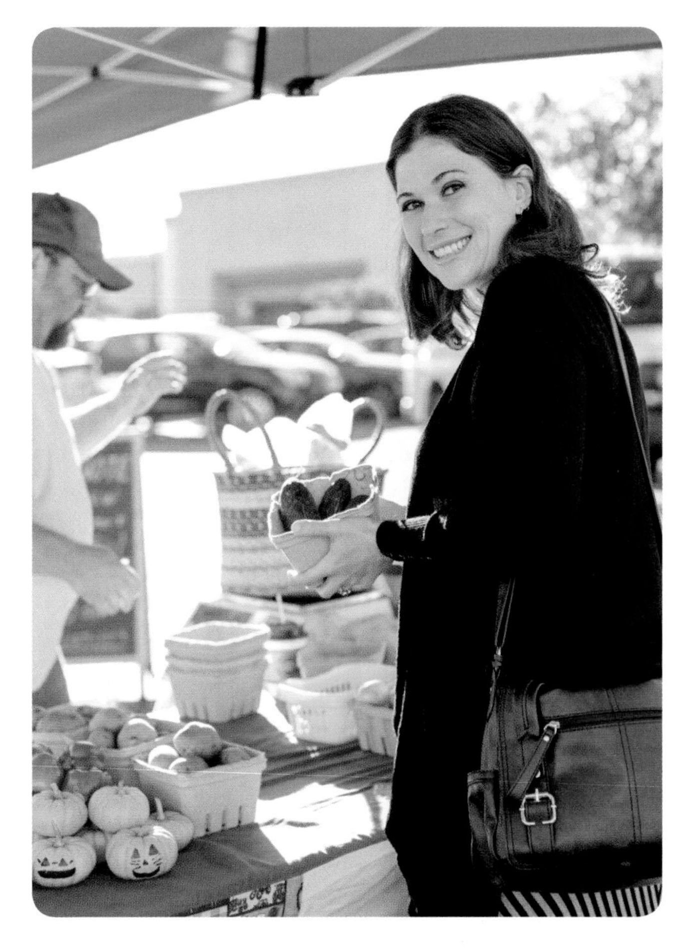

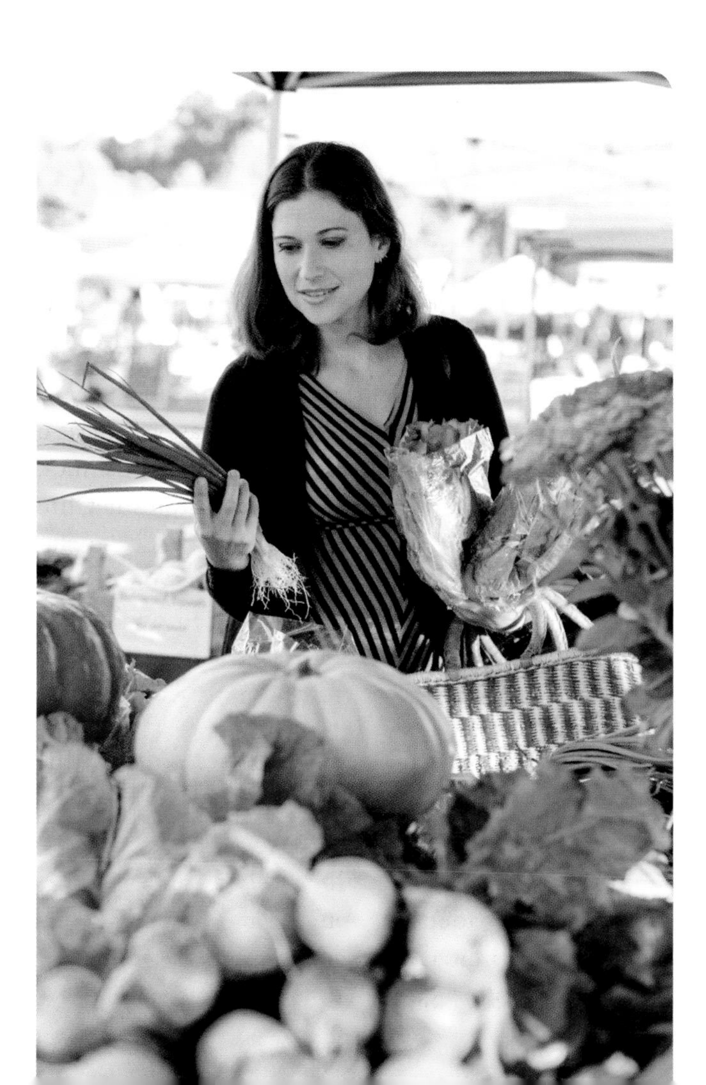

Local farmers (farmer's markets, farm stands, pick-your-own farms, farm shares, community-supported agriculture, and co-ops): Sourcing food from local farmers is one of the best ways to maximize the quality of your food (short of hunting, gathering, and growing your own) and can be a vital tool for getting high-quality food on a tight budget. It's also a great way to get organ meat, buy a half or whole butchered animal, and source vegetables and fruits that you might not be familiar with. There are many ways to get food from local farmers. Shopping at a farmer's market is convenient and gives you access to several local farmers in one place. It's also a great way to get to know the local food scene and form relationships with local farmers, other local food producers, and other shoppers who are passionate about food quality. Many farms also sell their products at farm stands either at the farm or in a more central location. (Some farmers share a stand, so one stand will give you access to the products from several local farms.) Some farms offer pick-your-own produce for a reduced price (the tradeoff is that you're the one laboring in the field), at least for peak-season produce.

Many farms offer a farm share program or community-supported agriculture (CSA), where you subscribe to get a box of each week's harvest (sometimes paying each week, sometimes paying for the entire season in advance), typically for reduced prices but also without much say in what will be in your box (which is actually a really fun way to challenge yourself to eat new foods). Some farm share programs will deliver to your door, whereas others have a pickup location and time for you to get your box each week. In many towns and cities, you can also join co-ops that source food from local farmers.

Need some help finding a local farmer, farmer's market, CSA, or pick-your-own farm near you? Try these great online directories:

- **www.eatwellguide.org**
- **www.localharvest.org**
- **www.pickyourown.org**

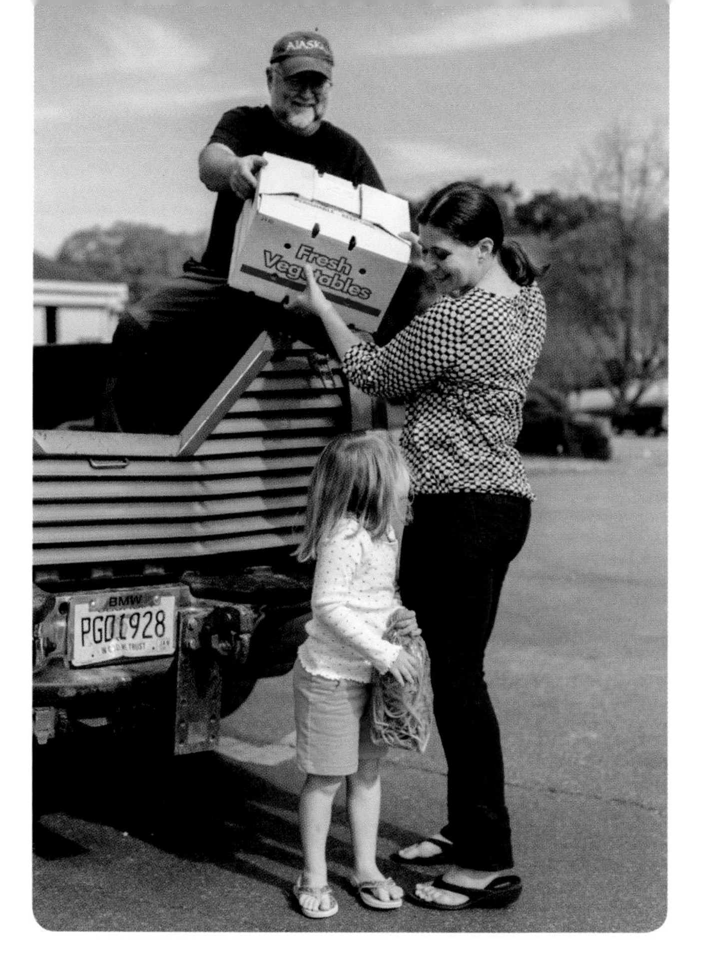

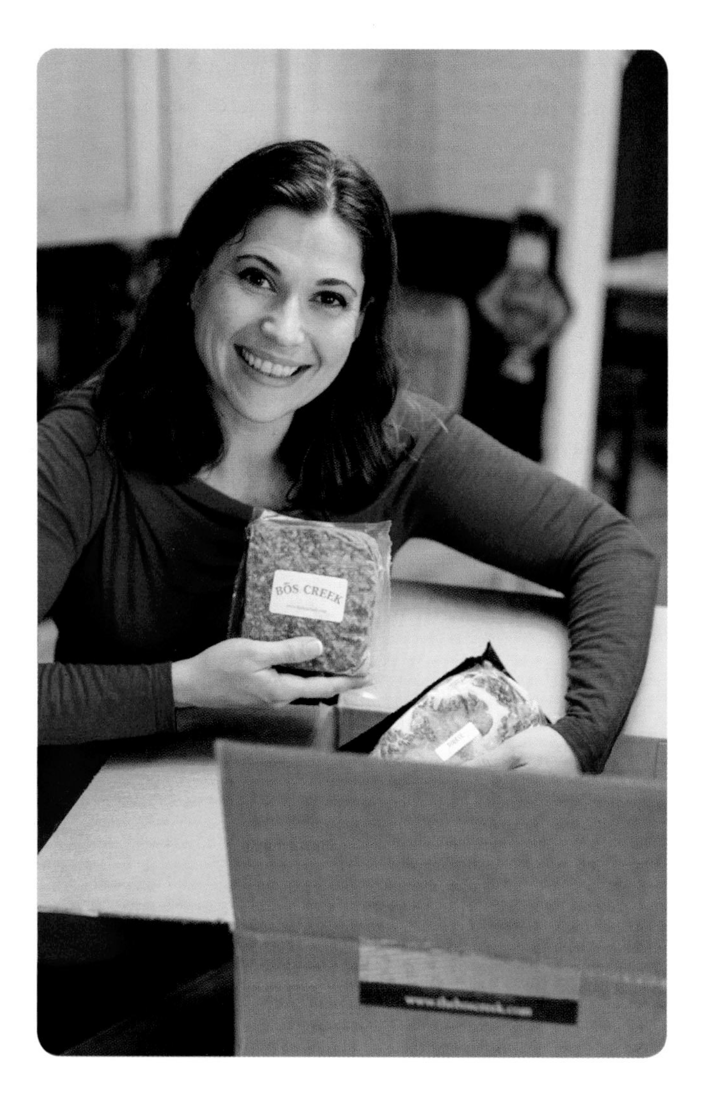

Online (oh, Amazon, how I love thee): The full range of unusual ingredients listed in this cookbook are available online. In fact, these foods are often cheaper online than in stores (though not always, so make sure to compare prices!). And there's something about the convenience of having foods delivered to your door that can't be beat. Yes, I fully admit to quite the penchant for online shopping. But it's not just nonperishable specialty foods that are available online. You have a dizzying array of grass-fed and pasture-raised meat producers to choose from, all ready to ship high-quality fresh or frozen meat right to your door. Some producers offer subscription services, and from others you order à la carte. Some establish minimums (weight, cost, or both) in order to get free shipping. Sometimes shipping costs vary by the time of year (typically higher in the summer when shipping frozen foods is more challenging). Some offer preseasoned or uncured deli meats (make sure to read the ingredients lists closely). Some offer a huge variety of organ meats, too! There's even a growing number of online options for farm-fresh produce (typically available only during peak season, and only for those crops that ship well) and other fresh foods.

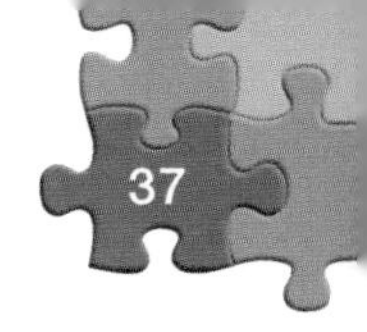

"How Do I Eat This Way on a Budget?"

Following a restricted diet on a budget requires the same tools as doing anything else on a budget—namely knowing your prices, comparison shopping, taking advantage of sales and coupons, buying in bulk, and knowing how to get the best bang for your buck.

Knowing your prices doesn't require a photographic memory for numbers or an uncanny ability to convert the per-banana price at one store to the per-pound price at another store (although that skill would be handy!). You can use a simple notebook to list your most commonly purchased items at each store you frequent, or use an app like Out-of-Milk to keep track for you. When you're getting used to eating this way, shop around, not only at different grocery stores and specialty markets (you'd be surprised how often the specialty markets with a reputation for being more expensive are actually cheaper for the specialty items you'll be looking for) but also online (factor in the cost of shipping, of course!). Before long you'll have your regular stops for different types of foods: perhaps your local warehouse club for seafood, a local farm stand for some produce and grass-fed meat, a regular grocery store for the rest of your produce and meat, and online sources for cooking fats and flavoring ingredients.

Almost everything goes on sale. Even online retailers have sales and coupons. Subscribing to a company's newsletter is typically the best way to find out about discounts. Having freezer space is useful when it comes to taking advantage of sales, but even if your freezer space is limited, you can benefit.

Buying in bulk is a great way to save money. The price per pound often decreases as you buy more. Many local farmers will give you a deal when you buy a quarter, half, or whole cow or pig. For example, you might pay $7 per pound for grass-fed ground beef, but if you buy a quarter or half a cow, you get a variety of cuts, from ground beef to prime rib, for $4 or $5 per pound (or less!). If you don't have the freezer space for half a cow, find some friends or family members to share a quarter cow with.

It's helpful to know what you can get at heavily discounted prices. You know those foods that jumped out at you as being "weird"? Well, when lots of people think that a food is too weird to eat, there typically isn't as much of a market for it, so prices are lower. So, yes, organ meat can be some of the cheapest meat available. Sometimes local farmers will give it to you for free (or at a heavy discount) because they can't find anyone to buy it. It also helps to know what is typically thrown away. If you ask, a butcher will put aside the grass-fed beef trimmings for you so that you can render your own tallow (and typically will give it to you for free or at a heavy discount). Fish heads might normally be thrown away, but if you ask at the fish counter, the fishmonger may give them to you for free (and you can make soup or cook them in other ways).

It's also helpful to know which meats tend to be cheaper per pound and which vegetables and fruits will stretch a meal further. Depending on where you live, chicken may be cheaper than pork, which is cheaper than beef. And when buying high-quality meat, it's helpful to know that in most places, grass-fed beef is cheaper than pasture-raised pork, which is cheaper than pasture-raised chicken. Tougher cuts of meat, like chuck roast, stew meat, pork shoulder, shanks, and short ribs, are usually less expensive (and very flavorful). Certain vegetables give you great bang for your buck. Cabbage, for example, is typically extremely inexpensive as compared with baby greens. In fact, cruciferous vegetables in general, except perhaps for the most common cauliflower and broccoli, tend

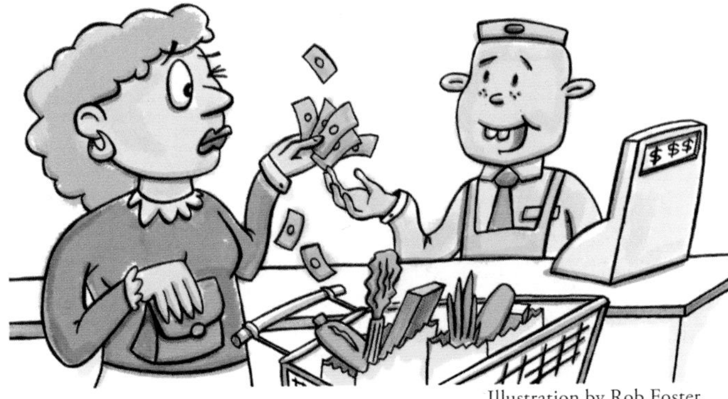

Illustration by Rob Foster

to be very inexpensive. Using root vegetables and plantains is a fantastic way to stretch a meal. Bananas tend to be much cheaper than apples, which tend to be much cheaper than grapes or berries. And when you can buy vegetables in bulk, you'll save even more.

Food that you have to put more time into also tends to be cheaper. For example, a whole chicken is typically cheaper per pound than a chicken cut into parts. A beef roast is cheaper per pound than steaks, and a pork roast is cheaper per pound than chops. Vegetables that require peeling and chopping tend to be cheaper than those that can be thrown straight into a pot or onto a plate, which are cheaper than preprepared or prewashed vegetables in plastic containers or microwave-safe bags.

Canned and frozen foods are often cheaper than fresh. While you probably won't want to buy canned vegetables because of additives, canned fish and shellfish are fantastic inexpensive options for increasing your seafood intake. (Look for BPA-free cans!) Canned seafood is typically cheaper than frozen, which is typically cheaper than fresh. However, when fish and shellfish are in season, they tend to go on sale, so knowing when your favorite types of seafood are in peak season can be a great way to save money. Frozen vegetables are a fantastic way to increase nutrient density since they are typically picked at their peak and frozen soon after. In fact, frozen vegetables tend to have more nutrients that fresh vegetables from the grocery store because the ones in the produce aisle tend to be picked before they are ripe and lose nutrients during shipping and storage before they make it into your grocery cart.

When foods do go on sale or are offered in bulk, you can save money by freezing your own. You can freeze the raw food right in the package you bought it in, preprepare the food so that it saves you time when you're ready to use it (like chopping or blanching veggies before freezing; some vegetables are best when blanched before being frozen, but not all), or cook and freeze meals for convenience on a busy weeknight. You can also ferment fruits and vegetables as an alternative to freezing them. For example, when cabbage is in season, you can make a large batch of sauerkraut to take advantage of both peak-season produce and the typically cheaper peak-season prices. Buying what's on sale is also a great way to buy in-season produce, since spikes in supply are one of the major reasons for drops in price.

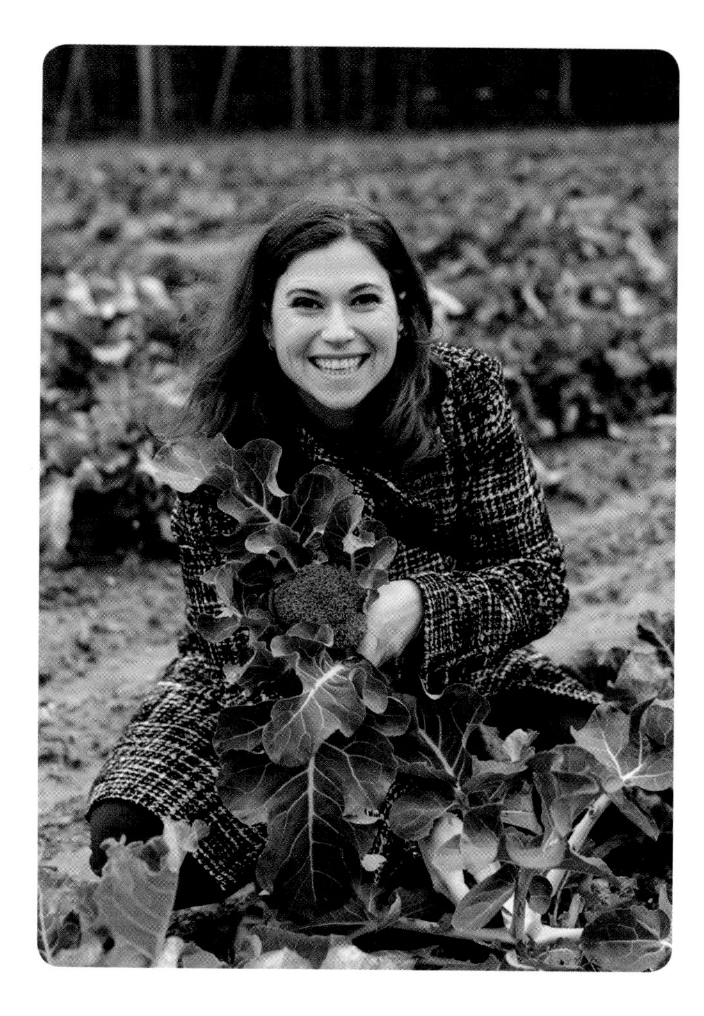

It's really helpful to know the people who grow your food. If you arrive at the farmer's market or your local farm stand at closing time, you will often be rewarded with good deals on whatever didn't sell. Bruisies (or seconds), the produce that has some flaws like bruises or bird beak holes, can often be purchased heavily discounted (the tradeoff is that they tend not to keep for long, so plan on eating or freezing them as soon as you get home). Joining a farm share or CSA is typically a great way to save on farm-fresh produce. Doing some of the work for your vegetables and fruits is another way to save money. In addition to pick-your-own farms, some farmers will trade your labor on the farm (weeding, harvesting, etc.) for produce if you ask. Do you have something else to trade? Don't be afraid to barter! Your local farmers are also a helpful resource for knowledge on what you can most easily grow in your climate in your backyard.

Probably the most helpful tool I can give you to stay within your means is to help you prioritize which foods are worth spending a little more on and which ones are okay to purchase in the conventionally produced, non-organic varieties.

The Dirty Dozen and the Clean Fifteen

The Environmental Working Group (EWG; www.ewg.org) is an environmental health research and advocacy group that analyzes the USDA and FDA pesticide test results of four dozen common vegetable and fruit crops every year. From this analysis, the EWG puts together two lists: the Dirty Dozen is a list of the top twelve fresh produce items most contaminated with pesticides, and the Clean Fifteen are the fifteen with the least pesticide residues.

While the Dirty Dozen list is updated yearly, it's important to note that leafy greens, berries, stone fruits, and fruits from the apple family are frequent flyers on this list. It's also important to remember that the benefits of a diet high in vegetables and fruit far outweigh the risks of pesticide exposure from eating the conventionally grown versions.

2014 Dirty Dozen*

- Apples
- Celery
- Cucumbers
- Grapes
- Kale/collard greens
- Nectarines
- Peaches
- Spinach
- Strawberries

2014 Clean Fifteen*

- Asparagus
- Avocados
- Cabbage
- Cantaloupe
- Cauliflower
- Grapefruit
- Kiwi
- Mangoes
- Onions
- Papayas
- Pineapples
- Sweet potatoes

* These lists include only those Dirty Dozen and Clean Fifteen foods that are also Paleo Approach friendly. For the complete and most current Dirty Dozen and Clean Fifteen lists, visit the Environmental Working Group website, www.ewg.org.

When your budget is tight, the single best place to spend a few extra pennies is on your cooking and dressing fats. The best, most nutrient-dense choices are grass-fed tallow, pasture-raised lard, extra-virgin coconut oil, red palm oil, extra-virgin olive oil, and extra-virgin avocado oil. Tallow and lard can be rendered very inexpensively at home (you can get quality fats from local meat farmers and butchers and online), whereas coconut, red palm, olive, and avocado oils tend to be cheapest when bought in bulk and online. Refined or semirefined fats (like refined coconut oil, palm oil, palm shortening, and virgin olive oil) contain fewer vitamins and antioxidants but are still good options in a pinch.

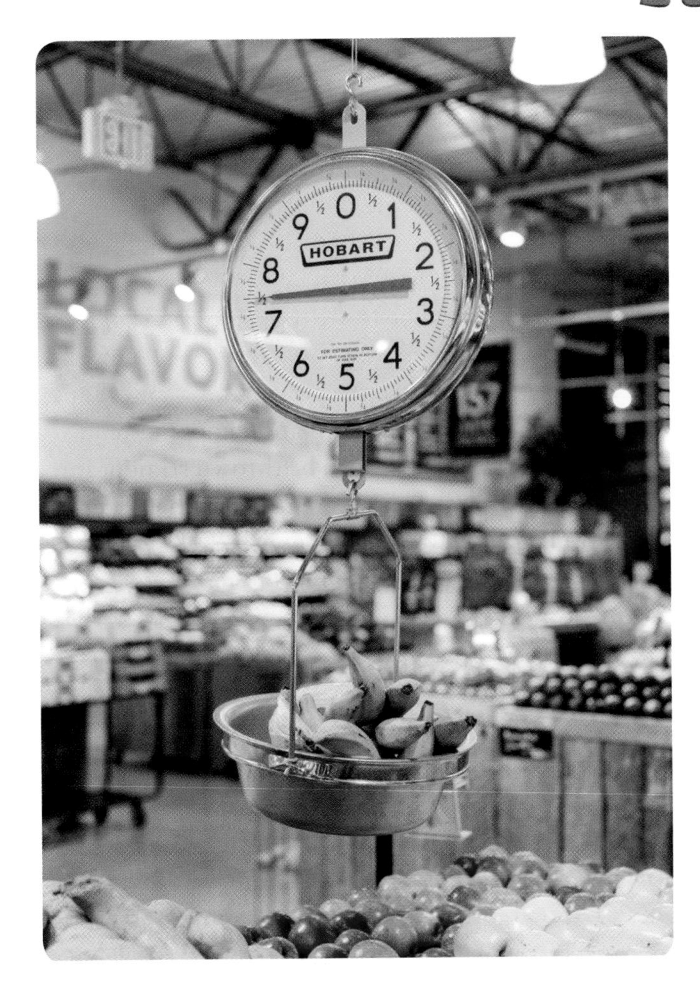

Even if the only food you can afford or source is the conventionally produced meat, seafood, and produce on sale at your local grocery store, that's okay. The point is to make you aware of the differences so that you can make the best choices within your means—not to bankrupt you! Many people find that as they progress on their health journey, they are able to dedicate more funds to quality foods. This might reflect money saved by avoiding restaurants, fast food, and prepackaged foods. Or it might reflect reduced medical expenses once you start feeling better. Sometimes it just reflects a shift in priorities and a choice to reduce expenses or go without in some other area of life in order to free up funds for local, grass-fed meat.

Meat Priorities

Best

- **Organ meat from grass-fed and pasture-raised animals:** Organ meat is densely packed with just about every vitamin and mineral, and the fat content is also extremely healthy.
- **Wild-caught fish and shellfish:** Wild-caught fatty fish can be found fresh, canned, or frozen. Look for sales in the late summer and early fall.
- **Grass-fed beef, bison, lamb, venison, and goat:** Ground meat is always the cheapest. Some local farmers sell bulk meat at a steep discount.
- **Wild game:** You can buy wild game if you do not hunt.

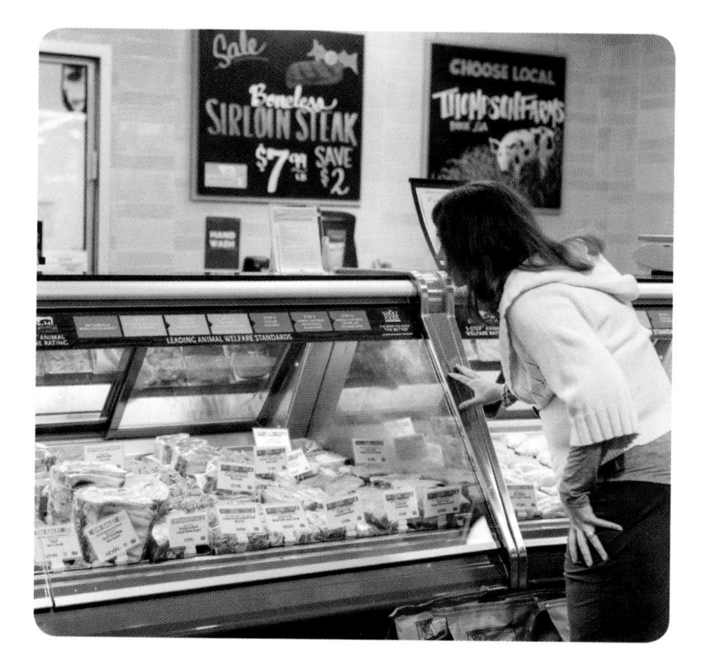

Better

- **Organ meat from organic and conventionally raised animals:** The fat profile is less favorable, but the organs still contain denser nutrition than muscle meat.
- **Farmed fish and shellfish:** Even farmed fish contains extremely beneficial fats and is rich in amino acids, vitamins, and minerals that aren't as easy to get from meat and poultry.
- **Pasture-raised pork and free-range poultry:** Look for meat from animals that are not fed soy.

Good

- **Organic meat and conventionally raised lamb and veal:** These animals do spend some time on pasture and eat at least some grass.
- **Lean cuts of beef:** Marbled steaks typically contain ten to fifteen times more omega-6 than omega-3 fatty acids.
- **Lean pork:** Usually, the lighter colored the meat, the lower the fat content.

Moderate or avoid

- **Fatty cuts of conventional beef and pork:** Ideally, this meat would be only an occasional treat.
- **Conventional chicken and turkey:** Conventionally raised chicken can have some of the highest omega-6 levels of any meat.

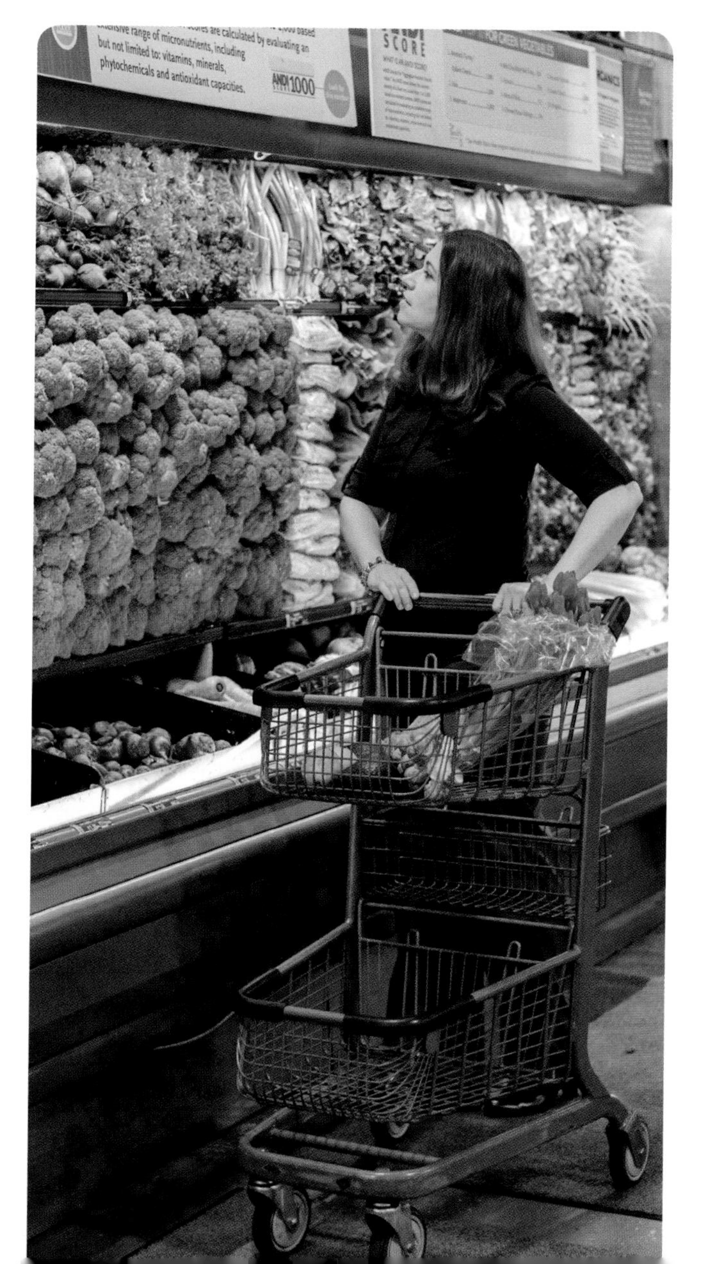

Vegetables and Fruit Priorities

Best

- **Wild edibles:** Wild varieties of mushrooms, alliums, leafy greens, and berries are some of the most nutrient-dense foods on the planet. Learn which edible plants grow near you so that you can forage (or get to know a local farmer who forages and sells the bounty at a nearby farm stand or farmer's market). Be careful of wild mushrooms, since misidentifying them can be very dangerous.
- **Local, organic, in-season fresh produce:** Next to wild plants, this is the most nutrient-dense produce you can get. Look for a farmer who is passionate about the quality of her soil.
- **Home-grown vegetables, fruits, and herbs:** Even if your space is limited, many edible plants grow well in flowerpots. You'll notice the savings just from growing fresh herbs.
- **Organic frozen produce:** Picked at the peak of ripeness and frozen soon after harvest, organic frozen produce can be more nutrient dense than fresh.
- **Organic fresh herbs and spices:** Herbs and spices tend to pack quite a nutrient punch. Including more herbs in your cooking, in salads, and even in green smoothies is a great way to increase nutrient density.

Better

- **Local, non-organic, in-season fresh produce:** Local, in-season produce is still nutrient dense even if it is not certified organic or naturally grown. Avoid non-organic produce from the Dirty Dozen list (see page 39) unless you can talk to the farmer about pesticide policies. Some farms use pesticides very sparingly, but enough that they are unable to be certified organic. Produce from these farms is usually a good option.
- **Organic fresh or frozen produce off the Dirty Dozen list:** When buying produce off the Dirty Dozen list, buy organic whenever possible, preferably in season (see page 39).
- **Conventional fresh or frozen produce off the Clean Fifteen list:** When buying off the Clean Fifteen list, conventional produce, preferably in season, is a great option (see page 39).
- **Organic dried or frozen herbs and spices:** While fresh herbs are more nutrient dense (and typically more flavorful), dried organic herbs and spices are still great options. Using frozen herbs is a great way to get the flavor of fresh herbs in your cooking while preserving nutrients. You can freeze your own when herbs are in season (see page 54).

Good

- **All other conventional produce:** It's important to eat lots of vegetables, even if your budget or location limits you to conventional store-bought options. Peeling fruits and vegetables is a very good way to limit your exposure to pesticides and produce waxes (some of which contain soy or gluten). If you are limited to conventional produce, choose those on the Dirty Dozen list less often, wash thoroughly, and peel if possible.
- **Additive-free vegetables and fruits in BPA-free cans:** Canning does preserve nutrients, though not as well as freezing. As long as these products don't contain preservatives or other additives, they are good options.
- **Non-organic herbs and spices:** As already mentioned, fresh herbs are very nutrient-dense foods. Using frozen herbs is a great way to get the flavor of fresh herbs in your cooking while preserving nutrients. You can freeze your own when herbs are in season. Dried spices are also great options for flavoring foods and are great to include in your diet even if you can't afford or source organic versions.

Moderate or avoid

- **Conventional produce off the Dirty Dozen list:** If you do buy conventional produce off the Dirty Dozen list, wash it thoroughly and peel it whenever possible.
- **Canned vegetables or fruits with preservatives, additives, added sugars, or salts or in BPA-lined cans:** Many of the preservatives and additives in canned vegetables and fruits are antinutrients or gut irritants.

Know Where Your Food Comes From

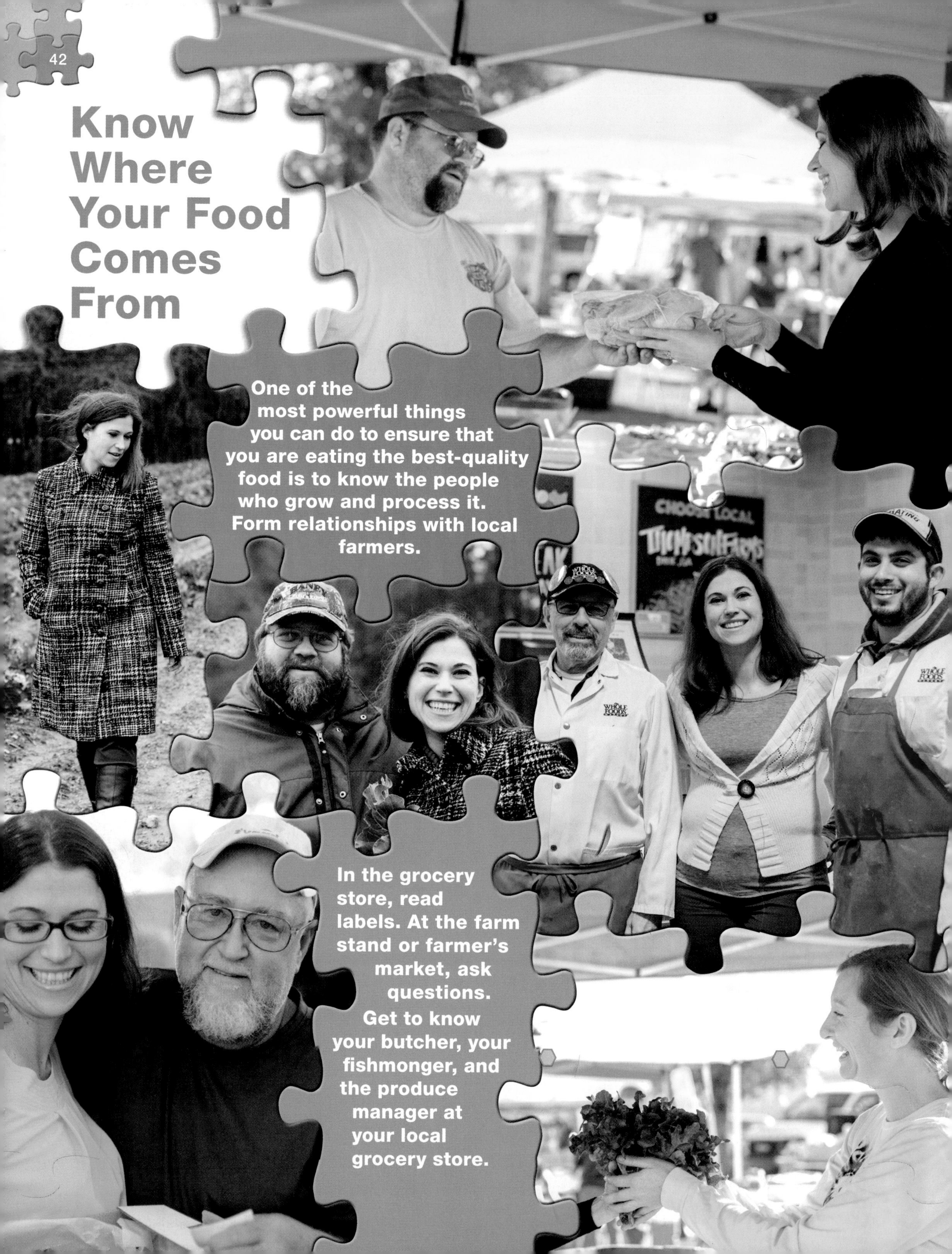

One of the most powerful things you can do to ensure that you are eating the best-quality food is to know the people who grow and process it. Form relationships with local farmers.

In the grocery store, read labels. At the farm stand or farmer's market, ask questions. Get to know your butcher, your fishmonger, and the produce manager at your local grocery store.

Visit your local farm. Volunteer to help with harvesting or weeding (this labor often brings rewards of fresh produce to take home).

Meet your meat. Know how the animals you plan to eat are treated. Know what they eat.

Being connected to your food system is important for knowing the quality of the food you are eating and also appreciating that food.

Some Gray Areas

Some foods are excluded from the Paleo Approach diet but are probably okay for most people. These gray-area foods include legumes with edible pods, like green beans, sugar snap peas, snow peas, scarlet runner beans, and peas; sprouted legumes, like mung beans; cultured grass-fed ghee (the culturing process degrades any trace proteins); pasture-raised egg yolks; spices derived from berries and fruits, like pepper, caraway, and cardamom; spices derived from seeds, like anise, cumin, coriander, and mustard; and nut and seed oils (especially macadamia nut oil and walnut oil, which contain very healthy fats). All these foods are potentially problematic for very sensitive individuals (and let's face it, if you have an autoimmune disease, chances are pretty high that you qualify), so I recommend eliminating them when you first adopt the Paleo Approach.

None of these ingredients are used in this cookbook because of the possibility that they will cause problems for some of you. They are generally considered Stage 1 Reintroduction Foods—that is, the first foods you should attempt to reintroduce once you begin to see improvements. Cultured grass-fed ghee and pasture-raised egg yolks are particularly nutrient-dense foods, which is a compelling reason to attempt to reintroduce them before other options. *The Paleo Approach* discusses the process of reintroduction in detail.

Other gray areas include nuts and seeds used to make herbal teas (for example, cardamom as an ingredient in chai tea), algae other than chlorella and spirulina (both of which are potential immune stimulators and are best avoided, whereas other algae might be okay, although they have not been as thoroughly studied), grass-fed dairy that has been fermented for an extended period (for example, 24-hour kefir), white rice, and traditionally prepared pseudograins like buckwheat (properly soaked, sprouted, and cooked). These are all candidates for self-experimentation but are not included in this cookbook.

There are a few foods that are gray areas but *are* included in this cookbook. These include wine and distilled alcohols where most, but perhaps not all, of the alcohol will be cooked off (see page 82), wild mushrooms that are sources of immune-modulating extracts (like

How Much Coconut Is Too Much Coconut?

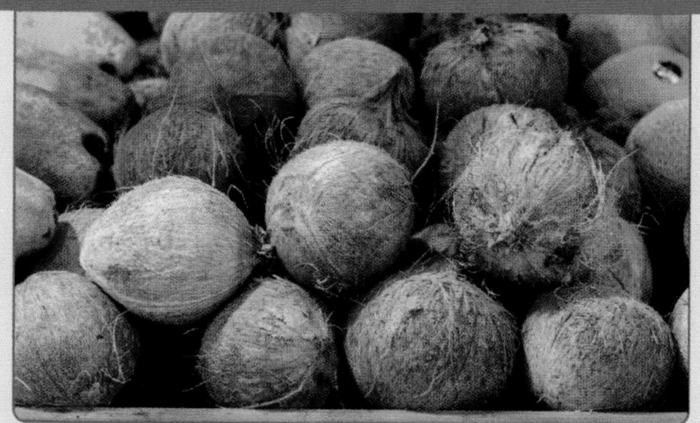

Coconut has many health benefits, but there are some compelling reasons to moderate your consumption. While the pros and cons of coconut are discussed in detail in *The Paleo Approach,* it's important to reiterate how much is reasonable here.

The following guide should be considered a starting place. When you consume coconut products, be on the lookout not only for gastrointestinal symptoms—bloating, nausea, constipation, diarrhea, tummyache, heartburn, changes in bowel habits, increased or decreased stool frequency, gas, undigested or partly digested food particles in stool—but also for symptoms of your disease worsening, fatigue, headache, mood issues, dry skin, acne or rashes, aches and pains, and trouble sleeping. Typically, the higher the fiber content of the coconut product, the more likely it is to be poorly tolerated. Often coconut oil is tolerated, but other coconut products are not. (I personally tolerate coconut oil, coconut milk, and coconut cream, but that's it.) And if coconut just doesn't work for you, that's okay. There is no minimum daily intake, after all. If you do great with coconut and feel better the more you consume, that's terrific. As previously mentioned, the number-one goal is to find what works for you.

Coconut Product	Suggested Maximum Daily Intake
Coconut sugar (aka palm sugar or nectar)	1 tablespoon
Coconut flour	1 to 2 tablespoons
Coconut butter (aka coconut cream concentrate, creamed coconut)	2 to 4 tablespoons
Unsweetened dried coconut (shredded, flakes, chips)	2 to 4 tablespoons (avoid sweetened dried coconut)
Fresh coconut flesh	4 to 6 tablespoons
Coconut cream	½ to 1 cup
Coconut milk (full fat or light)	1 cup
Coconut water	1 to 2 cups
Coconut oil (extra-virgin or refined)	Unlimited

shiitake mushrooms), and herbs from which immune-modulating extracts can be made (like lemon balm and turmeric). It's important to be aware that these foods may not work for you. Substitution options are generally included in the recipes that use these ingredients.

As much as the recommendations in *The Paleo Approach* are steeped in science, one overarching rule trumps them all: if you know beyond a shadow of a doubt that a food (or supplement or medication or activity) works for you, then you should feel free to continue to consume it; and if you know beyond a shadow of a doubt that a food (or supplement or medication or activity) is problematic for you (regardless of how highly praised it may be within these pages or those of *The Paleo Approach*), then you shouldn't eat it. My goal is to provide guidelines that give you the best possible chance of success, but this is not a one-size-fits-all approach, and you should feel at liberty to experiment. And at no time should a recommendation in *The Paleo Approach* replace the advice of your healthcare providers.

⚠ FODMAP Intolerance

For those with gastrointestinal symptoms, FODMAP intolerance (sometimes called fructose malabsorption or FODMAP sensitivity) is a distinct possibility. FODMAP is an acronym for "fermentable oligosaccharides, disaccharides, and monosaccharides and polyols," which are basically a group of highly fermentable, short- and medium-chain carbohydrates (typically high in fructose or lactose) and sugar alcohols. These carbohydrates are inefficiently absorbed in the small intestine, even in very healthy people, and gut bacteria love them (which is what makes them highly fermentable).

Symptoms of FODMAP intolerance include a variety of digestive symptoms, most typically bloating, cramps, diarrhea, constipation, indigestion, and sometimes excessive belching. If you have not been definitively diagnosed with FODMAP intolerance, it's up to you whether you start the Paleo Approach diet with or without high-FODMAP foods. Even if you have been diagnosed, most people find that as little as two to three weeks on a low-FODMAP diet is sufficient for them to be able to reintroduce FODMAPs into their diets successfully.

The key to following a low-FODMAP diet is to reduce or eliminate high-FODMAP foods. Some people are more sensitive to one type of FODMAP, so it's helpful to know whether a food is considered a high-FODMAP food due to fructose content, fructan content, or polyol content.

A variety of fruits make it onto the high-FODMAP food list either because they contain more than 0.5 grams of free fructose in excess of free glucose per 100-gram serving or because they contain more than 3 grams of free fructose per 100-gram serving.

⚠ The following fruits are considered FODMAPs due to fructose content:

- all canned fruit
- all dried fruit
- all fruit juices
- apples
- bananas (ripe)
- blueberries
- cherries
- dates
- figs
- grapes
- guavas
- kiwis
- mangoes
- pears
- plums
- watermelon
- large servings of any fruit

⚠ These fruits and vegetables are high FODMAP because they contain more than 0.2 grams of fructans per 100-gram serving:

- artichokes, globe
- artichokes, Jerusalem*
- asparagus**
- beets
- broccoli**
- brussels sprouts
- bulb onions*
- butternut squash**
- cabbage**
- chicory root
- coconut (except coconut oil)
- dandelion greens
- fennel bulb**
- garlic*
- grapefruit
- green onions (white part only)
- honeydew melon
- leeks (white part only)*
- longons
- nectarines
- okra
- onions
- peaches, white
- persimmons
- rambutan
- shallots*
- sweet potatoes**
- watermelon
- zucchini

*Denotes very high fructan content.

**Conflicting measurements; some say no fructans.

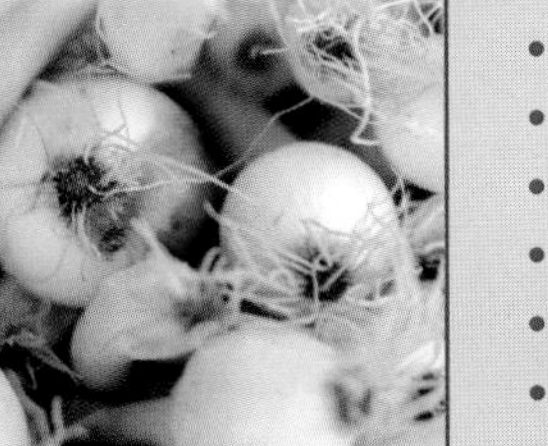

⚠ These fruits and vegetables contain significant amounts of polyols:

- apples
- apricots
- avocados
- blackberries
- cauliflower
- celery
- cherries
- longons
- lychees
- mushrooms
- nashi pears
- nectarines
- peaches
- pears
- plums
- prunes
- snow peas
- sweet potatoes
- watermelon

Where Do These Diet Recommendations Come From?

The Paleo Approach provides detailed scientific rationale including more than 1,200 citations for every aspect of the Paleo Approach, including why some foods need to be avoided and why it's important to eat more of others, and why it's important to get more sleep, manage stress, and get the right amounts of the right kinds of activity. Though it's not essential to understand the science behind these recommendations in order to implement and benefit from them, many people find motivation in the knowledge that these recommendations have a firm scientific foundation. Here are some of the highlights:

Nutrient Density

▶ A nutrient-poor diet is one of the biggest risk factors for autoimmune disease. Autoimmune diseases have been linked to dietary insufficiencies of a staggering number of vitamins and minerals, as well as to insufficiencies in antioxidants, fiber, and essential fatty acids.

▶ The immune system requires micronutrients (water-soluble and fat-soluble vitamins, minerals, and antioxidants), plus essential fatty acids and amino acids, to function normally.

▶ Eating fat is good for you. The healthiest fats are saturated and monounsaturated fats, and it is essential to consume a balanced ratio of omega-6 to omega-3 polyunsaturated fatty acids (ideally between 1:1 and 4:1).

▶ Eating fat is necessary for the absorption of fat-soluble vitamins.

▶ Eating a nutrient-dense diet based on quality meats, seafood, vegetables, and fruits is the healthiest and most effective way to ensure that your body is getting all the nutrients it needs for optimal health.

▶ Increasing nutrient density can increase your resilience to stress, meaning that stressors in your life have less of an impact on your well-being, and help regulate important hormones and neurotransmitters.

Gut Health

▶ A leaky gut is necessary for autoimmune disease to develop.

▶ A variety of proteins in grains—including prolamins, such as gluten, and agglutinins, such as wheat germ agglutinin—cause increased intestinal permeability (gut leakiness) and feed bacterial overgrowth in the gut.

▶ Digestive enzyme inhibitors in grains, legumes, nuts, seeds, and dairy products cause increased intestinal permeability and feed bacterial overgrowth in the gut.

▶ A high dietary intake of phytates or phytic acid—found in grains, legumes, nuts, and seeds—causes increased intestinal permeability.

▶ Types of saponins called glycoalkaloids, found in vegetables of the nightshade family, cause increased intestinal permeability. Other saponins found in legumes may also be problematic.

▶ Alcohol consumption causes increased intestinal permeability, damages the gut, and feeds bacterial overgrowth and dysbiosis.

▶ Excessive fructose intake (more than 20 grams per day) may cause increased intestinal permeability and damage to the liver.

▶ All sugar substitutes have negative health effects, and many of them cause increased intestinal permeability.

▶ Too much omega-6 fatty acids cause gut dysbiosis. Increasing omega-3 fatty acid intake helps correct gut dysbiosis.

▶ A diet rich in vegetables, including plenty of nonstarchy vegetables and some starchy vegetables, supports a healthy variety and amount of probiotic gut organisms.

▶ Probiotic-rich foods support a healthy gut microbiome.

▶ Foods rich in vitamin A, vitamin D, vitamin K_2, and the amino acids glutamine and glycine can help restore gut barrier function.

▶ The medium-chain triglycerides in coconut oil may help restore gut barrier function.

▶ Reducing and managing stress is critical for gut health.

Hormone Regulation

▶ High-carbohydrate diets cause insulin resistance and leptin resistance.

▶ Following a low-carbohydrate diet is not essential, but avoiding a high-carbohydrate diet is.

▶ Regulating blood glucose levels and insulin release by eating low- to moderate-glycemic-load foods is important. This approach helps regulate insulin and insulin sensitivity as well as leptin and leptin sensitivity.

▶ Fructose causes insulin resistance and leptin resistance. Fructose also doesn't suppress ghrelin levels after eating. Dietary fructose should be maintained in the 10- to 20-grams-per-day range.

▶ Hunger hormones are intricately linked to the immune system. Eating large, balanced meals that contain protein, fat, and low- to moderate-glycemic-load vegetables and fruits and minimizing snacking is the best way to regulate hunger hormones.

▶ Cortisol levels may rise as a result of skipping meals or intermittent fasting and stimulate the immune system.

▶ Dietary fiber, especially insoluble fiber, from whole-food sources such as vegetables helps regulate ghrelin levels and may regulate peristalsis by increasing gastrointestinal melatonin production.

▶ Reducing and managing stress, getting plenty of low- and moderate-intensity activity, and getting adequate sleep help regulate critical hormones.

Immune Health

▶ A variety of proteins in grains—including prolamins, such as gluten, and agglutinins, such as wheat germ agglutinin—stimulate the immune system.

▶ Gluten may be an important trigger in all autoimmune diseases.

▶ Digestive enzyme inhibitors in grains, legumes, nuts, seeds, and dairy products cause inflammation.

▶ Types of saponins called glycoalkaloids, found in vegetables of the nightshade family, significantly stimulate the immune system. Other saponins found in legumes may also be problematic.

▶ Alcohol consumption stimulates inflammation.

▶ Proteins found in egg whites act as carrier molecules for bacterial proteins to cross the gut barrier, which then stimulate the immune system.

▶ Excessive fructose intake (more than 20 grams per day) causes inflammation.

▶ Eating too much omega-6 fatty acids causes inflammation, whereas increasing omega-3 fatty acid intake helps reduce inflammation and modulate the immune system. Moderate consumption of monounsaturated fats and saturated fats is healthy.

▶ Reducing and managing stress and getting plenty of sleep are critical for normal immune function.

A Few Last Food Rules

> *There is no sincerer love than the love of food.*
> —George Bernard Shaw

You've read through the food lists and know what to eat and what to avoid, and you're sold on the importance of quality and variety. You've even figured out where you're going to buy some of these new foods and are working on priorities to stay within your budget. You're almost ready to get cooking!

I want to recap a few more guidelines from *The Paleo Approach*. I'll spare you the science, as promised, but know that these recommendations come from maximizing the essential nutrients and regulating important hormones that your immune system needs to function normally.

- **Eat large portions of nonstarchy vegetables with every meal. Aim for 10 to 14 cups per day.**
- **Eat some starchy vegetables.**
- **Eat the rainbow: aim to eat a variety of different vegetables every day.**
- **Eat some fruit, but make sure that your total fructose consumption is below 20 grams per day.**
- **Eat offal (organ meat and other unusual cuts) at least four or five times per week.**
- **Eat snout to tail: eat as much variety in cuts of meat as possible. Also vary the animals your meat is coming from.**
- **Eat seafood at least three times per week if you are eating grass-fed meat and very little poultry.**
- **Eat seafood daily if the quality of the meat you are buying is lower or if you are eating a lot of chicken and turkey.**
- **Eat shellfish at least once per week.**
- **Eat sea vegetables at least once per week.**
- **Eat both animal foods and plant foods with every meal.**
- **Eat probiotic foods.**
- **For most people, it's better to eat bigger meals less frequently. Aim for two or three large meals per day (and maybe one snack).**

If you're just starting out on your journey to better health, it's important to know that, because the damage to your gut is very likely affecting your body's ability to absorb nutrients from your food, nutrient density is paramount. As your gut heals, your ability to absorb and use the nutrients from your food will increase, and so will your body's rate of healing. Sleep, stress management, physical activity, and support of your circadian rhythms also speed up healing. (It's not all about food!) Supporting digestion is also important; practicing good meal hygiene and taking supplements may be extremely beneficial, at least initially (discussed in detail in *The Paleo Approach*).

As you move into the rest of this cookbook, I want to emphasize that change doesn't have to happen overnight. If it's easier for you to take baby steps, then that's the way you should approach this transition. I also want to emphasize that it will get easier. Yes, it takes effort to make broad, sweeping changes to your diet; and even when those changes make you feel better, it isn't always easy. But old favorites will eventually lose their hold on you, and new healthy favorites will take their place. Initially, you will find yourself spending more time in the kitchen, but as you gain comfort and confidence in cooking with these new ingredients, you will find efficiency in the kitchen once more. And yes, some of these new foods will taste foreign to you, and you may not like some of them; but your taste buds will adapt. Two years ago, I would wax on about how kidney was the only organ meat that I refused to eat because I disliked it so strongly. Now it's my favorite breakfast. The same goes for sauerkraut and raw kale salad. Yes, taste buds really do change, and it's a magical moment when you start finding that the most nutrient-dense and healing foods have become the most delicious to you. In the meantime, it's okay to hide liver even from yourself.

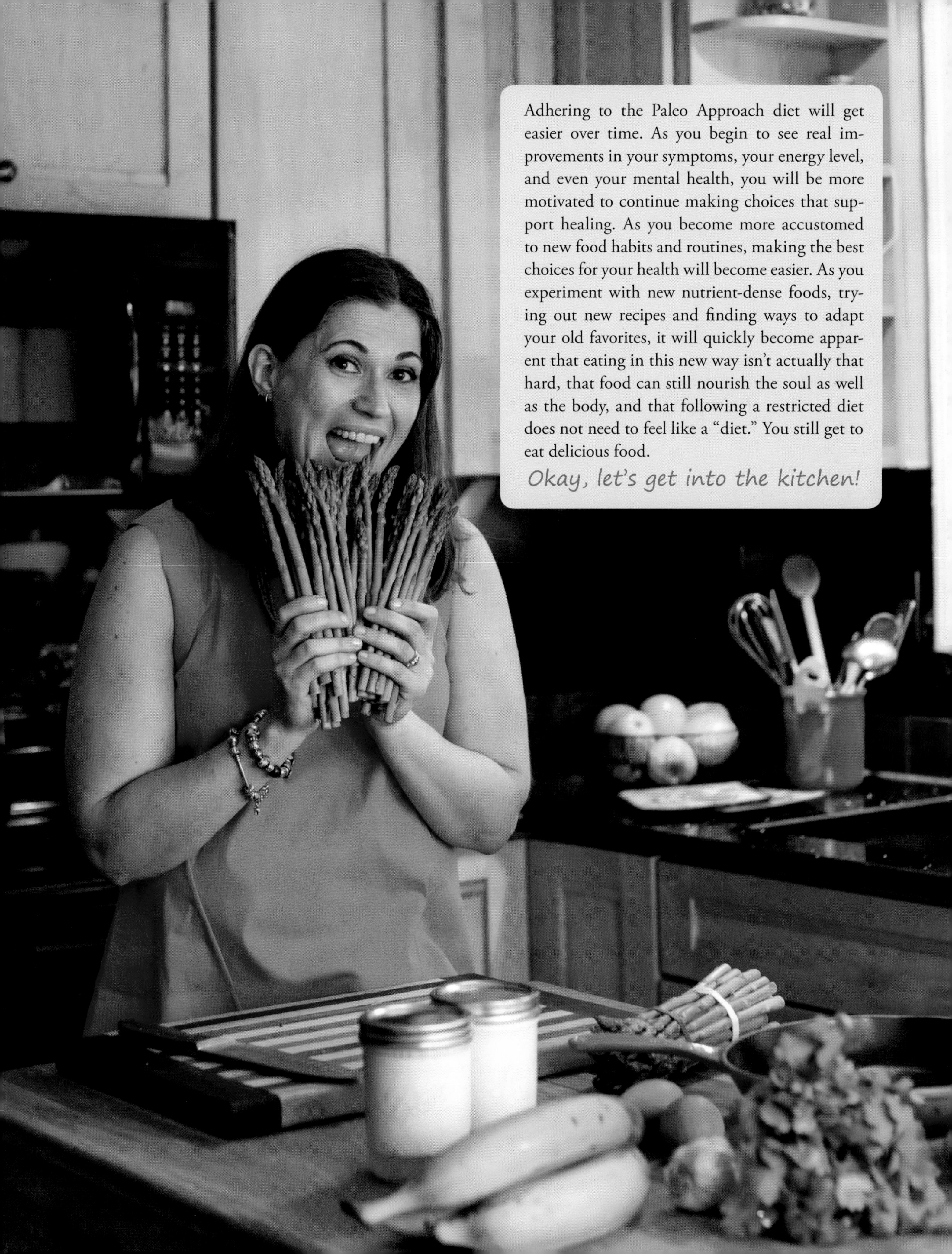

Adhering to the Paleo Approach diet will get easier over time. As you begin to see real improvements in your symptoms, your energy level, and even your mental health, you will be more motivated to continue making choices that support healing. As you become more accustomed to new food habits and routines, making the best choices for your health will become easier. As you experiment with new nutrient-dense foods, trying out new recipes and finding ways to adapt your old favorites, it will quickly become apparent that eating in this new way isn't actually that hard, that food can still nourish the soul as well as the body, and that following a restricted diet does not need to feel like a "diet." You still get to eat delicious food.

Okay, let's get into the kitchen!

Chapter 2
In the Kitchen

> *To eat is a necessity, but to eat intelligently is an art.*
>
> —Duc de La Rochefoucauld

One of the unfortunate effects of dramatically changing how you eat is that convenience foods are mostly a thing of the past. No longer are you able to quickly pick something up from the drive-thru or dial a number to have a meal delivered to your door (with a few exceptions, depending on where you live). Even grabbing a box of something preprepared out of your freezer for a meal that is just three minutes on high away is no longer an option (unless that preprepared meal is one that you prepared yourself!).

The Paleo Approach diet is definitely an adjustment. But spending more time in the kitchen doesn't need to be a hardship. As you reevaluate your priorities, you may find that food preparation becomes an opportunity to unwind or visit with your spouse or your kids. Maybe you'll use the time to catch up on your favorite podcast or audiobook or talk to a long-lost friend on the phone. Maybe it will be an opportunity to fit some activity into your day (lunges while the meat is browning, prisoner squats while the food processor is running, wall push-ups or dips using the kitchen counter between chopping vegetables). Maybe it will become a time to be in your own thoughts, to contemplate and reflect and appreciate. Maybe it'll just be about the food and the enjoyment of creating delicious, nourishing meals. My point is that cooking is a chore only if you approach it as one.

This chapter is about getting organized, getting more comfortable in the kitchen, and adjusting to spending more time preparing food. You'll find lists of essential pantry items, explanations of basic cooking and food preparation techniques, useful guides, ideas for substitutions, and tips on time management. You can think of this as the "how to get started" chapter.

This chapter is also designed for those of you who don't cook (notice that I didn't use the word *can't*—because you can, even if you haven't done much cooking until now). This chapter will bring you up to speed on everything you need to know to be successful in the kitchen, from the essential tools with which to stock your cabinets to the vocabulary you need to follow recipes.

I learned how to cook largely by just doing it. I helped my mom in the kitchen as a kid, and by my mid-teens I was responsible for cooking simple meals whenever her schedule made it difficult for her to do it. When I moved out on my own in my late teens, I began collecting cookbooks and experimenting with different flavors and cooking techniques. Over the years, I developed keen instincts in the kitchen by trying new recipes and being forced to improvise when midway through a recipe I found that I was missing an ingredient or had followed a step incorrectly. (This happened a lot.) One of my favorite cookbooks at that time, and the one that gave me the knowledge base I needed to salvage a meal when I found myself short a crucial component, was Julia Child's *The Way to Cook.* Julia's recipes are designed not to give you a formula to follow, but to teach you how to cook, to find flavors that work well together, and to know what to watch for at each stage of the process. This chapter is my nod to Julia Child, because it not only prepares you for the recipes and meal plans provided in this book, but also prepares you to go beyond *The Paleo Approach Cookbook.* Yes, before we even get to the recipes, I'm preparing you for life beyond them.

The recipes in this cookbook give you a formula to follow to help you succeed with the monumental task of changing your diet. In addition, these recipes very often suggest variations or substitutions. Not only are these variations opportunities to increase variety and expand your cooking repertoire, but they also are starting points for your own experimentation in the kitchen. As you gain experience with these new foods, you may want to add some of your favorite flavoring ingredients or herbs or remove an ingredient that just isn't your cup of tea. Eventually, you'll feel confident winging it in the kitchen, maybe even tackling adaptations of some of your old favorite dishes. Perhaps you will graduate completely from following recipes, and this book will collect dust on your bookshelf. But even though I use *The Way to Cook* infrequently (and yes, it does get a bit dusty), I still treasure it. Even two decades later, I find it a tremendous resource and a source of inspiration—and I hope that *The Paleo Approach Cookbook* fills this role for you.

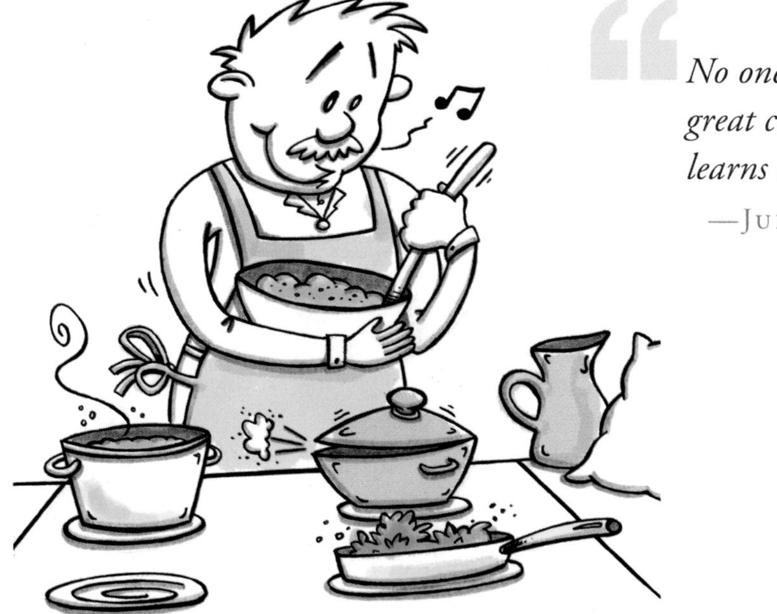

Illustration by Rob Foster

> *No one is born a great cook, one learns by doing.*
> —Julia Child

Stocking the Pantry

> *Even the most resourceful housewife cannot create miracles from a riceless pantry.*
>
> —Chinese Proverb

Stereotypes and rice aside, it really is true that a well-stocked pantry, fridge, and freezer is your best tool for creating flavorful and healthful meals in the shortest time and with the least stress. You have so many more options for quick meals if you have broth in your freezer, a selection of healthy cooking fats in your cupboard, an abundance of fresh vegetables in the crisper drawer of your fridge, and fresh herbs growing in pots on your kitchen windowsill.

The essential foods to have on hand are probably fairly different from what you're used to, although the general categories are the same: common base ingredients, cooking fats, oils for dressing foods, herbs and spices, and other flavoring ingredients. Having at least some of these foods on hand before you adopt the Paleo Approach diet will definitely make the transition easier. Of course, there's lots of room for expanding on the basics to have a wide variety of ingredients handy for your cooking adventures.

I made a concerted effort to use a great diversity of ingredients in these recipes, in part to introduce you to new foods and in part to build variety right into this book. This chapter includes some of the most fundamental pantry items to shop for initially; but, while stocking up on some basics beforehand can make a huge difference, you don't need to go out and buy all of these exotic foods at once. Instead, buy a few new pantry items each week and slowly build up your supply. You can prioritize which pantry items to buy each week by following the meal plans in Chapter 3 or simply by choosing which new recipes you want to try in the coming week before you head to the stores. By comparing the ingredients required for the coming week with what you already have stocked, you can add to your pantry slowly over time.

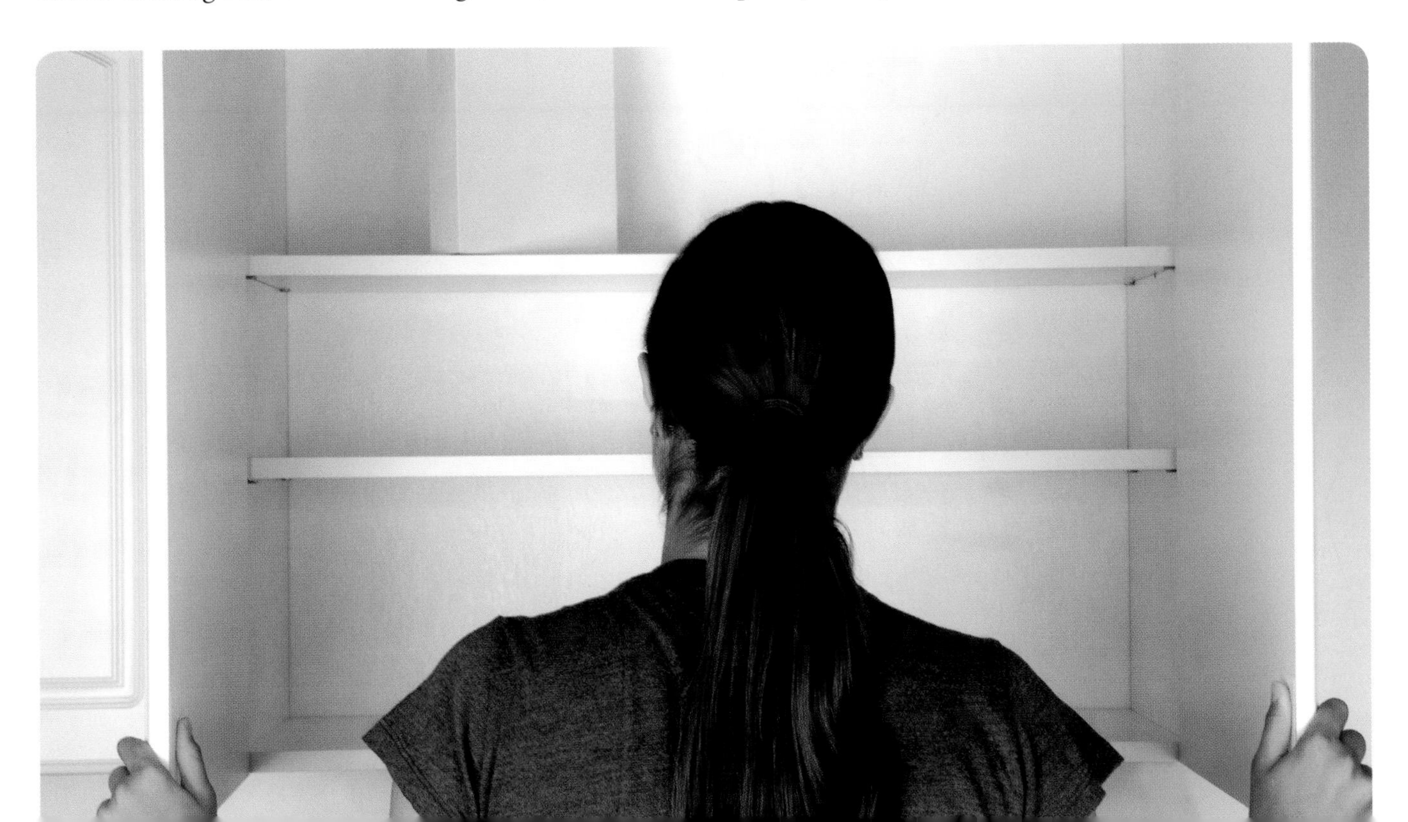

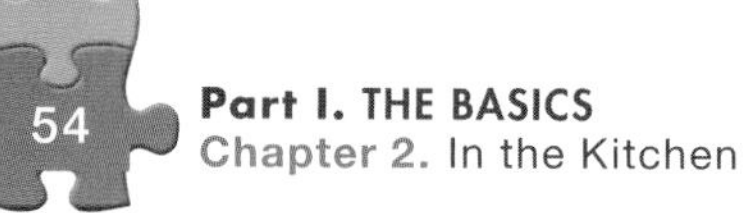

Nonperishables to Have on Hand

Cooking fats

- coconut oil
- tallow or lard

Dressing fats

- avocado oil
- extra-virgin olive oil

Basic herbs and spices

- bay leaves
- cinnamon
- mace
- rosemary
- sage
- salt (pink or gray sea salt)
- tarragon
- thyme

Flavoring ingredients

- apple cider vinegar
- balsamic vinegar
- coconut water vinegar
- fish sauce
- white wine vinegar

Other basics

- arrowroot powder
- coconut milk (homemade [page 116] or guar gum–free and in BPA-free cans)
- gelatin
- kuzu starch

Perishable Foods to Keep Stocked

Bacon

Bone Broth (page 110)

Fresh herbs: basil, cilantro, mint, parsley

Garlic

Ginger

Aromatic fruits and vegetables

- carrots
- celery
- onions
- lemons

Staple vegetables

- broccoli
- cabbage
- cauliflower
- leafy greens
- plantains
- root vegetables
- winter squash

Illustration by Rob Foster

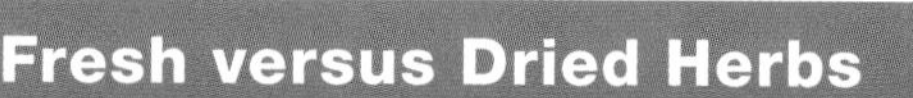

Fresh versus Dried Herbs

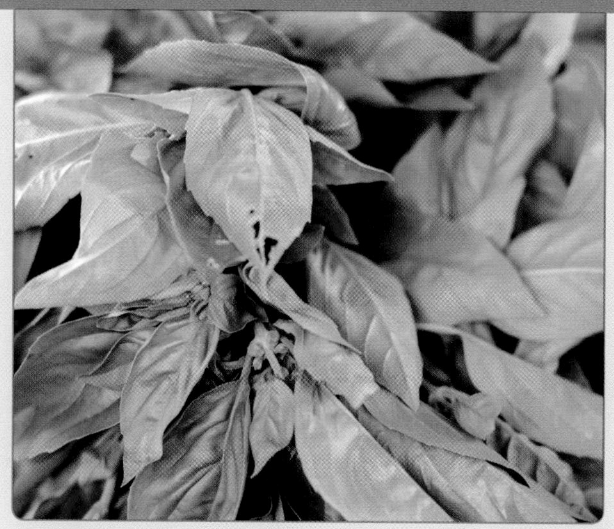

Without exception, the flavor of fresh herbs trumps dried. But you just can't beat the convenience of having an assortment of dried herbs in your pantry. Some herbs—like oregano, rosemary, sage, and thyme—retain their flavor well when dried. Other herbs, including basil, cilantro, mint, and parsley, taste better fresh—so much better, in fact, that I think it's pointless to buy the dried versions.

You can freeze fresh herbs when they're in season in your garden or when you buy a bunch from your local farmer's market or grocery store, so you retain the flavor and convenience of having them on hand without having to buy them every week.

To freeze fresh herbs:

- For every 2 cups packed fresh herb leaves, add ⅓ cup olive oil, avocado oil, or melted and cooled coconut oil.
- Pulse in a food processor, scraping down the sides of the bowl from time to time, until you get a chunky paste and all the leaves are chopped.
- Spoon 1 tablespoon into each well of an ice cube tray (1 tablespoon or "cube" of this mixture is equivalent to 1 tablespoon of chopped fresh herbs).
- Cover your ice cube tray with plastic wrap or aluminum foil and store in the freezer. These frozen spice cubes can be added directly to a pot or quickly thawed to season meat before cooking.
- Freeze fresh herbs individually (an ice cube tray of cilantro, another of mint, etc.) or freeze your favorite combinations (rosemary and thyme together, basil and oregano together, etc.).

The Wonderful World of Squash

There is such an enormous variety of squash that it must be impossible to ever get bored. Grocery stores typically stock more varieties than they used to, but the best source of new squash varieties is your local farm or farmer's market.

Summer and winter squash come from the same family of plants. Summer squash are harvested when immature, while the rinds are still tender and edible. Winter squash are harvested in the mature fruit stage, once the seeds have matured fully and the skins have hardened into tough rinds. Winter squash has a long shelf life and can typically be stored all winter. It also tends to be much starchier than summer squash and is generally cooked before eating.

The following are varieties of winter squash (and this list is by no means exhaustive):

- acorn squash
- ambercup squash
- Arikara squash
- Atlantic giant
- autumn cup squash
- autumn gold pumpkin
- baby bear pumpkin
- baby pam pumpkin
- banana squash (aka pink banana squash)
- Bushkin pumpkin
- buttercup squash
- butternut squash
- calabaza
- carnival squash
- cushaw (aka winter crookneck squash)
- delicata squash (aka peanut squash)
- fairytale pumpkin squash (aka Musquee de Provence)
- gem squash
- Georgia candy roaster
- Giraumon
- gold (or golden) nugget squash
- harvest moon pumpkin
- heart of gold squash
- hubbard squash
- Jarrahdale pumpkin
- kabocha
- Lakota squash
- Long Island cheese squash
- Lumina pumpkin
- Marina di Chioggia
- Mooregold squash
- Queensland blue pumpkin
- red kuri squash (aka hokkaido squash or baby red Hubbard squash)
- rouge vif d'Estampes
- spaghetti squash
- sugar loaf squash
- sugar pumpkin
- sweet dumpling squash
- turban squash
- winter luxury pumpkin

The following are varieties of summer squash:

- cousa squash
- pattypan squash (aka scallop squash)
- Pygon squash
- tromboncino (aka zucchetta)
- yellow crookneck squash
- yellow summer squash
- zucchini (aka courgette)

Fun Ingredients for Extra Flavor

Flavoring ingredients

- blackstrap molasses
- coconut aminos
- honey
- pomegranate molasses
- tamarind paste
- umeboshi paste
- wine

Cooking fats

- duck fat
- palm shortening (look for ethically and sustainably sourced)
- red palm oil (look for ethically and sustainably sourced)

Herbs and spices

- cloves
- curry leaves
- kaffir lime leaves
- lemongrass
- savory
- truffle salt (aka flavor powder)
- turmeric

Other kitchen basics

- coconut cream (guar gum–free and in BPA-free cans)
- nutritional yeast (make sure that it's gluten-free)
- tapioca starch

Ingredients for Special Treats

One of the great challenges of the Paleo Approach diet is that it omits the majority of ingredients used to make even typical gluten-free and Paleo baked goods. While desserts and replicas of breads and muffins should be reserved for special occasions, here is a list of ingredients you may wish to have on hand for those times when a treat is called for.

Baking fats

- avocado oil
- extra-virgin coconut oil
- lard
- leaf lard
- palm shortening

Flours and starches

- arrowroot powder
- coconut flour (see page 44)
- cricket flour or other insect flours
- fresh plantains (green or ripe)
- fresh vegetables and fruits (puréed or mashed)
- green banana flour
- konjac flour
- kuzu starch
- plantain flour (check the ingredients list; it is sometimes mixed with potato starch)
- sweet potato flour or starch
- tapioca starch (caution: common sensitivity)
- vegetable powders (pumpkin, sweet potato, spinach, beet)
- water chestnut flour

Binders (egg substitutes)

- agar agar
- applesauce
- coconut butter
- coconut cream
- coconut milk
- gelatin
- mashed bananas
- puréed pumpkin
- other vegetable and fruit purees

Leavening agents

- baker's yeast (caution: common sensitivity)
- baking soda
- cream of tartar

Flavorings

- carob powder (caution: high sugar content)
- cinnamon
- citrus juice and zest
- cloves
- distilled gluten-free alcohols (rum, sherry, cognac—if the alcohol will be cooked off)
- dried fruit
- flavoring extracts (check the ingredients list)
- freeze-dried fruit
- fresh or puréed fruits and vegetables
- ginger, fresh or ground
- mace
- nutritional yeast (caution: common sensitivity)
- salt
- spices (see page 27)
- tea (black, green, or herbal)
- vanilla extract (if the alcohol will be cooked off)
- vanilla powder (check the ingredients list)
- wine (if the alcohol will be cooked off)

Sugars and sweeteners

- carob powder
- coconut sugar (see page 44)
- date sugar
- dried fruit
- evaporated cane juice (aka sucanat—look for organic)
- fresh fruits or vegetables
- fruit or vegetable purees
- honey (raw; local preferred)
- maple sugar
- maple syrup (grade B preferred)
- molasses (blackstrap preferred)
- muscovado sugar (aka Barbados sugar)
- pomegranate molasses

Texture ingredients

- shredded coconut
- coconut chips
- unsweetened banana chips
- plantain chips (store-bought or homemade; pages 168 and 170)
- dried fruits and vegetables
- mashed fresh vegetables
- cut-up or grated fresh fruits and vegetables

Convenience Foods

In addition to the pantry items already mentioned, there are some great prepackaged foods that can make life easier. Some of them make great snacks or travel foods, others are easy lunches, and others are handy ingredients for a quick meal.

- canned or pouched fish (salmon, tuna, sardines, herring, kippers)
- canned shellfish (shrimp, crab, oysters, clams, mussels)
- caviar and roe (usually have a long shelf life in the fridge before opening; check ingredients)
- chutneys (check ingredients and look for raw, fermented versions)
- coconut milk kefir (check ingredients)
- coconut wraps
- deli meats (gluten-, nightshade-, and seed-free; uncured or naturally cured; and made with grass-fed and pasture-raised meats). Deli meats that are typically Paleo Approach friendly are bacon, prosciutto, pancetta (typically pepper and juniper berries are used in the curing process), ham (but not Black Forest ham unless explicitly labeled gluten-free), and Canadian bacon (that isn't coated with cornmeal). Sometimes roast beef and turkey breast are Paleo Approach friendly, but check the ingredients.
- dried fruit (dehydrated or freeze-dried)—in moderation
- dried vegetables (dehydrated or freeze-dried)
- fresh fruits and vegetables
- frozen fruits and vegetables
- jerky (look for brands that use salt as the only seasoning; many contain nightshades)
- kelp noodles
- kombucha
- nori
- olives (check ingredients)
- pemmican (including a growing number of nonperishable protein bars that use meat as a base)
- pickled herring and mackerel
- pickles (check ingredients; raw preferred)
- plantain chips
- root vegetable chips (check ingredients)
- sauerkraut (check ingredients; raw preferred)
- seaweed snacks (check ingredients)
- smoked fish (salmon, trout, kippers, etc.; can be hot smoked or cold smoked [lox]; check ingredients)
- sweet potato chips (check ingredients)
- sweet potato noodles (aka dangmyeon)
- wakame noodles
- water kefir

Plantains

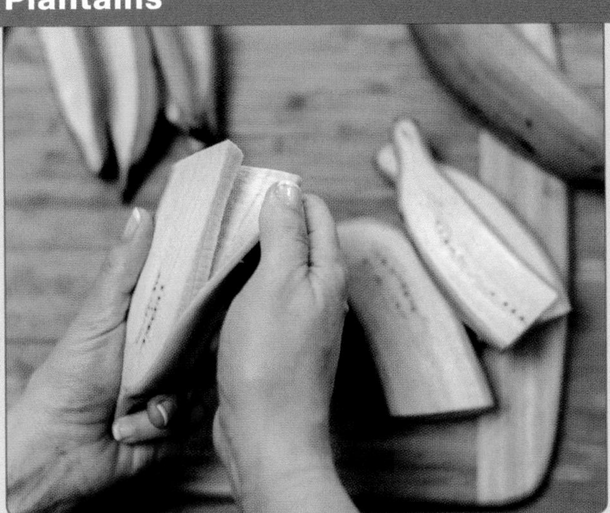

The plantain is a member of the banana family, sometimes called a cooking plantain or raw banana. While plantains technically can be eaten raw, they are typically cooked (this is the dominant differentiating factor between plantains and bananas).

Green plantains should be dark to light green and firm. The peel can be challenging to remove; it helps to quarter the plantain first, then pry the peel off. Green plantains have a high starch content and a neutral flavor and can be used as a potato substitute or as a flour substitute in grain-free baking. When you buy green plantains, you can store them in the crisper drawer of your fridge for up to two weeks, or peel and freeze them (either in large pieces or puréed). Keeping plantains in the fridge slows down the ripening process, but note that the peel will continue to yellow in the crisper drawer even though the inside is still green.

Ripe plantains have a lower starch content and a higher sugar content than green plantains, as well as a lovely apple-meets-banana flavor. They should be nearly all black. They can be prepared in a variety of ways, and their natural sweetness lends itself well to desserts. Plantains take a long time to ripen from green, typically three to four weeks. Ripe plantains can be stored in the crisper drawer of your fridge for up to five days or peeled and then frozen.

Storing Foods

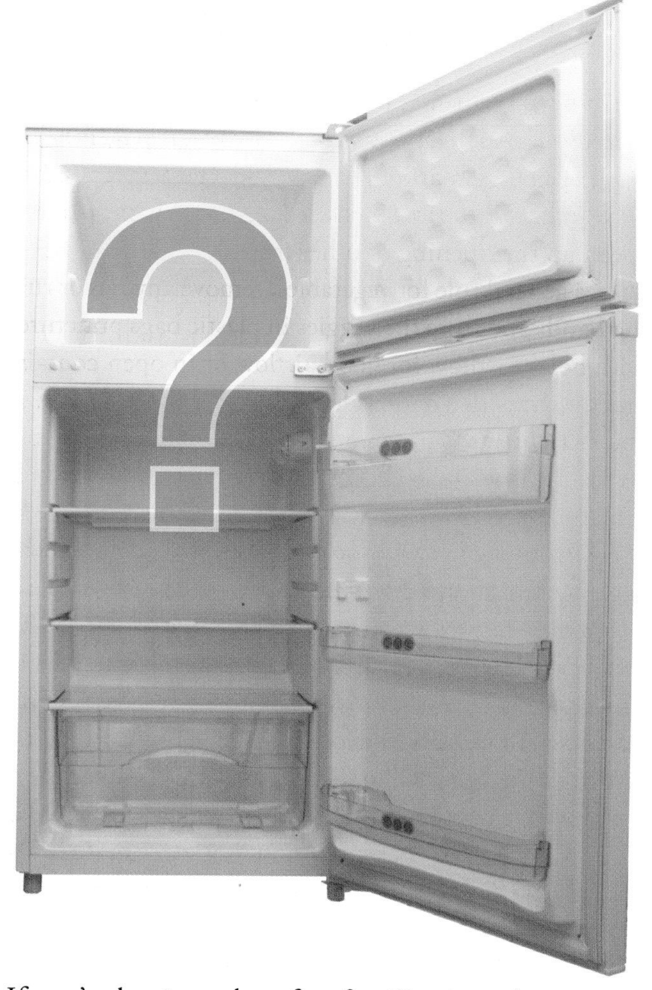

If you're buying a lot of unfamiliar ingredients, you may be wondering how best to store them. As a general rule, any product that you purchase from a refrigerated display case or that is shipped to you with ice packs in the packaging should be stored in the fridge at home. For products that you buy off store shelves or that are shipped to you in regular packaging, check the labels. If a product needs to go directly into the fridge, the label will say so. Other products may be fine in your cupboard until you open them, after which time refrigeration is required. If a label has no storage instructions, the product is typically fine at room temperature. If you're buying products from local manufacturers, ask when you purchase them how to store them.

Fats and oils deteriorate with exposure to light, heat, and oxygen. To increase the longevity of your cooking fats, store them in the refrigerator or freezer in tightly closed containers. Rendered tallow and poultry fat will keep for about six weeks in the refrigerator and for a year in the freezer. Lard has a longer shelf life; it will keep for one year in the refrigerator and for two years in the freezer. Solid plant oils like coconut oil and palm shortening should be stored in a cool, dry place. An opened jar will keep for about a year, and an unopened one will keep for up to two years. Olive and avocado oils should be stored at room temperature in a dark cupboard. They will retain their flavor and quality for up to a year after being opened.

When it comes to meat, poultry, and seafood, you'll probably find that you buy it frozen more often than fresh, because farmers and online grass-fed meat producers typically sell their meat frozen. Store frozen meat in the original packaging for up to six months for best quality (but pretty much indefinitely in terms of safety).

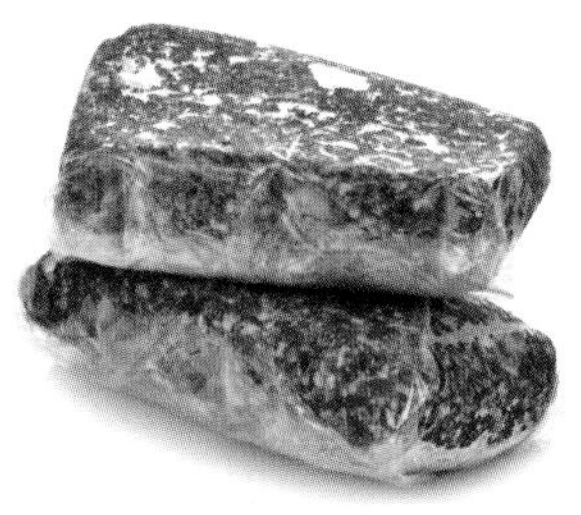

When buying fresh meat and poultry, keep it in the original packaging and store it in the coolest part of your refrigerator (typically at the back on the bottom shelf). Most fresh meat will keep for two to three days in the fridge before being cooked (ground meat and meat cut into small pieces, like stewing beef, will keep for two days, and larger cuts like steaks, chops, and roasts will typically keep for three days). I like to store meat on a rimmed baking sheet to prevent the juices from leaking onto other foods. When buying fresh seafood, keep it in its original packaging if possible and store it in a bowl of ice in the refrigerator. However, live shellfish (like clams) should not be put on ice; instead, open or poke holes in the packaging and store it on a rimmed baking sheet or plate in the fridge.

Looking for more tips on choosing and storing foods to preserve nutrient density?
Check out *Eating on the Wild Side*, by Jo Robinson.

Eating on the Wild Side
Jo Robinson

If you want to freeze meat, poultry, or seafood that you buy fresh, place the entire package in a resealable freezer bag. (Better yet, use a home vacuum sealer if you have one.) If you plan to store it in the freezer for several months, unpack any meat or seafood that isn't in a vacuum-sealed package and wrap the pieces individually in plastic wrap before placing them in a resealable freezer bag to help prevent freezer burn. (If your meat is vacuum sealed, there's no need to do so.)

The bigger challenge with freezing meat, poultry, and seafood is thawing it safely. There are three safe ways to thaw frozen food:

- **In the refrigerator:** The best and safest way to thaw is in the refrigerator. A small package of meat typically defrosts overnight, but most foods require a day or two, so plan ahead. Large roasts and whole turkeys will take even longer—approximately one day for every 5 pounds of weight.
- **In cold water:** For faster thawing, place the food package in a leak-proof plastic bag and immerse it in cold water. Check the water frequently to make sure that it stays cold, and change the water every thirty minutes. Small packages can thaw in as little as one hour with this method, and larger items will thaw in four to six hours (turkeys and very large roasts may take twenty-four hours to thaw using this method, which usually means that the several-days-in-the-fridge plan is a more practical way to go). Once it's thawed, cook the meat, poultry, or seafood immediately.
- **In the microwave:** Thawing meat in the microwave is perfectly safe (see page 70), although it's difficult to achieve even thawing without starting to cook the edges, which sometimes leads to overcooking those same edges when you go to prepare your meat. Follow your microwave's directions for thawing meat (since the optimal time and power setting will depend on your microwave). If you thaw meat, poultry, or seafood in the microwave, cook it immediately.
- **Cooking without thawing:** Cooking frozen meat, poultry, or seafood without thawing it first is perfectly safe to do; however, note that the cooking time will increase by approximately 50 percent. Always check the internal temperature with a meat thermometer (see pages 77 to 79) to make sure that your meat, poultry, or seafood is thoroughly cooked.

Another storage-related challenge is that farm-fresh organic produce often doesn't keep as well as its grocery store counterparts. So knowing the optimal way to store different types of vegetables and fruit is even more important!

Do not store fruits and vegetables together. Fruits that give off high levels of ethylene (a ripening agent), like apples, can prematurely ripen and spoil surrounding vegetables. (You can take advantage of this property to speed up the ripening of other fruits.)

As a general rule for vegetables, remove any ties or rubber bands and store the veggies in plastic bags punctured with holes to allow for good airflow or in open containers covered with a damp towel. Pack vegetables loosely in the refrigerator. Some vegetables, like leafy greens, can be soaked in a sink full of cool water before being stored, while others, like mushrooms and herbs, should not be washed until just prior to use. See the list on the following page for storage information for specific vegetables.

Fruits generally will continue to ripen if left sitting out on the countertop. Once perfectly ripe, these fruits can typically be refrigerated for at least a few days. (Even bananas can be refrigerated once ripened to your liking, although the peels will darken in the fridge.) Exceptions are grapes, citrus fruits, and berries, which will only deteriorate on the counter and should be refrigerated. The list on page 61 provides storage information for specific fruits. All fruits and vegetables stored at room temperature should be stored out of direct sunlight.

If you find yourself with a surplus of produce, nearly all fruits and vegetables can be stored in the freezer. Freeze them in small pieces on a baking sheet, and then place the frozen pieces in an airtight container or resealable freezer bag for use later.

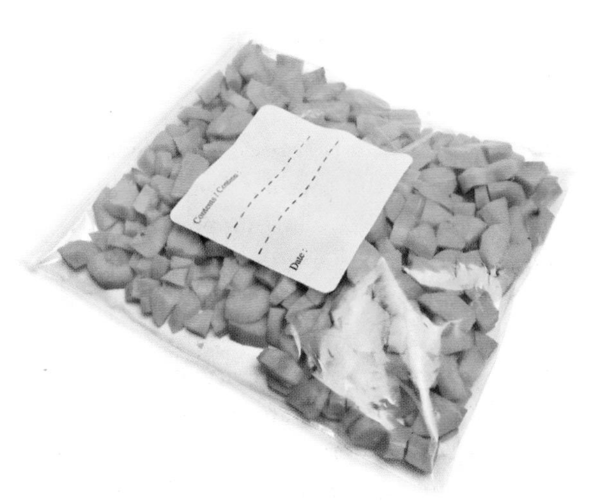

Storing Common Vegetables

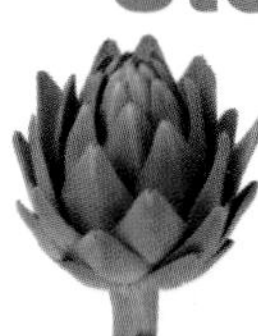

Artichokes: Store in the fridge in an airtight container with a damp piece of paper towel inside.

Asparagus: Store upright in a glass or bowl filled with water at room temperature for up to a week, or store in the fridge.

Basil: Store on the counter loosely packed in a jar with a small piece of damp paper towel inside.

Beets: Wash and store in an open container with a wet towel on top. Cut off any tops and store them separately.

Broccoli: Wrap in a damp towel and place in an open container in the fridge. Use as soon as possible.

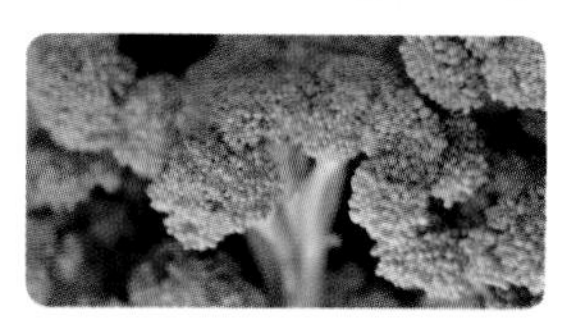

Brussels sprouts: If on the stalk, store the entire stalk in the fridge. If loose, store in an open container with a damp towel on top.

Cabbage: Store on the counter for up to a week, or in the crisper drawer of the fridge. Peel off the outer leaves if they start to wilt.

Carrots: Wrap in a damp towel and store in a closed container in the fridge. Cut off the tops and store them separately.

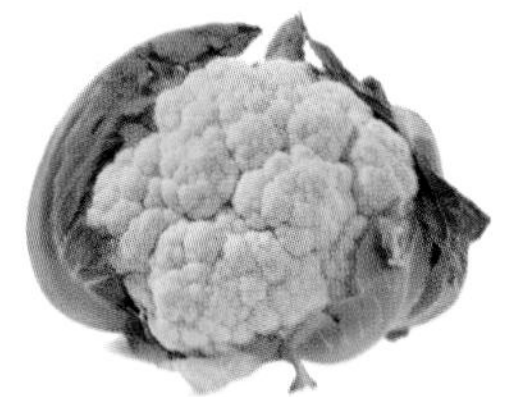

Cauliflower: Store in a closed container in the fridge. Use as soon as possible.

Celery: Store in a cup or bowl of shallow water on the counter for up to a week. For longer-term storage, wrap in aluminum foil and place in the fridge.

Celery root: Wrap in a damp towel and store in the crisper drawer of the fridge.

Fennel: Store in a cup or bowl of shallow water on the counter for up to several days. For longer-term storage, place in the fridge in a closed container with a little water.

Garlic: Store in a cool, dark place.

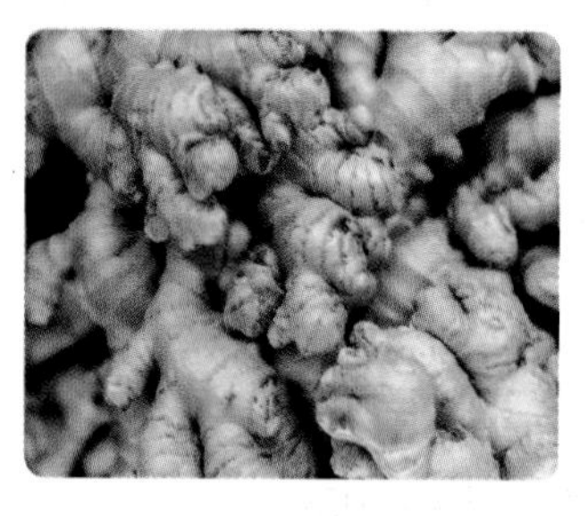

Ginger: Store unpeeled ginger in a plastic bag in the crisper drawer of the fridge. Ginger roots can also be frozen and microplaned directly from frozen.

Green garlic: Store in an airtight container in the fridge.

Herbs: Store in a glass or vase full of water in the fridge.

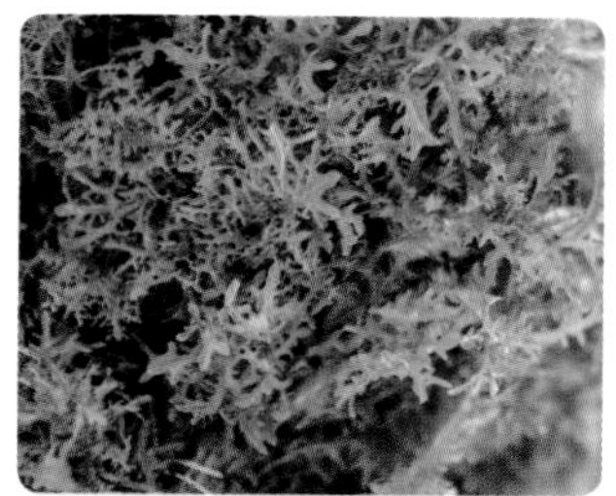

Leafy greens: Remove any bands or twist ties and store in an airtight container with a damp cloth.

Leeks: Store in a shallow cup of water on the counter (so that only the very bottoms of the stems have water), or wrapped in a damp towel in the crisper drawer of the fridge.

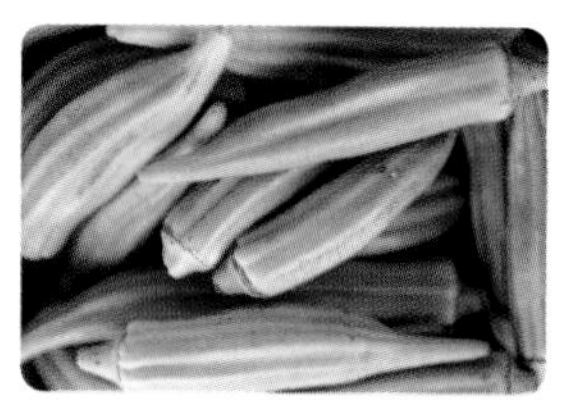

Okra: Store with a dry towel in an airtight container in the fridge. Use as soon as possible.

Onion: Store in a cool, dark, dry place.

Mushrooms: Keep in the fridge in their original packaging or in a paper bag.

Parsnips: Wrap in a damp cloth and store in an open container in the crisper drawer of the fridge.

Radishes: Store in an open container in the fridge with a wet towel placed on top. Remove the greens and store them separately.

Rhubarb: Wrap in a damp towel and place in an open container in the fridge.

Rutabagas: Store in a closed container in the crisper drawer of the fridge.

Spinach: Store loose in an open container in the crisper drawer, and refrigerate as soon as possible. Spinach loves to stay cold.

Spring onions: Remove any bands or twist ties and store in the crisper drawer of the fridge.

Sweet potatoes: Store in a cool, dark, well-ventilated place.

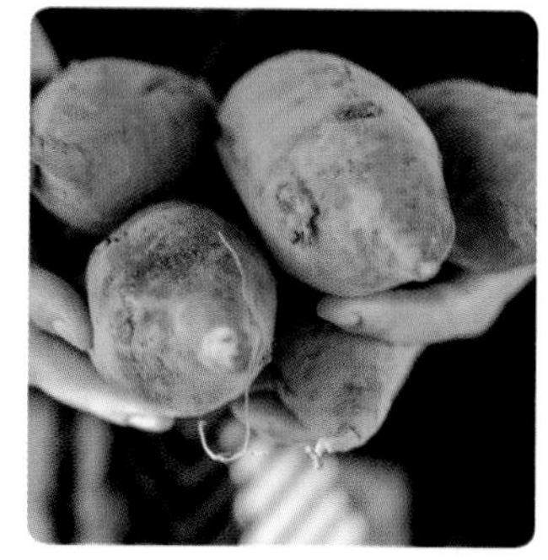

Turnips: Store in an open container covered with a moist cloth. Remove the greens and store them separately.

Storing Common Fruits

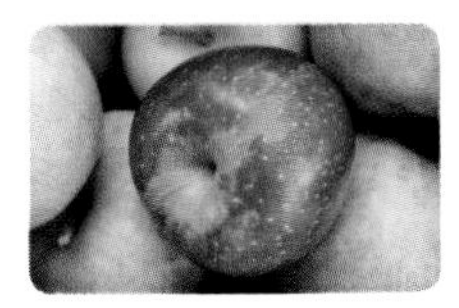

Apples: Store in a bowl or basket with good airflow at room temperature. For longer storage, keep in a cardboard box in the fridge.

Apricots: Store in a bowl or basket with good airflow at room temperature. Store in the fridge when fully ripe.

Avocados: Store in a bowl or paper bag at room temperature. To speed up ripening, place in a paper bag with an apple.

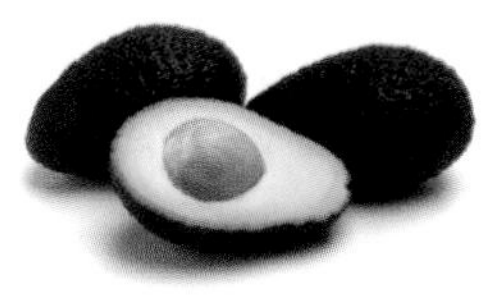

Bananas: Store in a basket with good airflow or hang on a banana holder at room temperature. To slow down ripening, take them apart and store them spaced apart.

Berries: Store in the refrigerator and wash right before you eat them.

Citrus: Store in a cool place with good airflow.

Cherries: Store in an airtight container in the fridge and wash right before you eat them.

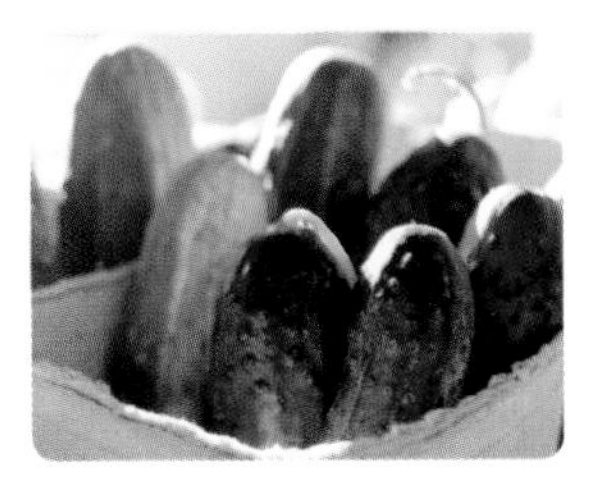

Cucumbers: Store wrapped in a moist towel in the fridge.

Dates: Drier dates (like Deglet Noor) can be stored in the original packaging in a cupboard. Moist dates (like Medjool) should be refrigerated in a container that allows airflow.

Figs: Store in the fridge in a paper bag or a container that allows airflow.

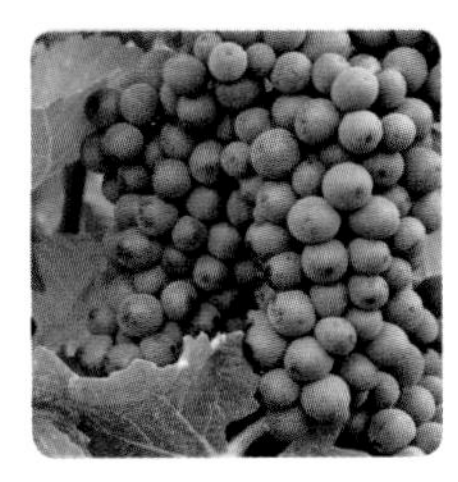

Grapes: Store in a bag or a container that allows airflow in the crisper drawer of the fridge, and wash right before you eat them.

Kiwis: Keep at room temperature until ripe, then refrigerate.

Lemons and limes: Store on the counter in a bowl that allows airflow. For longer storage, keep in the refrigerator (but note that they can absorb the odors of foods stored beside them).

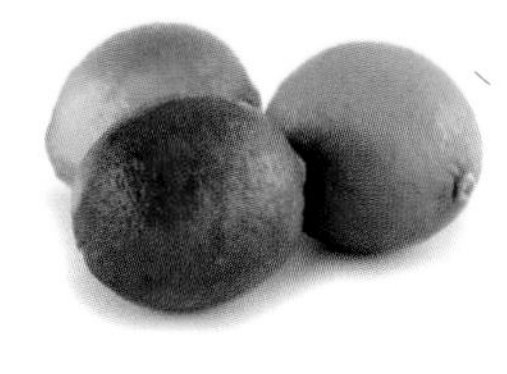

Mangoes: Store on the counter until ripe, then move to the refrigerator.

Melons: Store uncut in a cool, dry place, out of the sun, for up to a couple of weeks. Softer melons like cantaloupe should be moved to the fridge when ripe. Cut melon should be kept in the fridge with the cut side covered with plastic wrap or cut side down on a plate.

Nectarines: Store in a bowl that allows airflow on the counter, and refrigerate only when fully ripe. To hasten ripening, place in a paper bag with an apple.

Oranges: Store at room temperature in a bowl or basket that allows airflow. For longer-term storage, move to the refrigerator.

Peaches: Store on the counter in a bowl that allows airflow, and refrigerate only when fully ripe. To hasten ripening, place in a paper bag with an apple.

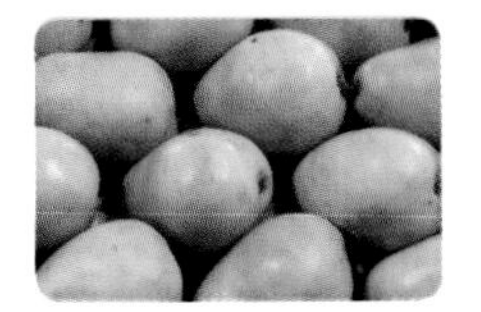

Pears: Store in a bowl or basket that allows airflow or in a paper bag. To hasten ripening, place in a paper bag with an apple.

Persimmons: Store at room temperature until fully ripe, and then move to the refrigerator. To hasten ripening, place in a paper bag with an apple.

Pineapples: Whole pineapples can be stored on the counter until ripe. Once ripe, pineapple can be stored whole or peeled and cut in an airtight container in the fridge.

Plums: Store at room temperature until fully ripe, and then move to the refrigerator.

Pomegranates: Store in a cool, dry place.

Raspberries: Wash in a solution of 1 part vinegar to 3 parts water and drain well. Place the berries in the fridge in a bowl lined with a dry paper towel, replacing the paper towel when it gets damp.

Strawberries: Store in a paper bag in the fridge and wash right before you eat them.

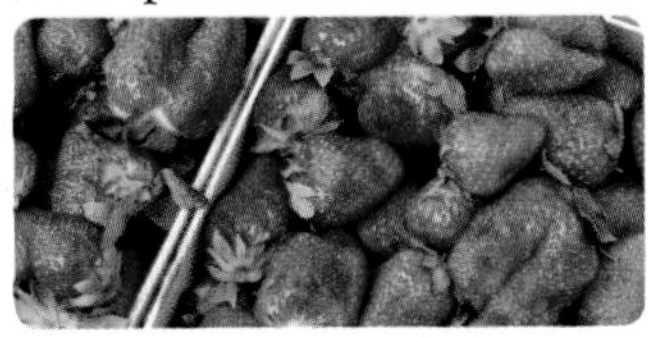

Watermelon: Keep uncut watermelon on the counter at room temperature. After cutting, store in the fridge with the cut side covered with plastic wrap.

Winter squash: Store in a cool, dark, well-ventilated place.

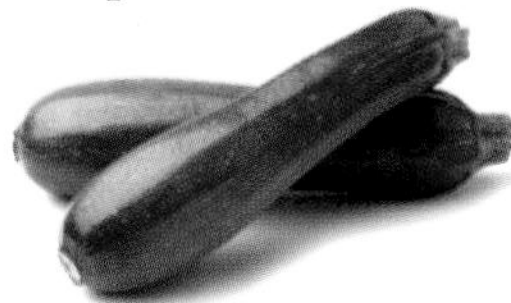

Zucchini and other summer squash: Wrap in a damp cloth and store in the fridge.

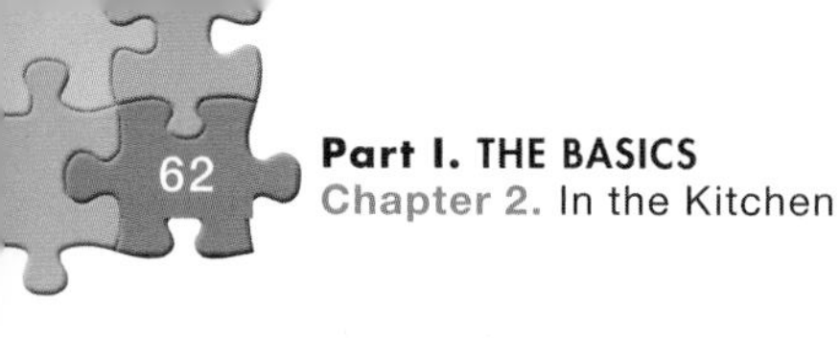

The Language of Cooking

If you aren't a cookbook fanatic like I am and don't while away the hours watching cooking shows on TV, then you might find yourself intimidated or confused by cooking terminology. What is the difference between sautéing and frying? What does it mean to braise? What's the difference between chopping a vegetable and dicing it? And what's the difference between a skillet and a frying pan?

Cooking is like love . . . it should be entered into with abandon or not at all.
—JULIA CHILD

I would be lying if I said that I didn't have to look up the answers to some of these questions in order to write this chapter. I've been cooking successfully for three decades without knowing the meanings of all of these cooking terms. And, really, if a recipe calls for chopped carrots and you dice them instead, chances are pretty good that you won't know the difference in the finished product. But it's helpful for following recipes (and writing them!) to have these terms straight, so here we go.

AL DENTE: An Italian term used to describe the texture of a food that is cooked until it offers a slight resistance to the bite.

BAKE: To cook by dry heat in the oven.

BARBECUE: To cook outdoors over a propane or charcoal grill or over a wood fire.

BASTE: To moisten a food during cooking with pan drippings or a special sauce to add flavor and prevent drying.

BATTER: A mixture containing flour (or a flour substitute) and liquid that is thin enough to pour.

BEAT: To mix rapidly in order to incorporate as much air as possible, which makes a mixture smooth and light.

BLANCH: To immerse in rapidly boiling water and allow to cook only slightly.

BLEND: To incorporate two or more ingredients thoroughly.

BOIL: To heat a liquid until bubbles break continually on the surface.

BOUQUET GARNI: Various stems of herbs tied together with string or butcher's twine and added to a pot in which a dish such as a stew is being cooked. Using a bouquet garni makes it easier to remove the tough stems after the dish is cooked.

BREAD: To dredge or coat with bread crumbs or other ingredients that have a similar texture.

BRAISE: To cook using a combination of moist and dry heat, typically searing at a high temperature in a cooking fat and then cooking in a covered pot with a liquid at a lower temperature.

BRINE: A mixture of salt and water.

BROIL: To cook under strong, direct heat, typically in the oven.

BROWN: To cook briefly in hot fat, allowing a crust to form on all sides and seal in the juices. This method also enriches flavor.

BRUSH: To lightly coat with a liquid using a pastry or basting brush.

CARAMELIZE: To heat a sugar, fruit, or vegetable such as an onion in order to brown it and give it a special taste.

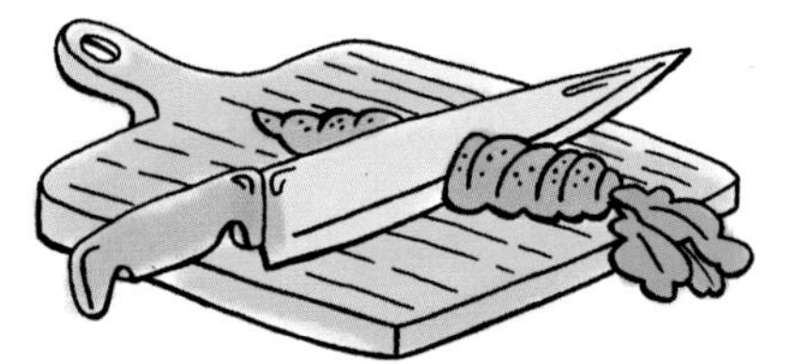

CHOP: To cut a solid food into pieces with a sharp knife or other cutting tool.

CLARIFY: To separate and remove the solids from a liquid, thus making it clear.

COAT: To cover the surface of a food with another substance.

CREAM: To soften a fat by beating it at room temperature.

CRUSH: To smash into tiny pieces with a rolling pin, mallet, mortar and pestle, or garlic press.

CURDLE: To cause minute solids to separate from a liquid by adding acid or heating too quickly. Curdling can be intentional or a kitchen accident.

CUBE: To cut into cube-shaped pieces, typically ½ to 1 inch in size.

CURE: To preserve meat by drying and salting and/or smoking.

DASH: A very small quantity; a scant ⅛ teaspoon.

DEBONE: To remove the bones from a cut of meat or fish. Used interchangeably with *bone.*

DEGLAZE: To dissolve the thin glaze of juices and brown bits on the surface of a pan in which food has been fried, sautéed, or roasted. To do so, you add liquid and stir and scrape over high heat, thereby adding flavor to the liquid for use as a sauce.

DEGREASE: To remove fat from the surface of a stew, soup, or stock. The dish is usually cooled in the refrigerator first so that the fat hardens and becomes easier to remove. Used interchangeably with *defat.*

DEVEIN: To remove the dark vein that runs along the back of a shrimp by using a sharp knife or special deveining tool.

DICE: To cut into small cubes of uniform size and shape, usually ⅛ to ¼ inch.

DIP: To briefly plunge bite-sized foods into a liquid mixture.

DISSOLVE: To cause a dry substance to become part of a liquid.

DOLLOP: A very small amount, usually a teaspoonful.

DOUGH: A combination of wet and dry ingredients that can be shaped but not poured.

DRAIN: To remove liquid or fat, often by placing a food in a colander or strainer or on a paper towel.

DREDGE: To sprinkle or coat with flour or another fine substance.

DRIZZLE: To sprinkle drops of liquid lightly over a food in a casual manner.

DRY RUB: A dry mixture composed of salt, herbs, and/or spices that is rubbed into meat, poultry, or seafood to flavor it.

DUST: To sprinkle with dry ingredients, typically using a strainer, sieve, or shaker.

FILLET: As a verb, to remove the bones from meat or fish. A fillet (or filet) is a piece of deboned flesh.

FLAKE: To break lightly into small pieces.

FLAMBÉ: To flame a food by dousing it in potable alcohol and setting it alight.

FOLD: To incorporate a delicate substance into another substance without releasing air bubbles.

FRICASSEE: To cook by braising; usually applies to fowl or rabbit.

FRY: To cook in hot fat. To cook in a small amount of fat is called *pan-frying* or *sautéing;* to cook in a 1- to 2-inch layer of hot fat is called *shallow fat-frying;* to cook in a deep layer of hot fat is called *deep fat-frying.*

GARNISH: To decorate a dish in order to enhance its appearance and/or add flavor.

GLAZE: To coat with a glossy substance, typically a thin sugar syrup cooked to about 300°F; the mixture may be thickened slightly.

GRATE: To rub a food on a grater that separates it into bits or shreds.

GRATIN: From the French word for "crust." This term is used to describe an oven-baked dish—usually cooked in a shallow oval gratin dish—on which a golden brown crust of crumbs or sauce forms.

GREASE: To lightly coat a pan with cooking fat or oil in order to prevent cooked food from sticking to it.

GRILL: To cook directly over intense heat on a rack over hot coals, natural wood, or gas. Often used interchangeably with *barbecue.*

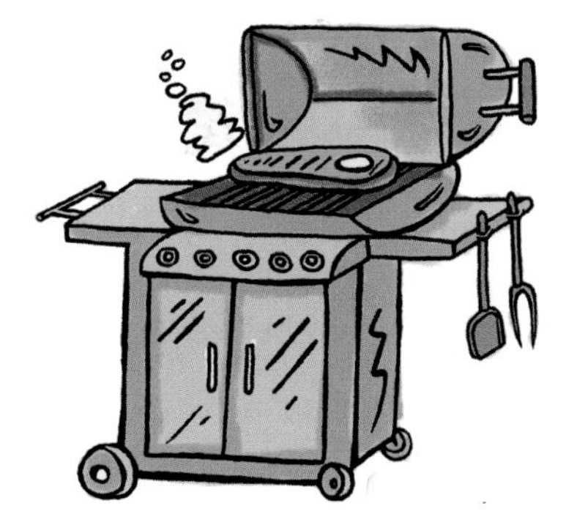

GRIND: To turn a solid piece of food into fine pieces or a powder by using a mortar and pestle, food processor, or meat grinder.

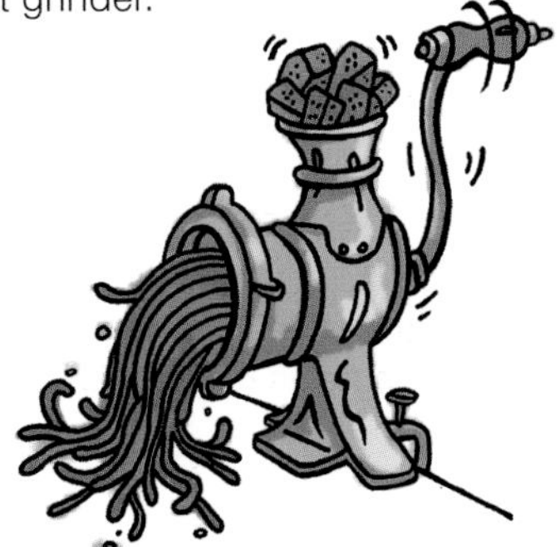

HALF MOON: To cut a food, typically an onion, into semicircles.

JULIENNE: To cut into thin strips.

KNEAD: To work and press dough with the palms of your hands.

LUKEWARM: Neither cool nor warm; approximately body temperature.

MARINATE: To flavor meat, poultry, seafood, or vegetables by soaking them in a liquid mixture of seasonings known as a marinade.

MASH: To crush, beat, or squeeze food into a soft state using a fork or masher.

MATCHSTICK CUT: To cut vegetables or fruits into thin strips approximately 2 inches long. Often used interchangeably with *julienne.*

MELT: To dissolve a solid or semisolid over low heat.

MEUNIÈRE: A French term used to describe a food that has been dredged with flour and sautéed in butter. (There isn't much meunièring going on in this book, but I think dredging with tapioca starch and sautéing in lard comes pretty close.)

MINCE: To cut or chop into tiny pieces, typically ⅛ inch or smaller.

MIX: To combine ingredients, usually by stirring.

PAN-BROIL: To cook uncovered in a hot frying pan, pouring off the fat as it accumulates.

PAN-FRY: To cook in a small amount of fat. Used interchangeably with *sauté.*

PARBOIL: To cook in a liquid just below the boiling point, often cooking only partially. This procedure is usually followed by final cooking in a seasoned sauce.

PARE: To cut away the outermost skin of a fruit or vegetable. This job is typically done with a paring knife.

PEEL: To remove the peel from a fruit or vegetable. This job is typically done with your hands, as in peeling an orange, or with a vegetable peeler, as in peeling an apple.

PICKLE: To preserve meat, vegetables, or fruits in brine.

PINCH: The trifling amount you can hold between your thumb and forefinger. Approximately 1⁄16 teaspoon.

PIT: To remove the pit from a fruit.

PLANKED: Cooked on a thick hardwood plank.

PLUMP: To soak dried fruits or mushrooms in liquid until they swell.

POACH: To cook very gently in a hot liquid kept just below the boiling point.

POT-ROAST: To braise meat, especially a tough cut with substantial connective tissue.

POUND: To flatten meat or poultry, often between sheets of wax paper, using a heavy mallet or frying pan. Pounding helps tenderize the meat.

PRICK: To pierce a food with the tines of a fork or other sharp point to prevent it from bursting or rising during baking.

PURÉE: To mash a food until perfectly smooth. Puréeing can be done by hand, by using a food mill, or by whirling in a blender or food processor.

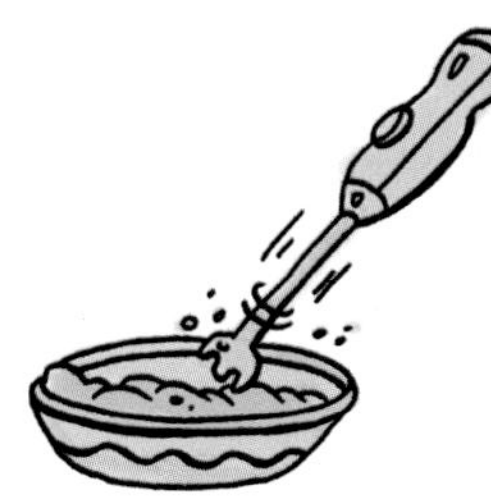

RECONSTITUTE: To rehydrate a dry food by soaking it in liquid.

REDUCE: To boil down a liquid in order to lessen the volume and concentrate the flavor.

REFRESH: To run cold water over a food that has been parboiled in order to stop the cooking process quickly; used interchangeably with *shock*. Also, to make limp salad ingredients crisp again by letting them stand in cold water.

RENDER: To melt and clarify hard animal fat for cooking purposes.

REST: To let meat sit after being removed from the heat before slicing or serving. The rest time allows the muscle fibers to relax so that less juice is released when the meat is sliced.

ROAST: To cook by dry heat in an oven. The difference between roasting and baking is mostly one of convention: breads, cakes, pies, and casseroles are typically baked, while meats and vegetables are roasted.

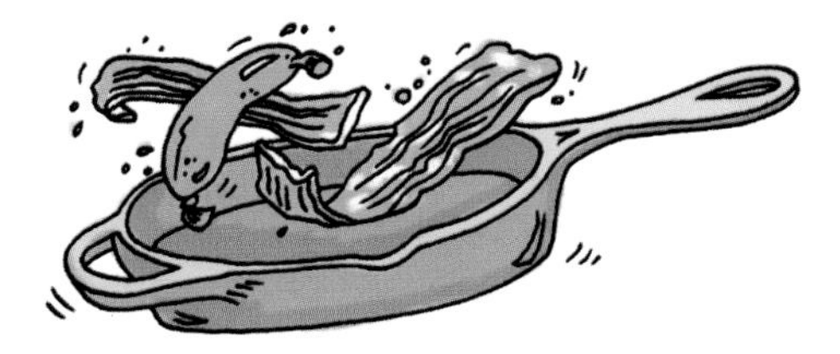

SAUTÉ: To cook and/or brown a food in a small amount of hot fat.

SCALD: To heat a liquid, typically dairy, to a temperature just below the boiling point.

SCALLOP: To bake a food, usually in a casserole dish, with a sauce or other liquid. Crumbs often are sprinkled on top.

SCORE: To cut narrow grooves or gashes in the outer surface of a food.

SEAR: To brown very quickly over intense heat. This method increases shrinkage but develops flavor and improves appearance.

SEASON: To add flavoring to enhance a food's taste. Also, to prepare a metal surface for cooking by adding oil and then heating it, which seals the tiny pits in the metal and prevents food from sticking.

SHRED: To cut or tear into long, narrow pieces.

SIFT: To put one or more dry ingredients through a sieve or sifter to remove large pieces and incorporate air.

SIMMER: To cook slowly in a liquid over low heat, at an approximate temperature of 180°F. The surface of the liquid should be barely moving, broken from time to time by slowly rising bubbles.

SKIM: To remove impurities, whether scum or fat, from the surface of a liquid during cooking, resulting in a clear, cleaner-tasting final product.

SLICE: To cut into even slices, usually across the grain and ⅛ to ⅜ inch thick.

SLIVER: To cut into extra-thin strips.

SMOKE: To preserve a food by exposing it to smoke.

SPIRAL SLICE: To cut vegetables or fruits into long, noodlelike strips by using a spiral slicer.

STEAM: To cook in steam in a pressure cooker, deep well cooker, double boiler, or steamer basket fit into a pot. A small amount of boiling water is used, with more water added during the steaming process if necessary.

STEEP: To extract color, flavor, or other qualities from a substance (such as tea leaves) by soaking it in water that is just below the boiling point.

STERILIZE: To destroy micro-organisms by boiling, exposing to dry heat, or steaming.

STEW: To simmer slowly in a small amount of liquid for a long time.

STIR: To mix ingredients with a circular motion until well blended or of uniform consistency.

STIR-FRY: A cooking method developed by the Chinese that involves quickly moving food around in a small amount of oil in a wok or frying pan over high heat.

STRAIN: To remove solids from a liquid by pouring it through a sieve, strainer, or colander.

STUFF: To fill a cavity (such as the inside of a turkey or a hollowed-out pepper) with a mixture.

TO TASTE: To your liking. This term is usually used to describe adding salt or other spices slowly, mixing and tasting with each addition until a food is perfectly seasoned.

TOSS: To combine ingredients with a lifting motion.

TRUSS: To secure poultry or a roast with string or skewers so that it holds its shape as it cooks.

WEDGE: To cut into large slices, typically pie-shaped or larger at one end or in the middle and narrower at the other end(s).

WHIP: To beat rapidly to incorporate air and produce expansion, as with heavy cream or egg whites.

WHISK: To mix a sauce, dressing, eggs, or other liquid using a swift circular motion, usually with a balloon-shaped wire instrument called a whisk.

ZEST: The outer colorful skin of a citrus fruit. When finely grating the zest of a fruit, be careful not to include the bitter white pith found just underneath the surface of the skin (both components of the peel of the fruit). You can use a grater, vegetable peeler, or zester (a special tool used just to remove or grate zest) to accomplish this task.

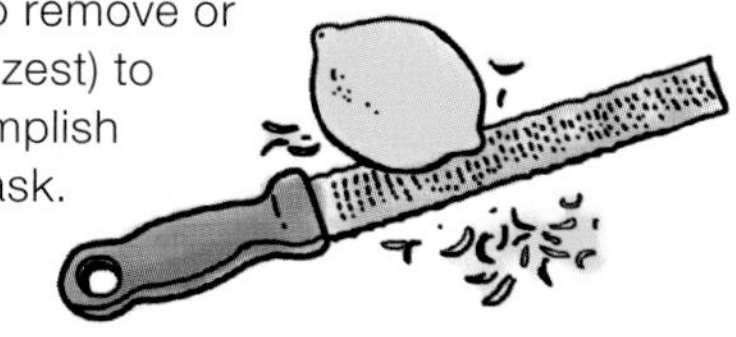

Cooking Tools

Cooking tools can be divided into two categories: essential and nonessential but awesome. The essentials list contains basic implements—a few pots and pans, a good knife or two, a cutting board, various spatulas and stirring spoons, and a can opener—basically higher-quality versions of what probably graced the shared kitchen in your college dorm. The nonessentials list includes a variety of gadgets and small appliances that, while not absolute necessities, save an amazing amount of time and energy in the kitchen.

Essentials

If you're starting from scratch, here are the barest essentials:

Baking pan: A large metal, glass, or ceramic pan, either 9 inches square or 13 by 9 inches, with 2-inch-high sides. This versatile pan can be used for a variety of dishes.

Can opener: Even though you won't be eating many canned foods, a can opener is still a necessity. A safe-cut, or smooth-edge, model cuts around the outside of the can rather than the lid, produces smooth edges, and won't lower the lid into your food.

Casserole dish: A glass, ceramic, or enameled metal baking dish, sometimes with higher sides. Casserole dishes come in a variety of shapes and sizes and often come with lids. They are typically more aesthetically pleasing than baking pans, so they can be used for both baking and serving.

Chef's knife: A knife with a large triangular blade, typically 6 to 9 inches long, used for chopping, slicing, dicing, and mincing.

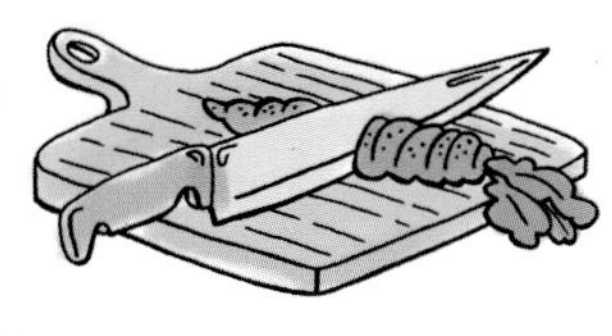

Dutch oven: This versatile pot can be used on the stovetop or in the oven. Heavy enameled pans are best, but a small stockpot with ovenproof handles and a tight-fitting lid will also do the job. A 7-quart or 8-quart Dutch oven is the most useful size.

Garlic press: Whenever a recipe calls for crushed garlic, a garlic press is a required tool. Look for one that includes a reverse-side matching grid of blunt pins to clean out the holes of the press.

Grater: A flat or box-shaped tool that typically can be used to zest (or finely grate), coarsely grate, shred, or slice many different foods. The easiest type to use is a box grater, which gives you the most versatility.

Ladle: Look for a large bowl that makes it easy to serve soups. A bent handle at the top enables you to hook the ladle on the side of a pot to keep it from falling in.

Measuring cups and spoons: Having a way to measure your ingredients is essential for following any recipe! You will need a variety of sizes, from ¼ teaspoon to 1 tablespoon for measuring spoons, from ¼ cup to 1 cup for dry measuring cups, and from 1 cup to 8 cups for liquid measuring cups.

Meat thermometer: Look for an oven-safe meat thermometer so that you can stick the probe into your meat at the beginning of cooking and monitor the internal temperature throughout the cooking process. Digital thermometers (with an oven-safe probe and a display that remains outside the oven) often have an alarm that you can set to go off when your meat reaches the desired temperature.

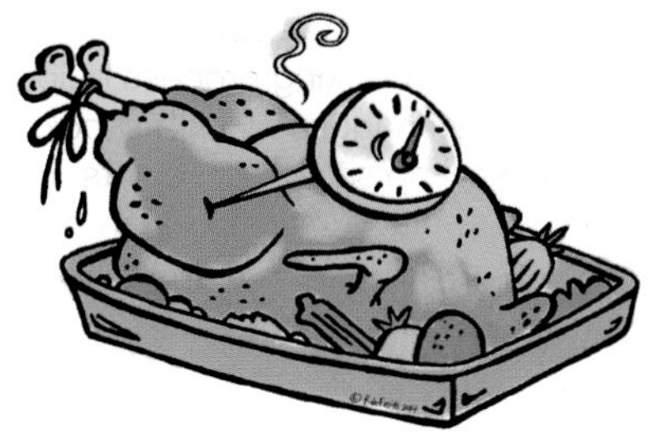

Metal spatula: Often called a flipper, a metal spatula is a necessity for turning foods. A thin offset blade allows you to get under delicate items like pancakes. A medium-length blade keeps you from having to pick up foods at an awkward angle.

Paring knife: A knife with a small triangular blade, typically 3 inches long, used for paring and cutting fruits and vegetables.

How to Care for Your Pots and Pans

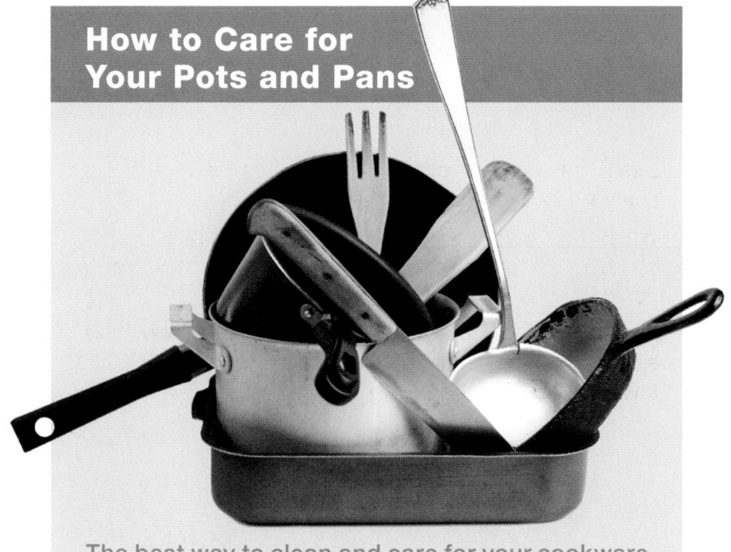

The best way to clean and care for your cookware depends on the material it's made of.

Aluminum: Soak in hot, soapy water and use a scouring pad, sponge, or cloth to scrub clean. If the pan has darkened, fill it with water and vinegar or lemon juice (5 parts water to 1 part vinegar) and boil for 15 minutes. Avoid steel wool.

Cast iron: Clean cast iron with hot water (no dish soap!) and a scouring pad, sponge, or cloth. It's easier to clean while the pan is still warm after cooking. Dry immediately. Avoid steel wool.

Ceramic, glass, and porcelain: Soak in hot, soapy water and use a scouring pad, sponge, or cloth to scrub clean. These materials are typically dishwasher safe.

Copper: Wash in hot, soapy water and dry immediately. Avoid steel wool. Copper tarnishes quickly, so use polish to brighten it (wash with dish soap after polishing and prior to using). Most copper pans are lined with tin. If you can see tin through the copper, it's time to send your pan away for relining.

Enameled metal or cast iron: Soak in hot, soapy water, and use a sponge or cloth to clean (no scouring pads or other abrasives).

Nonstick surfaces: Never use a metal implement such as a metal spatula or spoon with nonstick cookware. It's also very important not to heat it above 500°F, at which point chemicals from the nonstick coating can leach into your food. Clean with a sponge or cloth and warm, soapy water. Avoid anything abrasive, such as a scouring pad or steel wool. Replace nonstick pans as soon as you see any kind of scratch or flaking on the surface.

Stainless steel: Wash in hot, soapy water with a scouring pad, sponge, or cloth. Special stainless-steel cleaners can help remove stubborn stains (but wash with dish soap before using). You can also fill with vinegar or lemon juice and water (1 part vinegar to 5 parts water) and boil for 15 minutes. Avoid steel wool.

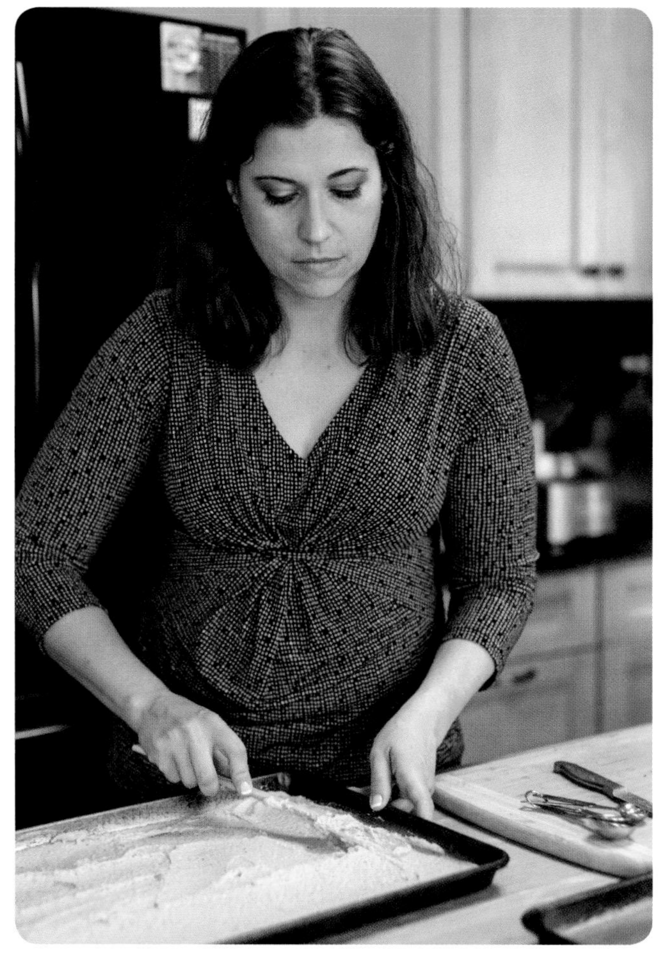

Rimmed baking sheet: Also known as a jellyroll pan, a rimmed baking sheet has a low lip on all four sides to keep juices from dripping into your oven and is very versatile.

Roasting pan: A large, deep pan typically made of stainless steel, enameled steel, or aluminum. A low, open roasting pan with a rack is the most versatile type.

Rubber spatula: Very useful for mixing and folding batters and scraping the sides of a bowl or pot to make sure that all the contents get poured into the target container. Silicone models are heat resistant and can be used in hot pots.

Saucepan: A small pot ranging in size from 1 quart to 4 quarts (it's nice to have couple of different sizes) and typically about 4 inches deep, with a tight-fitting lid. Look for saucepans with ovenproof handles.

Saucepot: A deep, wide, and fairly light pot used for making soups and stews. A pot between 5 quarts and 8 quarts with a tight-fitting lid will be the most useful.

How to Season Cast-Iron Cookware

Cast-iron cookware generally needs to be seasoned (even if you buy it preseasoned) unless it's enamel coated. You season cast iron by heating a fat in the pan until it polymerizes on the surface and creates a slippery coating. Every time you cook with fat, you will add a little to this coating (that is, continuing to season your pan); however, cooking with liquid, salt, or anything with a bit of sugar content removes the coating.

When you first get your cast-iron pan, or if your pan starts looking dull or rusty or food starts sticking to it more than usual, follow these steps to season it:

- Place the pan in the oven and heat it to 200°F.
- Remove the pan from the oven (turn off the oven for now) and coat it inside and out with organic flax oil.
- Remove the excess oil with a paper towel. Put the pan back in the oven upside down and turn on the oven to 500°F.
- Once the oven is to temperature, let the pan "bake" for 1 hour. Turn off the oven and let the pan sit in there until the oven is cool (about 2 hours). Don't open the door before that point unless you want to fill your kitchen with toxic smoke.
- With a new pan, repeat this process about six times before your first use. After that, season it as needed, anytime the surface needs to be recoated.

Once you have a good seasoning built up, it's easier to maintain. To maintain seasoning:

- Use plenty of good-quality cooking fat whenever you use your cast-iron pan.
- Wash the pan while it's still warm with a gentle scrubber (brush or scouring pad) and hot water. Never use dish soap!
- Dry the pan immediately and thoroughly after washing, either by gently heating it on the stovetop or with a towel.

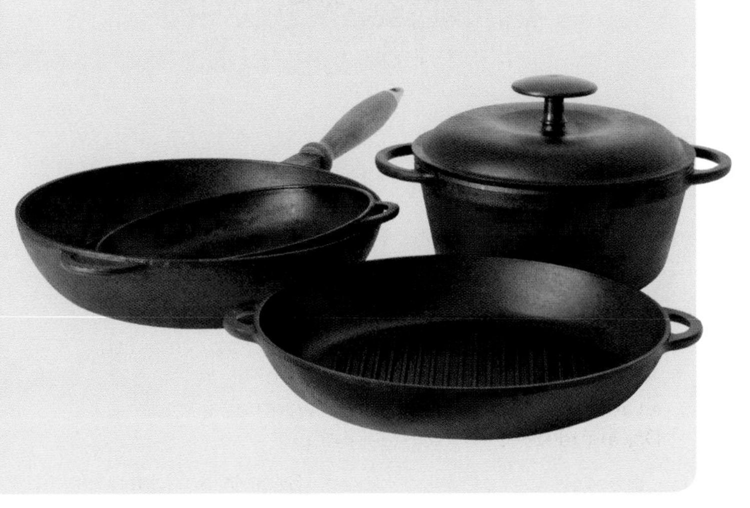

Scissors and shears: A good pair of kitchen scissors comes in handy for opening food packages, cutting strings, snipping fresh herbs, cutting bacon, and trimming artichoke leaves—to name just a few uses! Shears, which are larger and spring loaded, make sectioning poultry and cutting pork skins much simpler. Look for sturdy models that are easy to clean.

Sieve or strainer: This tool can be used to sift dry ingredients (like coconut flour) and to strain liquids (like broth). It's handy to have a few different sizes.

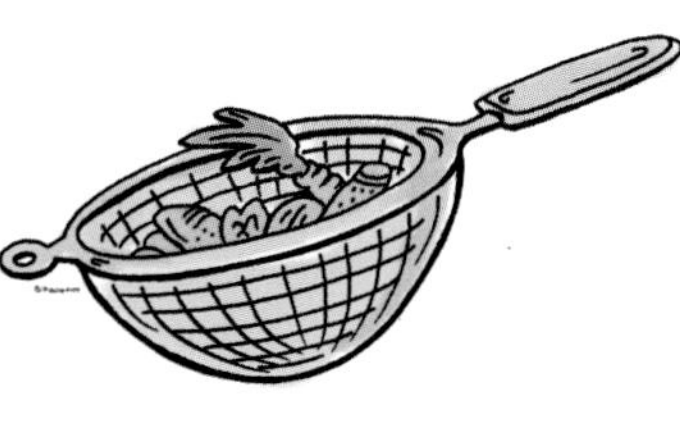

Skillet: A 10-inch or 12-inch cast-iron skillet is a wonderful investment. Enamel-lined skillets are more expensive but have the benefit of not requiring seasoning. It's also useful to have a 10-inch or 12-inch stainless-steel pan, which is great for browning meat and then deglazing.

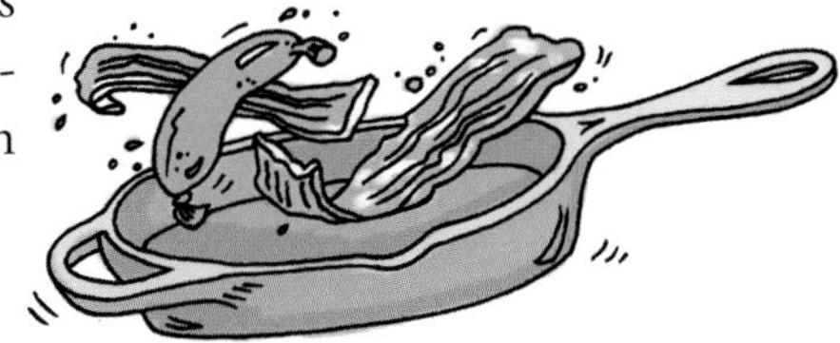

Slotted spoon: A large spoon with holes in the bowl that is used for scooping solid foods out of a liquid. Choose a sturdy spoon with a stainless-steel handle that won't get too hot.

Steamer: While you can "steam" veggies in a regular pot with just a little water, a steamer basket or insert does a much better job of retaining nutrients and preserving taste and texture. A collapsible-style metal steamer basket can fit into pots and pans of various sizes. A two-tier steamer pan looks like a double boiler (in which you boil water in the bottom pan to heat the top pan, which fits inside it), but the steamer insert has holes in the bottom and sides to let steam through. A bamboo steamer fits into a wok or over a pot of simmering liquid.

Stir spoons: Having a variety of sturdy spoons for stirring soups, stews, batters, sautéed vegetables, and other similar items is a must.

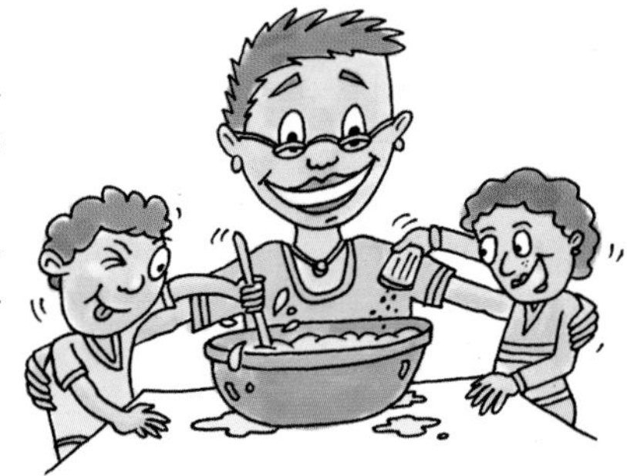

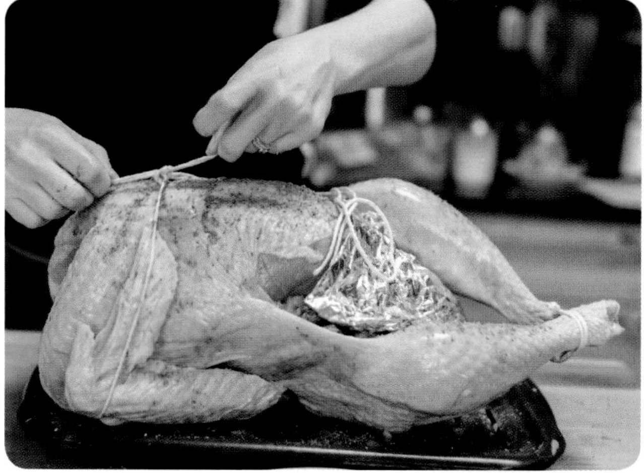

Stockpot: A tall, narrow, and very large pot used for cooking soups and stocks as well as bulky foods like lobster. Look for at least a 10-quart size. (12 quarts or 16 quarts is even better.)

Tongs: Useful for picking up slippery, hot, or messy foods to flip, move, or serve them without piercing them (especially useful for flipping and serving meat). Select a style with nonslip handles and scalloped tips for a firm grip.

Vegetable peeler: While you can use a paring knife to peel vegetables, a vegetable peeler is an inexpensive tool that saves so much time in the kitchen that it makes the essentials list. A swivel blade removes less peel than a fixed blade since it conforms to the shape of the vegetable; however, a fixed blade gives you more control.

Whisk: A tool that has thick wire loops attached to a handle, a whisk can be used to mix sauces, batters, gravies, salad dressings, and dips. Different sizes are best for different tasks, but a medium to large whisk will get most of these jobs done.

Zester (or microplane grater): If your box grater doesn't have a side for very fine grating (or zesting), then a zester is a must. When pulled across citrus fruit, it removes only the peel, leaving the bitter pith underneath. A microplane grater can also be used to grate garlic, ginger, and spices like nutmeg.

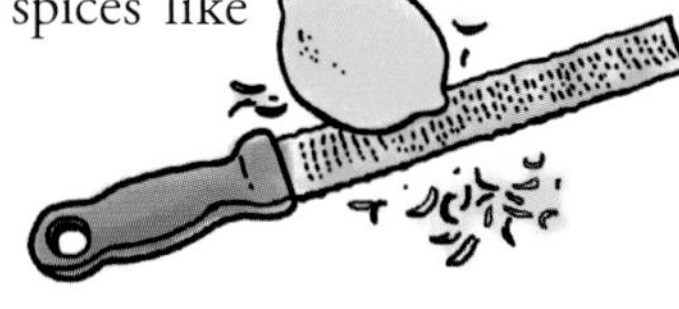

How to Hone a Blade

When it comes to kitchen safety and sanity, well-sharpened knives are a must. Sharp knives are less likely to slip than dull blades, and they get the job done more quickly and easily. For most people, it's probably simplest to take the blades to a local kitchen store to get them sharpened, but honing your blades at least a few days a week, if not daily, will keep them sharp between professional treatments.

You need a sharpening steel to hone a blade. To use a sharpening steel, rest one end of the steel on your countertop. Position the heel of the knife (the widest part of the blade) at a 20-degree angle (yes, it's okay to break out the protractor to make sure) on the underside of the sharpening steel near the finger guard, with the sharp end of the blade facing downward (away from you!). Draw the knife downward while pulling the handle toward you (no rush; slow and steady wins the race). Once you have sharpened the full length of the blade, repeat the process on the other side. Continue alternating sides of the blade with each stroke until sharp.

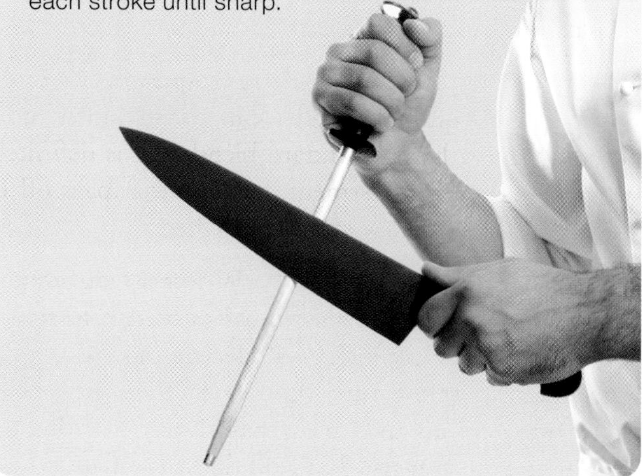

Of all these basic kitchen tools, I would emphasize the importance of having a couple of high-quality, sharp knives. Sharp knives are much safer than dull ones—not only are you less likely to cut yourself, but should you accidentally slice a finger, a wound from a sharp blade will heal much faster than one from a dull blade. I would also emphasize the importance of having a good meat thermometer. Grass-fed and pasture-raised meat tends to cook more quickly than conventionally raised meat, and the time it takes the meat to reach the target internal temperature can vary by farm and by season. Using a meat thermometer ensures that you don't overcook your meat, which is definitely a tear-worthy event!

Nonessentials (But Awesome Tools to Have)

Really, you can cook glorious meals with very simple tools. There are, however, a variety of additional kitchen gadgets and small appliances that, though nonessential, save time and energy in the kitchen. And when you are embarking on a diet and lifestyle change that requires you to prepare all your own food, any time-saver is hugely appreciated.

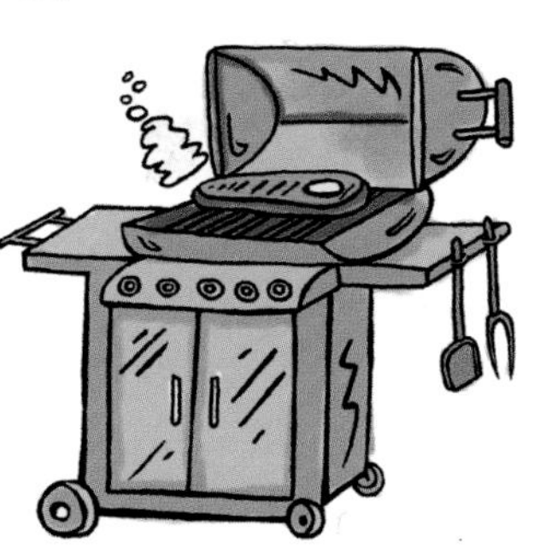

Barbecue or indoor grill: Let's be honest: food cooked on a barbecue is just plain delicious. Whether you opt for a gas grill or a charcoal grill is a matter of personal choice. An electric indoor grill will do all the same jobs, typically with less hassle, but the flavor it imparts is not quite the same.

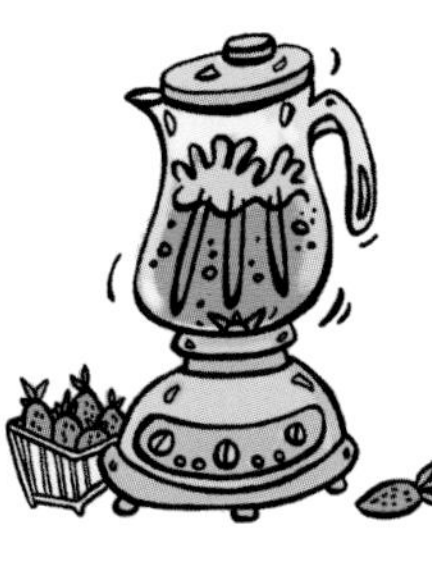

Blender: A high-powered, high-quality blender can do so much more than a standard blender. It is definitely an investment, but one that pays off in time saved in the kitchen.

Citrus juicer: Whether you choose a simple glass mold on which to smash citrus halves or a sophisticated electric model, a citrus juicer is much more efficient at extracting juice, especially from lemons and limes, than simply crushing the fruit with your fingers. *Tip:* Roll the whole fruit on the countertop while applying some pressure with your palm before slicing it in half to juice it. This breaks up the fibers of the fruit and makes juicing easier, faster, and more efficient.

Countertop deep-fryer: If you plan to deep-fry, you have two options: a large, heavy-bottomed stovetop pot with an oil thermometer or a countertop deep-fryer that controls the temperature for you. Countertop deep-fryers tend to make less of a mess than a pot on the stove due to their built-in vented lids, and the temperature control feature ensures that the fat comes back up to temperature as quickly as possible after you add your food without heating it above the smoke point. There are many options in terms of size and amount of fat required. Models with the heating element under the fat compartment (as opposed to submerged in the fat) tend to require less fat for the same volume of food. See page 82 for deep-frying basics.

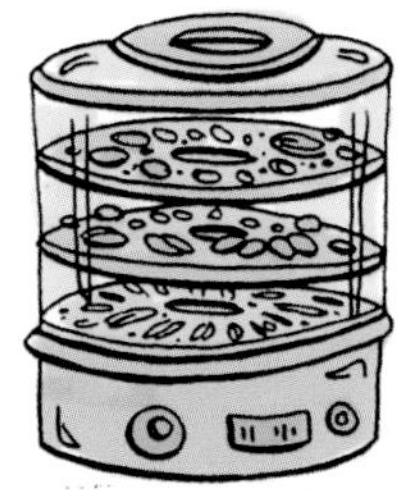

Dehydrator: Dehydrators range from simple, low-powered, on/off-switch, inexpensive versions to very sophisticated programmable models. They open up a whole new range of cooking options, from drying your own fruits and vegetables (for snacks or to use as ingredients in soups and stews) to making your own vegetable flours and jerky.

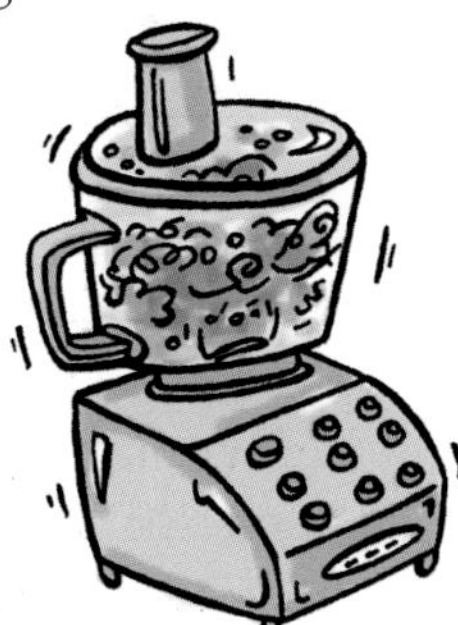

Food processor: A food processor with a few different blades, especially grating and slicing in addition to processing, is a tremendous time-saver. Certain jobs, like puréeing plantains, shredding cabbage for coleslaw, or slicing root vegetables extra thin to make potato chips, are so much faster with a good food processor; the time saved is extraordinary. Look for a model that comes with different-sized bowls for versatility.

Freezer: A freezer isn't really a cooking tool, but it's such a handy appliance when you're making all your own food from scratch, buying meat by the quarter or half animal, and batch-cooking for quick meals that it deserves a spot on the list. Look for one that isn't frost-free. While you'll have to sacrifice some time to thaw your freezer to defrost it every year or two, the food you store in your freezer will have double or triple the storage life (the temperature swings of a frost-free freezer cause freezer burn). Bonus: A freezer without the frost-free feature is typically much cheaper. Chest freezers tend to be the least expensive, whereas upright freezers are much easier to keep organized.

Grill pan: An alternative to using a barbecue or an electric indoor grill, this combination griddle/grill provides a versatile way to cook foods with less cooking fat than frying to better replicate the dry heat of a barbecue. The bottom surface is ridged, allowing fat to drip away. Use a grill pan over high heat for best results.

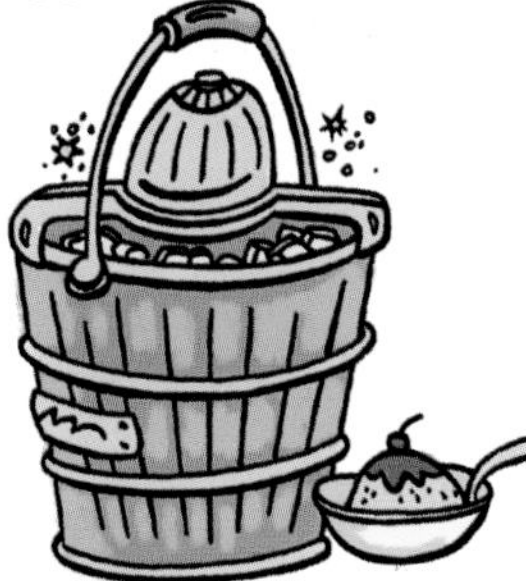

Ice cream maker: One of the simplest and healthiest treats you can make on the Paleo Approach diet is ice cream or sorbet. Ice cream makers range from hand-crank options that use ice and rock salt in an outer compartment to freeze your mix to electric models with a chamber that lives in your freezer until ready to use to fully automated and programmable models with a self-refrigerating compressor.

Microwave Safety

As discussed in *The Paleo Approach,* you don't have to give up the convenience of microwave cooking. And yes, it's okay to dance with joy at this good news! There are, however, some basic safety precautions and general rules that you should follow when using the microwave:

- Never put metal in the microwave. Microwave energy excites the electrons in metal and causes sparks. This goes for the obvious metal pans and dishes, but also twist ties and metal around the rims of glass jars, in some ceramic glazes, embedded in food labels, and even in plates (like your grandmother's Royal Doulton china with the gold rim). If you see sparks, turn off the microwave immediately!
- Use paper products only for cooking less than ten minutes, or they could ignite. Don't use recycled paper in the microwave, since recycled paper can contain tiny specks of metal. Also avoid using dyed paper products, since the dye can leach into your food.
- Don't use plastic containers in the microwave. Even microwave-safe plastics can leach chemicals (many of them estrogen-mimicking compounds) into your food, especially if the food you are microwaving has a high fat content.
- Don't use plastic wrap in the microwave. Yes, there are "microwave-safe" versions out there, but these are still plastics and are best avoided.
- Always remove a tight cover carefully, opening it away from your face, because steam can build up under the cover. Better yet, never use a dish with a tight cover in the microwave.
- Glass and ceramic are the two best materials for microwave-safe dishes. Look for a variety of sizes of bowls and dishes with glass or ceramic lids (instead of plastic lids) for microwave cooking.
- Always use a dish that is bigger than you think you need, large enough for stirring and boiling. Think of how you would fill a saucepot and not how you'd fill a casserole dish.
- Remember that the size of the food affects the cooking time. Small or thin pieces cook faster than large or thick ones.
- You can use microwave to thaw frozen meats and seafood in a pinch, but the quality of the meat can be affected. Those edges that cook while you're still thawing the middle won't have the same flavor and texture as if you thawed the meat using one of the methods discussed on page 59.
- The easiest and safest way to clean a microwave is to microwave a wet cloth for ten to twenty seconds. The steam helps loosen any food bits stuck to the inside, and you can use the now-hot cloth (be careful!) to wipe the inside of the microwave clean.

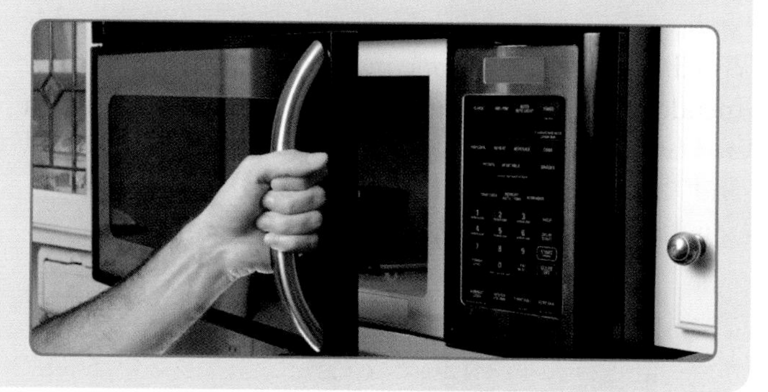

Juicer: While I hope you are eating whole vegetables rather than juicing to get your greens, an inexpensive home juicer can be a useful tool. It can replace a citrus juicer in addition to being used to make the vegetable juices called for in some of this book's recipes. You probably won't use a juicer often, so look for a cheap one that will get the job done.

Kitchen scale: Some foods vary so much in size or density that the only accurate way to measure them for a recipe is to weigh them. A digital scale that you can place a bowl or measuring cup on top of and reset to zero between each ingredient addition to your bowl is a very useful tool.

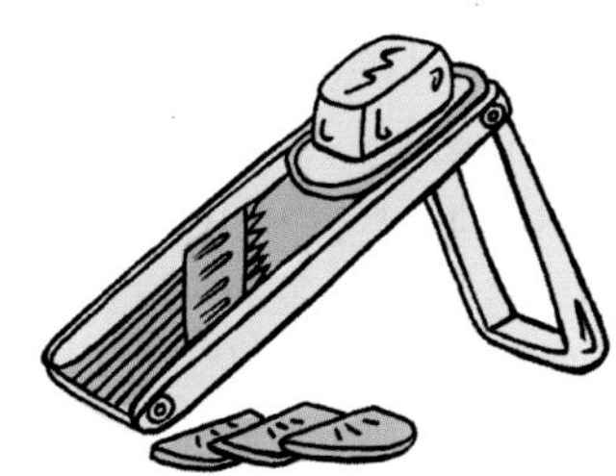

Mandoline slicer: This gadget speeds things up in my kitchen like no other tool. It slices, minces, and juliennes, and for small to medium-sized jobs it is often much faster to clean than a food processor (which can't make long slices or julienne like a mandoline can). Look for a mandoline with several different blade options for the most versatility. And always use the finger guard!

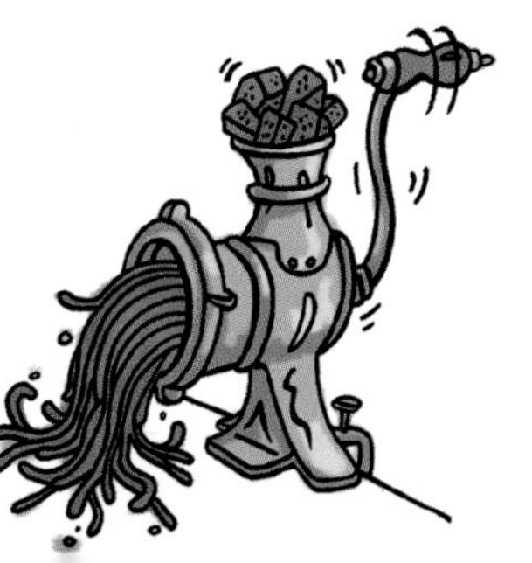

Meat grinder: You will likely find yourself grinding meat at home when adopting the Paleo Approach, mainly as a strategy to camouflage organ meat. While you can grind meat in a food processor, a meat grinder yields a better texture. You can find manual and electric countertop models or attachments for a stand mixer.

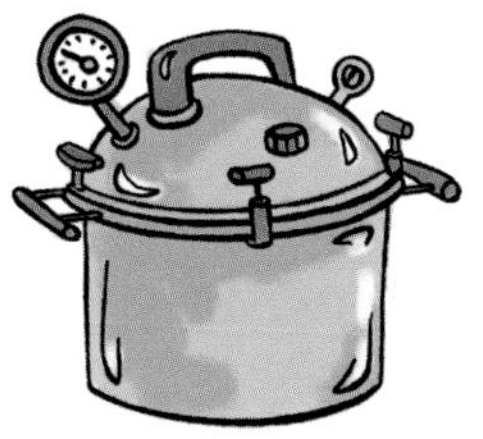

Pressure cooker: While stovetop pressure cookers are less expensive, look for a digital countertop model. A programmable pressure cooker gives you the flexibility of setting a timer and has many built-in safety features. There are also all-in-one models that enable you to sear meat and steam vegetables and even have slow-cooker and yogurt-maker functions.

Salad spinner: While a colander and paper towel can do a great job of removing excess water from leafy greens, a salad spinner does a better job more quickly. Look for one with a solid bowl for both swishing greens clean and serving them.

Sausage stuffer: Typically an attachment for a meat grinder (although standalone models do exist), a sausage stuffer is a must-have if you intend to stuff sausage mix into casings.

Silicone bakeware: If you plan to bake from this cookbook, having silicone muffin and cake pans is tremendously useful. Gluten-free, egg-free baking has a bad habit of being hard to remove even from greased and "floured" (with arrowroot powder) pans, but silicone bakeware makes it a snap!

Silicone baking pan liners: Lining a baking pan with parchment paper or aluminum foil can make a huge difference in terms of cleanup. Silicone liners are reusable and very versatile.

Smoker: While smoking your food isn't the healthiest method for day-to-day cooking, it's a pretty fantastic treat; you just can't beat the taste of some foods cooked in a smoker! Look for one with a built-in thermometer and a method for controlling the temperature. There are also smoker-barbecue hybrids, which give you the benefit of having two great cooking tools in one.

Spice grinder or mortar and pestle: The fresher your spices, the better their flavor. Freshly grinding whole spices like mace arils, cloves, cinnamon sticks, and pink rock salt in an electric or manual spice grinder (including mashing with a mortar and pestle) can have a huge positive impact. You can also use an electric spice grinder to make your own coconut flour, pumpkin flour, and plantain flour. A mortar and pestle can be used to crush fresh herbs to form a paste for seasoning meat.

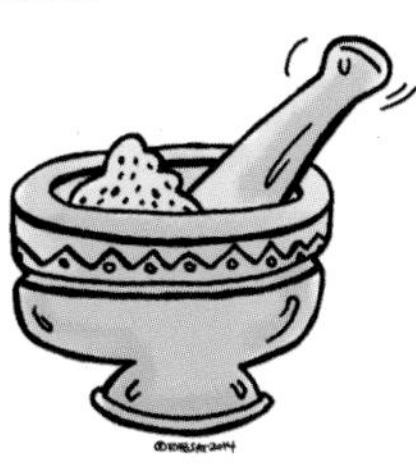

Spiral slicer: Spiral-cut vegetables are a fun and nutrient-dense replacement for pasta. Look for a spiral slicer with several different-sized blades for more flexibility in the shape of your finished product.

Stand mixer: A stand mixer probably won't see as much action in your kitchen while you follow the Paleo Approach diet as it might otherwise, but there are some tasks for which a stand mixer is very useful. Some mixers come with a slot for attachments like meat grinders, sausage stuffers, and ice cream makers! It's always useful to have a tool that can do more than one thing.

Yogurt maker: This inexpensive kitchen gadget is a must-have if you intend to make homemade coconut milk yogurt. Simple models have just an on/off switch, whereas more sophisticated models include a timer.

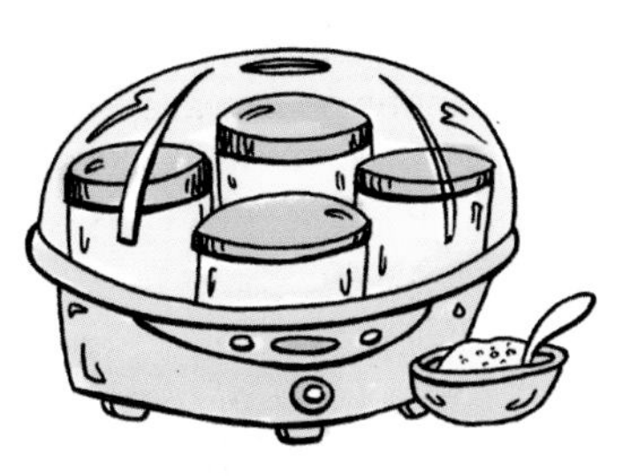

Wok: A wok is a pan with a rounded bottom that is used for frying and steaming in Asian cooking. Woks are available in different materials and sizes, are relatively simple to use, and have advantages over flat-bottom frying pans or skillets, namely a large cooking surface area and the ability to take advantage of both the hot area at the bottom of the pan to sear food and the lower temperature at the sides of the pan for slower cooking.

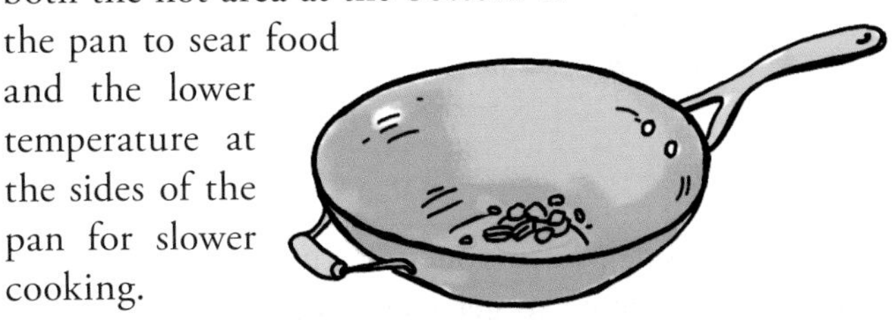

Certainly, there are lots more fun time-saving gadgets that you may find useful. If you're anything like me, visiting a kitchen supply store is even better than shoe shopping! This list represents those tools that are suggested in this book's recipes. Feel free to expand on your current supply of kitchen gadgets with anything you think will save you time or make a task easier and/or safer.

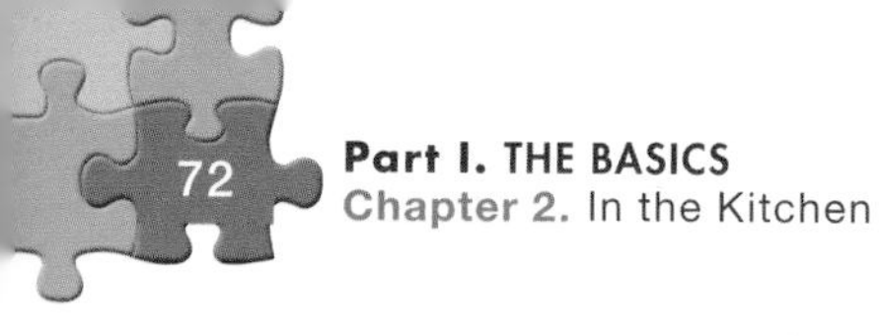

Managing Your Time in the Kitchen

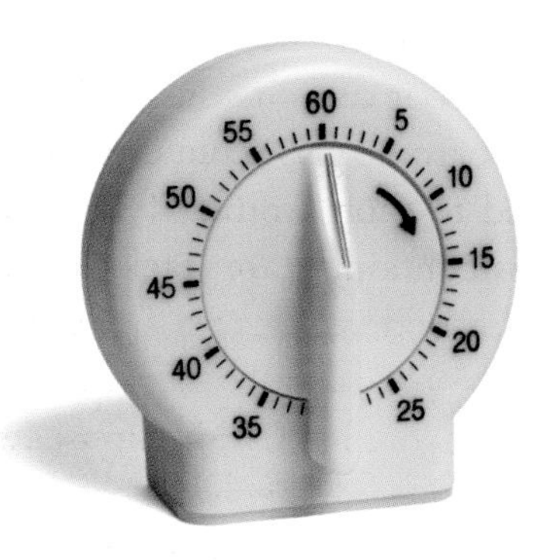

> *When poets write about food it is usually celebratory. Food as the thing-in-itself, but also the thoughtful preparation of meals, the serving of meals, meals communally shared: a sense of the sacred in the profane.*
>
> —Joyce Carol Oates

An important topic to cover is how to manage (and save) time in the kitchen. If you aren't used to cooking elaborate meals or making dishes from scratch, the transition to spending more time preparing food may be even harder than the transition to eating different foods.

It's important to emphasize that this new way of cooking and eating will get easier. As you spend more time in the kitchen, you will naturally become more proficient and efficient. As you cook different recipes, you will find favorites and develop a repertoire of quick meals that you can prepare either on the fly or in advance so that the time commitment still fits into your busy workday. Remember that you are learning a new skill. Whether you've never cooked anything that didn't come in a box or microwaveable bag before or you're already a big fan of home cooking, cooking with new techniques, tools, and ingredients is going to put you on a steep learning curve. It's okay to feel a little overwhelmed. Take a deep breath and do the best you can. And, to pull out the biggest cliché ever: practice makes perfect. Or, as I like to remind myself every time I tackle change in my life, it's only effort until it's routine.

Several strategies are just plain essential for minimizing the time you spend in the kitchen. While every person will need to figure out the best approach to fit her schedule and lifestyle, these are some of the techniques that I use to minimize my time toiling over a hot stove.

Batch Cooking

You can approach batch cooking either as "cooking for the freezer" or as "cooking for leftovers," or as both simultaneously. Batch cooking simply means that you are cooking a larger quantity of food than you would make for a single meal. Even though it may take a little longer to cook a double or triple batch of a recipe, the time you save over cooking that recipe on two or three separate occasions can be significant.

Having a freezer full of already-cooked meals, ready to be reheated in a flash, can be a life-saver. On those busy weeknights when you arrive home starving, you can simply pull a meal out of the freezer and throw it directly into the microwave (see page 70). Think of your freezer as your own fast-food restaurant. And having a variety of ready-made meals in your freezer means that there's always more than one thing on the menu!

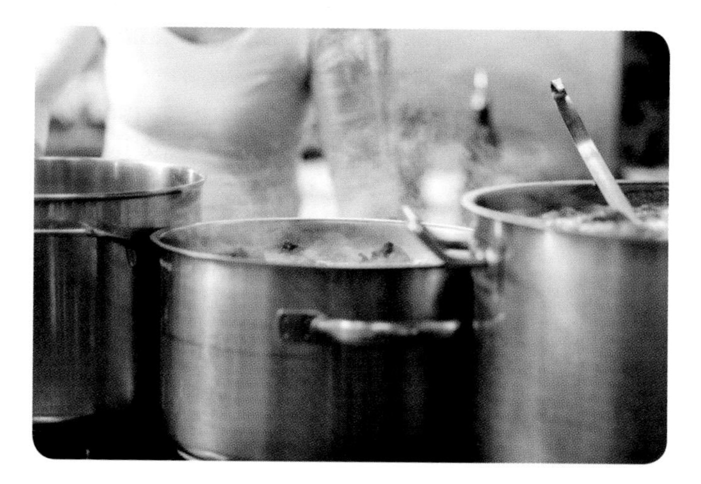

When freezing foods, let them cool prior to placing them in freezer-safe containers (unless you're using something like mason jars, in which case placing hot foods in your jars and loosely securing the lids allows you to get a seal prior to freezing and extends the freezer storage life). Foods such as muffins and sausage patties and ingredients such as berries are best frozen on a baking sheet, separated so they aren't touching, and then placed in a freezer bag or other freezer-safe container once frozen; this prevents them from sticking to each other and makes it easier to grab what you need out of a large batch. When choosing a freezer container, think about how many servings you want to freeze in each container. A large container is great for freezing a family meal's worth of food, whereas smaller containers are handy for individual portions or items that you will use as ingredients in smaller quantities, like broth.

Contrary to popular belief, refreezing previously frozen foods is actually safe to do most of the time. If you thawed an item in the refrigerator, it is safe to refreeze it without cooking it, although there may be a loss of quality due to the moisture lost through thawing. After cooking raw foods that were previously frozen, it is safe to freeze the cooked foods. If previously cooked and then frozen foods are thawed in the refrigerator, you may refreeze the unused portion. If you purchased frozen meat, poultry, or seafood, you can refreeze it if it has been handled properly (meaning that it's been kept cold). Do not refreeze any foods that are left outside the refrigerator for longer than two hours or that have spent more than an hour in temperatures above 90°F. Do not refreeze meat that was thawed in a microwave without cooking it first. Always freeze leftovers within three to four days of cooking.

Thawing food in the fridge is the safest method and preserves food quality the best. You can also use the water bath method described on page 59, even for soups, stews, broth, and other frozen prepared-ahead-of-time meals, provided that they are in sealed containers or bags. However, if you use the water bath method to thaw a food, don't refreeze the leftovers. If you're reheating cooked foods, you can typically skip thawing, especially if you are reheating them in the microwave or oven. (Frozen foods can burn on the stovetop, so if you choose this method, use low heat and watch it carefully.)

If you are cooking for leftovers, think about what will save you time when you reheat your meal. Will it help if you slice the entire roast tonight so that it's presliced and easy to serve tomorrow? Will it help if you refrigerate your leftovers as full dinner plates as opposed to putting the chicken in one container and the veggies in another?

I recommend investing in good containers for storing your leftovers, whether in the fridge or the freezer. Glass is great because it can go straight from the fridge to the microwave (some glass containers are ovenproof, but you'll need to shop around if that's a priority), and square glass containers are stackable (a feature that should not be underestimated in terms of handiness). Some glass containers are also freezer safe, adding even more functionality. Wide-mouthed mason jars are great for storing leftovers, and some sizes are freezer safe. These also have some stacking ability and seal tightly enough that they can go from freezer to water bath to microwave—and that means fewer dishes! A mason jar can even be packed in an insulated lunch box for an easy meal at work or school.

When it comes to reheating leftovers or thawed frozen foods, you can use the microwave (see page 70), the oven, or the stovetop, depending on the type of food you are reheating. Cooked food can be reheated from frozen—while it takes longer than reheating thawed food, it takes less time than thawing and then reheating. Reheating from frozen can affect texture, so it's not always the best choice in terms of food quality, but sometimes it is the only choice in terms of getting food into your mouth when you're ravenous!

If you find cooking in large batches too challenging during the week, dedicate one or both days on the weekend to cooking a large quantity of food, whether for your freezer or for leftovers during the week. While broth, soups, and stews are the most obvious choices, you can also batch-cook meats and vegetables. Try roasting two chickens or two legs of lamb instead of one and freezing the sliced cooked meat in small containers. These small portions are great for adding to salads or soups or using as your dinner protein during the week. Vegetables can get a bit mushy if cooked and then frozen, thawed, and reheated, but this won't matter much if you're freezing a mashed vegetable. And if you have Garlic and Rosemary Roast Beef (page 205) and Kufu (page 318) in the freezer, you are just some steamed broccoli away from a wonderful meal.

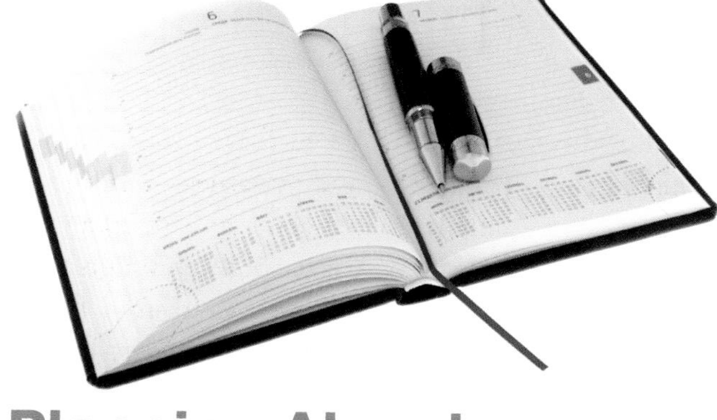

Planning Ahead

The best tool you have for making this transition is to plan ahead. It's important to know in advance what you're going to eat on a rushed weeknight, how you're going to handle getting out the door in a hurry in the morning, and what you'll do when the rest of your family is enjoying a tempting treat.

This is where batch cooking comes in handy. Batch cooking itself is a way of planning ahead, but it's not the only way. You can put ingredients in a slow cooker in the morning so that dinner will be ready when you get home. Maybe planning ahead just means that you take some meat out of the freezer to thaw the night before you'll be ready to cook it. Maybe planning ahead means ordering some ingredients online. Planning ahead can be as simple as making a shopping list and sticking to it!

This technique doesn't just encompass the mental planning of what you're going to make/eat and when; it also encompasses food prep that can be done ahead of time. Beyond the more obvious example of slow-cooking, planning ahead might mean chopping some vegetables when you have a few spare minutes. Or it might mean combining the ingredients for a sauce or dressing or putting a meat into a marinade in the fridge before you leave for work. Every minute you invest ahead of time is a minute less that it will take you to get dinner on the table when you're in a rush.

Do you normally hurry to get out the door in the morning? Having some leftovers or precooked sausage on hand can make a huge difference in terms of actually eating breakfast before leaving the house. A rushed morning may be a good time for a Superfood Smoothie (page 141), in which case planning ahead means ordering some Paleo Approach–friendly protein powders online and having an assortment of nutrient-dense ingredients to add.

If you know that you're going to be tempted by a treat that your family is enjoying or a dessert at a potluck, make use of the Sweet Treats and Beverages chapter in this cookbook. Many of the treats can be frozen so that you have them in case of an emergency (you know, the if-I-don't-get-to-eat-a-treat-right-now-I'm-going-to-go-certifiably-insane kind of emergency). Having a special indulgence that is just for you can be the difference between feeling a sense of deprivation that drives you to fall off the wagon and feeling pampered and content.

Using the Right Tools

As simple as it sounds, having the right kitchen tools can make all the difference in the world. Whether it means having sharp knives as opposed to dull ones, or using an immersion blender instead of a wire potato masher, or having a pair of tongs to flip slippery foods instead of struggling with a spatula, the right tools can have a significant impact on the amount of time it takes you to accomplish any task in the kitchen. Consider splurging on higher-end tools, gadget, utensils, and small appliances if you can. You typically (but not always) get what you pay for; a more expensive kitchen tool often does the job better and faster and is easier to clean.

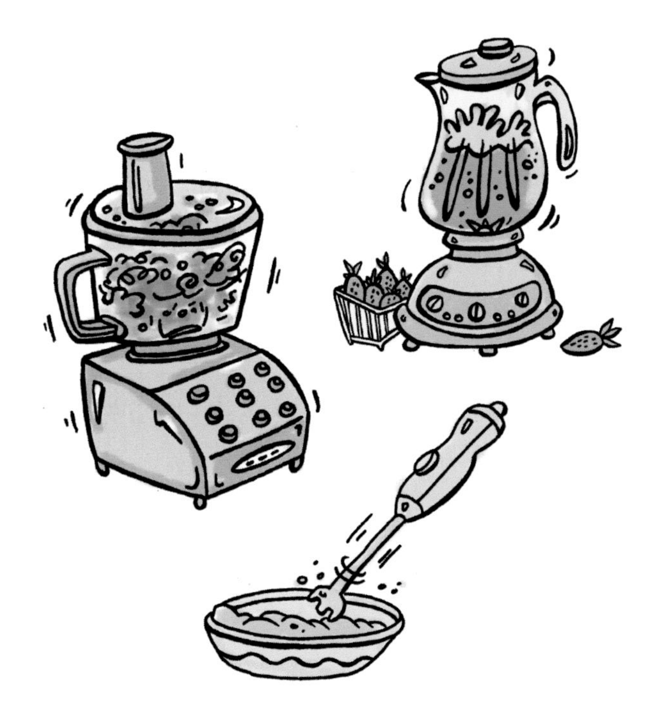

Pulling Together Quick Meals

Having a solid repertoire of quick meals that you can pull together in a pinch is an absolute must. Quick meals come in several flavors (pardon the pun):

1. ***"Oops, I forgot to pull some meat out of the freezer, so I'll make ______."*** Fill in the blank with a meal from your big-batch cooking day on the weekend, or some poached fish (my personal favorite food to cook from frozen), or some frozen precooked shrimp that can be force-thawed under cold water, or even individually wrapped pork chops or steaks that will thaw in less than an hour in a sink full of water and broil in about 8 minutes. It could even be a "naked" rotisserie chicken from the hot bar at your local natural food store.

2. ***"I have the benefit of planning ahead, but I'm going to have only 15 minutes to cook."*** In this case, using a slow cooker or programmable pressure cooker is super handy. But that's not the only way to plan ahead for this scenario. If you're going to have some time in the morning for food prep, you can chop or even precook vegetables, season meat, assemble sauces and dressings, and make a salad. Then it might just be a matter of throwing everything into a frying pan or under the broiler at dinnertime. Many recipes in this cookbook have very short cook times if you've done the food prep ahead of time.

3. ***"I don't have time to prepare AND I don't have time to cook."*** There are premade foods that will work in a pinch, like the aforementioned naked rotisserie chicken, canned fish, and raw veggies. That said, if you find that you just can't ever make time to cook, it's time to reevaluate your schedule and your priorities. Maybe you can do some batch cooking on the weekend so that meals during the week are composed of leftovers and frozen favorites. And if you consistently struggle to find time to cook and you are battling an autoimmune disease, you need to read Chapters 4 and 7 of *The Paleo Approach.*

Leftovers, Leftovers, Leftovers!

I've already covered cooking for leftovers, but I want to reiterate just how useful—and versatile!—having leftovers can be. Eating leftovers doesn't have to mean that you eat the same meal night after night (although it can if you enjoy it). There are lots of ways to use leftovers and not feel bored by repetition in your meals.

One simple way is to cook a large batch of meat—for example, a large roast, a leg of lamb, or a whole chicken or two—while switching up your side dishes every night. One night you might make Braised Greens (page 300) and Roasted Sweet Potato (page 313), the next night you might have steamed broccoli and Wild Mushrooms and Tarragon (page 305), and the next night you might have leftover sweet potatoes but change it up with a salad and some Cauliflower Gravy (page 123). Maybe one night you serve burgers with Guacamole (page 171), the next night with Barbecue Sauce (page 124), and the third night with sautéed onions and mushrooms and Arugula Pesto (page 310). Even leftover vegetables can be changed up by adding a dressing (page 126), tossing them with some chopped fresh herbs, or simply mixing together two different dishes of leftover veggies.

You can also completely reinvent your leftovers. Cooked meat can be added to stir-fries, salads, and soups to radically change their flavor, texture, and appearance. Try mixing cooked meat or seafood with some veggies and wrap in coconut wraps or nori (the Paleo Approach–friendly version of leftover sandwiches!). And when in doubt, freeze a meal of leftovers. Even though you'll be eating the same meal when you do reheat it, you can enjoy several days, weeks, or months of different meals before you get to it.

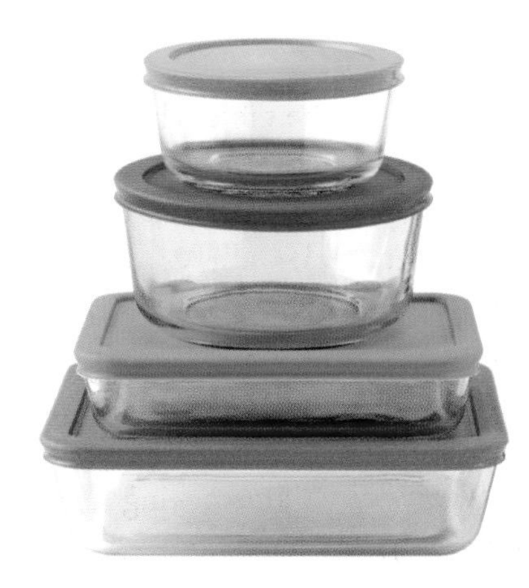

Using Convenience Foods

If you're struggling to make absolutely everything from scratch, there is no shame in taking advantage of some convenience foods. Precut veggies in microwavable steamer bags, prewashed salad greens, precut fruits and raw veggies that don't require any preparation, packaged sweet potato chips and plantain chips, and frozen vegetables ready to be added to a pot are all great ways to save time. Meat that your butcher has already sliced (usually for no extra fee), fish that your fishmonger has already filleted (sometimes for a higher price per pound), and Paleo Approach–friendly preprepared meats, like the twice-mentioned naked rotisserie chicken, as well as precooked shrimp, canned or smoked fish, and some deli meats, can save you a ton of time when it comes to getting quality protein on your plate. Canned coconut milk or cream, specialty flours, and other specialty foods like coconut wraps, nori wraps, and seaweed snacks can all save you time and help you pull together a meal when your schedule is packed. See page 57 for other convenience foods to stock up on.

Sharing the Joy

If you're going to spend substantially more time in the kitchen, finding a helper or two or three can make a huge difference. Whether you recruit your spouse to chop some vegetables or get your kids to set the table, having someone else do even a small proportion of the work can relieve a large proportion of the burden of food preparation. And having someone else do a large proportion of the work is even better! This is also an opportunity to turn a chore into quality family time. Beyond the fact that many hands make light work, many mouths make good conversation. After all, the best house parties always end up in the kitchen . . . why not make that party a daily event?

What do you do if you live on your own? Or if your spouse works a schedule that doesn't allow him to help? Or if your kids are too young to provide assistance that reduces rather than amplifies your stress? Try inviting a friend or family member over on the weekend during your batch-cooking day. Beyond an extra pair of hands in the kitchen, visiting with a friend makes the time spent cooking much more fun.

Food should be enjoyed rather than endured.
—Steve Hamilton

The same goes for cooking.
—Sarah Ballantyne

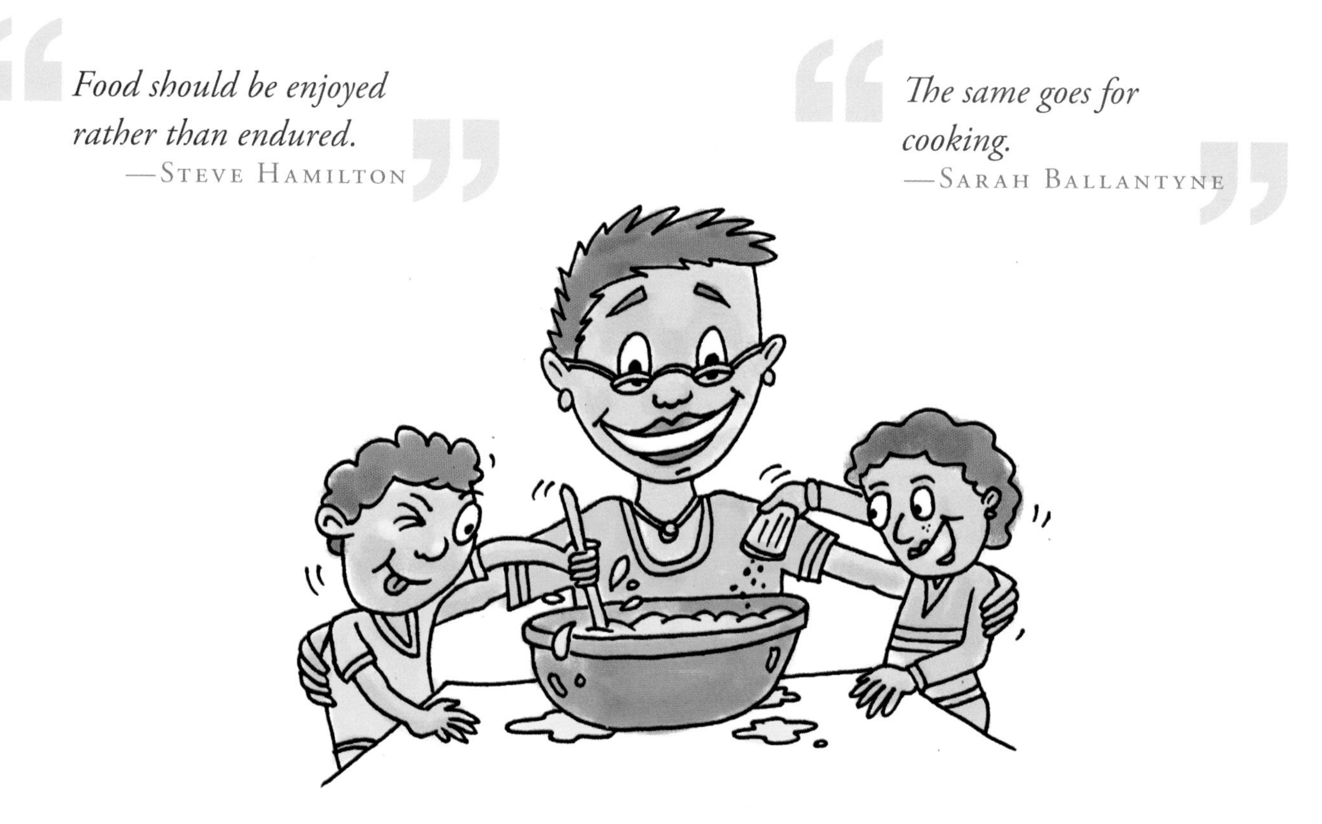

Illustration by Rob Foster

Useful Guides

Need to know what temperature to set the oven to when you're cooking a leg of lamb? Need help converting imperial units to metric? Want to look up the smoke point of a fat to figure out what temperature to set your deep-fryer to? I've got you covered.

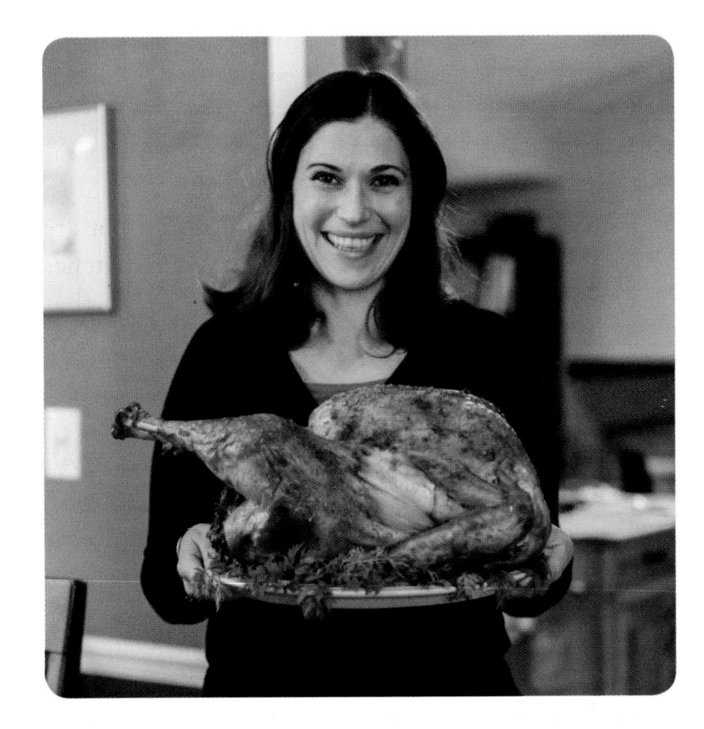

Meat Cooking Times and Temperatures

The single most important kitchen tool when it comes to cooking meat is an oven-safe meat thermometer. Grass-fed and pasture-raised meat often cooks much more quickly than conventionally produced meat, and many factors can influence just how much more quickly. For example, two years ago the pasture-raised turkey I bought for Thanksgiving dinner cooked in 3¼ hours. Last year, it cooked in 2¾ hours. Both years, the turkey weighed 15 pounds and, stuffed, should have taken at least 4 hours to cook. If I hadn't had a meat thermometer in place, my family would have been eating very dry, overcooked turkey.

The following list is based on USDA recommendations and should be considered a general guide and starting place. It is often recommended to reduce the oven temperature by 25°F when cooking grass-fed and pasture-raised meat.

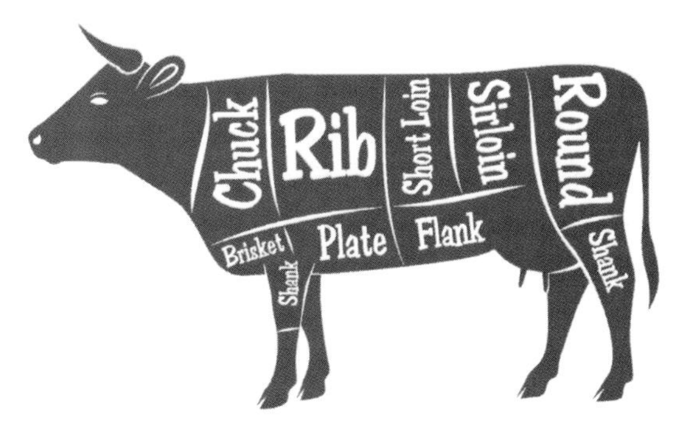

Beef

Cut	Size	Cooking Method	Cooking Time
Hamburger patties, fresh	4 oz.	Grill, broil, or fry, turning halfway through	6–10 minutes
Chuck roast, brisket	3–4 lbs.	Braise at 325°F	2–3 hours
Rib roast, bone-in	4–6 lbs.	Roast at 325°F	23–25 minutes per lb.
Rib roast, boneless, rolled	4–6 lbs.	Roast at 325°F	28–33 minutes per lb.
Round or rump roast	2½–4 lbs.	Roast at 325°F	30–35 minutes per lb.
Steaks	¾ inch thick	Broil or grill, turning halfway through	8–10 minutes
Stew or shank cross-cuts	1–1½ inches thick	Cover with liquid and simmer	2–3 hours
Short ribs	4 inches long and 2 inches thick	Braise at 325°F	1½–2½ hours
Tenderloin, whole	4–6 lbs.	Roast at 425°F	45–60 minutes

Hamburger patties: Internal Temperature **160°F**

All other cuts: Internal Temperature **145°F** for medium-rare | **160°F** for medium. Let rest for at least **3 minutes.**

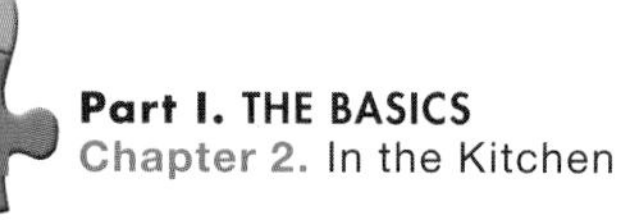

Lamb

Cut	Size	Cooking Method	Cooking Time
Ground lamb patties	2 inches thick	Broil or grill, turning halfway through	10–16 minutes
Breast, rolled	1½–2 lbs.	Braise at 325°F	1½–2 hours
Chops, rib, or loin	1–1½ inches thick	Broil or grill, turning halfway through	7–11 minutes
Cubes, for kabobs	1–1½ inches	Broil or grill, turning halfway through	8–12 minutes
Leg, bone-in	5–7 lbs.	Roast at 325°F	20–25 minutes per lb.
	7–9 lbs.	Roast at 325°F	15–20 minutes per lb.
Leg, boneless, rolled	4–7 lbs.	Roast at 325°F	25–30 minutes per lb.
Leg steaks	¾ inch thick	Broil or grill, turning halfway through	14–18 minutes
Shoulder roast or shank leg half	3–4 lbs.	Roast at 325°F	30–35 minutes per lb.
Stew meat, pieces	1–1½ inches	Cover with liquid and simmer	1½–2 hours
Shanks	¾–1 lb.	Cover with liquid and simmer	1½–2 hours

Ground lamb patties: Internal Temperature 160°F

All other cuts: Internal Temperature 145°F for medium-rare | 160°F for medium. Let rest for at least 3 minutes.

Pork

Cut	Size	Cooking Method	Cooking Time
Ground pork patties	½ inch thick	Fry, turning halfway through	8–10 minutes
Ground pork patties (direct heat)	½ inch thick	Broil or grill	8–10 minutes
Boston butt	3–6 lbs.	Roast at 350°F	45 minutes per lb.
Crown roast	10 lbs.	Roast at 350°F	12 minutes per lb.
Leg, (fresh ham) half, bone-in	5–8 lbs.	Roast at 350°F	22–25 minutes per lb.
Leg, (fresh ham) whole, bone-in	18–20 lbs.	Roast at 350°F	15 minutes per lb.
Loin chops or cutlets	¼ inch	Fry, turning halfway through	3–4 minutes
	¾ inch	Fry, turning halfway through	7–8 minutes
Loin chops, bone-in or boneless	¾ inch	Broil or grill, turning halfway through, or braise	6-9 minutes
	1½ inches	Broil or grill, turning halfway through	12–16 minutes
Loin cubes and tenderloin medallions	½–1 inch	Braise	8–10 minutes
Loin kabobs	1-inch cubes	Broil or grill, turning halfway through	10–15 minutes
Loin or shoulder cubes	1-inch cubes	Stew	45–60 minutes
Loin roast, bone-in or boneless	2–5 lbs.	Roast at 350°F	20 minutes per lb.
Ribs (baby back, country style, or spareribs)	2–4 lbs.	Roast at 350°F	1½–2 hours
Ribs, all types	2–4 lbs.	Braise	1½–2 hours
Ribs, all types (indirect heat)	2–4 lbs.	Broil or grill, turning halfway through	1½–2 hours
Shoulder, boneless	3–6 lbs.	Braise	2–2½ hours
Tenderloin	½–1½ lbs.	Broil or grill, turning halfway through	20 minutes
		Roast at 425°F–450°F	20–27 minutes
Tenderloin medallions	¼–½ inch thick	Fry, turning hallway though	4–8 minutes

Ground pork patties: Internal Temperature 160°F

All other cuts: Internal Temperature 145°F for medium | 160°F for well-done. Let rest for at least 3 minutes.

Poultry

Type of Chicken	Size	Cooking Method	Cooking Time
Breast halves, bone-in	6–8 oz.	Roast at 350°F	30–40 minutes
		Simmer	35–45 minutes
		Grill, turning halfway through	20–30 minutes
Breast halves, boneless	4 oz.	Roast at 350°F	20–30 minutes
		Simmer	25–30 minutes
		Grill, turning halfway through	12–16 minutes
Drumsticks	4 oz.	Roast at 350°F	35–45 minutes
		Simmer	40–50 minutes
		Grill, turning halfway through	16–24 minutes
Legs or thighs	4–8 oz.	Roast at 350°F or simmer	40–50 minutes
		Grill, turning halfway through	20–30 minutes
Whole broiler-fryer*	3–4 lbs.	Roast at 350°F	1¼–1½ hours
		Simmer or grill	1–1¼ hours**
Whole roasting hen*	5–7 lbs.	Roast at 350°F	2–2¼ hours
		Simmer	1¾–2 hours
		Grill	18–25 minutes per lb.**
Whole capon*	4–8 lbs.	Roast at 350°F	2–3 hours
		Grill	15–20 minutes per lb.**
Whole Cornish hens*	18–24 oz.	Roast at 350°F	50–60 minutes
		Simmer	35–40 minutes
		Grill	45–55 minutes**
Wings or wingettes	2–3 oz.	Roast at 350°F	30–40 minutes
		Simmer	35–45 minutes
		Grill	8–12 minutes per side
Type of Turkey	**Size**	**Cooking Method**	**Cooking Time**
Breast	4–6 lbs.	Roast at 325°F	1½–2¼ hours
	6–8 lbs.		2¼–3½ hours
Whole turkey, unstuffed	8–12 lbs.		2¾–3 hours
	12–14 lbs.		3–3¾ hours
	14–18 lbs.		3¾–4¼ hours
	18–20 lbs.		4¼–4½ hours
	20–24 lbs.		4½–5 hours
Whole turkey, stuffed	8–12 lbs.		3–3½ hours
	12–14 lbs.		3½–4 hours
	14–18 lbs.		4–4¼ hours
	18–20 lbs.		4¼–4¾ hours
	20–24 lbs.		4¾–5¼ hours

Internal Temperature 165°F

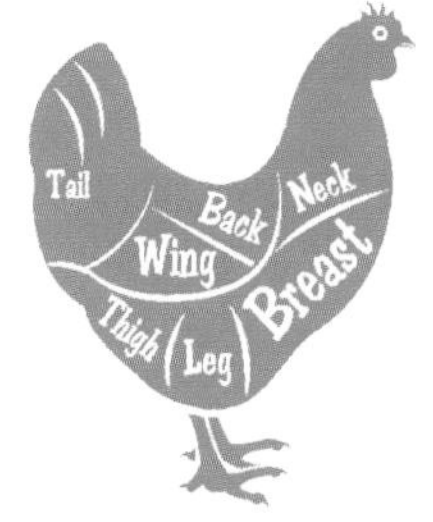

* Unstuffed. If stuffed, add 15–30 minutes.

**Indirect method using drip pan.

Grilling Basics

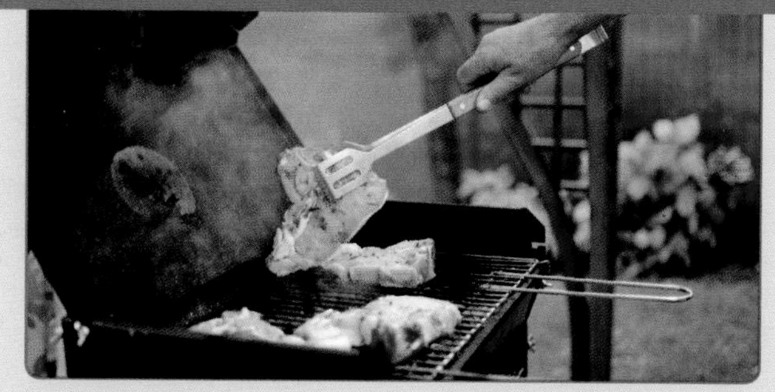

Grilling is as much an art as it is a science. While there are general rules to follow, grilling requires intuition, which is generally gleaned from experience, and the ability to improvise. I fully admit to being merely a competent griller myself; but the good news is that grilling is a very forgiving cooking technique—you don't need to be an expert to make great food on a grill.

Grilling—or, more technically, direct-heat grilling—involves cooking food directly over a hot flame, whether from a campfire, a gas grill, or a charcoal barbecue. The exact procedure for grilling depends on the equipment (or lack thereof) you're using, and it's always best to follow the manufacturer's recommendations for lighting your grill and adjusting the temperature.

Gas grills generally need to preheat for 10 to 15 minutes with the burners on high and the cover closed before you adjust the temperature and put your food on the grill. For charcoal grills, light the coals with the cover off 30 to 45 minutes before you plan to start cooking. How hot you want your grill will depend on what you plan to cook. In general, larger pieces of meat that need to be cooked longer will require a lower temperature, or else the outside will burn.

A grill thermometer is the most foolproof way to gauge the heat of your grill, but if you don't have one, you can always use the hand test. Carefully hold your hand, palm side down, about 2 inches above the cooking grate. Count the number of seconds you can hold your hand in that position before the heat forces you to pull it away. Then use this table to determine the approximate temperature:

Seconds	Temperature Classification	Approximate Temperature
1	Too hot (food will burn)	>425°F
2	Hot	375°F to 425°F
3	Medium-hot	350° to 375°F
4	Medium	300° to 350°F
5	Low	200° to 300°F

Controlling the temperature on a gas grill is simply a matter of adjusting the knob settings. When cooking with charcoal, lower the temperature by spreading the coals farther apart or by raising the cooking grate. To raise the cooking temperature, lower the grate or move the coals closer together and tap off the ash. When the temperature needs to be adjusted quickly, whether using a gas or charcoal grill, raise or lower the lid.

Some general grilling tips:

- Have the proper grill tools to do the job. These include long-handled tongs (if using charcoal, one pair for food and one pair for coals), a long-handled basting brush, a long-handled metal spatula, a meat thermometer, a grill thermometer, heavy-duty oven mitts, metal or disposable foil drip pans, and a wire brush to clean the grate. There are lots of additional accessories for specific grilling applications, but these basics will get you started.
- Keep your grill a safe distance away from anything flammable, like lighter fluid, fences, trees, and your house. A good general rule is at least 10 feet, although the building code in some areas is less.
- Always keep your grill grate clean to prevent sticking and for better taste and general safety. Scrub the grate with a wire brush while the grill is warm but not hot.
- Oil the food, not the grate. Avocado oil has a very high smoke point and, because it's liquid at room temperature, is very handy for coating food in preparation for grilling.
- Always keep an eye on what you're grilling. Besides the fact that you have an open flame probably not too far from your house, food can burn quickly, so be on your guard and check it frequently.
- It's easier to fix undercooked food than overcooked. When in doubt, remove the food from the grill, test for doneness (either by thermometer or by taste test), and return it to the grill if undercooked.
- Soak bamboo skewers in water for at least 20 minutes before making kabobs to prevent the skewers from burning. Soak cedar planks for at least an hour before placing them on the grill.
- Season your food at least an hour prior to grilling. It's generally best not to apply sauces prior to grilling since they can burn before the meat is fully cooked. Most recipes suggest basting with sauces for only the last 5 minutes of cooking.
- Cook vegetables and fruits at the outer, cooler edges of the grill, as they tend to burn more quickly than meat.
- Do not use a spray bottle of water to control flare-ups. Flare-ups are caused by too much fat (or sugar from a sauce) and too much heat. If you have a fatty cut of meat, trim the excess fat before grilling or use a drip pan so that any fat dripping off doesn't land directly on the hot coals or flame.
- Turning food is essential for even cooking and to prevent burning. It's okay to turn your food more than once, but food typically tastes better the less it's turned (in other words, don't get flip happy).
- Once it's cooked, place grilled food on a clean plate.

Cooking Fish

In general, fish is cooked when it just begins to flake easily when tested with a fork and loses its translucent or raw appearance. To be thoroughly cooked, fish should reach a minimum internal temperature of 145°F.

One helpful guideline is the 10-minute rule for cooking finfish. Apply it when baking, broiling, grilling, steaming, and poaching fillets, steaks, or whole fish. (Do not apply the 10-minute rule to microwave cooking or deep-frying.)

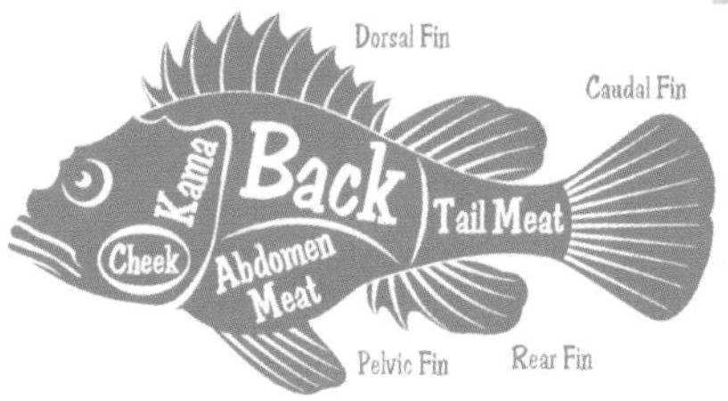

Here's how to use the 10-minute rule:

1. Measure the fish at its thickest point. If it is to be stuffed or rolled, measure it after stuffing or rolling.
2. Cook the fish at 450°F for 10 minutes per inch of thickness, turning the fish halfway through the cooking time. For example, a 1-inch fish steak should be cooked for 5 minutes per side for a total cooking time of 10 minutes. Pieces of fish that are less than ½ inch thick do not have to be turned.
3. Add 5 minutes to the total cooking time if you are cooking the fish in foil or in a sauce.

Measurement Conversions

Liquid or Volume Measurements (Approximate)			
1 teaspoon		⅓ tablespoon	5 ml
1 tablespoon	½ fl. oz.	3 teaspoons	15 ml or 15 cc
2 tablespoons	1 fl. oz.	⅛ cup or 6 teaspoons	30 ml or 30 cc
¼ cup	2 fl. oz.	4 tablespoons	59 ml
⅓ cup	2⅔ fl. oz.	5 tablespoons plus 1 teaspoon	79 ml
½ cup	4 fl. oz.	8 tablespoons	118 ml
⅔ cup	5⅓ fl. oz.	10 tablespoons plus 2 teaspoons	158 ml
¾ cup	6 fl. oz.	12 tablespoons	177 ml
7/8 cup	7 fl. oz.	14 tablespoons	207 ml
1 cup	8 fl. oz. or ½ pint	16 tablespoons	237 ml
2 cups	16 fl. oz. or 1 pint	32 tablespoons	473 ml
4 cups	32 fl. oz.	1 quart	946 ml
1 pint	16 fl. oz. or 2 cups	32 tablespoons	473 ml
2 pints	32 fl. oz.	1 quart	946 ml or 0.946 liter
1 liter	1.057 quarts		1000 ml
8 pints	128 fl. oz.	4 quarts	3785 ml or 3.78 liters
4 quarts	128 fl. oz.	1 gallon	3785 ml or 3.78 liters
1 gallon	128 fl. oz.	4 quarts	3785 ml or 3.78 liters

Dry or Weight Measurements (Approximate)		
1 oz.		30 g
2 oz.		55 g
3 oz.		85 g
4 oz.	¼ lb.	125 g
8 oz.	½ lb.	240 g
12 oz.	¾ lb.	375 g
16 oz.	1 lb.	454 g
32 oz.	2 lbs.	907 g
¼ lb.	4 oz.	125 g
½ lb.	8 oz.	240 g
¾ lb.	12 oz.	375 g
1 lb.	16 oz.	454 g
2 lbs.	32 oz.	907 g
1 kg	2.2 lbs. or 35.2 oz.	1000 g

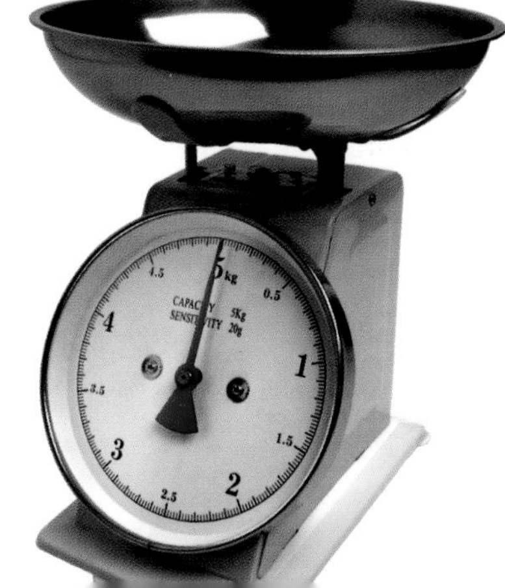

Smoke Points of Fats and Oils

Fat/Oil	Temperature
Avocado oil, refined	520°F
Avocado oil, virgin	375°F
Coconut oil, extra-virgin	350°F
Coconut oil, refined	450°F
Lard	370°F
Leaf lard	370°F
Macadamia nut oil	410°F
Olive oil, extra-virgin	250°F–320°F*
Olive oil, refined	450°F
Olive oil, virgin	375°F
Palm oil	450°F
Palm shortening	450°F
Poultry fat/schmaltz	375°F
Red palm oil	425°F
Salo	370°F
Strutto	370°F
Tallow	400°F
Walnut oil, semirefined	400°F
Walnut oil, virgin	320°F

* The smoke point of olive oil varies. Unless a manufacturer specifically tells you the smoke point of its olive oil, it's best to assume 250°F.

Alcohol Cook-off Times

If you are very sensitive to alcohol, it's helpful to know how much might be left over after using different cooking techniques. You can also almost always substitute broth, water, or fruit juice for wine in a recipe or substitute vanilla powder for vanilla extract.

Preparation Method	Percentage of Alcohol Retained
Added to boiling liquid and removed from heat	85%
Flamed	75%
No heat; stored overnight	70%
Baked for 25 minutes, not stirred into mixture	45%
Baked or simmered, stirred into mixture:	
15 minutes	40%
30 minutes	35%
1 hour	25%
1½ hours	20%
2 hours	10%
2½ hours	5%

Deep-Frying Basics

Deep-frying can be done in fat that is anywhere between 320°F and 400°F, but the ideal temperature for most foods is 350°F to 375°F. Deep-frying in this temperature range allows less absorption of fat into the food while searing the outside to lock in moisture and create that wonderful crispy outer layer. However, it's important to keep your fat below its smoke point (at least 5°F lower to be safe). So, if you're deep-frying in coconut oil, keep the temperature at 345°F. If you're using lard, go ahead and keep the temperature at 360°F. This is most easily accomplished with a countertop deep-fryer, which regulates the temperature for you and can be purchased quite inexpensively. You can also use a large heavy-bottomed pan and an oil thermometer, but because controlling the temperature of your fat can be tricky, you will want to aim to keep it at least 20°F below its smoke point (even if this is less than ideal from a cooking chemistry standpoint).

The best fats for deep-frying are those with higher smoke points, such as palm shortening, tallow, and lard (or a combination). Each fat gives its own flavor, which may influence your choice. Palm shortening has very little flavor, whereas beef tallow and lard are just plain tasty! Also, when you mix fats, you average their smoke points. So if you want to use lard for higher-temperature deep-frying, try mixing it with an equal amount of palm shortening (which has a higher smoke point).

A few rules for deep-frying:

- Never drop your food into the hot fat—this can cause a dangerous splatter. Instead, bring the food right to the surface and let it slide into the hot fat.
- Make sure to drain or pat dry any excess moisture. Water or other liquids will cause the fat to bubble and splatter more.
- Don't overcrowd the pan. Make sure that there's plenty of space between items in your deep-fryer to ensure that they cook evenly.
- Always use a deep-fry basket or strainer to remove food from the fat—don't be tempted to use a fork or chopsticks!

You can reuse the same fat many times as long as it never goes above its smoke point. When you're done, let the fat cool slightly, and then pour it through a very fine sieve or paper towel–lined sieve to filter out any food crumbs. Store your fat in a cool, dark place. The next time you deep-fry, top it up with some fresh fat. Change your fat when it doesn't taste good anymore or has darkened in color considerably.

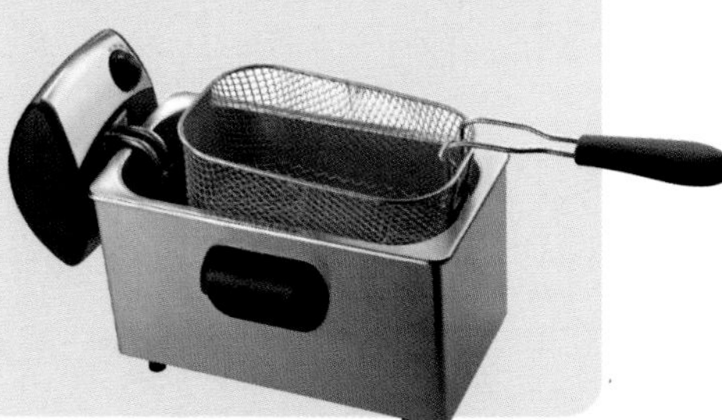

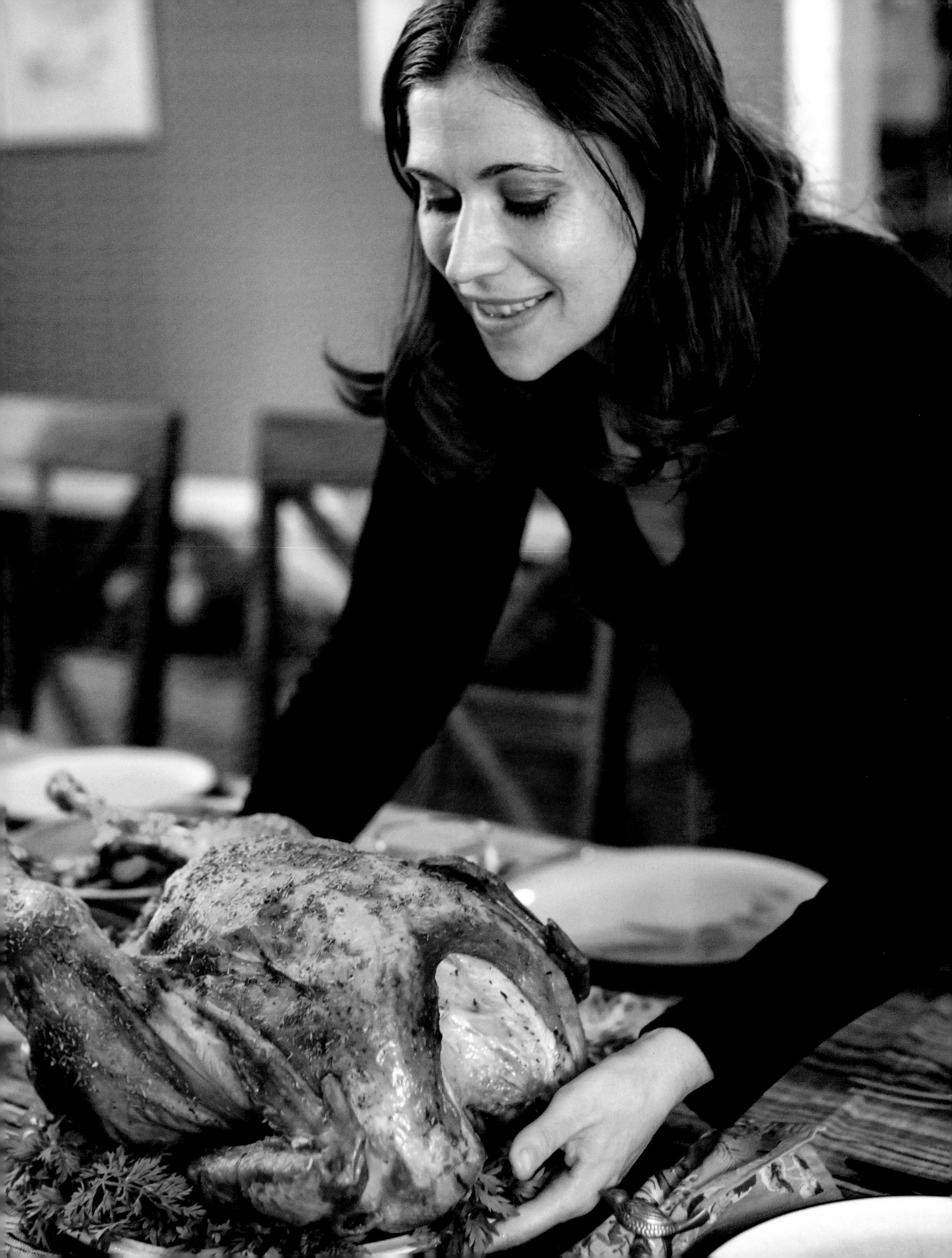

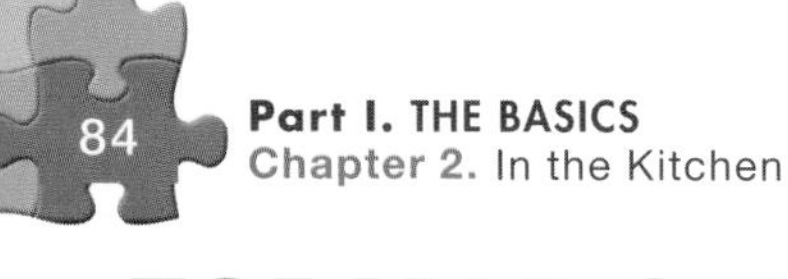

FODMAP Substitutions

Most of the time, you can simply omit a high-FODMAP ingredient from a recipe. With garlic and onions, however, substituting is more difficult since they are often an important part of a dish's flavor. While caramelizing onions and garlic greatly reduces the FODMAP content, it may not be sufficient for many people with FODMAP intolerance. Here are some ways to substitute:

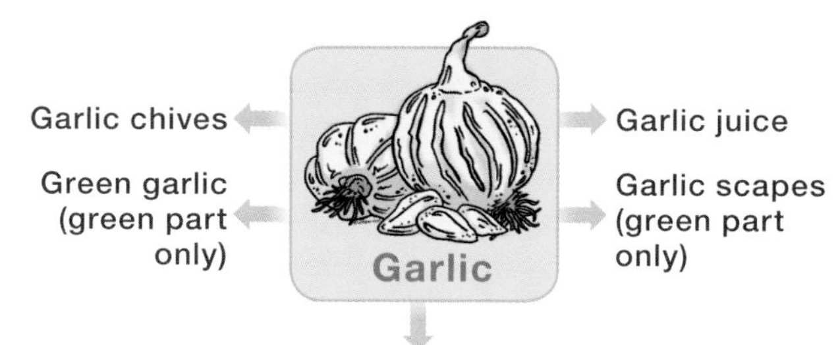

Onion
Asafetida powder (check ingredients)
Chives
Leek (green part only)
Onion juice
Green onion (green part only)

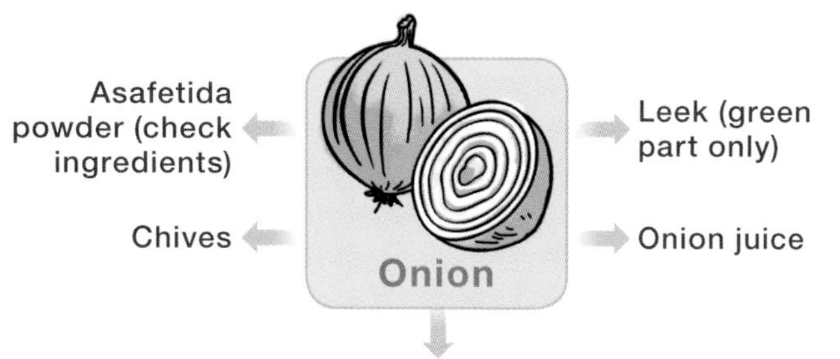

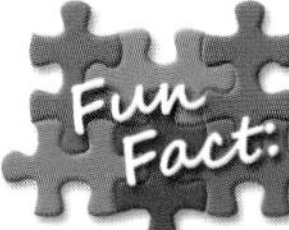

There are five categories of taste: sweet, salty, bitter, sour, and umami. The term umami comes from the Japanese scientist Dr. Kikunae Ikeda, who identified this taste classification. The word is pronounced "oo-MA-mee" and is aptly made up of two distinct words:

- *Umai, which means delicious*
- *Mi, which means essence*

Simple Cooking Substitutions

As you begin to tackle modifying your old favorite recipes, it helps to have a starting point for substitutions. If a recipe calls for tomato paste, what can you use instead? What are your options to replace flour or cornstarch to thicken a sauce? And what if you're allergic to an ingredient in one of the recipes in this book and need to find a replacement? Though this list is not exhaustive, here are the most useful cooking substitutions. See the baking ingredients list on page 56 for more substitution options.

Umami (a flavor that wheat, soy, chilies, and tomatoes impart to cooking)

Anchovies
Anchovy paste
Capers
Fish sauce
Wine
Truffles
Truffle salt
Shrimp paste
Mushrooms
Nutritional yeast
Olives

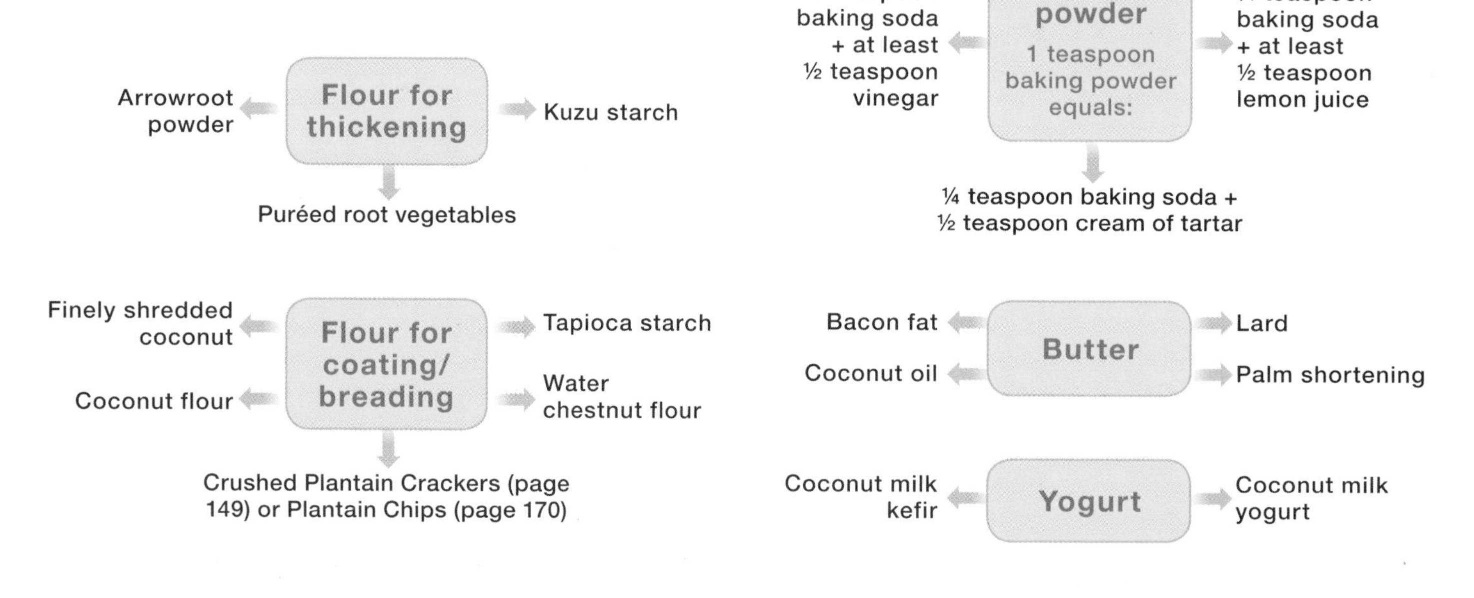

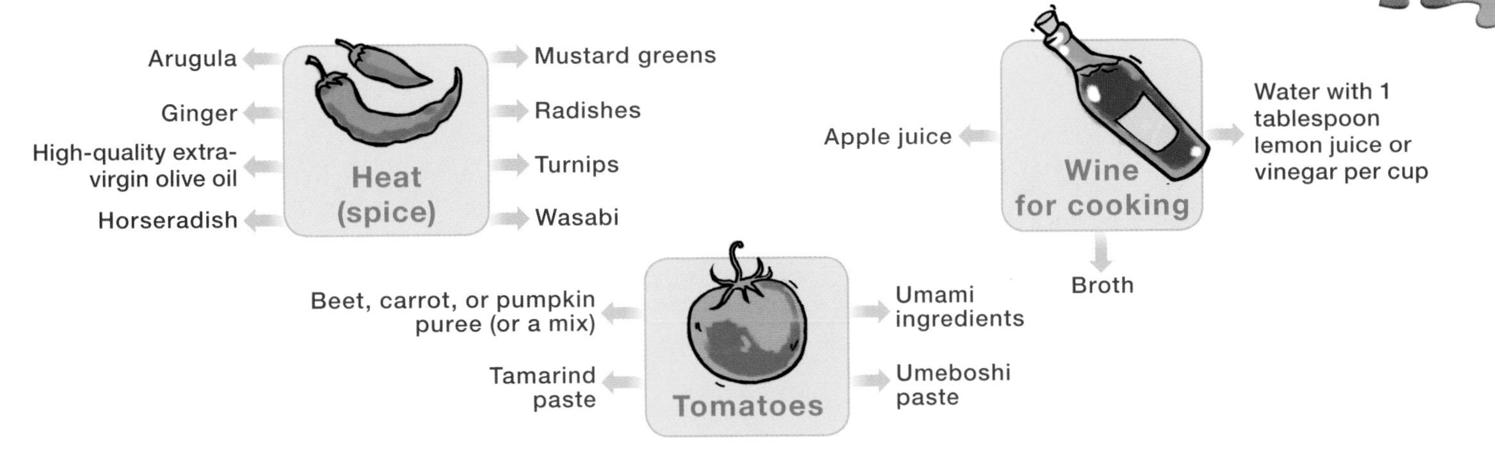

Meal Component Substitutions

Trying to figure out how to make a Paleo Approach meal look like an old favorite? Want to know the best options for replacing that hamburger bun or those pasta noodles? Here are some substitution ideas:

Bread or buns
Coconut wraps
Collard leaves
Lettuce leaves/ wraps
Portobello "Buns" (page 228)
Sliced kohlrabi or turnips
Russ' Flatbread (page 326)
Swiss chard leaves
Root Vegetable Biscuits (page 328)
Pasta noodles
Broccoli slaw
Julienned vegetables (carrots, broccoli stems, cucumbers)
Kelp noodles
Wakame noodles
Sweet potato noodles (dangmyeon)
Spaghetti squash
Spiral-sliced vegetables (sweet potato, butternut squash, kohlrabi, turnip, rutabaga, large radish, zucchini)
Crackers
Belgian endive leaves
Celery sticks
Cucumber slices
Plantain Chips (page 170)
Plantain Crackers (page 149)
Slices of kohlrabi, turnip, or large radish
Tortilla wraps
Blanched cabbage leaves
Coconut wraps
Collard leaves
Lettuce leaves
Nori
Swiss chard leaves
Mashed potatoes
Cauliflower Mash (page 295)
Mashed plantain (Mofongo, page 210, or Kufu, page 318)
Mashed sweet potato
Other mashed root vegetables
Roasted or baked potatoes
Roasted or baked sweet potato (page 313)
Roasted Parsnips (page 325)
Roasted plantains
Roasted Taro (page 320)
Chips
Plantain Chips (page 170)
Sweet Potato Chips (page 168)
Raw vegetables
Rice
Cauliflower Rice (page 298)

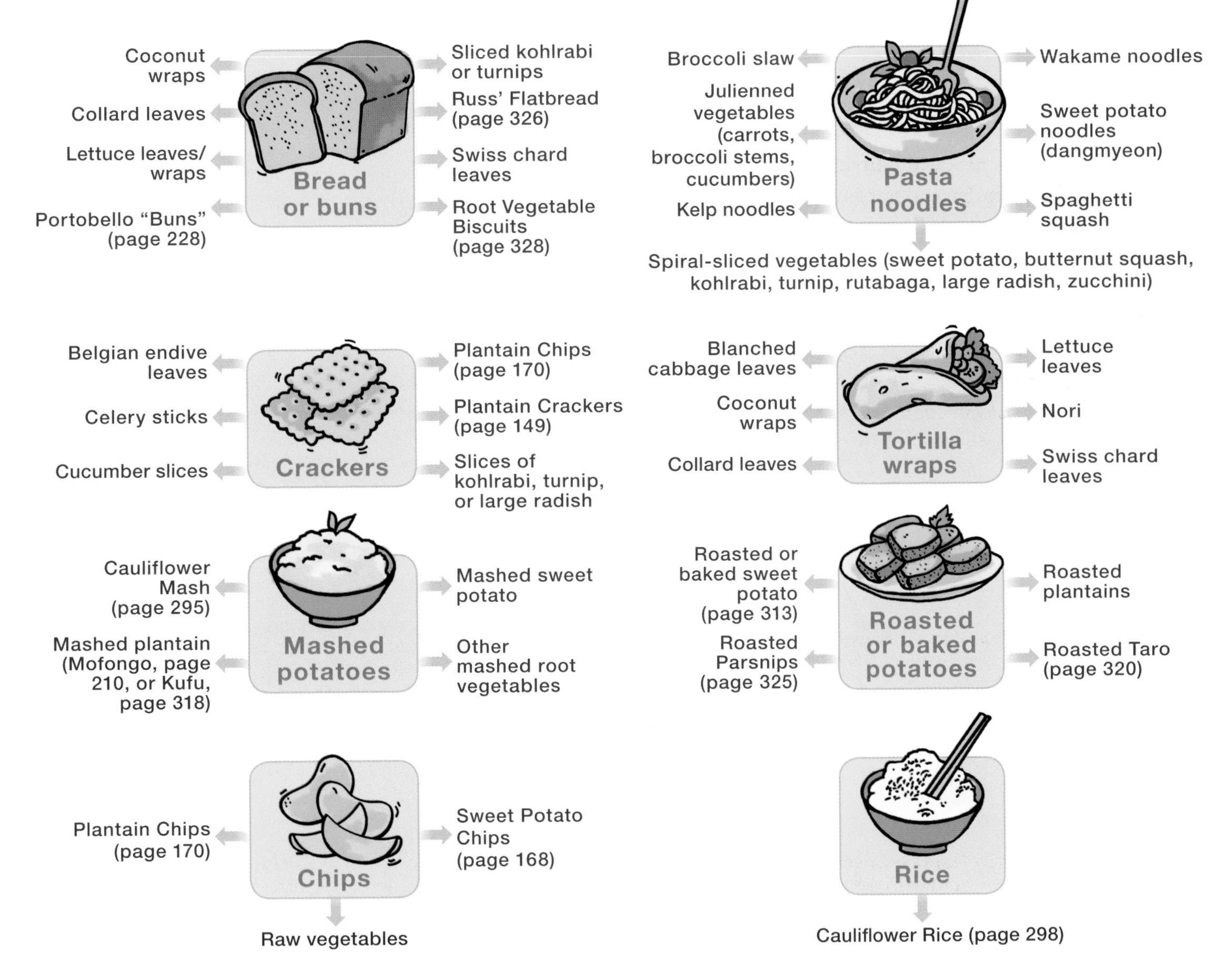

Chapter 3

Meal Plans and Shopping Lists

To help you plan ahead and manage your time in the kitchen, this chapter includes six one-week meal plans. You don't need to follow a meal plan to see results when following the Paleo Approach diet or to enjoy using this cookbook, but if you're the kind of person who has difficulty planning ahead (and staying on plan because of it), or if you're worried that your diet won't be nutritionally balanced if you choose what to eat on your own, then these meal plans are for you.

As you navigate each plan, first read through the recipes for the week. You'll notice that the weekend recipes are more involved than the weekday ones. This assumes that you have more time for food preparation on weekends than you do during the week. There are suggestions for what to make ahead of time to help you navigate a busy work/school week. You'll also notice several meals composed of leftovers. The meal plan also provides a couple of meals worth of leftovers for your freezer.

Once you've read through the meals for the week, have a look at the recipes and the shopping list. If any food jumps out at you as being a strong dislike or sensitivity, plan a substitute for either that ingredient or the entire dish. If you know that you'd rather just have a can of salmon with some salad for lunch than a meal that requires preparation, that's fine, too. There are also opportunities to customize your meals. For example, you can chose any veggie to steam or any green to braise—or have a salad. Also have a look at the suggested variations for each meal in the plan. If you know that it's going to be hard to get blood oranges when they aren't in season, for example, you can choose another fruit for your salsa. Or maybe you know that your local farmer will have Brussels sprouts this week, so you can swap Bacon-Braised Brussels Sprouts for Easy Broiled Asparagus. You can also follow any of the suggested variations of a recipe listed in your meal plan. Figure out if and how you want to modify the plan, and update the shopping list to reflect those modifications.

Next, compare the items on your shopping list with what's actually in your pantry, fridge, and freezer. Strike off the list any foods that you already have in the house. Also figure out if you will need to order any items online. For those items, you'll want to order well in advance to make sure that they arrive in time. Finally, make a plan of which items you are going to buy from which stores, farm stands, or farmer's markets.

These meal plans were constructed assuming that you are feeding two people (or one very hungry person). If you'll simply be feeding yourself, you may either halve the recipes or freeze the extra portions. If you're cooking for a family of more than two, you'll want to double or triple each recipe when you make it in order to have enough for the leftover meals that are built into each meal plan.

Don't like eating leftovers and don't mind spending more time in the kitchen? Or cooking for a horde so that even a triple batch is unlikely to provide leftovers? Go ahead and substitute new meals instead of leftover meals in the plans. Remember to adjust the quantities of your recipes and your shopping list accordingly.

Most of the meals included in the plans avoid the more unusual ingredients that you might have to put some effort into sourcing, as well as the more overt offal recipes. I encourage you to substitute meals that include these ingredients once you're feeling more at ease with this way of eating and cooking.

If you are following a low-FODMAP Paleo Approach diet, make sure that you follow the FODMAP ALERT modifications for the recipes listed in the two low-FODMAP meal plans. If you aren't eating a low-FODMAP diet, you can still enjoy these two weeks of meal plans, but you don't need to bother with the modifications.

You don't need to follow the weeks in order. If Week 3 looks more exciting to you than Week 1, or if the pumpkin powder needed as an ingredient for Week 2 won't arrive on time, then mix it up. The idea is to give you a guide, not an inflexible rule book.

Now you're ready to go shopping. The meal plans assume that you will shop either on Friday or early on Saturday. Though the shopping lists are designed for one big weekly shopping trip (which may or may not include more than one stop), you can break it up into two or more trips to the grocery store if that makes more sense for you. You may want to do a bigger shop on Saturday morning and another smaller shop on Wednesday afternoon, for example. This is actually a better way to organize your week from a nutrient density standpoint, because your produce will be fresher. Have a look at which fresh vegetables and fruits are used in the recipes later in the week and save those for midweek top-up shopping.

After you are done with your shopping, have a look at the "Plan Ahead" list. This list includes whole recipes and parts of recipes that can be made ahead of time on the weekend to save you time during the week. It's not essential to do all or any of these tasks during a big cook-up afternoon, but if you typically find yourself tight on time on weekdays, you will appreciate the effort you put in on the weekend.

Snack Suggestions

It is generally healthier to eat large meals spaced well apart (about 5 to 6 hours) and avoid snacking. But this isn't necessarily the best choice for everyone. For example, if you have a history of metabolic syndrome or adrenal insufficiency (adrenal fatigue), if you have difficulty managing chronic stress, or if your schedule forces you to go more than 6 hours between meals, you may find yourself in need of a snack. If you aren't sure whether a snack is appropriate for you, read about hunger hormones in Chapters 2 and 3 of *The Paleo Approach.*

While you will likely find yourself satisfied with three square meals a day, if you do need to snack, the recipes in Chapter 6 are great options, as are many of the convenience foods listed on page 57. When choosing a snack food, I urge you to consider nutrient-dense options. For example, opt for oysters (On the Half Shell, page 263, or canned), sardines, mussels (Steamed, page 253, or canned), clams (Steamed, page 253, or canned), Pâté (page 152), liverwurst or other organ meat sausages (check ingredients), veggies and Guacamole (page 171), Kale Chips (page 166), or Dehydrator Plantain Chips (page 170). As with your meals, think of snack time as an opportunity to get essential nutrients rather than just another time to eat.

If you go through all six weeks of meal plans and then choose to start again at the beginning, you'll be able to compare the meals in each meal plan with what you have stored in your freezer from the first time around. For example, you'll likely have enough sausage to get you through a week (or even two or three) without making a new batch. This is also an opportunity to mix things up. Maybe a certain recipe wasn't your cup of tea. Pick something new to take its place! Challenge yourself with additional offal recipes or recipes that use ingredients you've never tried.

Most important, have fun. These meal plans are designed to make things easier for you. If they aren't achieving that goal, nothing is forcing you to stick with them. Go ahead and devise your own meal plans. Or skip the meal plans altogether, buy whatever inspires you at the farmer's market on Saturday morning, and then figure out what to make from those ingredients when you get home. The point is to figure out how to make this approach work for you, and meal plans are only one tool in your toolbox.

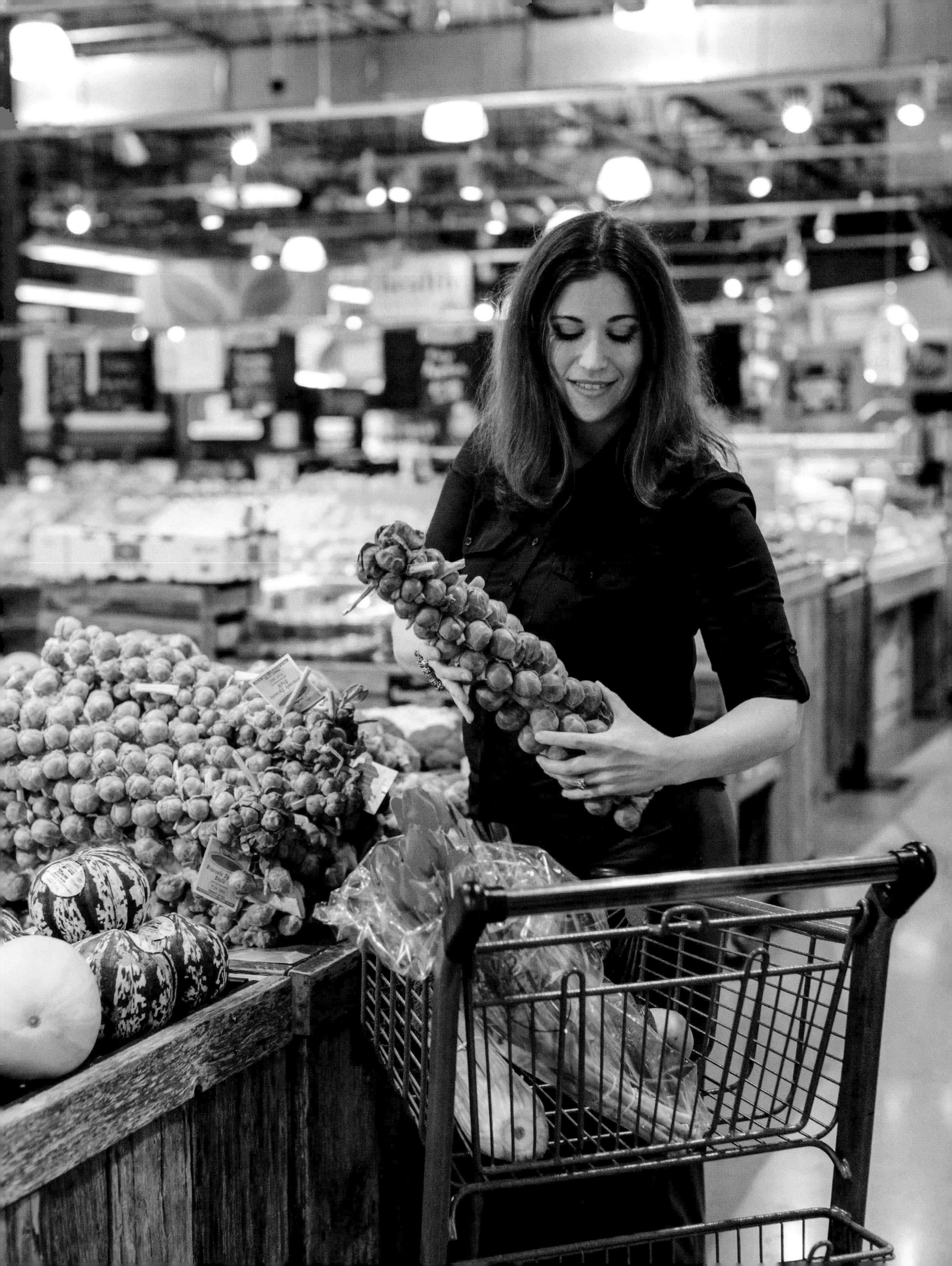

Week 1

Shopping List

Meat
bacon (10–16 oz.)
beef tongue (2½–3 lbs.)
ground beef (1 lb.)
ground pork (5 lbs.)
top sirloin or rib roast (3–4 lbs.)

Seafood
hake (2½ lbs. of fillets)
oysters (2 lbs., shucked)
salmon (4–6 [6–8 oz.] fillets)
whole fish, gutted and scaled (such as red snapper, 3–5 lbs.)

Fruits
avocados (3)
banana (1)
berries, melon, or other fruit (1 cup for Bacon Fruit Cups)
blood oranges (2 lbs.)
grapefruit (1–2)
lemons (3–4)
lime (1)

Nonperishables
albacore tuna (5 oz. can)
capers
raisins (½ cup)
ingredients for your favorite salad dressing (oil, vinegar, herbs, etc.)

Vegetables
asparagus (2 lbs.)
broccoflower (4–5 heads, enough for 8 cups of florets and stems)
broccoli (2 lbs.)
butternut squash (2 lbs.)
cabbage or other vegetable for fermenting (3 lbs.)
carrots (1½ lbs.)
cauliflower (2½ heads)
celery root (1 large)
celery (1 head or heart)
cilantro (fresh)
dill (fresh)
fennel (2 small bulbs)
garlic (2–3 heads)
ginger root
golden beets (2–3 medium)
green plantains (6–8 medium)
mushrooms (wild, 1½ lbs.)
onions (2 large)
parsley (fresh)
portobello mushroom caps (4–6)
red onion (1)
rosemary (fresh)
shallot (1 large)
sweet potatoes (2 lbs.)
tarragon (fresh)
thyme (fresh)
zucchini (1 medium)
greens for braising (for 7 meals)
leafy greens plus add-ons for salads (for 5 meals)
leafy greens and superfood add-ons for Superfood Smoothie (for 1 meal)
large lettuce leaves (such as romaine or butterleaf) for Tuna Salad Wraps
seasonings for Cauliflower Rice (garlic, herbs, lemon, etc.)
veggies for steaming (for 3 meals)

Pantry Items
apple cider vinegar
avocado oil
baking soda
balsamic vinegar
bay leaf powder, or make your own using dried bay leaves
bay leaves
Bone Broth (9¼ cups, or ingredients to make 1 batch—page 110)
cinnamon (ground)
cinnamon stick
cloves (whole)
coconut oil (extra-virgin)
gelatin
lard
lemon juice (or additional fresh lemons to make your own)
mace
maple syrup (grade B)
marjoram (dried)
muscovado sugar or evaporated cane juice
olive oil (extra-virgin)
protein powder for Superfood Smoothie
pumpkin powder (½ cup, or 2 cups puréed pumpkin to make your own)
saffron
sage (dried)
salt (pink or gray)
tallow, bacon fat, and/or duck fat
thyme (dried)
truffle salt (optional)
turmeric (dried)
white wine (1¾ cups) or more broth

Other
casings for sausage (optional)
pickles (raw fermented, or ingredients to make your own—page 114)
sauerkraut (raw fermented, if not making your own)
vegetable juice (8–16 oz., or veggies to make your own)

Plan Ahead

- Bacon Bits: ¼ cup for Scalloped Hake and Oysters—make some extra bacon on Saturday morning
- Broth
- Carrot-Raisin Muffins
- Coconut Milk Yogurt
- English Bangers: Either precook sausage patties or stuff sausage into casings and then parboil; let cool and then freeze
- Green Tea and Garlic Pickles for Tuna Salad Wraps—or you can buy pickles if you prefer
- Plantain Crackers (double batch)
- Pumpkin powder for Carrot-Raisin Muffins (or buy online)
- Salad Dressing
- Sauerkraut: Note that this needs to ferment, typically for a week

Tip: If you bake a big enough whole fish on Saturday, you can use it for making the Scalloped Hake and Oysters on Sunday and for leftovers on Monday.

Meal Plan

	Breakfast	Lunch	Dinner
SATURDAY	Bacon Fruit Cups (page 136)	Baked Whole Fish (page 240)	Garlic and Rosemary Roast Beef (page 205)
	Braised Greens (page 300)	Maple-Braised Butternut Squash (page 309)	Perfect Steamed Vegetables (page 296)
	Sauerkraut (page 112)	Garden Salad (page 160)	Cauliflower Mash (page 295)
		Easy Broiled Asparagus (double batch; page 306)	
SUNDAY	English Bangers (page 132)	Beef Tongue with Celery Root and Fennel Slaw (page 270)	Scalloped Hake and Oysters (page 248)
	Braised Greens (page 300)	Plantain Crackers (double batch; page 149)	Braised Greens (page 300)
	Cinnamon Broiled Grapefruit (page 143)	Vegetable Terrine (page 316)	Roasted Broccoflower (page 302)
MONDAY	English Bangers (leftover)	Scalloped Hake and Oysters (leftover)	Baked Whole Fish (leftover)
	Maple-Braised Butternut Squash (leftover)	Braised Greens (page 300)	Roasted Sweet Potato (page 313)
	Roasted Broccoflower (leftover)	Cauliflower Mash (leftover)	Garden Salad (page 160)
	Sauerkraut (leftover)		Vegetable Terrine (leftover)
TUESDAY	Garlic and Rosemary Roast Beef (leftover)	Beef Tongue with Celery Root and Fennel Slaw (leftover)	Scalloped Hake and Oysters (leftover)
	Roasted Sweet Potato (leftover)	Plantain Crackers (leftover)	Easy Broiled Asparagus (leftover)
	Perfect Steamed Vegetables (page 296)	Garden Salad (page 160)	Wild Mushrooms and Tarragon (page 305)
	Cinnamon Broiled Grapefruit (page 143)	Roasted Broccoflower (leftover)	
WEDNESDAY	English Bangers (leftover)	Garlic and Rosemary Roast Beef (leftover)	Beef Tongue with Celery Root and Fennel Slaw (leftover)
	Carrot-Raisin Muffins (page 140)	Plantain Crackers (leftover)	Roasted Sweet Potato (leftover)
	Vegetable Terrine (leftover)	Braised Greens (page 300)	Garden Salad (page 160)
	Sauerkraut (leftover)	Wild Mushrooms and Tarragon (leftover)	"Cream" of Broccoli Soup (page 183)
THURSDAY	Superfood Smoothie (page 141)	Tuna Salad Wrap (page 260)	Lemon and Thyme Broiled Salmon with Blood Orange Salsa (page 242)
		"Cream" of Broccoli Soup (leftover)	Plantain Crackers (leftover)
			Braised Greens (page 300)
			Cauliflower Rice (page 298)
FRIDAY	English Bangers (leftover)	Lemon and Thyme Broiled Salmon with Blood Orange Salsa (leftover)	Burgers with Caramelized Onions and Portobello "Buns" (page 228)
	Carrot-Raisin Muffins (leftover)	Garden Salad (page 160)	Roasted Sweet Potato (leftover)
	Braised Greens (page 300)	Cauliflower Rice (leftover)	Perfect Steamed Vegetables (page 296)
	Sauerkraut (leftover)		

Week 2

Shopping List

Meat

- bacon (16–20 oz.)
- ground beef (1 lb.)
- ground lamb (4 lbs.)
- ground pork (1 lb.)
- liver (1 lb., ground preferred)
- pork ribs (7–8 lbs.)

Seafood

- mahi mahi (4–6 [6 oz.] fillets)
- whitefish (3–4 [6–8 oz.] fillets)
- lox (2–3 oz.)

Fruits

- apples (4)
- avocado (1)
- banana (1)
- berries (½–1 cup for Coconut Milk Yogurt)
- cranberries (½ cups fresh or frozen)
- ingredients for your favorite fruit salad (for 3 meals)
- lemons (3)
- mango (1)

Nonperishables

- capers
- clams (3 [5–6 oz.] cans)
- coconut milk yogurt (1⅔ cups, or ingredients to make your own—page 118)
- ingredients for your favorite dip (avocado or coconut milk yogurt plus herbs—page 172)
- ingredients for your favorite salad dressing (oil, vinegar, herbs, etc.)
- nori sheets (2)
- olives (whole green or black, ¾ cup)
- sardines (2 [4 oz.] cans)

Vegetables

- artichoke hearts (12 oz.)
- arugula or mustard greens (6–10 cups)
- basil (fresh)
- beets (6–8)
- Brussels sprouts (1 lb.)
- butternut squash (2 lbs.)
- carrots (2 lbs.)
- cauliflower (1½ heads)
- celery (1 head or heart)
- chives (fresh)
- cucumber (1)
- garlic (1½–2 heads)
- ginger root
- green onion (1)
- onions (4)
- oregano (fresh)
- parsley (fresh)
- parsnips (2 lbs.)
- plantains (1 green and 2 ripe)
- radishes (8 oz.)
- red cabbage (1 lb.)
- red onion (1)
- rosemary (fresh)
- sage (fresh)
- savoy cabbage (1 head)
- sunflower sprouts (½ cup)
- taro root (1 lb.)
- tarragon (fresh)
- thyme (fresh)
- turmeric root
- turnip (1 large)
- zucchini (1 medium)
- greens for braising (for 3 meals)
- leafy greens plus add-ons for salads (for 3 meals)
- leafy greens and superfood add-ons for Superfood Smoothie (for 2 meals)
- starchy root vegetable for French Fries (1 lb.)
- veggies for steaming (for 4 meals)
- your favorite veggies to dip (for 2 meals)

Pantry Items

- apple cider vinegar
- avocado oil
- balsamic vinegar
- bay leaves (dried)
- Bone Broth (12–12½ cups, or ingredients to make 1½ batches—page 110)
- cinnamon (ground)
- coconut aminos
- coconut oil (extra-virgin)
- coconut water vinegar
- fish sauce
- gelatin
- honey
- lard
- lemon juice (or additional fresh lemons to make your own)
- mace
- marjoram (dried)
- molasses (blackstrap)
- olive oil (extra-virgin)
- oregano (dried)
- pomegranate molasses
- protein powder for Superfood Smoothie
- red palm oil
- rosemary (dried)
- sage (dried)
- salt (pink or gray)
- savory (dried)
- tallow, bacon fat, and/or duck fat
- tarragon (dried)
- thyme (dried)
- truffle salt (optional)
- turmeric (ground)

Other

- casings for sausage (optional)
- coconut cream (2 cups, or ingredients to make your own—page 116)
- lactobacillus-based probiotic supplement (if making homemade Coconut Milk Yogurt)
- vegetable juice (16–24 oz., or veggies to make your own)

Plan Ahead

- Barbecue Sauce for Pork Ribs
- Broth
- Coconut Cream (if making your own)
- Coconut Milk Yogurt
- Herbes de Provence for mahi mahi
- Hidden Liver Meatloaf
- Lamb Sausage: Either precook sausage patties or stuff sausage into casings and then parboil; let cool and then freeze
- Salad Dressing

Meal Plan

	Breakfast	Lunch	Dinner
SATURDAY	Lamb Sausage (page 132)	New England Clam Chowder (page 196)	Hidden Liver Meatloaf (page 272)
	Taro Hash (page 138)	Garden Salad (page 160)	French Fries (page 323)
	Perfect Steamed Vegetables (page 296)		Bacon-Braised Brussels Sprouts (page 321)
			Cauliflower Mash (page 295)
SUNDAY	Lamb Sausage (leftover)	New England Clam Chowder (leftover)	Simple Baked Whitefish (page 244)
	Taro Hash (leftover)	Garden Salad (page 160)	Balsamic-Roasted Beets (page 304)
	Bacon-Braised Savoy Cabbage and Apple (page 314)		Perfect Steamed Vegetables (page 296)
	Coconut Milk Yogurt (page 118) and fresh berries		Cauliflower Mash (leftover)
MONDAY	Superfood Smoothie (page 141)	Sardine Salad (page 163)	New England Clam Chowder (leftover)
		French Fries (leftover)	Garden Salad (page 160)
TUESDAY	Hidden Liver Meatloaf (leftover)	Simple Baked Whitefish (leftover)	BBQ Pork Ribs (page 216)
	Plantain and Apple Fritter (page 139)	Fruit Salad (page 336)	Balsamic-Roasted Beets (leftover)
	Braised Greens (page 300)	Veggies and Dip (page 172)	Cran-Apple Coleslaw (page 164)
	Cauliflower Mash (leftover)		Bacon-Braised Brussels Sprouts (leftover)
WEDNESDAY	Lamb Sausage (leftover)	BBQ Pork Ribs (leftover)	Mediterranean Mahi Mahi (page 246)
	Plantain and Apple Fritter (leftover)	Fruit Salad (leftover)	Roasted Butternut Squash (page 308)
	Perfect Steamed Vegetables (page 296)	Cran-Apple Coleslaw (leftover)	Braised Greens (page 300)
	Coconut Milk Yogurt (leftover)	Veggies and Dip (leftover)	Garlicky Artichoke Hearts (page 303)
THURSDAY	Crispy Bacon (page 120)	Mediterranean Mahi Mahi (leftover)	BBQ Pork Ribs (leftover)
	Plantain and Apple Fritter (leftover)	Fruit Salad (leftover)	Roasted Parsnips (page 325)
	Bacon-Braised Savoy Cabbage and Apple (leftover)	Perfect Steamed Vegetables (page 296)	Cran-Apple Coleslaw (leftover)
		Garlicky Artichoke Hearts (leftover)	Carrot-Ginger Soup (page 189) with bacon
FRIDAY	Superfood Smoothie (page 141)	Smoked Salmon and Mango Salsa Nori Wraps (page 175)	Mediterranean Mahi Mahi (leftover)
		Roasted Butternut Squash (leftover)	Roasted Parsnips (leftover)
		Cran-Apple Coleslaw (leftover)	Braised Greens (page 300)
			Carrot-Ginger Soup with bacon (leftover)

Week 3

Shopping List

Meat
bacon (8 oz.)
beef heart (3 lbs., ground preferred)
ground beef (1 lb.)
ground chicken or turkey (4 lbs.)
ground lamb (1 lb.)
ground pork (2 lbs.; or 1 lb. each ground pork and pork fat))
lamb chops (2 lbs.)
whole chickens (2, 4–6 lbs. each)

Seafood
littleneck clams (4–5 lbs.)
salmon (3-4 [6–8 oz.] fillets)
whitefish (1½–2 lbs.)

Fruits
apples (4–5)
avocados (4–5)
banana (1)
Granny Smith apples (2)
grapefruit (1)
ingredients for your favorite fruit salad (for 3 meals)
lemons (4)

Nonperishables
black olives (4 oz.)
ingredients for your favorite salad dressing (oil, vinegar, herbs, etc.)
raisins (2 tablespoons)

Vegetables
acorn squash (2 large)
asparagus (1 lb.)
basil (fresh)
Brussels sprouts (1 lb.)
cabbage or other veggies for fermenting (3 lbs.)
carrots with greens (2 lbs.)
cauliflower (2 heads)
cilantro (fresh)
dill (fresh)
garlic (6–8 heads)
kale (2 bunches)
kohlrabi (½ cup)
leeks (4)
mint (fresh)
mushrooms (any type, ½ lb.)
mushrooms (wild, 1½ lbs.)
onions (2)
oregano (fresh)
parsley (fresh)
radishes (1 lb.)
spaghetti squash (1 large or 2 small)
spinach (2 cups)
sweet potatoes (1–2)
taro root (2 lbs.)
tarragon (fresh)
turnip (½ cup)
zucchini (2 lbs.)
greens for braising (for 4 meals)
leafy greens plus add-ons for salads (for 4 meals)
leafy greens and superfood add-ons for Superfood Smoothie (for 1 meal)
seasonings for Cauliflower Rice (garlic, herbs, lemon, etc.)
veggies for steaming (for 4 meals)

Pantry Items
avocado oil
Bone Broth (9 cups, or ingredients to make 1 batch—page 110)
cinnamon (ground)
coconut oil (extra-virgin)
fish sauce
garlic powder
kuzu starch
lard
lemon juice (or additional fresh lemons to make your own)
marjoram (dried)
olive oil (extra-virgin)
onion powder
protein powder for Superfood Smoothie
red wine (1 cup) or substitute (see page 85)
rosemary (dried)
sage (dried)
salt (pink or gray)
savory (dried)
tallow, bacon fat, and/or duck fat
thyme (dried)
truffle salt (optional)
white wine (½ cup, or additional broth and lemon juice)

Other
casings for sausage (optional)
sauerkraut (raw fermented, if not making your own)
vegetable juice (8–16 oz., or veggies to make your own)

Plan Ahead

- Apple-Chicken Sausage for Vegetable Soup: Either precook sausage patties or stuff sausage into casings and then parboil; let cool and then freeze
- Applesauce
- Beef Heart Sausage: Either precook sausage patties or stuff sausage into casings and then parboil; let cool and then freeze
- Broth
- Kale Chips
- Maître D' "Butter"
- Poultry Seasoning for Roasted Chicken
- Salad Dressing
- Sauerkraut: Note that this needs to ferment, typically for a week
- Sweet Potato Chips

Meal Plan

	Breakfast	Lunch	Dinner
SATURDAY	Beef Heart Sausage (page 132)	Vegetable Soup with Chicken Sausage (page 194)	Greek-Inspired Lamb Chops (page 217)
	Applesauce (page 122)	Garden Salad (page 160)	Mashed Acorn Squash with Forty Cloves of Garlic (page 307)
	Perfect Steamed Vegetables (page 296)		Braised Greens (page 300)
	Sauerkraut (page 112)		Cauliflower Rice (page 298)
SUNDAY	Vegetable Soup with Chicken Sausage (leftover)	Greek-Inspired Lamb Chops (leftover)	Roasted Chicken (page 209)
	Garden Salad (page 160)	Mashed Acorn Squash with Forty Cloves of Garlic (leftover)	Whole Carrot "Tabouleh" (page 315)
		Braised Greens (page 300)	Mint Pesto Zucchini "Pasta" (page 310)
		Cauliflower Rice (leftover)	Roasted Radishes (page 322)
MONDAY	Beef Heart Sausage (leftover)	Steamed Clams (page 253)	Bacon-Braised Whitefish and Brussels (page 254)
	Cinnamon Broiled Grapefruit (page 143)	Mashed Acorn Squash with Forty Cloves of Garlic (leftover)	Garden Green Vichyssoise (page 188)
	Perfect Steamed Vegetables (page 296)	Mint Pesto Zucchini "Pasta" (leftover)	
	Sauerkraut (leftover)	Roasted Radishes (leftover)	
TUESDAY	Roasted Chicken (leftover)	Steamed Clams (leftover)	"Spaghetti" (page 224)
	Applesauce (leftover)	Sweet Potato Chips (page 168)	Fruit Salad (page 336)
	Perfect Steamed Vegetables (page 296)	Garden Green Vichyssoise (leftover)	Garden Salad (page 160)
	Sauerkraut (leftover)		
WEDNESDAY	Beef Heart Sausage (leftover) or Apple Chicken Sausage (leftover)	Roasted Chicken (leftover)	Salmon with Maître D' "Butter" (page 245)
	Garden Green Vichyssoise (leftover)	Fruit Salad (leftover)	Savory Roasted Taro (page 320)
		Kale Chips (page 166)	Braised Greens (page 300)
		Whole Carrot "Tabouleh" (leftover)	Wild Mushrooms and Tarragon (page 305)
THURSDAY	Superfood Smoothie (page 141)	Salmon with Maître D' "Butter" (leftover)	Bacon-Braised Whitefish and Brussels (leftover)
		Fruit Salad (leftover)	Wild Mushrooms and Tarragon (leftover)
		Kale Chips (leftover)	
		Easy Broiled Asparagus (page 306)	
FRIDAY	Beef Heart Sausage (leftover)	"Spaghetti" (leftover)	Roasted Chicken (leftover)
	Applesauce (leftover)	Sweet Potato Chips (leftover)	Savory Roasted Taro (leftover)
	Perfect Steamed Vegetables (page 296)	Garden Salad (page 160)	Braised Greens (page 300)
	Sauerkraut (leftover)		Easy Broiled Asparagus (leftover)

Week 4

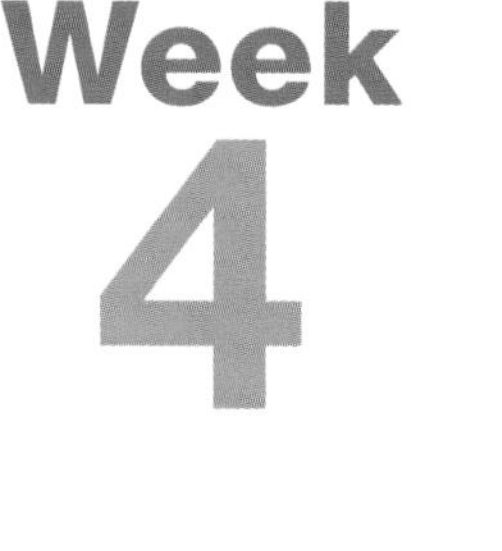

Shopping List

Meat
bacon (2½ lbs.)
bison liver (1 lb.)
ground beef (1 lb.)
ground chicken or turkey (2–2½ lbs.)
lamb chops (2 lbs.)
pork roast (4–5 lbs.)
steaks (2 [4–8 oz.])

Seafood
salmon (4–6 [6–8 oz.] fillets)
trout (3–4 [6–8 oz.] fillets)

Fruits
apples (3)
avocados (7)
banana (1)
berries, melon, or other fruit (1 cup for Bacon Fruit Cups)
blood oranges (2 lbs.)
cranberries (2 cups, fresh or frozen)
lemons (3–4)
limes (2–3)
orange (1)

Nonperishables
albacore tuna (1 [5 oz.] can)
sardines (2 [4 oz.] cans)
capers
ingredients for your favorite salad dressing (oil, vinegar, herbs, etc.)

Vegetables
arugula or mustard greens (6–10 cups)
broccoflower (4–5 heads, enough for 8 cups of florets and stems)
broccoli (2 lbs.)
butternut squash (2 lbs.)
cabbage or other veggies for fermenting (3 lbs.)
cauliflower (2 heads)
celery (1 head or heart)
cilantro (fresh)
garlic (3 heads)
ginger root
green onion (1)
mint (fresh)
onions (2)
oregano (fresh)
parsley (fresh)
plantains (2–4 green)
portobello mushroom caps (4–6)
red onion (1)
rhubarb (8 oz.)
rosemary (fresh)
sweet potatoes (2 lbs.)
taro root (1 lb.)
tarragon (fresh)
thyme (fresh)
zucchini (2 lbs.)
greens for braising (for 1 meal)
large lettuce leaves (such as romaine or butterleaf) for Tuna Salad Wraps
leafy greens plus add-ons for salads (for 4 meals)
leafy greens and superfood add-ons for Superfood Smoothie (for 2 meals)
raw vegetables for dipping (2 meals)
seasonings for Cauliflower Rice (garlic, herbs, lemon, etc.)
starchy root vegetable for French Fries (1 lb.)
veggies for steaming (for 4 meals)

Pantry Items
avocado oil
balsamic vinegar
Bone Broth (4 cups, or ingredients to make ½ batch—page 110)
cinnamon (ground)
coconut aminos
coconut oil (extra-virgin)
coconut water vinegar
cloves (ground)
garlic powder
lard
lemon juice (or additional fresh lemons to make your own)
lime juice (or additional fresh limes to make your own)
mace
maple syrup (grade B)
olive oil (extra-virgin)
onion powder
oregano (dried)
protein powder for Superfood Smoothie
salt (pink or gray)
tallow, bacon fat, and/or duck fat
tarragon (dried)
truffle salt (optional)
turmeric (ground)
white wine (½ cup) or more broth

Other
casings for sausage (optional)
pickles (raw fermented, or ingredients to make your own, page 114)
sauerkraut (raw fermented, if not making your own)
vegetable juice (16–32 oz., or veggies to make your own)

Plan Ahead

- Broth
- Green Tea and Garlic Pickles for Tuna Salad Wraps—or you can buy pickles if you prefer
- Plantain Chips or Crackers
- Rhubarb Chutney
- Salad Dressing
- Sauerkraut: Note that this needs to ferment, typically for a week
- Steak Spice

Meal Plan

	Breakfast	Lunch	Dinner
SATURDAY	Bacon Fruit Cups (page 136)	Bacon-Apple Chicken Burgers with Maple-Cranberry Sauce (page 222)	Teriyaki-Poached Trout (page 250)
	Garden Salad (page 160)	Roasted Butternut Squash (page 308)	Cauliflower Rice (page 298)
		Roasted Broccoflower (page 302)	Perfect Steamed Vegetables (page 296)
SUNDAY	Bacon-Apple Chicken Burgers with Maple Cranberry Sauce (leftover)	Tuna Salad Wrap (page 260)	Tarragon Roasted Pork (page 208)
	Roasted Broccoflower (leftover)	Plantain Chips (page 170) or Crackers (page 149)	Roasted Butternut Squash (leftover)
	Sauerkraut (page 112)	"Cream" of Broccoli Soup (page 183)	Braised Greens (page 300)
MONDAY	Superfood Smoothie (page 141)	Teriyaki-Poached Trout (leftover)	50/50/50 Burgers (page 289) with Portobello "Buns" (page 228)
		Cauliflower Rice (leftover)	French Fries (page 323)
		Garden Salad (page 160)	Guacamole (page 171)
			Raw Veggies
TUESDAY	Bacon-Apple Chicken Burgers with Maple Cranberry Sauce (leftover)	Tarragon Roasted Pork (leftover)	Simple Grilled Steak with Rhubarb Chutney (page 218)
	Roasted Butternut Squash (leftover)	Plantain Chips or Crackers (leftover)	Roasted Sweet Potato (page 313)
	Perfect Steamed Vegetables (page 296)	Garden Salad (page 160)	Perfect Steamed Vegetables (page 296)
WEDNESDAY	50/50/50 Burgers (leftover)	Tarragon Roasted Pork (leftover)	Lemon and Thyme Broiled Salmon with Blood Orange Salsa (page 242)
	Taro Hash (page 138)	French Fries (leftover)	Garden Salad (page 160)
	Sauerkraut (leftover)	Guacamole (leftover)	"Cream" of Broccoli Soup (leftover)
		Raw Veggies	
THURSDAY	Superfood Smoothie (page 141)	Sardine Salad (page 163)	Greek-Inspired Lamb Chops (page 217)
		Plantain Chips or Crackers (leftover)	Mint Pesto Zucchini "Pasta" (page 310)
			Roasted Sweet Potato (leftover)
FRIDAY	50/50/50 Burgers (leftover)	Greek-Inspired Lamb Chops (leftover)	Lemon and Thyme Broiled Salmon with Blood Orange Salsa (leftover)
	Taro Hash (leftover)	Mint Pesto Zucchini "Pasta" (leftover)	"Cream" of Broccoli Soup (leftover)
	Sauerkraut (leftover)	Roasted Sweet Potato (leftover)	Perfect Steamed Vegetables (page 296)

Week 5 (Low FODMAP)

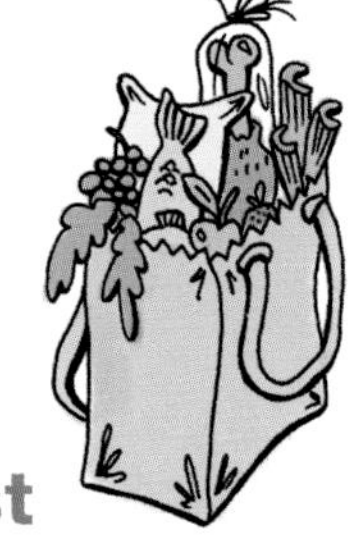

Shopping List

Meat
bacon (1 lb.)
beef heart (2 lbs.)
bison chuck roast (3–4 lbs.)
ground beef (4 lbs.)
ground pork (4 lbs.)
leg of lamb (4–6 lbs.)
liver (½ lb.)

Seafood
salmon (2–3 [6–8 oz.] fillets)
sea scallops (1 lb. frozen, or buy fresh midweek)
shrimp (1 lb.)
squid (1 lb.)

Nonperishables
bamboo shoots (2 [5 oz.] cans)
sardines (2 [4 oz.] cans)
water chestnuts (2 [5 oz.] cans)
ingredients for your favorite salad dressing (oil, vinegar, herbs, etc.)
kelp noodles (1 lb.)

Vegetables
arugula or mustard greens (6–10 cups)
baby bok choy (6–8 oz.)
bok choy (1 bunch)
butternut squash (2 lbs.)
cabbage or other veggies for fermenting (3 lbs.)
carrots (1½ lbs.)
celery (2 stalks)
cucumber (1–2, if making Tzatziki)
dill (fresh, if making Tzatziki)
ginger root
green garlic (2–3 stalks)
green onions (12–15)
kale (1 bunch)
leeks (2–3)
mint (fresh)
oyster mushrooms (4 oz.)
parsley (fresh)
parsnips (3 lbs.)
plantains (2–4 green)
rosemary (fresh)
sage (fresh)
shiitake mushrooms (3 fresh or dried)
spaghetti squash (3–4 lbs.)
tarragon (fresh)
thyme (fresh)
zucchini (2 lbs.)
greens for braising (for 5 meals)
leafy greens and superfood add-ons for Superfood Smoothie (for 1 meal)
leafy greens plus add-ons for salads (for 5 meals)
starchy root vegetable for French Fries (1 lb.)
veggies for steaming (for 6 meals)

Fruits
banana (1 green)
ingredients for your favorite fruit salad (for 2 meals)
lemons (2)

Pantry Items
arrowroot powder
bay leaves (dried)
Bone Broth (10½–12½ cups, or ingredients to make 1½ batches—page 110)
cloves (ground)
coconut oil (extra-virgin)
coconut water vinegar or white wine vinegar
fish sauce
lard
lemon juice (or fresh lemons to make your own)
mace (ground)
marjoram (dried)
olive oil (extra-virgin)
oregano (dried)
protein powder for Superfood Smoothie
red wine (½ cup) or more broth
rosemary (dried)
sage (dried)
salt (pink or gray)
savory (dried)
tallow, bacon fat, and/or duck fat
tapioca starch
thyme (dried)

Other
casings for sausage (optional)
coconut milk yogurt (½ cup, or ingredients to make your own—page 118; if making Tzatziki)
sauerkraut or other fermented veggies (raw fermented, if not making your own)
vegetable juice (8–16 oz., or veggies to make your own)

When following a low-FODMAP meal plan, remember to check recipes for FODMAP ALERT modifications.

Plan Ahead

- Broth
- Farmer's Sausage: Either precook sausage patties or stuff sausage into casings and then parboil; let cool and then freeze
- Kale Chips
- Plantain Crackers or Chips
- Salad Dressing
- Sauerkraut or other fermented veggies

Meal Plan

	Breakfast	Lunch	Dinner
SATURDAY	Farmer's Sausage (page 132)	Calamari with Tzatziki Sauce (page 258)	Rustic Bison Pot Roast (page 212)
	Braised Greens (page 300)	French Fries (page 323)	Perfect Steamed Vegetables (page 296)
	Sauerkraut or other fermented veggies (page 112)	Garden Salad (page 160)	
SUNDAY	Rustic Bison Pot Roast (leftover)	"Wonton" Soup (page 184)	Hidden Offal Swedish Meatballs (page 282)
	Perfect Steamed Vegetables (leftover)	Plantain Chips (page 170) or Crackers (page 149)	Zucchini Noodles (page 310)
		Kale Chips (page 166)	Garden Salad (page 160)
MONDAY	Hidden Offal Swedish Meatballs (leftover)	"Wonton" Soup (leftover)	Leg of Lamb with Mint Vinegar (page 206)
	Zucchini Noodles (leftover)	Garden Salad (page 160)	Roasted Butternut Squash (page 308)
	Kale Chips (leftover)		Braised Greens (page 300)
TUESDAY	Rustic Bison Pot Roast (leftover)	Calamari with Tzatziki Sauce (leftover)	Beef Heart "Chow Mein" (page 278)
	Roasted Butternut Squash (leftover)	French Fries (leftover)	Perfect Steamed Vegetables (page 296)
	Braised Greens (leftover)	Garden Salad (page 160)	
WEDNESDAY	Farmer's Sausage (leftover)	Hidden Offal Swedish Meatballs (leftover)	Leg of Lamb with Mint Vinegar (leftover)
	Roasted Butternut Squash (leftover)	Zucchini Noodles (leftover)	Roasted Parsnips (page 325)
	Perfect Steamed Vegetables (leftover)	Fruit Salad (page 336)	Braised Greens (page 300)
	Sauerkraut or other fermented veggies (leftover)		
THURSDAY	Farmer's Sausage (leftover)	Sardine Salad (page 163)	Asian-Inspired Salmon en Papillote (page 262)
	Roasted Parsnips (leftover)	Plantain Chips or Crackers (leftover)	Spaghetti Squash Noodles (page 224)
	Braised Greens (leftover)	Fruit Salad (leftover)	Perfect Steamed Vegetables (page 296)
	Sauerkraut or other fermented veggies (leftover)		
FRIDAY	Superfood Smoothie (page 141)	Bacon-Wrapped Scallops (page 155)	Leg of Lamb with Mint Vinegar (leftover)
		Plantain Chips or Crackers (leftover)	Spaghetti Squash Noodles (leftover)
		Perfect Steamed Vegetables (leftover)	Garden Salad (page 160)
		Kale Chips (leftover)	

Week 6 (Low FODMAP)

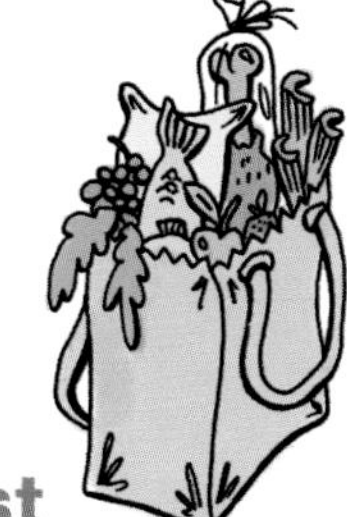

Shopping List

Meat
bacon (4 slices)
ground pork (6 lbs.)
oxtail (2 lbs.)
pork chops (2 lbs.)
steaks (3–4, 4–8 oz. each)

Seafood
mahi mahi (4–6 [6 oz.] fillets)
mixed shellfish (1 lb.)
salmon (5–6 [6–8 oz.] fillets)
whitefish (3–4 [6–8 oz.] fillets)

Fruits
banana (1 green)
ingredients for your favorite fruit salad (for 4 meals)
lemons (5)
limes (2–3)
orange (1) or orange juice (¼ cup)

⚠ When following a low-FODMAP meal plan, remember to check recipes for FODMAP ALERT modifications.

Vegetables
arugula or mustard greens (6–10 cups)
butternut squash (1 lb.)
cabbage or other veggies for fermenting (3 lbs.)
carrots (1 lb.)
celery (2 stalks)
cilantro (fresh)
fiddlehead ferns (3 cups)
ginger root
green garlic (1–2 stalks)
green onions (5–6)
kabocha squash (1 large)
kale (1 bunch)
kohlrabi (2 lbs.)
leeks (3 lbs.)
mixed greens (12 cups collards, mustard greens, turnip greens, etc.)
oregano (fresh)
parsley (fresh)
parsnips (2 lbs.)
plantains (2–4 green)
radishes (8 oz.)
rosemary (fresh)
sage (fresh)
taro root (3 lbs.)
tarragon (fresh)
thyme (fresh)
turmeric root
turnips (2 lbs.)
zucchini (1 medium)
greens for braising (for 6 meals)
leafy greens and superfood add-ons for Superfood Smoothie (for 1 meal)
leafy greens plus add-ons for salads (for 6 meals)
veggies for steaming (for 5 meals)

Nonperishables
capers
ingredients for your favorite salad dressing (oil, vinegar, herbs, etc.)
olives (whole green or black, ¾ cup)
sardines (2 [4 oz.] cans)

Pantry Items
avocado oil
Bone Broth (10 cups and 6 cups fish, or ingredients to make 1 batch of each—page 110)
cloves (whole)
cinnamon (ground)
coconut aminos
coconut oil (extra-virgin)
coconut water vinegar
fish sauce
ginger (ground)
lard
lemon juice (or additional fresh lemons to make your own)
mace
marjoram (dried)
olive oil (extra-virgin)
oregano (dried)
pomegranate molasses
protein powder for Superfood Smoothie
red palm oil
red wine (1 cup) or more broth
rosemary (dried)
sage (dried)
salt (pink or gray)
savory (dried)
tallow, bacon fat, and/or duck fat
tarragon (dried)
thyme (dried)
truffle salt
turmeric (ground)

Other
casings for sausage (optional)
sauerkraut or other fermented veggies (raw fermented, if not making your own)
vegetable juice (8–16 oz., or veggies to make your own)

Plan Ahead

- Broth
- Breakfast Sausage: Either precook sausage patties or stuff sausage into casings and then parboil; let cool and then freeze
- Herbes de Provence for mahi mahi
- Kale Chips
- Plantain Chips or Crackers
- Salad Dressing
- Sauerkraut or other fermented veggies

Meal Plan

	Breakfast	Lunch	Dinner
SATURDAY	Breakfast Sausage (page 132)	Pork Pad Thai (page 234)	Simple Baked Whitefish (page 244)
	Braised Greens (page 300)	Perfect Steamed Vegetables (page 296)	Savory Roasted Taro (page 320)
	Sauerkraut or other fermented veggies (page 112)		Garden Salad (page 160)
	Fruit Salad (page 336)		Fiddleheads (page 312)
SUNDAY	Pork Pad Thai (leftover)	Pomegranate Molasses–Glazed Salmon (page 239)	Mediterranean Mahi Mahi (page 246)
	Braised Greens (page 300)	Carrot-Ginger Soup, butternut squash variation (page 189)	Perfect Steamed Vegetables (page 296)
	Sauerkraut or other fermented veggies (leftover)	Garden Salad (page 160)	Kale Chips (page 166)
		Fiddleheads (leftover)	
MONDAY	Breakfast Sausage (leftover)	Sardine Salad (page 163)	Seafood and Leek Soup (page 190)
	Braised Greens (page 300)	Savory Roasted Taro (leftover)	Plantain Chips (page 170) or Crackers (page 149)
	Sauerkraut or other fermented veggies (leftover)	Perfect Steamed Vegetables (page 296)	Garden Salad (page 160)
TUESDAY	Superfood Smoothie (page 141)	Simple Baked Whitefish (leftover)	Lemon and Thyme Broiled Pork Chops (page 230)
		Carrot-Ginger Soup, butternut squash variation (leftover)	Oxtail-Braised Greens (page 284)
		Braised Greens (page 300)	Roasted Parsnips (page 325)
WEDNESDAY	Breakfast Sausage (leftover)	Pomegranate Molasses–Glazed Salmon (leftover)	Simple Grilled Steak (page 218)
	Roasted Parsnips (leftover)	Fruit Salad (leftover)	Spiced Kabocha Squash (page 324)
	Braised Greens (page 300)	Perfect Steamed Vegetables (page 296)	Garden Salad (page 160)
	Kale Chips (page 166)		
THURSDAY	Lemon and Thyme Broiled Pork Chops (leftover)	Seafood and Leek Soup (leftover)	Mediterranean Mahi Mahi (leftover)
	Oxtail-Braised Greens (leftover)	Plantain Chips or Crackers (leftover)	Perfect Steamed Vegetables (page 296)
	Fruit Salad (leftover)	Garden Salad (page 160)	Kale Chips (leftover)
FRIDAY	Breakfast Sausage (leftover)	Simple Grilled Steak (leftover)	Lemon and Thyme Broiled Pork Chops (leftover)
	Plantain Chips or Crackers (leftover)	Fruit Salad (leftover)	Oxtail-Braised Greens (leftover)
	Roasted Parsnips (leftover)	Garden Salad (page 160)	Spiced Kabocha Squash (leftover)
	Braised Greens (page 300)		Sauerkraut or other fermented veggies (leftover)

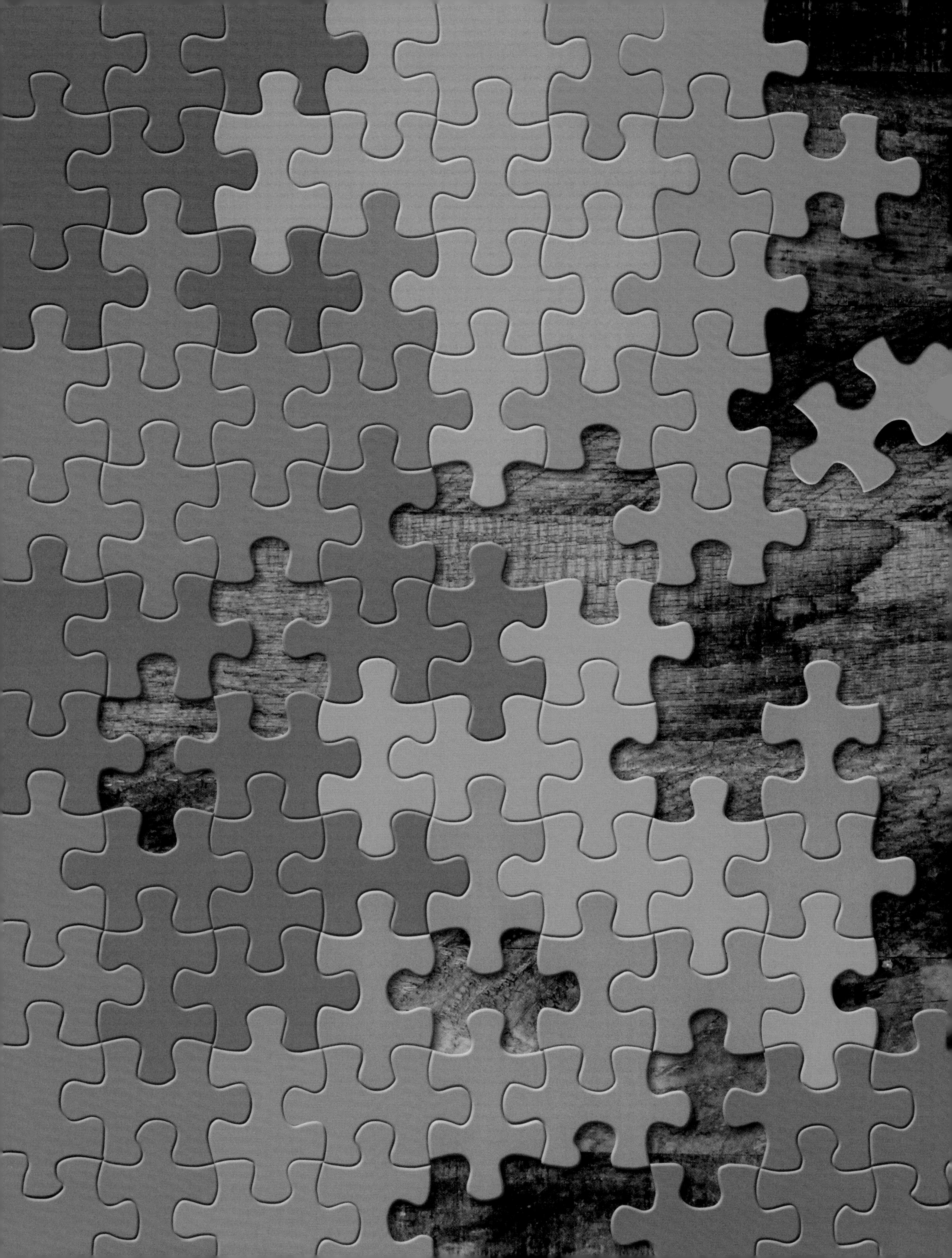

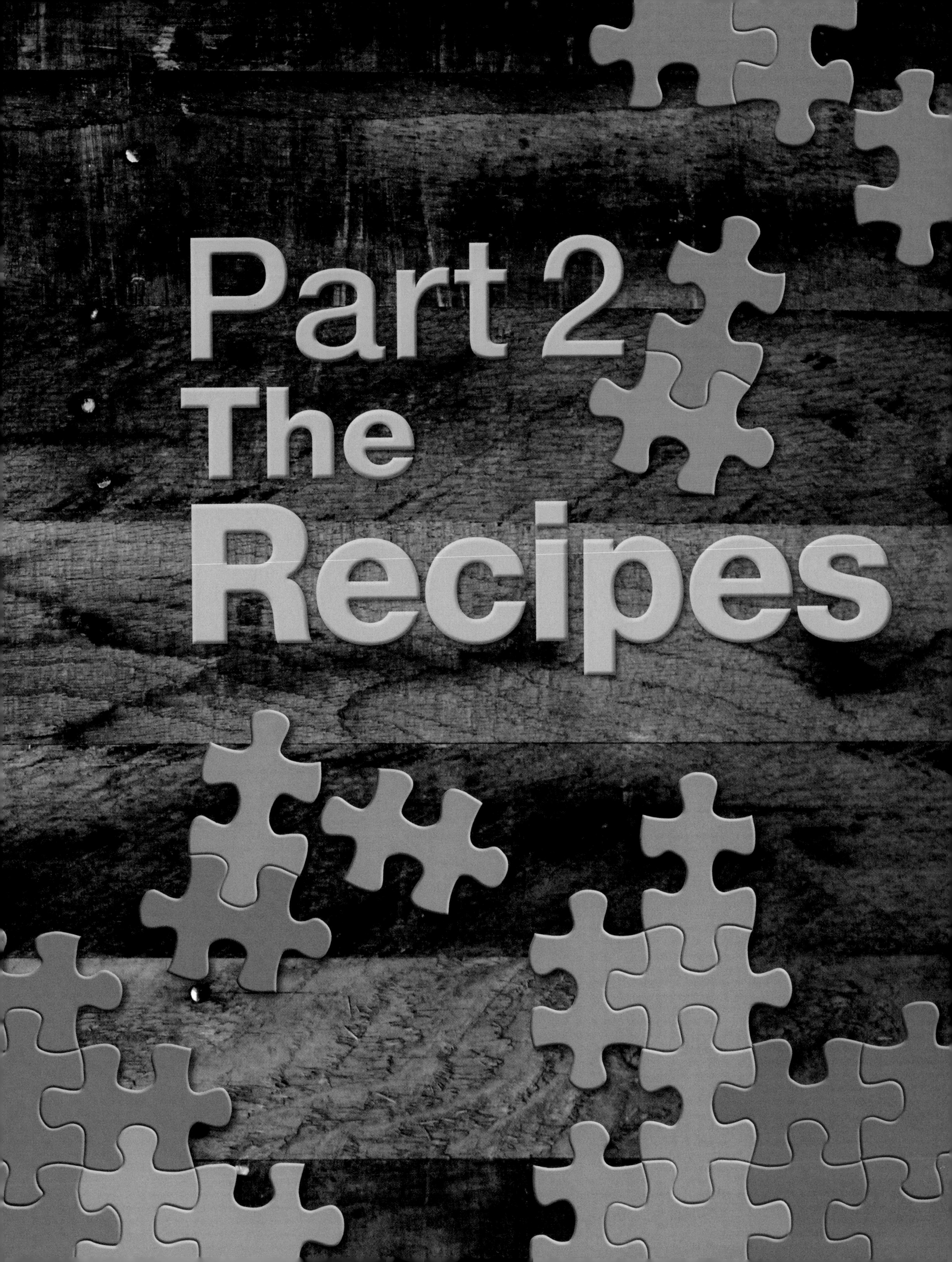
Part 2
The
Recipes

Chapter 4
Kitchen Staples

In this chapter you will find recipes for staples—foods that are used as components in other recipes throughout this book, though some of them can be enjoyed on their own, too. While some of these staples can be purchased premade, making them yourself tends to cost much less, while also typically being healthier. Store these staples in your pantry, fridge, or freezer to have on hand for other recipes or to use as is.

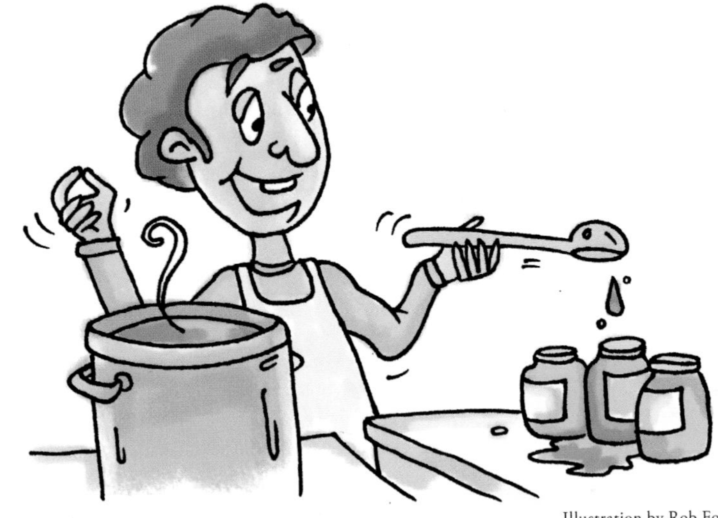

Illustration by Rob Foster

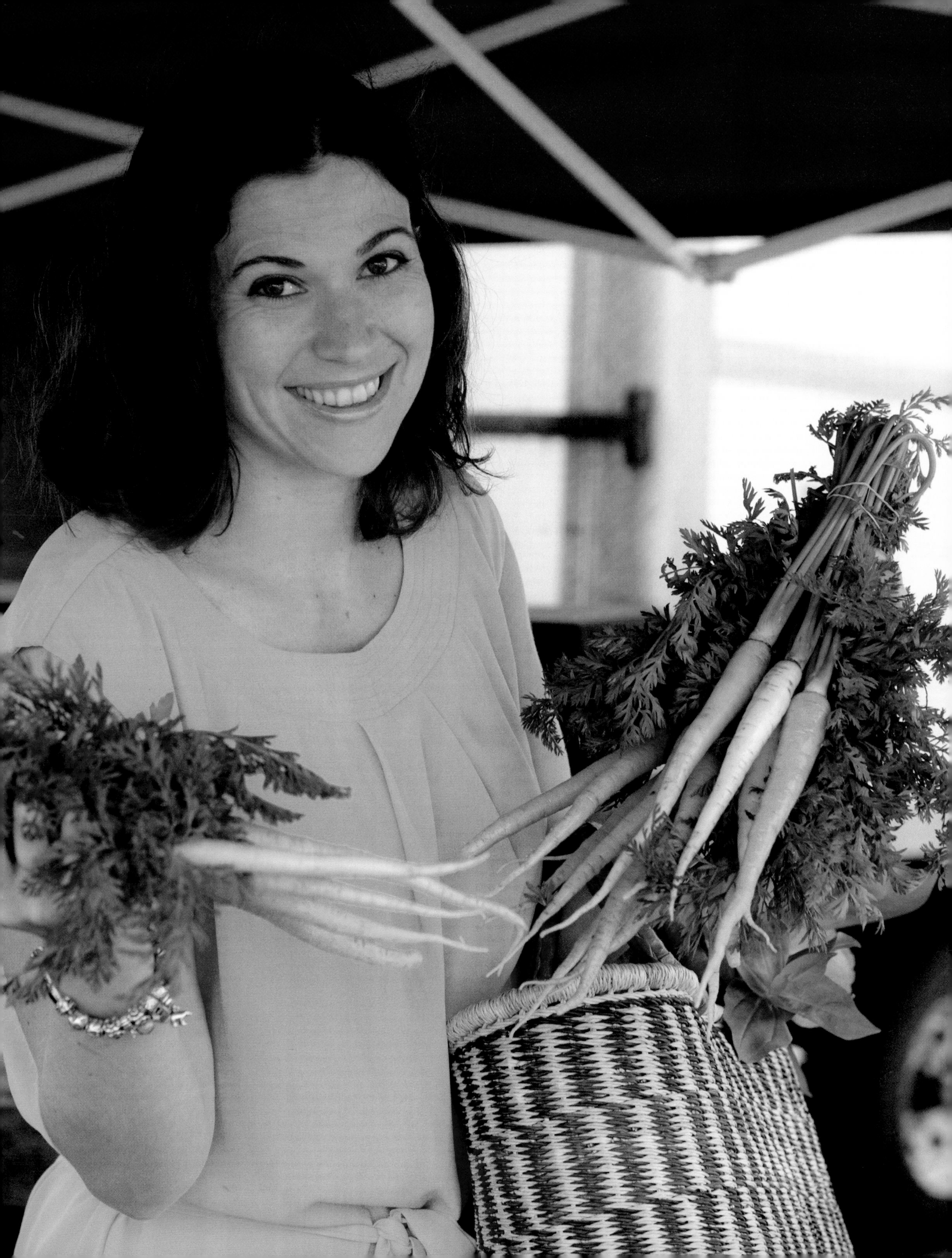

Tallow and Lard

Tallow and lard are two very important staples. They are great fats in which to cook just about anything. Tallow can be made with the fat from beef, bison, lamb, or venison. Lard can be made with the fat from pork or boar. Tallow and lard can be made with subcutaneous fat (trimmed from fattier cuts of meat or cut from close to the hide of the animals during processing) or from suet (the visceral fat from around the internal organs). It's important to get quality fat or suet from grass-fed, pasture-raised, or wild animals.

PREP TIME: 5 to 20 minutes
COOK TIME: 1 hour per pound of fat
YIELD: 1 pint per pound of fat

INGREDIENTS:

1 to 5 pounds animal fat, ground or cut into 1-inch cubes or smaller pieces

SPECIAL EQUIPMENT

- Strainer

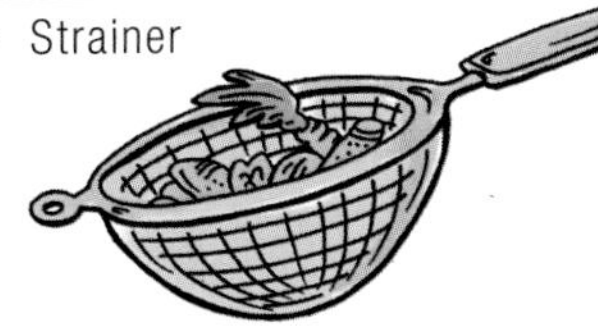

1. Place the fat in a large, heavy pot and cover with a lid. Place on the stovetop over low heat.
2. Stir every 30 to 45 minutes to dislodge any sticky bits from the bottom of the pot.
3. The tallow or lard is ready when all the fat has melted. (There will be some bits that look like little bits of ground beef as well.) This will take approximately 1 hour per pound of fat, varying by type of fat and how small the pieces are.
4. Place a metal strainer over a glass jar, bowl, or measuring cup. Line with a single sheet of paper towel. Pour the melted fat through the lined strainer into the jar. Let cool before putting on the lid.
5. Store at room temperature out of direct sunlight for up to 3 months, or in the fridge or freezer for up to 2 years.

TIPS:

It's easiest to grind (with either a meat grinder or a food processor) or chop fat into small pieces when it's very cold. The smaller the pieces, the more quickly the fat will render.

Those little bits that are filtered out of the rendered tallow or lard are delicious! You can crisp them up in a skillet, add a little salt, and eat them straight, or add them to Braised Greens (page 300) or mashed vegetables (pages 295 and 307) for a special treat.

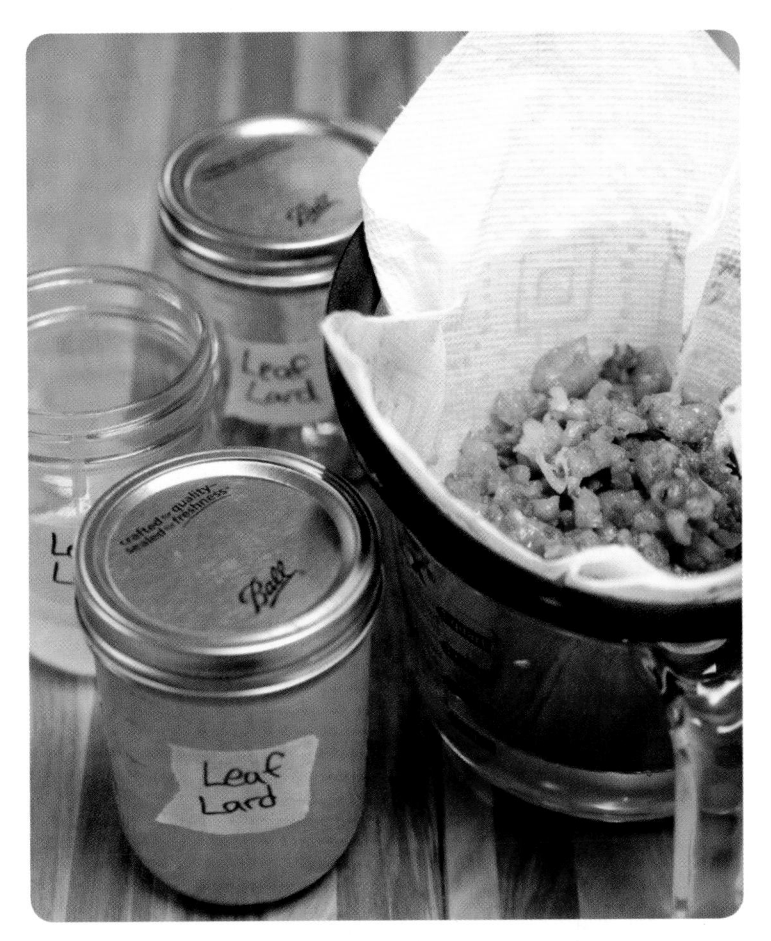

NUTRITION FACTS

Serving Size	26 g
Recipe Yields	410 g
Calories	**235**
Fats	**26 g**
MUFA	10.9 g
Omega-3	0.16 g
Omega-6	0.81 g
Saturated Fat	13 g
Carbohydrates	**0 g**
Fiber	0 g
Starch	0 g
Fructose	0 g
Glucose	0 g
Sucrose	0 g
Protein	**0 g**
Alanine	0 g
Arginine	0 g
Aspartic acid	0 g
Cystine	0 g
Glutamic acid	0 g
Glycine	0 g
Histidine	0 g
Isoleucine	0 g
Leucine	0 g
Lysine	0 g
Methionine	0 g
Phenylalanine	0 g
Proline	0 g
Serine	0 g
Threonine	0 g
Tryptophan	0 g
Tyrosine	0 g
Valine	0 g
Vitamins	
Vitamin B1	0 mg
Vitamin B12	0 mcg
Vitamin B2	0 mg
Vitamin B3	0 mg
Vitamin B5	0 mg
Vitamin B6	0 mg
Choline	20.8 mg
Folate	0 mcg
Vitamin A	0 mcg
Vitamin C	0 mg
Vitamin D	7.28 IU
Vitamin E	0 mg
Vitamin K	0 mcg
Minerals	
Calcium	0 mg
Copper	0 mg
Iron	0 mg
Magnesium	0 mg
Manganese	0 mg
Phosphorus	0 mg
Potassium	0 mg
Selenium	0.05 mcg
Sodium	0 mg
Zinc	0 mg

nutrition content estimated using the USDA database.

Handy-Dandy Spice Blends

Most of these spice blends are used in various recipes throughout this book. However, they are all versatile and really can be used with any meat or vegetable. Store in a spice shaker and keep on hand for quick weeknight meals—just grab some meat and vegetables and throw them into a pan to cook with one of these homemade spice blends.

INGREDIENTS:

Garlic Salt
(Makes 6 tablespoons)

¼ cup garlic powder

2 tablespoons pink or gray salt or truffle salt

Greek Seasoning
(Makes 6 tablespoons)

2 tablespoons dried lemon zest

2 tablespoons dried oregano leaves

2 tablespoons garlic powder

Italian Seasoning
(Makes 6 tablespoons)

1 tablespoon dried oregano leaves

1 tablespoon dried rosemary

1 tablespoon dried marjoram leaves

1 tablespoon dried thyme leaves

1 tablespoon dried savory

1 tablespoon garlic powder

Herbes de Provence
(Makes 10 tablespoons)

3 tablespoons dried marjoram leaves

3 tablespoons dried thyme leaves

3 tablespoons dried savory

1 teaspoon dried oregano leaves

1 teaspoon dried rosemary

1 teaspoon dried tarragon

½ teaspoon dried rubbed sage

Poultry Seasoning
(Makes 10 tablespoons)

3 tablespoons garlic powder

3 tablespoons dried savory

2 tablespoons dried thyme leaves

1 tablespoon dried marjoram leaves

1 tablespoon onion powder

Steak Spice
(Makes 5 tablespoons)

3 tablespoons truffle salt

1 tablespoon ground turmeric

1 teaspoon garlic powder

1 teaspoon onion powder

1 teaspoon dried oregano leaves

Tarragon Salt
(Makes 6 tablespoons)

¼ cup dried tarragon, ground to a powder

2 tablespoons pink or gray salt or truffle salt

SPECIAL EQUIPMENT

- Spice grinder (optional)

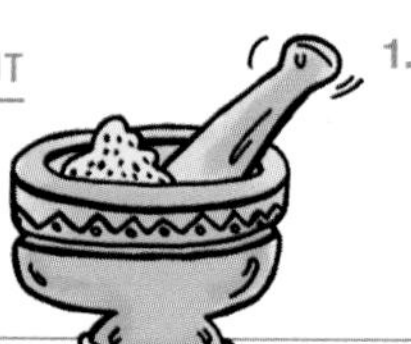

1. Combine the spices in a spice grinder or mini food processor and process until powdered, or place them directly in a spice shaker or spice jar. If you don't have a spice shaker, you can also sprinkle by hand or dust with a sieve. Store in the pantry or cupboard for up to 6 months or freeze for up to 2 years.

TIPS:

These spice blends don't need to be made with store-bought dried herbs and spices! Making your own is actually very simple.

Homemade Garlic Powder. *Peel the cloves from 3 to 4 heads of garlic. Slice the garlic thinly and dry in a food dehydrator on a fruit roll sheet until completely crisp—12 to 48 hours, depending on your dehydrator. (If you don't own a fruit roll sheet, use parchment paper to line the racks.) Alternatively, you can dry the garlic in the oven on the lowest temperature. Grind the dried garlic in a spice grinder or mini food processor until you have a fine powder. Makes 2 to 4 tablespoons.*

Homemade Onion Powder. *Thinly slice 2 to 3 onions into rounds and place on a tray in a food dehydrator. Dehydrate until completely crisp—12 to 48 hours, depending on your dehydrator. Alternatively, you can dry the onion slices in the oven at the lowest temperature. Grind the dried onion in a spice grinder or mini food processor until you have a fine powder. Makes 3 to 4 tablespoons.*

Homemade Dried Lemon Zest. *Slice the zest (just the outer colored portion of the rind) off of 7 to 8 lemons and place on a fruit roll sheet in a food dehydrator. (If you don't own a fruit roll sheet, use parchment paper to line the racks.) Dry until completely crisp—6 to 12 hours, depending on your dehydrator. Alternatively, you can dry the lemon zest in the oven at the lowest temperature. Grind the dried zest in a spice grinder or mini food processor until you have a fine powder. Makes 2 to 3 tablespoons.*

Homemade Dried Herbs. *You can dry fresh herbs in a dehydrator for several hours or by hanging bunches of herbs upside down in a cool place out of direct sunlight for several days.*

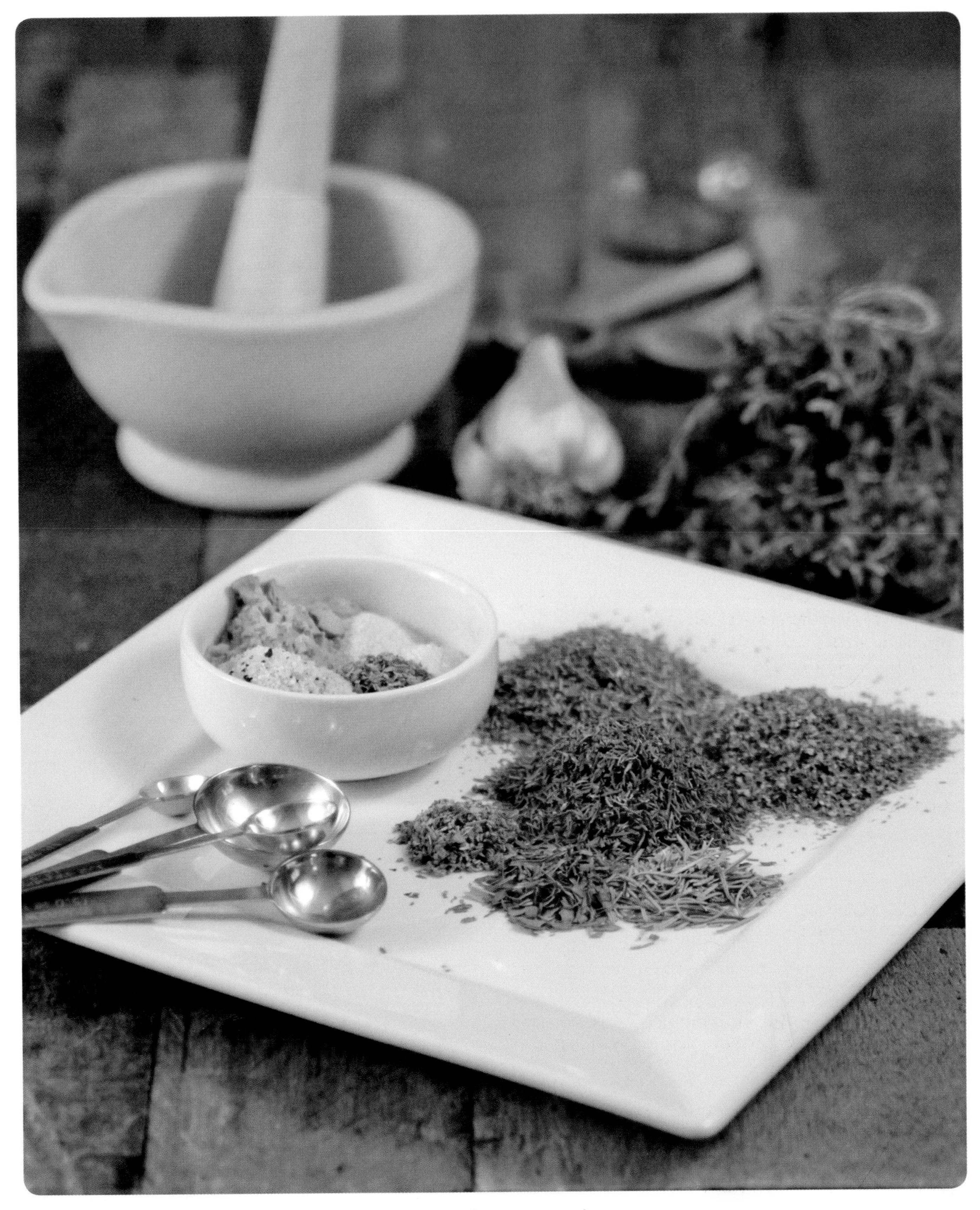

FODMAP ALERT *Omit the garlic, or replace with green garlic or garlic scapes (green part only) that are minced and then dried in a dehydrator or oven. Omit the onion, or replace with green onion or leek (green part only) or chives that are minced and then dried in a dehydrator or oven.*

Bone Broth

Homemade broth is rich in minerals and glycine and can be consumed straight, used in soups and stews, and used for braising meats and vegetables.

Bones (or feet or fish heads) for broth can be purchased from your farmer, butcher, or fishmonger (sometimes they will give them to you for free) or saved from various meals in your freezer until you have accumulated enough for a batch of broth.

In general, the longer you cook broth, the more you demineralize the bones and the higher the mineral content of your broth will be.

The collagen in broth (the glycine-rich protein that makes it gelatinous when chilled) comes from connective tissue around the bones. Chicken feet, pig's feet, beef knuckle bones, oxtail, and fish heads will each make your broth rich with collagen. You can also use a mix. For example, I use leftover bones from Roasted Chicken (page 209) to make chicken broth, but I like to throw in a handful of feet to make sure that it gels.

PREP TIME: 10 minutes
COOK TIME: 7 hours to 5 days
YIELD: 10 to 12 cups

INGREDIENTS:

Chicken or Turkey Broth:

- 2 to 3 pounds chicken or turkey bones (bones from 2 to 3 roasting chickens or from 1 turkey); include giblets and feet if desired
- 1 gallon water (or enough to cover the bones by 1 to 2 inches)
- 1 tablespoon apple cider vinegar
- 2 medium onions, roots cut off, quartered
- 4 or 5 carrots, cut in half
- 6 to 8 celery stalks, cut into thirds
- 6 to 8 cloves garlic
- 3 bay leaves
- 1 teaspoon salt

Beef, Bison, Lamb, or Pork Broth:

- 2 to 3 pounds beef bones (or use bison, lamb, or pork)
- 1 gallon water (or enough to cover the bones by 1 to 2 inches)
- 1 tablespoon apple cider vinegar
- 2 medium onions, roots cut off, quartered
- 3 bay leaves
- 1 teaspoon whole cloves (omit for pork broth)
- 1 teaspoon salt

POULTRY OR MEAT BONE BROTH:

1. Combine the bones, water, and vinegar in a large stockpot (or pressure cooker or slow cooker). Bring to a boil over high heat, then reduce the heat to maintain a simmer. Alternatively, cook under high pressure in a pressure cooker or bring to a boil and then reduce the heat to low in a slow cooker.
2. During the first hour of cooking, skim off any foam that has risen to the surface. (This improves the flavor of the final broth.) You don't need to do this step if you're using a pressure cooker.
3. Simmer, covered, for 24 to 48 hours (or 6 to 12 hours under high pressure in a pressure cooker or 2 to 5 days in a slow cooker). Periodically stir and check the water level. Top up with additional water if needed to make sure that the bones are covered by an inch or two of water.
4. Add the remaining ingredients. Simmer for an additional 4 to 6 hours (or 1 to 2 hours in a pressure cooker or 6 to 8 hours in a slow cooker).
5. Strain and discard the bones and vegetables. Store the broth in the fridge for up to 5 days or in the freezer for up to 6 months.

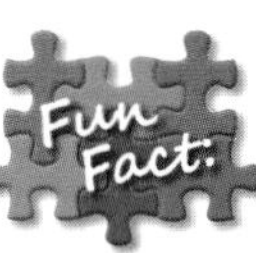

Adding a small amount of vinegar to a batch of broth increases bone demineralization so your finished product has a higher mineral content (and I promise it won't taste vinegary).

SPECIAL EQUIPMENT

- Large stockpot, slow cooker, or pressure cooker

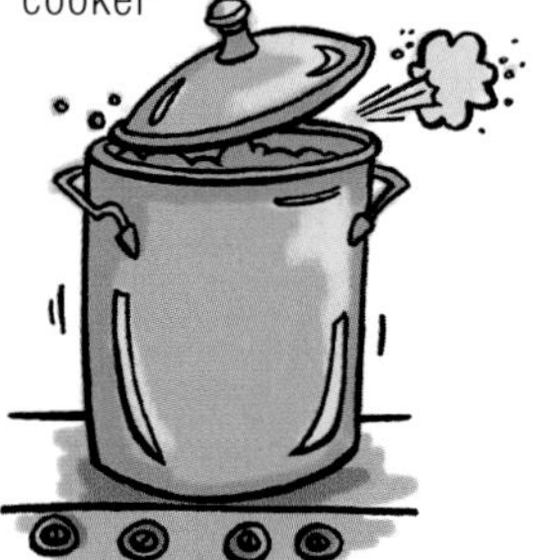

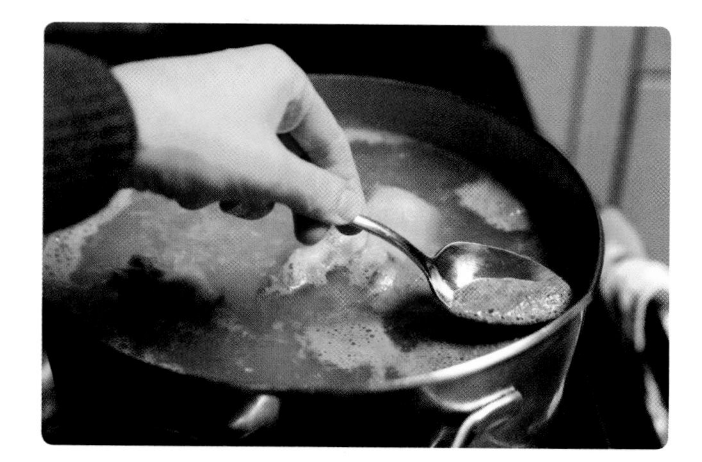

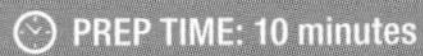

PREP TIME: 10 minutes
COOK TIME: 1 to 8 hours
YIELD: 10 to 12 cups

INGREDIENTS:

Fish Broth:

2 to 4 pounds fish heads, tails, and bones

1 gallon water (or enough to cover the bones by 1 to 2 inches)

1 tablespoon apple cider vinegar

1 medium onion or 2 medium leeks, roots cut off, quartered

3 or 4 celery stalks, cut into thirds

1 or 2 carrots, cut in half

Optional: substitute white wine for 1 cup of the water

FODMAP ALERT *Replace the garlic with green garlic or garlic scapes (green part only) or omit. Replace the onion with green onion or leek (green part only) or chives or omit.*

FISH BROTH:

1. Combine all the ingredients in a large stockpot (or pressure cooker or slow cooker). Bring to a boil over high heat, then reduce the heat to maintain a simmer. Alternatively, cook under high pressure in a pressure cooker or bring to a boil and then reduce the heat to low in a slow cooker.
2. During the first hour of cooking, skim off any foam that has risen to the surface. (This improves the flavor of the final broth.) You don't need to do this step if you're using a pressure cooker.
3. Simmer, covered, for 3 to 4 hours (1 to 2 hours in a pressure cooker or 6 to 8 hours in a slow cooker). Periodically stir and check the water level. Top up with additional water if needed to make sure that the ingredients are covered by an inch or two of water. Strain and discard the bones and vegetables. Store the broth in the fridge for up to 5 days or in the freezer for up to 6 months.

TIPS:

Every time you eat meat on the bone, save the bones. Label different containers in your freezer for different types of bones (chicken, beef, lamb, etc.) and continue to add to these containers until you have accumulated enough for making broth. You can also save fish heads, tails, and bones if you bake whole fish.

If you're making broth from pig's feet or chicken feet that haven't been blanched, boil them in a pot of water for 5 minutes, discard the water, rinse the feet, then make your broth as normal.

If you are making broth from very meaty bones or marrow bones (common for beef broth), you may wish to remove the meat from the broth while it still has flavor! After the first 6 to 12 hours of cooking, remove the bones from the broth. Once cool enough to handle, remove the meat, then return the bones to the pot for the remainder of the cooking time. You can enjoy this meat plain or add it to soups, stews, stir-fries, or braised vegetables.

If you are using bones from grass-fed, pasture-raised, or wild animals, there is no reason to skim the fat. However, if you used bones from conventionally raised animals or simply want leaner broth, the easiest way to skim the fat is to chill the broth in the fridge overnight and then scrape the solid fat layer off the top (keep for other cooking uses if you used good-quality bones, or discard).

Want to keep it simple? You don't need to add herbs and aromatic veggies. If you like it plain, feel free to stick with bones, water, vinegar, and salt!

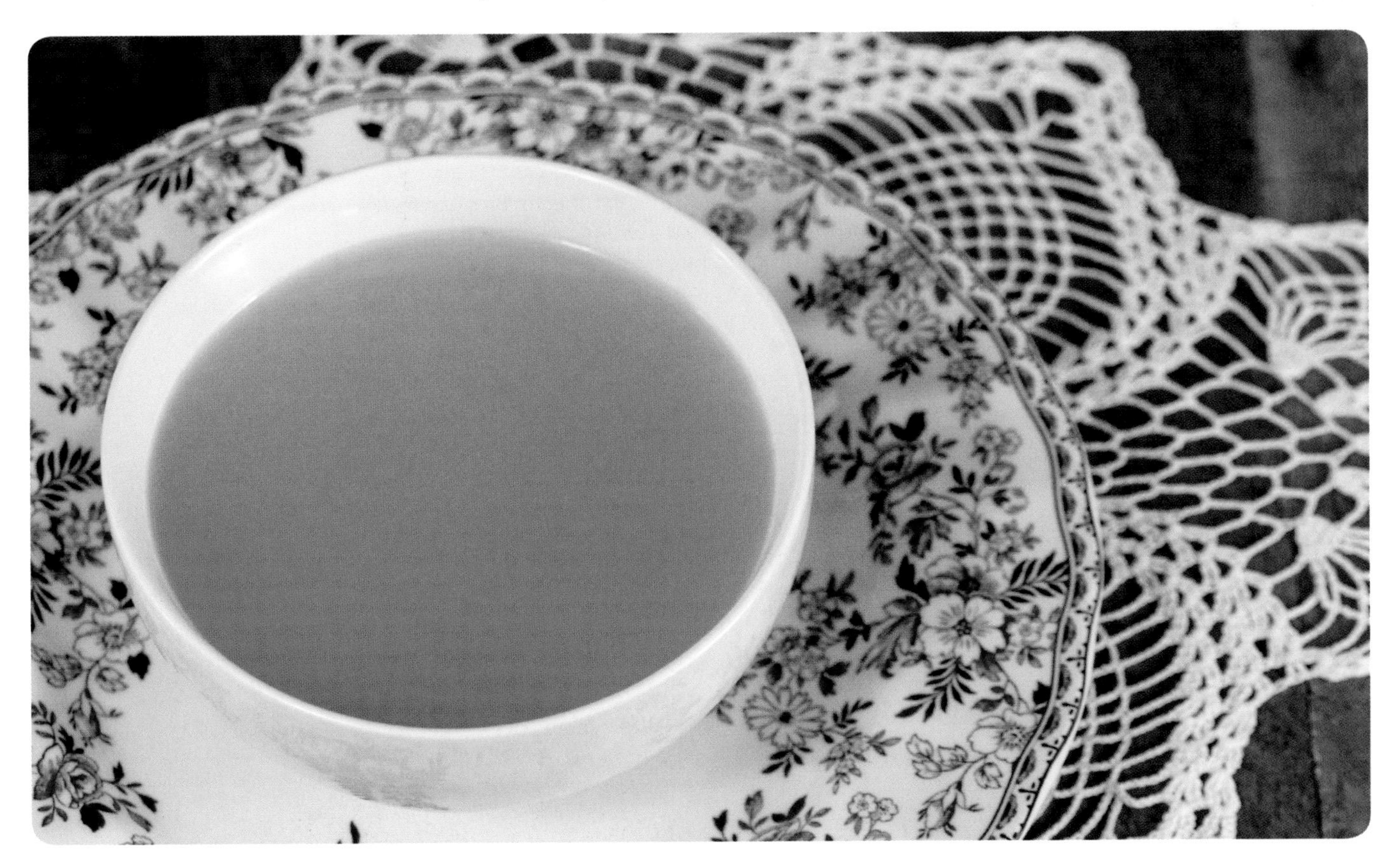

Sauerkraut

Homemade sauerkraut is a completely different experience than store-bought kraut. The flavor and texture are different, plus homemade sauerkraut is probably the richest food source of diverse probiotics available, with slightly different strains in every batch.

You don't need any special equipment to make sauerkraut. A large glass cracker or cookie jar with a wide mouth, a slightly smaller jar that fits inside the mouth of the larger jar, a tea towel, and a knife are really the only "equipment" you need. Of course, if you want a foolproof way to ferment vegetables and think that you will doing a lot of fermenting, investing in a fermentation crock is definitely worthwhile.

Certain types of cabbage just work better for sauerkraut. These are basically your "regular" cabbages (green or red/purple), although sui choy works as well (it softens quickly, so reduce the fermentation time). Sauerkraut works best with fresh, organic cabbage. The fresher the cabbage, typically the higher the water content, too, which means less fiddling with the liquid levels.

Unrefined sea salt, Himalayan salt, kosher salt, or pickling salt works well for fermenting vegetables. Do not use iodized table salt for making sauerkraut.

This recipe can easily be scaled up or down depending on how much kraut you want to make, or to match the size of your fermentation vessel. The general rule is 1½ teaspoons of salt per pound of cabbage or other vegetables. Three pounds of cabbage is about perfect for a 5-quart cracker jar.

PREP TIME: 20 minutes to 1 hour
COOK TIME: 5 days to 5 weeks or longer
SERVINGS: 30-plus

INGREDIENTS:

3 pounds cabbage (1 large head or 2 smaller heads)

1½ tablespoons unrefined sea salt, pink salt, pickling salt, or other noniodized salt

FODMAP ALERT *While fermentation decreases FODMAP content, some people still may be unable to consume sauerkraut. As an alternative to cabbage, use grated carrots, turnips, or winter squash. When fermenting other vegetables, you are more likely to have to top off with brine (check after 8 hours and again at 24 hours). Start tasting after 3 days, since these vegetables often ferment more quickly than cabbage.*

1. Peel a few of the outer leaves from each head of cabbage and set aside.
2. Slice the cabbage as thinly as possible using a food processor, mandoline slicer, or knife.
3. Place the cabbage in a large bowl. (If you don't have a bowl big enough for all 3 pounds, you can do this in batches.) Sprinkle with the salt.
4. Massage the cabbage with your hands to thoroughly distribute the salt and start the process of breaking down the cabbage. Massage until well wilted.
5. Make sure that your fermentation vessel is very clean (see above for vessel recommendations). Pack the sauerkraut into the vessel, handful by handful, pressing down firmly with each handful to make sure that it's tightly packed.
6. Place the large outer leaves over the top of the shredded cabbage (you may have to tear or fold them to cover the entire surface). This ensures that the shredded cabbage stays submerged.
7. Weight down the cabbage. A clean glass jar slightly smaller in diameter than the mouth of your fermentation vessel filled with water works well. If you are using a fermentation crock, use the weight that comes with it.
8. Cover with a breathable barrier (paint-straining bag, nut-milk bag, several layers of cheesecloth, coffee filter, linen towel, or even paper towels) and secure with a rubber band (unless using something like a paint-straining bag that has elastic around the opening). If using a fermentation crock, put on the lid.

TIPS:

How do you know that the sauerkraut is fermented "to your liking"? Just taste it! Starting on day 5, taste it every day; it's ready when you think it tastes good. Keep in mind that it will taste less sour after being in the fridge a few days.

NUTRITION FACTS	
Serving Size	46 g
Recipe Yields	1369 g
Calories	**11.5**
Fats	**0.05 g**
MUFA	<0.01 g
Omega-3	0 g
Omega-6	<0.01 g
Saturated Fat	0.02 g
Carbohydrates	**2.66 g**
Fiber	1.15 g
Starch	0.05 g
Fructose	0.67 g
Glucose	0.77 g
Sucrose	0.04 g
Protein	**0.59 g**
Alanine	0.02 g
Arginine	0.03 g
Aspartic acid	0.06 g
Cystine	<0.01 g
Glutamic acid	0.14 g
Glycine	0.01 g
Histidine	0.01 g
Isoleucine	0.01 g
Leucine	0.02 g
Lysine	0.02 g
Methionine	<0.01 g
Phenylalanine	0.01 g
Proline	0.02 g
Serine	0.02 g
Threonine	0.02 g
Tryptophan	<0.01 g
Tyrosine	<0.01 g
Valine	0.02 g
Vitamins	
Vitamin B1	0.03 mg
Vitamin B12	0 mcg
Vitamin B2	0.02 mg
Vitamin B3	0.11 mg
Vitamin B5	0.1 mg
Vitamin B6	0.06 mg
Choline	4.91 mg
Folate	19.8 mcg
Vitamin A	2.3 mcg
Vitamin C	16.8 mg
Vitamin D	0 IU
Vitamin E	0.07 mg
Vitamin K	34.9 mcg
Minerals	
Calcium	18.9 mg
Copper	<0.01 mg
Iron	0.5 mg
Magnesium	5.51 mg
Manganese	0.07 mg
Phosphorus	11.9 mg
Potassium	79.8 mg
Selenium	0.14 mcg
Sodium	56.8 mg
Zinc	0.08 mg

nutrition content estimated using the USDA database.

9. Check the level of the liquid over the next 24 hours. If it is not at least 1 inch above the top of the cabbage, dissolve 1 teaspoon salt into 1 cup water. Then pour the salty water into your fermentation vessel until the level of the water is at least 1 inch above the top of the cabbage.
10. The sauerkraut will be ready in as little as 5 days, but can ferment for up to 5 months (check the liquid level periodically and top up with salted water if needed). A little bubbling or foaming is normal.
11. Once the sauerkraut is fermented to your liking, transfer to smaller jars (if desired) and keep in the fridge for up to 6 months.

SPECIAL EQUIPMENT

- Mandoline slicer or food processor with a slicer attachment, or a knife and some patience
- Large glass jar with a wide mouth
- Smaller glass jar that fits inside the mouth of the larger jar
- Paint-straining bag, nut-milk bag, cheesecloth, or coffee filter and elastic band
- Or a fermentation crock

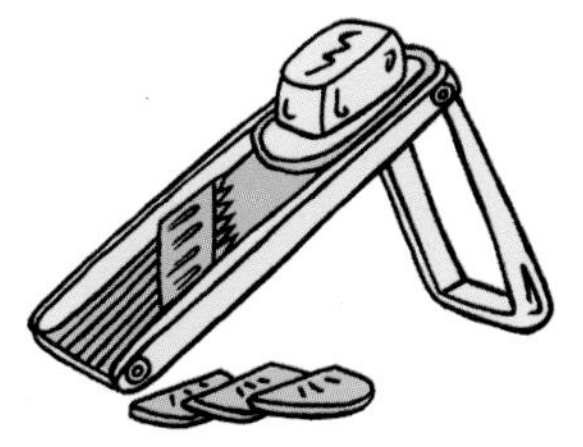

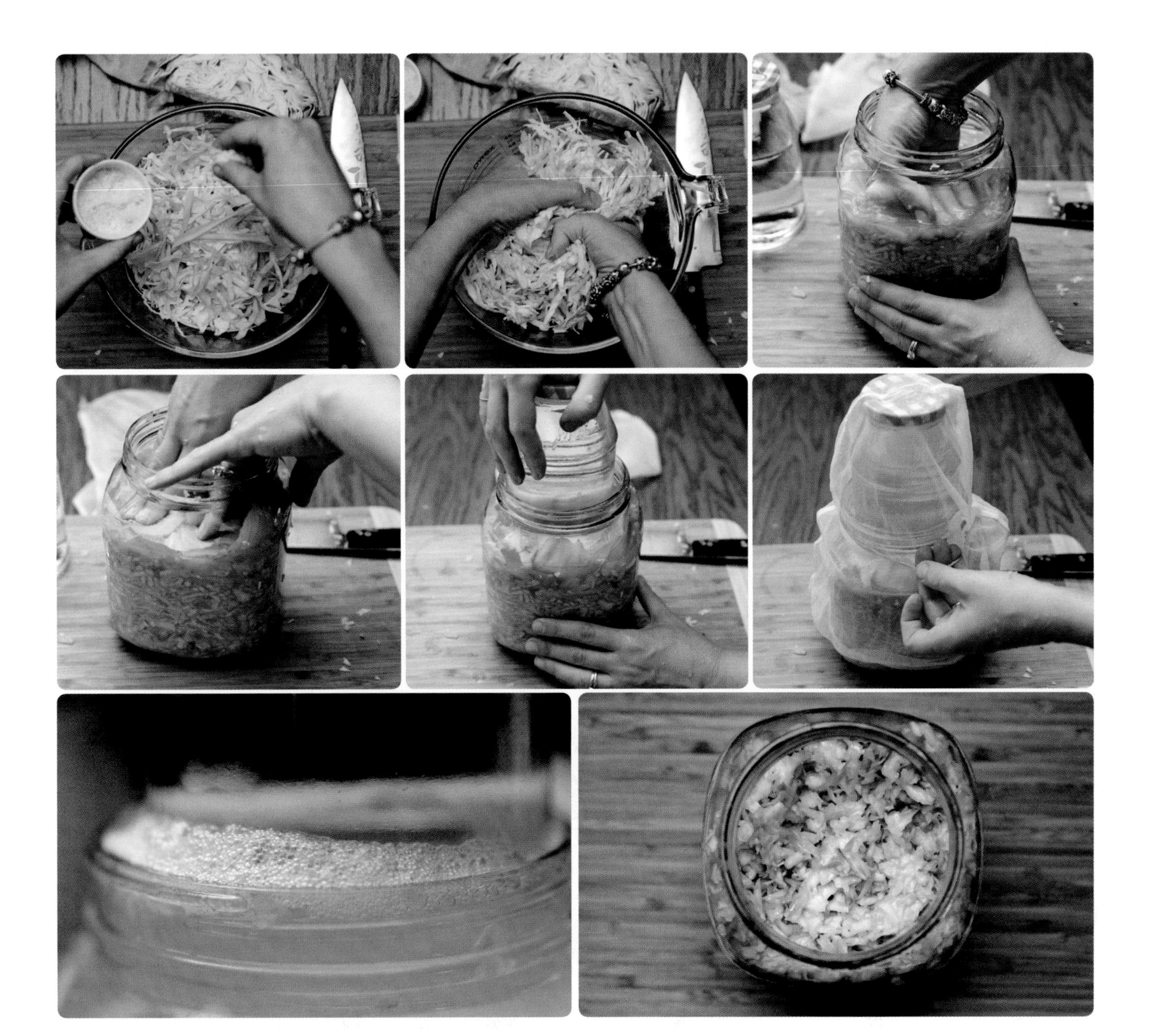

Green Tea and Garlic Pickles

Green tea, and more specifically its tannin content, is the secret to keeping these pickles crunchy. Alternatively, you can use a grape leaf to provide tannins to your pickle ferment.

Unrefined sea salt, Himalayan salt, or pickling salt works well for fermenting vegetables. Do not use iodized table salt.

This recipe can easily be scaled up or down depending on how many pickles you want to make, or to match the size of your fermentation vessel.

PREP TIME: 20 minutes
COOK TIME: 3 to 5 days sliced, 6 to 10 days whole
SERVINGS: 30-plus

INGREDIENTS:

- 6 teabags green tea or 6 teaspoons loose-leaf green tea
- ¼ cup unrefined sea salt, pink salt, pickling salt, or other noniodized salt
- 6 cups hot water (see Tips)
- 2 pounds pickling cucumbers
- 1 head garlic
- 2 sprigs fresh dill

FODMAP ALERT

Just don't eat the garlic.

SPECIAL EQUIPMENT

- Mandoline slicer, food processor with a slicer attachment, or a knife and some patience
- Large glass jar with a wide mouth
- Smaller glass jar that fits inside the mouth of the larger jar
- Paint-straining bag, nut-milk bag, cheesecloth, or coffee filter and an elastic band
- Or a fermentation crock

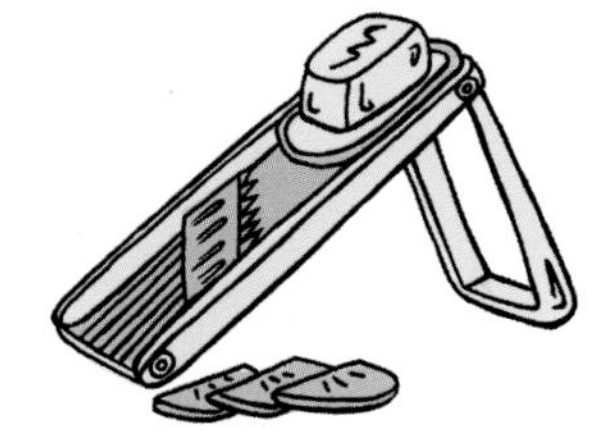

1. Put the teabags and salt in a heatproof bowl. Pour the hot water over the teabags and salt. Stir occasionally to make sure that the salt dissolves. Let cool to room temperature.
2. Slice the cucumbers ¼ inch thick (or slice into wedges or leave whole). Peel the garlic and leave the cloves whole. Mix the cucumbers and garlic together.
3. Place the dill at the bottom of a large glass jar or fermentation crock. Pile the garlic and cucumbers on top. Pour the cooled green tea over the top.
4. Place a glass jar, bowl, or the weight from your fermentation crock over the top of the cucumbers to keep them submerged. There should be at least 1 inch of liquid above the top of the cucumbers.
5. Cover with a breathable barrier (paint-straining bag, nut-milk bag, several layers of cheesecloth, coffee filter, linen towel, or even paper towels) and secure with a rubber band (unless using something like a paint-straining bag that has elastic around the opening). If using a fermentation crock, put on the lid.
6. The pickles will be ready in 3 to 5 days if sliced, and 4 to 10 days if wedged or whole. After 3 days, taste them to see if they are to your liking (they will soften as they get more sour). Transfer to smaller jars (if desired) and keep in the fridge for up to 2 months.

TIPS:

Green tea is traditionally made with water at 170°F to 185°F (as opposed to black tea, which is made with boiling water). Bring the water to a boil, remove it from the heat, and then let it sit for 1 to 2 minutes before pouring over the teabags.

The longer you ferment your pickles, the more sour and soft they will be. After 3 days, taste every day, and move them to the fridge once they are to your liking.

Keep the garlic! Yes, it's potent, but it's delicious to use in Salad Dressings (page 126) and in dips (see Veggies and Dip, page 172).

VARIATIONS:

Want to make just a jar of pickles? You can scale down this recipe and ferment directly in a mason jar with a clean, small, smooth rock to weigh down the cucumbers.

NUTRITION FACTS	
Serving Size	36 g
Recipe Yields	1093 g
Calories	**6.6**
Fats	**0.04 g**
MUFA	<0.01 g
Omega-3	<0.01 g
Omega-6	0.01 g
Saturated Fat	0.01 g
Carbohydrates	**1.49 g**
Fiber	0.24 g
Starch	0.6 g
Fructose	0.26 g
Glucose	0.23 g
Sucrose	<0.01 g
Protein	**0.27 g**
Alanine	<0.01 g
Arginine	0.02 g
Aspartic acid	0.02 g
Cystine	<0.01 g
Glutamic acid	0.07 g
Glycine	<0.01 g
Histidine	<0.01 g
Isoleucine	<0.01 g
Leucine	0.01 g
Lysine	0.01 g
Methionine	<0.01 g
Phenylalanine	<0.01 g
Proline	<0.01 g
Serine	<0.01 g
Threonine	<0.01 g
Tryptophan	<0.01 g
Tyrosine	<0.01 g
Valine	0.01 g
Vitamins	
Vitamin B1	0.01 mg
Vitamin B12	0 mcg
Vitamin B2	0.01 mg
Vitamin B3	0.04 mg
Vitamin B5	0.09 mg
Vitamin B6	0.03 mg
Choline	2.09 mg
Folate	2.38 mcg
Vitamin A	1.54 mcg
Vitamin C	1.22 mg
Vitamin D	0 IU
Vitamin E	<0.01 mg
Vitamin K	4.92 mcg
Minerals	
Calcium	7.45 mg
Copper	0.02 mg
Iron	0.36 mg
Magnesium	4.33 mg
Manganese	0.05 mg
Phosphorus	9.04 mg
Potassium	52 mg
Selenium	0.26 mcg
Sodium	44.9 mg
Zinc	0.07 mg

nutrition content estimated using the USDA database.

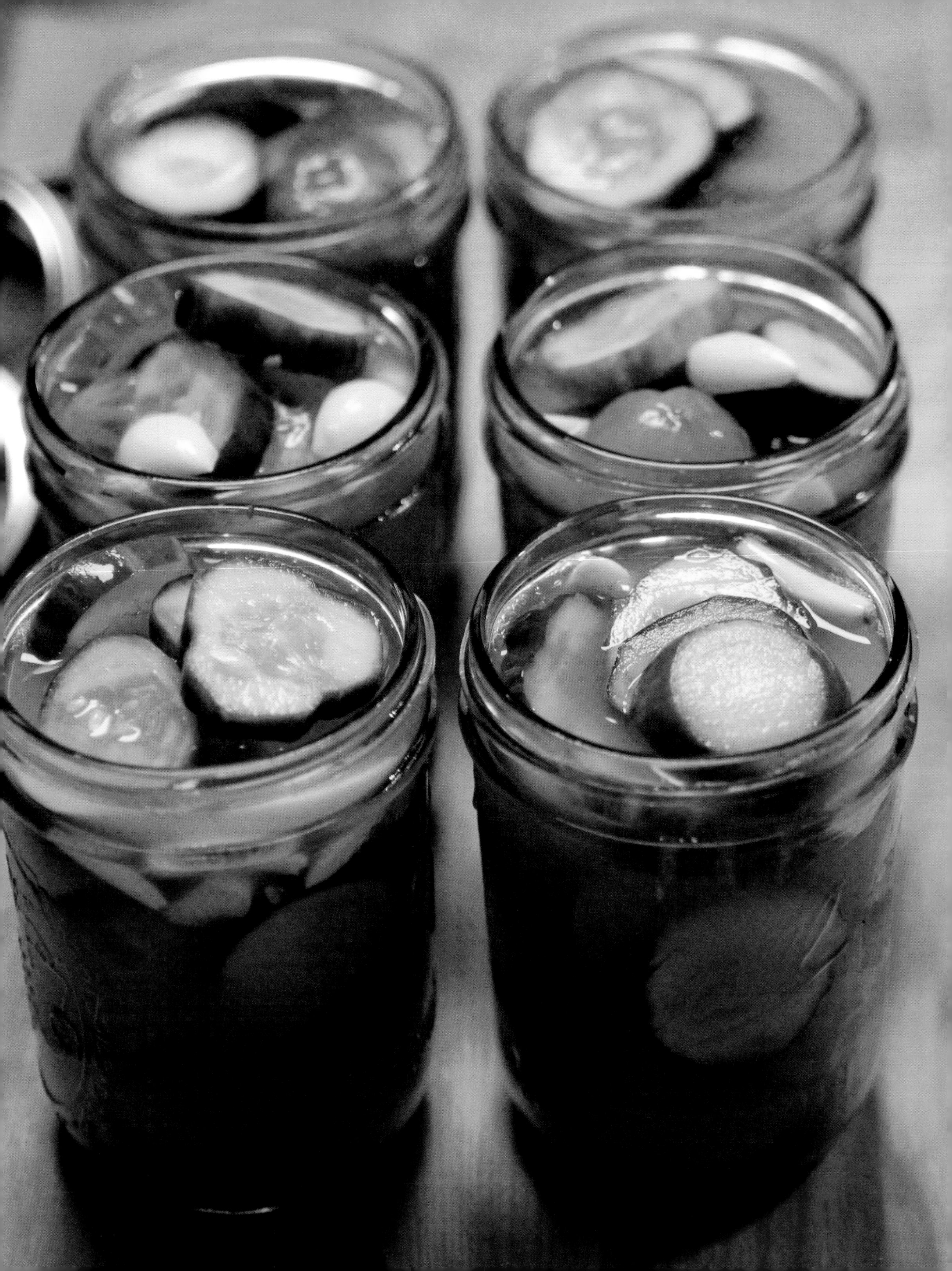

Coconut Milk, Cream, and Whipped Topping

It is getting easier and easier to purchase emulsifier-free full-fat coconut milk and coconut cream in BPA-free cans and tetra packs. (Please do not confuse coconut cream with creamed coconut or coconut cream concentrate, which are the same thing as coconut butter.) The convenience of packaged coconut milk and cream just can't be beat, but they can be expensive. If these high-quality products are beyond your food budget, or if you live in an area where sourcing them is a challenge, you can make you own from unsweetened dried coconut (shredded or flaked). If you buy shredded coconut in bulk, you'll find that the cost of making your own is anywhere between one-quarter and one-half the cost of buying it.

PREP TIME: 5 minutes
COOK TIME: 30 minutes
YIELD: 1⅔ cups coconut milk (equivalent to one 13½-ounce can) or ⅔ cup coconut cream or whipped topping

INGREDIENTS:

2 cups finely shredded unsweetened dried coconut

2¾ cups water

SPECIAL EQUIPMENT

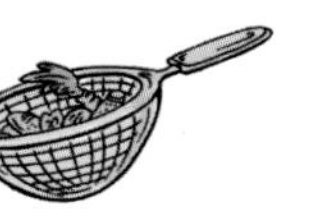

- Blender
- Nut-milk bag, paint-straining bag, or fine-mesh strainer

TIPS:

Because there are no emulsifiers, the coconut milk will naturally separate and be a little clumpy (the consistency of curdled milk with a very solid top layer) when chilled. If you want to drink the milk, blend in a blender right before drinking.

You can make large batches of coconut milk and freeze it in freezer-safe mason jars (leave an inch of headroom) so that you always have some handy.

Homemade Coconut Flour. Dehydrate the coconut pulp on fruit roll sheets in a dehydrator for 12 to 24 hours, then blend on high until it's a fine powder. (If you don't own a fruit roll sheet, use parchment paper to line the racks.)

Coconut Whipped Topping–Stuffed Strawberries. Remove the stems and cores from strawberries. Cut a deep X in the top of each berry and spread the quarters apart. Fill with chilled coconut whipped topping and refrigerate until serving.

1. Combine the coconut and water in a saucepan and bring to a full boil over high heat. Turn off the heat, cover, and let sit for 1 hour.
2. Pour the coconut and water into a blender. Blend on high for 2 to 5 minutes, until the texture is thick and only slightly granular.
3. Pour the pulp into a nut-milk bag, yogurt-cheese bag, paint-straining bag, or fine-mesh strainer suspended over a glass bowl, mason jar, or measuring cup. (If using a nut-milk bag or paint-straining bag, it is easier to handle if you place the bag inside a sieve or strainer.)
4. Either let the coconut milk strain out by gravity or squeeze the pulp through the nut-milk bag.
5. If not using immediately, store the coconut milk in a glass jar in the fridge for up to 2 weeks or in the freezer for up to 1 year. Shake well, blend, or gently warm before using.

COCONUT CREAM:

1. Follow the steps above for making coconut milk, and place in the fridge to chill thoroughly until the cream separates, at least 6 hours or overnight. Spoon the separated cream off the top. You can also do this with a can of coconut milk after it has sat in the fridge overnight.

WHIPPED TOPPING:

1. Follow the instructions above for making coconut cream. Place the cream in a blender and blend on high for 1 minute. Transfer to a jar and chill in the refrigerator for at least 1 hour.
2. Simply spoon off the top and use. Serve with berries or sliced peaches, or enjoy with your favorite dessert from Chapter 12.

VARIATIONS:

When rehydrating the dried coconut, you can use coconut water instead of water for even more coconut flavor.

FODMAP ALERT *Coconut milk has a much lower FODMAP content than other coconut products; however, some people with FODMAP intolerance may still need to avoid it.*

NUTRITION FACTS	
Serving Size	228 g
Recipe Yields	381 g
Calories	**461**
Fats	**47.4 g**
MUFA	2.02 g
Omega-3	0 g
Omega-6	0.52 g
Saturated Fat	42.1 g
Carbohydrates	**12.7 g**
Fiber	2.07 g
Starch	<0.01 g
Fructose	0 g
Glucose	0.66 g
Sucrose	9.48 g
Protein	**3.67 g**
Alanine	0.19 g
Arginine	0.6 g
Aspartic acid	0.36 g
Cystine	0.07 g
Glutamic acid	0.84 g
Glycine	0.17 g
Histidine	0.08 g
Isoleucine	0.14 g
Leucine	0.27 g
Lysine	0.16 g
Methionine	0.07 g
Phenylalanine	0.19 g
Proline	0.15 g
Serine	0.19 g
Threonine	0.13 g
Tryptophan	0.04 g
Tyrosine	0.11 g
Valine	0.22 g
Vitamins	
Vitamin B1	0.05 mg
Vitamin B12	0 mcg
Vitamin B2	0 mg
Vitamin B3	1.53 mg
Vitamin B5	0.37 mg
Vitamin B6	0.07 mg
Choline	19.4 mg
Folate	31.9 mcg
Vitamin A	0 mcg
Vitamin C	2.51 mg
Vitamin D	0 IU
Vitamin E	0.02 mg
Vitamin K	0.23 mcg
Minerals	
Calcium	9.12 mg
Copper	0.54 mg
Iron	1.85 mg
Magnesium	73 mg
Manganese	1.84 mg
Phosphorus	135 mg
Potassium	529 mg
Selenium	8.44 mcg
Sodium	27.4 mg
Zinc	1.35 mg

nutrition content estimated using the USDA database. values are based on Coconut Milk.

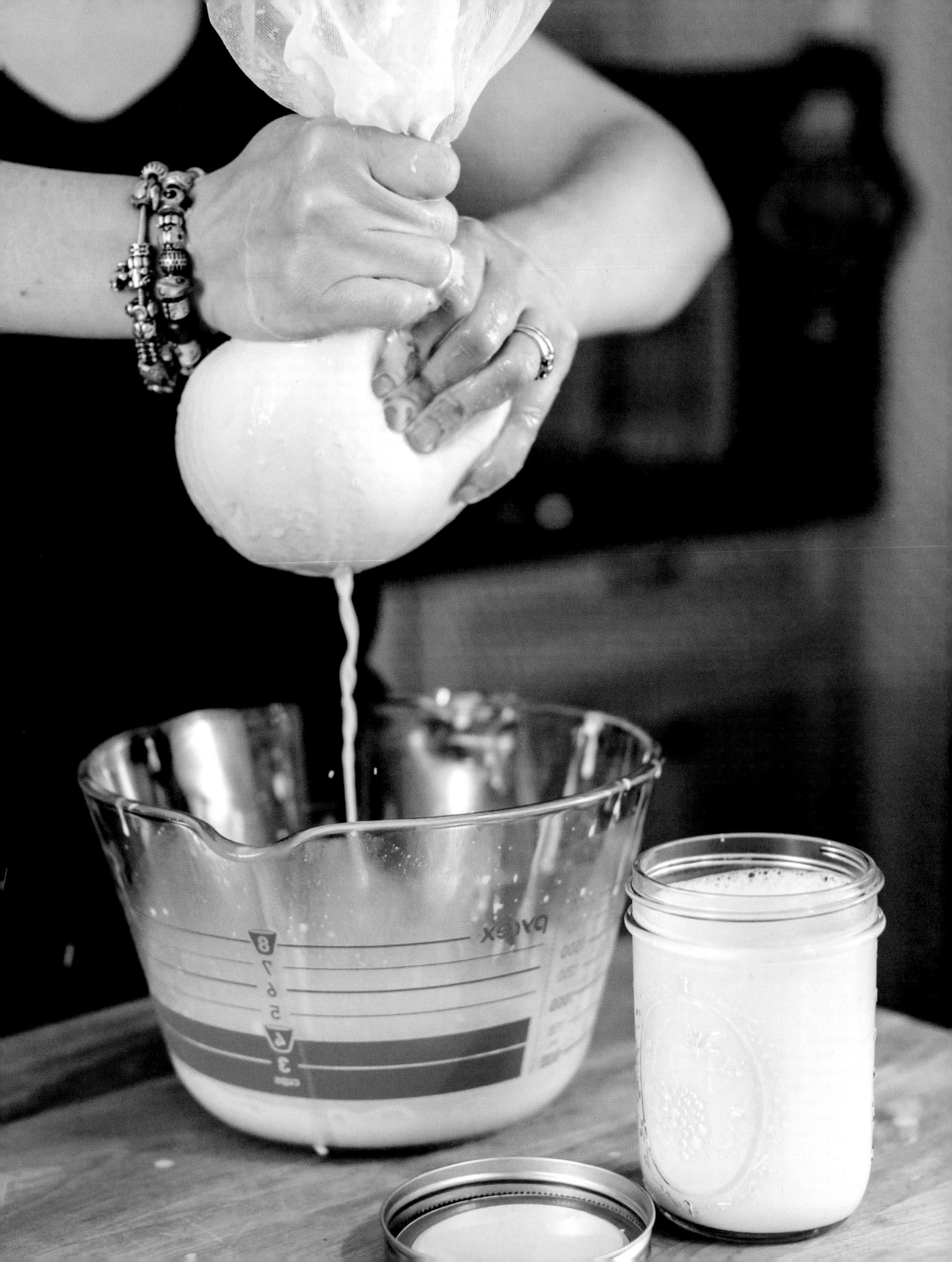

Coconut Milk Yogurt

By using a probiotic supplement instead of a yogurt starter or a spoonful of yogurt from either store-bought or a previous batch of yogurt, you have complete control over which probiotic organisms are in your yogurt. This means that you can have a yeast-free yogurt simply by using a yeast-free supplement. Look for a supplement that has lactobacillus strains (or one that contains both lactobacillus and bifidobacterium strains). Just as diversity is best for supplementation, the same is true for yogurt making. Look for a supplement that contains several different strains.

How many capsules of probiotic supplement you use to start your yogurt will depend on the amount of bacteria in each capsule. The label should specific how many CFU (colony forming units) or PFU (plaque forming units) are in each capsule (the terms are used interchangeably). Anywhere between 10 and 20 billion PFU will work, although this recipe is optimized when an amount closer to 20 billion is used. This might be 1 capsule or 5 capsules, depending on the brand of probiotic you are using.

Yogurt makers marketed for making homemade yogurt for baby food are inexpensive (typically under $20) and very convenient for small batches. You can also easily double or triple this recipe for a larger yogurt maker. If you don't have a yogurt maker, you can find a variety of tricks for incubating the yogurt (keeping it between 100°F and 105°F for an extended period) online.

PREP TIME: 20 minutes (15 of which is spent waiting for the coconut milk to cool)
COOK TIME: 10 to 14 hours for incubation, plus 2 to 3 hours to set
SERVINGS: 4

INGREDIENTS:

1¾ cups homemade Coconut Milk (page 116) or 1 (13½-ounce) can full-fat coconut milk

1¼ teaspoons gelatin

2 teaspoons honey

Lactobacillus-based probiotic supplement, 15 to 20 billion PFU (aka CFU)

SPECIAL EQUIPMENT

- Yogurt maker or other way to keep your yogurt culture warm
- Thermometer

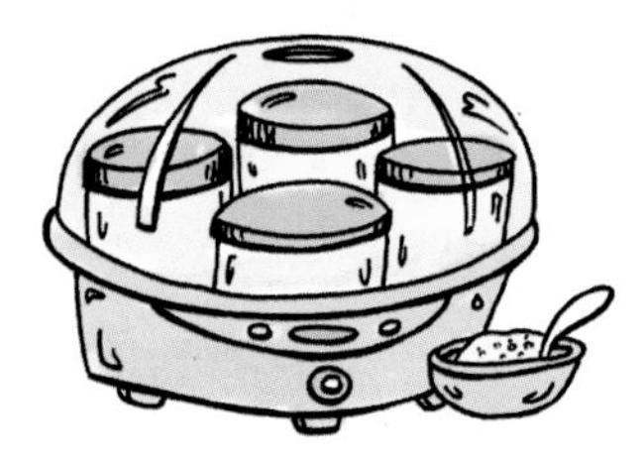

1. Thoroughly clean or sterilize the jar(s) you'll be using to make the yogurt.
2. Pour the coconut milk into a heatproof glass container if planning to heat it in the microwave, or into a saucepan if planning to heat it on the stovetop. Sprinkle the gelatin over the surface and wait 2 to 3 minutes for the gelatin to bloom (this just means that the gelatin is absorbing the liquid). Stir in the gelatin.
3. Heat the coconut milk to 120°F in the microwave or on the stovetop. (If you make this yogurt frequently, you'll quickly find out just how many seconds it takes your microwave to heat the milk perfectly—in my microwave, it's 75 seconds.)
4. Stir thoroughly to make sure that the gelatin has dissolved.
5. Let the milk cool to 105°F. (Anywhere between 100°F and 110°F will work, but don't add your probiotic until the coconut milk is below 110°F.)
6. Stir in the honey. Open the probiotic capsule(s) and sprinkle the contents into the milk. Stir well.
7. Pour into the sterilized jar(s) and incubate for approximately 12 hours (if the yogurt is too sour, incubate for a shorter period next time; if it's not sour enough, incubate longer).
8. Refrigerate the yogurt until the gelatin has set (2 to 3 hours). Stir and enjoy!

FODMAP ALERT *Culturing reduces the already moderate FODMAP content of coconut milk. However, some people with FODMAP intolerance still may not tolerate this yogurt.*

NUTRITION FACTS	
Serving Size	110 g
Recipe Yields	438 g
Calories	**255**
Fats	**25.1 g**
MUFA	1.07 g
Omega-3	0 g
Omega-6	0.27 g
Saturated Fat	22.2 g
Carbohydrates	**8.72 g**
Fiber	2.32 g
Starch	<0.01 g
Fructose	1.44 g
Glucose	1.26 g
Sucrose	0.03 g
Protein	**3.17 g**
Alanine	0.19 g
Arginine	0.45 g
Aspartic acid	0.28 g
Cystine	0.05 g
Glutamic acid	0.63 g
Glycine	0.28 g
Histidine	0.06 g
Isoleucine	0.11 g
Leucine	0.2 g
Lysine	0.14 g
Methionine	0.05 g
Phenylalanine	0.14 g
Proline	0.21 g
Serine	0.15 g
Threonine	0.1 g
Tryptophan	0.03 g
Tyrosine	0.08 g
Valine	0.16 g
Vitamins	
Vitamin B1	0.03 mg
Vitamin B12	0mcg
Vitamin B2	<0.01 mg
Vitamin B3	0.8 mg
Vitamin B5	0.2 mg
Vitamin B6	0.04 mg
Choline	9.35 mg
Folate	17.2 mcg
Vitamin A	0 mcg
Vitamin C	2.96 mg
Vitamin D	0 IU
Vitamin E	0.16 mg
Vitamin K	0.11 mcg
Minerals	
Calcium	17.5 mg
Copper	0.3 mg
Iron	1.75 mg
Magnesium	39.2 mg
Manganese	0.97 mg
Phosphorus	106 mg
Potassium	278 mg
Selenium	6.89 mcg
Sodium	17.6 mg
Zinc	0.71 mg

nutrition content estimated using the USDA database.

TIPS:

The honey in this recipe is to feed the bacteria, not to make the end product taste sweeter. This finished yogurt will be very similar in sweetness to plain dairy yogurt (or perhaps mildly sweeter).

If you don't like the flavor of the yogurt, try a different supplement as a starter.

If you make yogurt frequently, you can add 1 to 2 tablespoons of your previous batch of yogurt to the new batch instead of a probiotic supplement as a starter. However, if you have a yeast sensitivity, it's best to use probiotic supplements every time.

If your yogurt is lumpy when you go to stir it, blend for 20 to 30 seconds in a blender and then let it reset in the fridge.

VARIATIONS:

- *Fruit-Flavored Yogurt. Stir in 3 to 4 tablespoons puréed fresh fruit per cup of yogurt before you eat it. Alternately, stir in 1 to 2 tablespoons no-sugar-added organic jam or jelly per cup of yogurt.*
- *Vanilla Yogurt. Add 1 to 3 teaspoons vanilla extract or ¼ to 1 teaspoon vanilla powder when you heat the coconut milk.*
- *Greek-Style Yogurt. Use coconut cream instead of coconut milk for a creamier, thicker yogurt.*

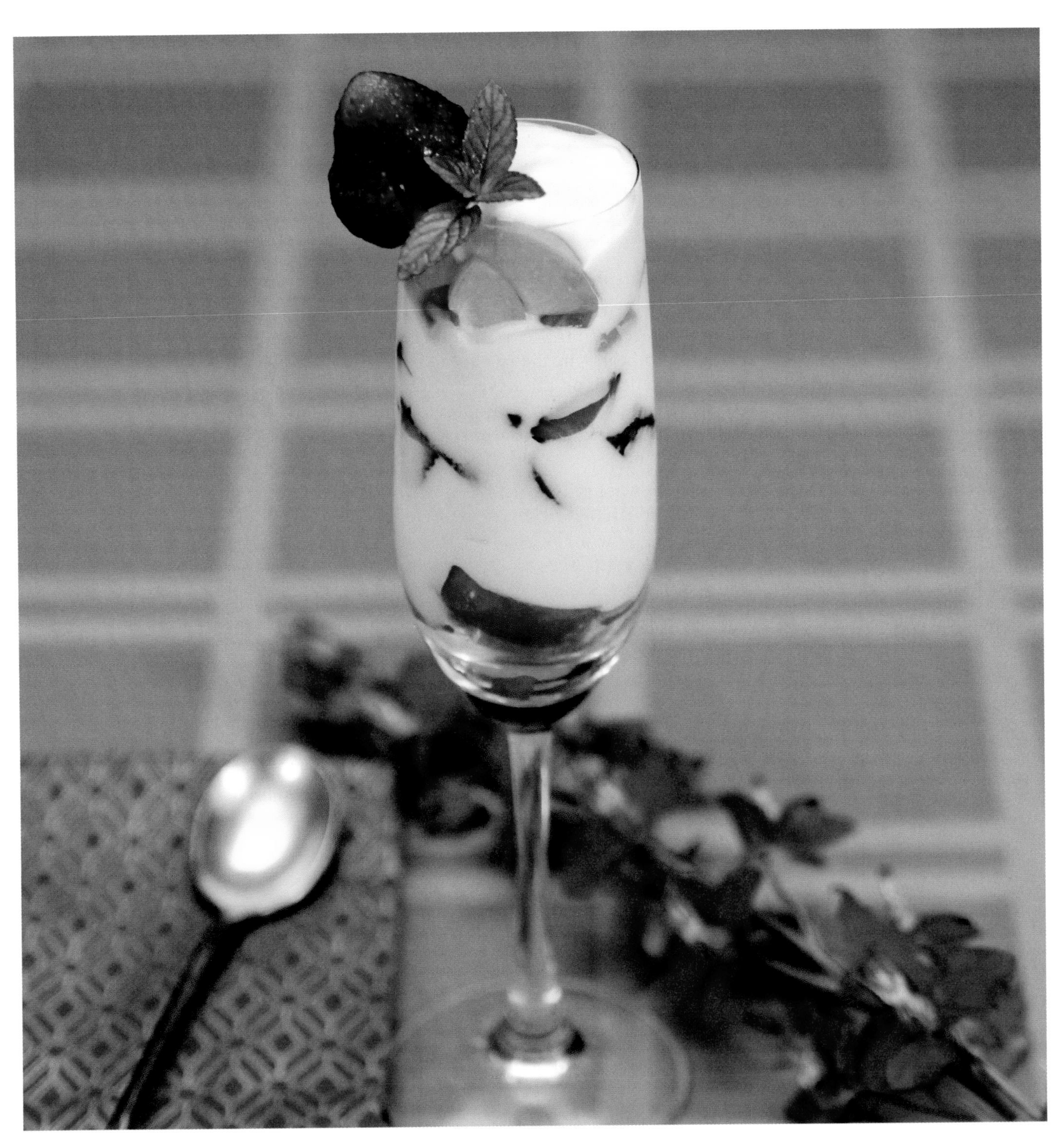

Crispy Bacon and Bacon Bits

As bacon becomes a more routine food in your home, being able to make larger quantities quickly and easily, and without grease splatters all over your kitchen, becomes important. Make sure to use a high-rimmed baking dish to keep grease from spilling over the side when you remove it from your oven!

NUTRITION FACTS	
Serving Size	8 g
Recipe Yields	varies
Calories	**43.3**
Fats	**3.34 g**
MUFA	1.48 g
Omega-3	0.02 g
Omega-6	0.34 g
Saturated Fat	1.1 g
Carbohydrates	**0.11 g**
Fiber	0 g
Starch	0 g
Fructose	0 g
Glucose	0 g
Sucrose	0 g
Protein	**2.96 g**
Alanine	0.2 g
Arginine	0.2 g
Aspartic acid	0.29 g
Cystine	0.03 g
Glutamic acid	0.45 g
Glycine	0.22 g
Histidine	0.12 g
Isoleucine	0.14 g
Leucine	0.24 g
Lysine	0.25 g
Methionine	0.07 g
Phenylalanine	0.12 g
Proline	0.17 g
Serine	0.12 g
Threonine	0.12 g
Tryptophan	0.03 g
Tyrosine	0.1 g
Valine	0.16 g
Vitamins	
Vitamin B1	0.03 mg
Vitamin B12	0.1 mcg
Vitamin B2	0.02 mg
Vitamin B3	0.89 mg
Vitamin B5	0.09 mg
Vitamin B6	0.03 mg
Choline	9.86 mg
Folate	0.16 mcg
Vitamin A	0.88 mcg
Vitamin C	0 mg
Vitamin D	3.36 IU
Vitamin E	0.02 mg
Vitamin K	<0.01 mcg
Minerals	
Calcium	0.88 mg
Copper	0.01 mg
Iron	0.12 mg
Magnesium	2.64 mg
Manganese	<0.01 mg
Phosphorus	42.6 mg
Potassium	45.2 mg
Selenium	4.96 mcg
Sodium	137 mg
Zinc	0.28 mg

nutrition content estimated using the USDA database.

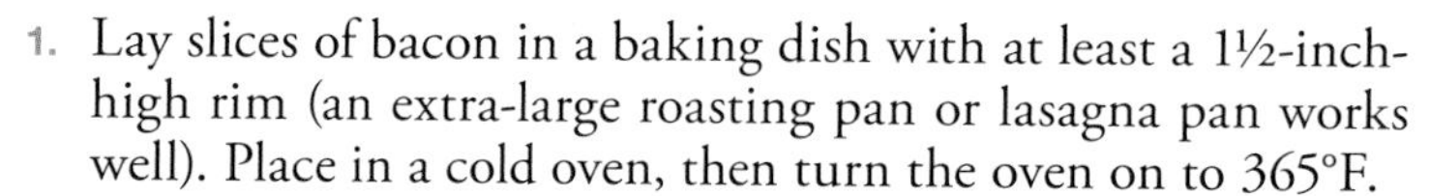

PREP TIME: 5 minutes
COOK TIME: 10 to 20 minutes
YIELD: variable

INGREDIENTS:

bacon

SPECIAL EQUIPMENT

- High-rimmed baking dish

1. Lay slices of bacon in a baking dish with at least a 1½-inch-high rim (an extra-large roasting pan or lasagna pan works well). Place in a cold oven, then turn the oven on to 365°F.
2. Most bacon will be perfectly cooked, lightly browned and crispy, around the time your oven has finished preheating. If your bacon is thinly sliced, watch it, because it may be done before your oven beeps to tell you that it has reached temperature. If you have very thick-cut bacon, it may need to cook for 3 to 5 more minutes after your oven comes to temperature. If you like your bacon on the soft side, simply remove it from the oven a few minutes earlier.
3. To make bacon bits, chop the crispy bacon with a knife or break it apart with your fingers. Store in an airtight container in the fridge until ready to use.

Fun Fact: The reason this works so well is that bacon is best when heated slowly. If you prefer to cook your bacon in a skillet on the stovetop, lay it in a cold skillet and then turn on the heat.

TIPS:

As you cook bacon more frequently, you will get to know exactly how long it takes in your oven to cook to your liking. You may want to set a timer the first few times you cook bacon this way, just to measure how long it takes. Then you can start using your timer to time bacon so it becomes something you don't have to watch anymore. Remember that if you switch brands, or even if your farmer uses a different meat processor, it will likely affect how long it takes the bacon to cook.

Some bacon, especially bacon cured with a lot of sugar or natural sweeteners like maple syrup, just doesn't crisp well; it is likely to burn before it goes crisp, even when cooked at a lower temperature. Save it for recipes like Bacon-Braised Brussels Sprouts (page 321) or Bacon-Apple Chicken Burgers with Maple-Cranberry Sauce (page 222).

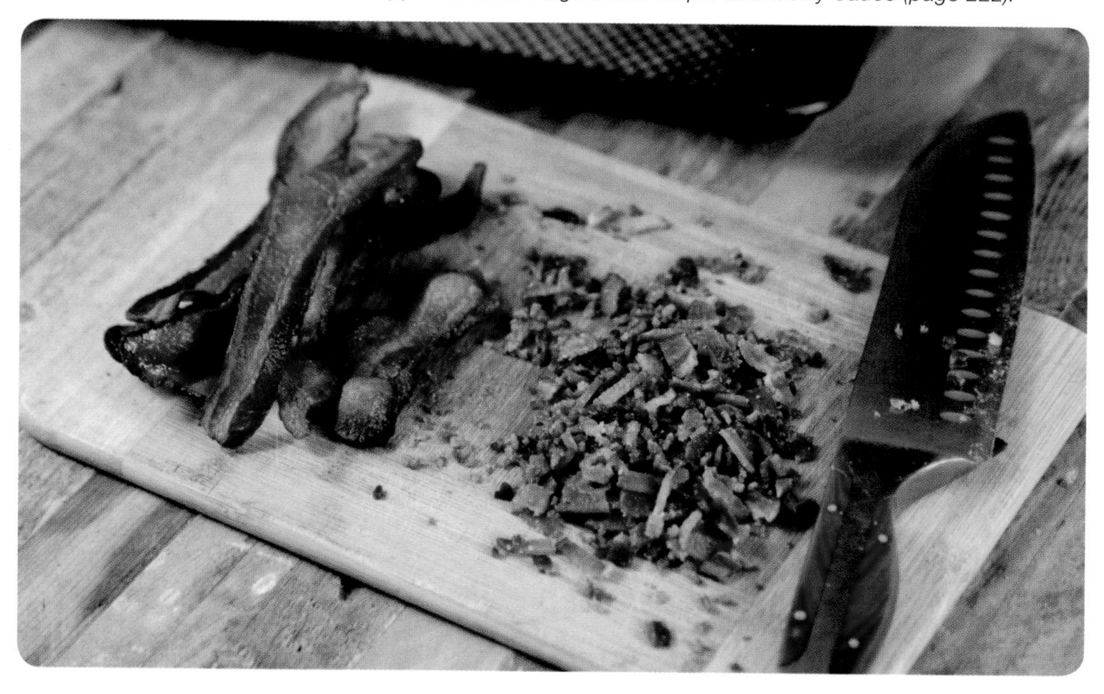

Homemade Fruit and Vegetable Flours

While many of the flour substitutes used in this book (such as arrowroot powder, coconut flour, and tapioca flour) are easily found in the baking section of most grocery stores, some will require ordering online or seeking out in specialty stores. If you're having trouble sourcing pumpkin flour, sweet potato flour, water chestnut flour, or plantain flour, don't worry, because you can make it at home!

You can actually make homemade vegetable powders from a wide array of vegetables. Many of these can be used in baking or added to soups, stews, and sauces to thicken them. Go ahead and be adventurous!

PREP TIME: 20 minutes
COOK TIME: 12 to 24 hours
YIELD: 4 to 6 tablespoons per 1 cup pumpkin puree or sweet potato mash, ⅓ to ½ cup plantain flour per large green plantain, 2 to 4 tablespoons per 5-ounce can water chestnuts

INGREDIENTS:

For Pumpkin Flour:

Mashed cooked pumpkin or canned pumpkin

For Sweet Potato Flour:

Mashed cooked sweet potato

For Plantain Flour:

Peeled and sliced raw green plantain

For Water Chestnut Flour:

Canned sliced water chestnuts, rinsed and drained

1. To make pumpkin or sweet potato flour, spread out the mash on one or two fruit roll sheets in a dehydrator (if you don't own a fruit roll sheet, use parchment paper to line the racks). To make plantain or water chestnut flour, lay the slices of plantain or water chestnut on the dehydrator racks.
2. Dehydrate until completely hard (12 to 24 hours, depending on the dehydrator).
3. Process in a food processor or blender until it's a fine powder.

TIPS:

Pumpkin Puree. *The easiest way to cook fresh pumpkins for pumpkin puree is to pierce the skin a couple of times with a fork or knife and place the whole pumpkins in a 350°F oven for about 1 hour (or longer if your pumpkins are big). Let cool. The seeds and rind will be easy to remove, and the flesh can easily be mashed with a fork, wire potato masher, or immersion blender.*

Sweet Potato Mash. *The easiest way to cook sweet potato for mashed sweet potato is to boil 2 or 3 whole sweet potatoes in a saucepot or stockpot with enough water to cover until the sweet potatoes easily slide off a knife when pierced, typically 40 to 50 minutes, depending on the size of your sweet potatoes. Rinse with cold water until cool enough to handle, and the peel will come off easily. Mash with a fork, wire potato masher, or immersion blender. To serve as a side dish, add a little lard or coconut oil and salt to taste.*

SPECIAL EQUIPMENT

- Dehydrator
- Food processor or blender

FODMAP ALERT

Do not use Sweet Potato Flour.

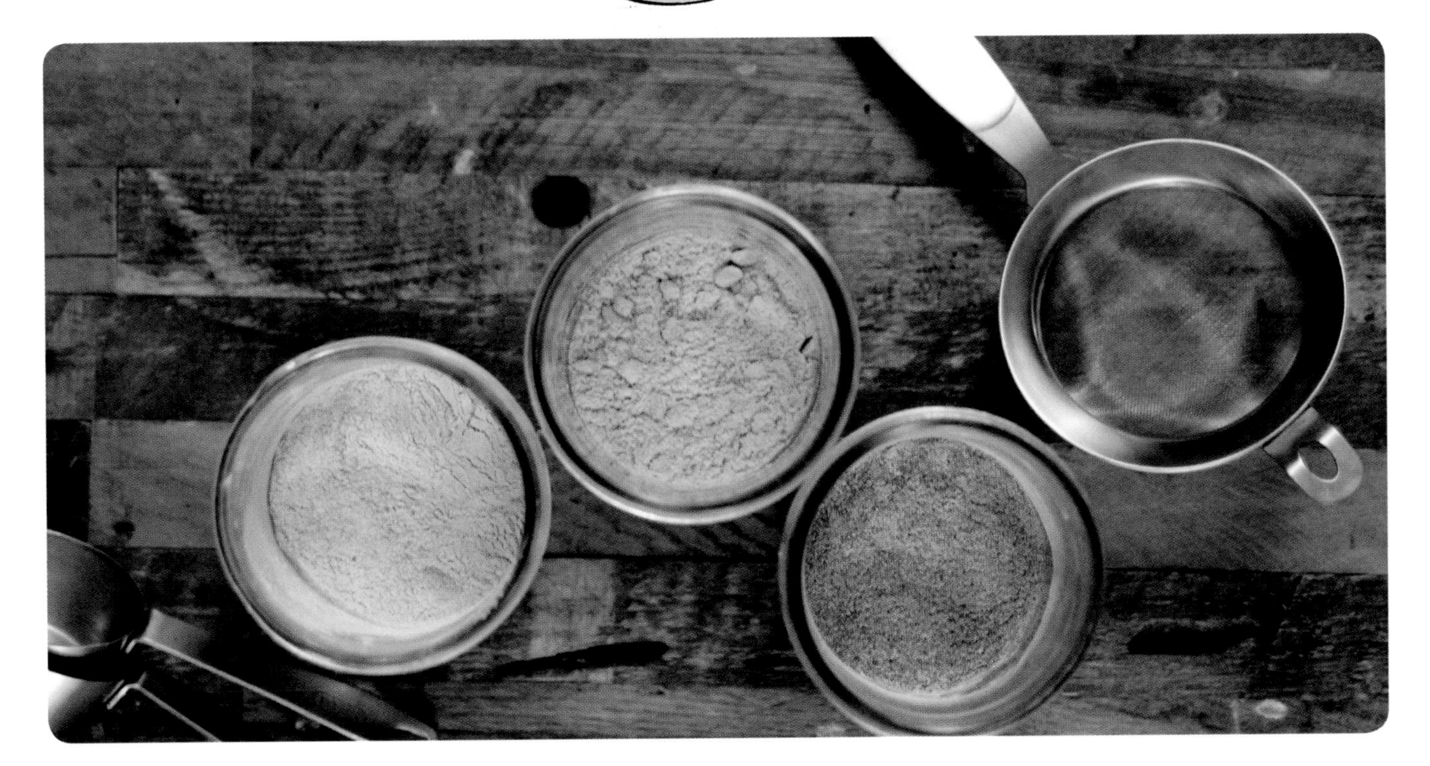

Applesauce

I like to keep plain applesauce in my freezer to serve with pork, spice up for a dessert on its own, or use as an ingredient in a variety of treats (see Applesauce Spice Cake on page 362).

This recipe can easily be scaled up or down depending on how many apples you have and how much applesauce you want to make.

PREP TIME: 10 to 30 minutes
COOK TIME: 20 minutes
YIELD: 3 cups

INGREDIENTS:

4 or 5 apples (about 2½ pounds)

¼ cup water

1. Peel and core the apples. There's no need to cut them up too small.
2. Place the apples and water in a large pot and cover. Bring to a simmer over high heat, then reduce the heat to medium.
3. Simmer until the apples are soft, about 20 minutes (less if your apple pieces are smaller, more if they are larger). The cooking time will also vary depending on the apple variety.
4. Let cool. Mash with a potato masher or fork for a lumpier consistency or with an immersion blender for a smoother consistency. Some varieties of apple won't need to be mashed at all.

FODMAP ALERT

This recipe cannot be made low-FODMAP.

SPECIAL EQUIPMENT

- Apple peeler (optional)
- Immersion blender or potato masher

VARIATIONS:

Spiced Applesauce. Add ½ to 1 teaspoon each ground cinnamon and mace, plus a pinch of ground cloves, to 1 cup applesauce.

Spiced Applesauce Sorbet. Put 4 cups spiced applesauce in an ice cream maker and churn following the manufacturer's instructions.

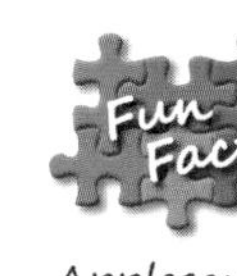

The best apple varieties for making applesauce are considered to be McIntosh, Jonathan, Winesap, Jonagold, Cortland, and Braeburn. However, any variety or combination of varieties will work. Applesauce is a great use for "bruisies" or "seconds," which can often be purchased at a heavy discount directly from the farmer.

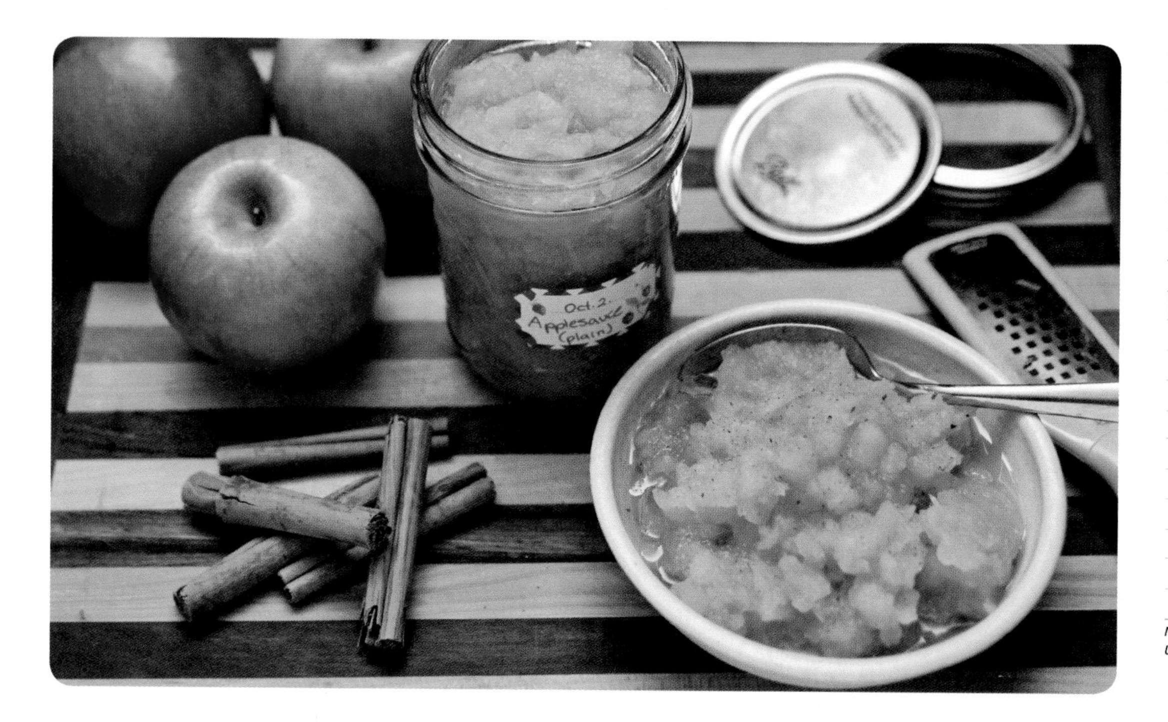

NUTRITION FACTS	
Serving Size	199 g
Recipe Yields	1194 g
Calories	**100**
Fats	**0.68 g**
MUFA	0.03 g
Omega-3	0.03 g
Omega-6	0.16 g
Saturated Fat	0.11 g
Carbohydrates	**25.8 g**
Fiber	4.54 g
Starch	0.43 g
Fructose	0 g
Glucose	0 g
Sucrose	0 g
Protein	**0.49 g**
Alanine	0 g
Arginine	0 g
Aspartic acid	0 g
Cystine	0 g
Glutamic acid	0 g
Glycine	0 g
Histidine	0 g
Isoleucine	0 g
Leucine	0 g
Lysine	0 g
Methionine	0 g
Phenylalanine	0 g
Proline	0 g
Serine	0 g
Threonine	0 g
Tryptophan	0 g
Tyrosine	0 g
Valine	0 g
Vitamins	
Vitamin B1	0.03 mg
Vitamin B12	0 mcg
Vitamin B2	0.02 mg
Vitamin B3	0.18 mg
Vitamin B5	0.09 mg
Vitamin B6	0.08 mg
Choline	6.43 mg
Folate	1.89 mcg
Vitamin A	3.78 mcg
Vitamin C	0.38 mg
Vitamin D	0 IU
Vitamin E	0.09 mg
Vitamin K	1.13 mcg
Minerals	
Calcium	9.45 mg
Copper	0.07 mg
Iron	0.36 mg
Magnesium	5.67 mg
Manganese	0.22 mg
Phosphorus	15.1 mg
Potassium	166 mg
Selenium	0.57 mcg
Sodium	1.89 mg
Zinc	0.08 mg

nutrition content estimated using the USDA database.

Cauliflower Gravy

This gravy is a welcome addition to any meal. While it qualifies as a vegetable side dish and is full of healing bone broth all on its own, I just had to include it in the Kitchen Basics chapter!

PREP TIME: 5 to 10 minutes
COOK TIME: 20 minutes
YIELD: 3 cups

INGREDIENTS:

- ½ head cauliflower, cut into florets
- 1½ cups Bone Broth (chicken or beef, page 110)
- 1 clove garlic
- Salt, to taste

1. Place the cauliflower in a saucepot with the broth and garlic. Bring to a boil, then reduce the heat to maintain a simmer. Simmer for 15 to 20 minutes, until the cauliflower is overcooked.
2. Pour the mixture into a high-speed blender. Blend for 1 minute, until completely smooth. Taste and season with salt if desired. If too thick, thin with additional broth or water.

VARIATIONS:

You can also use lamb or pork broth for this recipe.

Cream of Cauliflower Soup. Thin the gravy with ½ to 1 cup additional broth or coconut milk. Add 3 tablespoons chopped fresh parsley, chives, or a mix of tarragon and thyme. Enjoy warm or as a chilled soup with a dollop of Coconut Milk Yogurt (page 118).

FODMAP ALERT

This recipe cannot be made low-FODMAP.

SPECIAL EQUIPMENT

- Blender

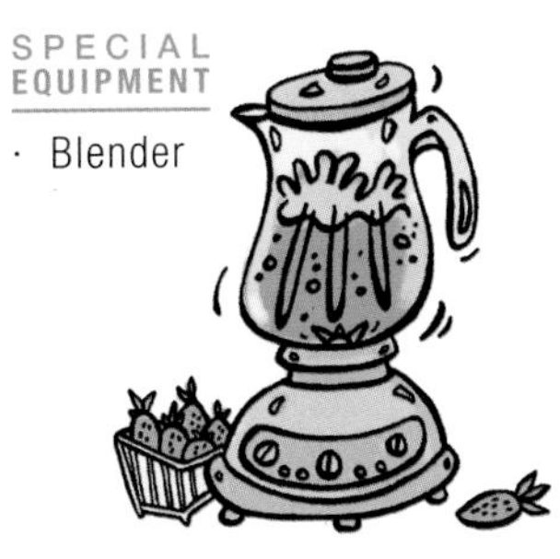

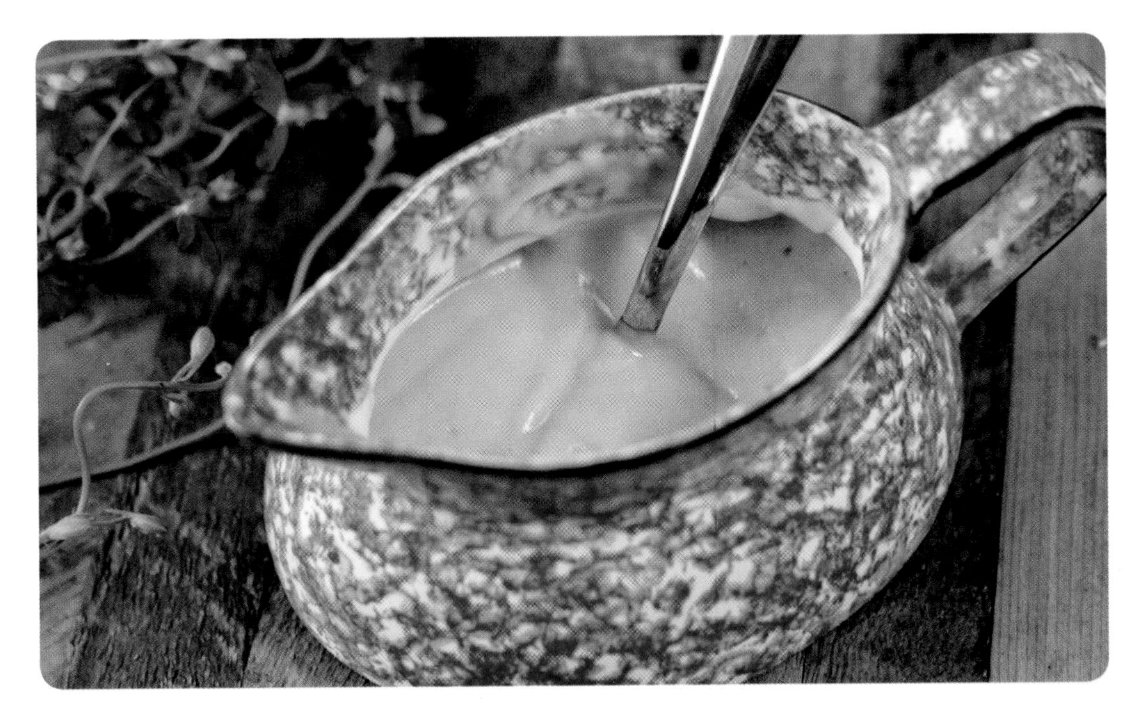

NUTRITION FACTS	
Serving Size	66 g
Recipe Yields	657 g
Calories	**13.6**
Fats	**0.3 g**
MUFA	0.1 g
Omega-3	<0.01 g
Omega-6	0.04 g
Saturated Fat	0.08 g
Carbohydrates	**2 g**
Fiber	0.6 g
Starch	0.4 g
Fructose	0.29 g
Glucose	0.28 g
Sucrose	0 g
Protein	**1.31 g**
Alanine	0.03 g
Arginine	0.03 g
Aspartic acid	0.05 g
Cystine	<0.01 g
Glutamic acid	0.08 g
Glycine	0.02 g
Histidine	0.02 g
Isoleucine	0.02 g
Leucine	0.03 g
Lysine	0.06 g
Methionine	<0.01 g
Phenylalanine	0.02 g
Proline	0.02 g
Serine	0.03 g
Threonine	0.02 g
Tryptophan	<0.01 g
Tyrosine	0.02 g
Valine	0.04 g
Vitamins	
Vitamin B1	0.02 mg
Vitamin B12	0.04 mcg
Vitamin B2	0.03 mg
Vitamin B3	0.65 mg
Vitamin B5	0.2 mg
Vitamin B6	0.06 mg
Choline	14.3 mg
Folate	16.8 mcg
Vitamin A	0 mcg
Vitamin C	14.3 mg
Vitamin D	0 IU
Vitamin E	0.02 mg
Vitamin K	4.58 mcg
Minerals	
Calcium	8.52 mg
Copper	0.03 mg
Iron	0.2 mg
Magnesium	4.87 mg
Manganese	0.05 mg
Phosphorus	24.3 mg
Potassium	121 mg
Selenium	0.22 mcg
Sodium	34.3 mg
Zinc	0.12 mg

nutrition content estimated using the USDA database.

Barbecue Sauce

Barbecue sauce without gluten or nightshades? Yes! This barbecue sauce is incredibly flavorful and versatile. Use it to season hamburgers, steak, chicken . . . any meat that you want to grill. It can be stored in the fridge for up to a week or in the freezer for up to two months. Go ahead and make a double or triple batch to have on hand!

PREP TIME: 20 minutes
COOK TIME: 25 to 30 minutes
YIELD: 2 cups

INGREDIENTS:

- 2 tablespoons red palm oil
- 1 large yellow onion, diced
- 1 apple, peeled, cored, and grated
- ¼ cup molasses
- ⅓ cup apple cider vinegar
- 1 tablespoon peeled and grated fresh ginger
- 1½ tablespoons fish sauce
- ¼ teaspoon ground mace
- 1 clove garlic, crushed
- 1 teaspoon ground turmeric
- Pinch of ground cinnamon

1. Heat the palm oil in a saucepan over medium-high heat. Add the onion and sauté for 10 to 15 minutes, until caramelized.
2. Add the remaining ingredients. Bring to a boil, then reduce the heat to maintain a simmer. Simmer uncovered for 15 minutes.
3. Remove from the heat and purée with an immersion blender.

TIPS:

This barbecue sauce tastes best on meat cooked on a charcoal grill or in a smoker. If you plan to use an indoor grill or bake your meat in the oven, consider adding a drop or two of liquid smoke to the sauce.

VARIATIONS:

Replace half to all of the molasses with tamarind paste or pomegranate molasses.

FODMAP ALERT

This recipe cannot be made low-FODMAP.

SPECIAL EQUIPMENT

- Immersion blender

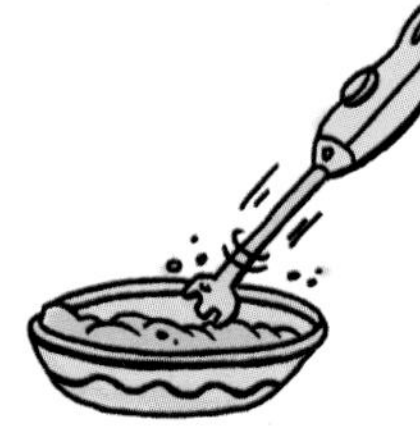

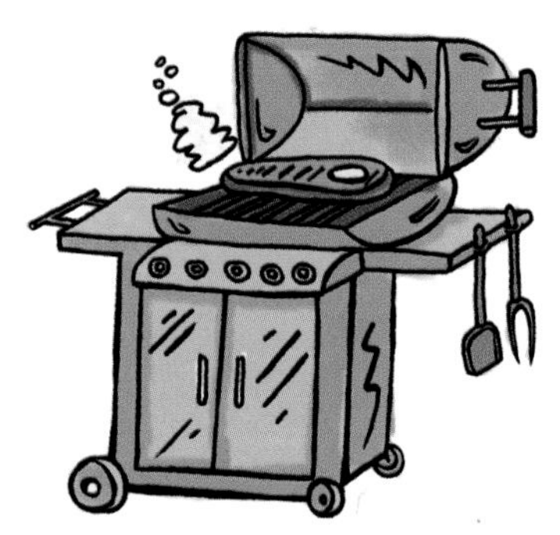

NUTRITION FACTS

Serving Size	32 g
Recipe Yields	519 g
Calories	**41.4**
Fats	**1.75 g**
MUFA	0.63 g
Omega-3	<0.01 g
Omega-6	0.17 g
Saturated Fat	0.84 g
Carbohydrates	**6.38 g**
Fiber	0.3 g
Starch	0.31 g
Fructose	1.41 g
Glucose	1.13 g
Sucrose	1.79 g
Protein	**0.25 g**
Alanine	0.01 g
Arginine	0.02 g
Aspartic acid	0.02 g
Cystine	<0.01 g
Glutamic acid	0.04 g
Glycine	0.01 g
Histidine	<0.01 g
Isoleucine	<0.01 g
Leucine	0.01 g
Lysine	0.02 g
Methionine	<0.01 g
Phenylalanine	<0.01 g
Proline	<0.01 g
Serine	<0.01 g
Threonine	<0.01 g
Tryptophan	<0.01 g
Tyrosine	<0.01 g
Valine	0.01 g
Vitamins	
Vitamin B1	<0.01 mg
Vitamin B12	<0.01 mcg
Vitamin B2	<0.01 mg
Vitamin B3	0.12 mg
Vitamin B5	0.06 mg
Vitamin B6	0.06 mg
Choline	2.04 mg
Folate	2.18 mcg
Vitamin A	0.29 mcg
Vitamin C	0.95 mg
Vitamin D	0 IU
Vitamin E	0.28 mg
Vitamin K	0.26 mcg
Minerals	
Calcium	15.1 mg
Copper	0.04 mg
Iron	0.37 mg
Magnesium	17.8 mg
Manganese	0.13 mg
Phosphorus	6.89 mg
Potassium	114 mg
Selenium	1.18 mcg
Sodium	135 mg
Zinc	0.05 mg

nutrition content estimated using the USDA database.

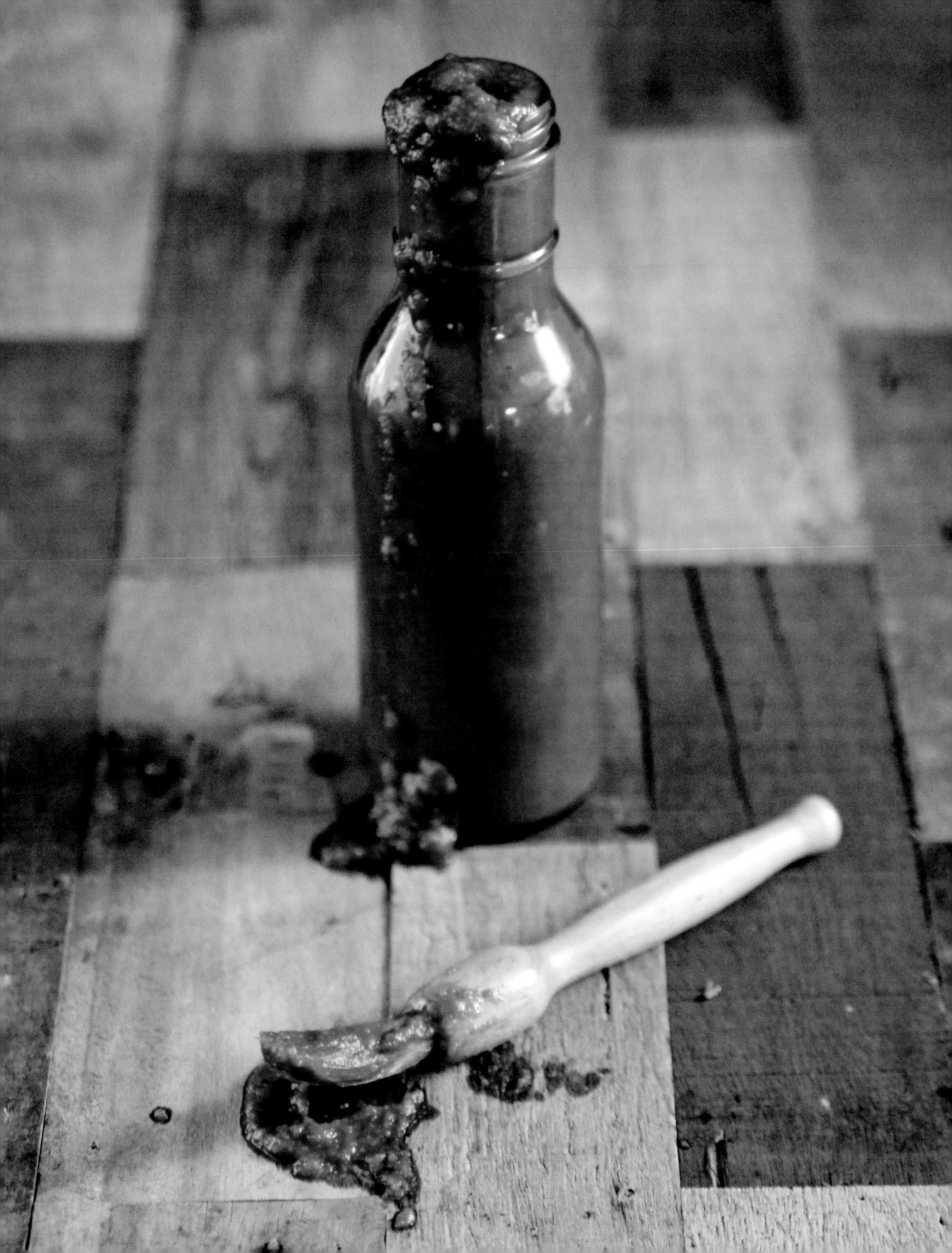

Salad Dressing

Finding salad dressings made with high-quality fats, acids, and herbs can be a challenge. Fortunately, it doesn't take much time to make your own, and most of these variations will keep for quite a while in the fridge.

These dressings are placed here in the Kitchen Basics chapter because while dressing salads may be their most common use, they can be used to flavor many different dishes. For example, use them as a marinade for your favorite meat, or pour them over Perfect Steamed Vegetables (page 296) to add a little pizzazz.

INGREDIENTS:

Basic Vinaigrette

3 tablespoons oil, such as extra-virgin olive oil, avocado oil, walnut oil, or macadamia nut oil

2 tablespoons acidic liquid, such as fresh lemon juice, fresh lime juice, apple cider vinegar, balsamic vinegar, coconut water vinegar, or white or red wine vinegar

Pinch of salt

Creamy Balsamic Dressing

¼ cup extra-virgin olive oil

½ cup balsamic vinegar

¼ medium avocado

Pinch of salt or truffle salt

Greek Salad Dressing

½ cup extra-virgin olive oil

2 tablespoons fresh lemon juice

⅓ cup apple cider vinegar or red wine vinegar

1 teaspoon dried oregano leaves

2 cloves garlic, crushed

1 teaspoon grated lemon zest

⅛ teaspoon salt

Thai Salad Dressing

¼ cup fresh lime juice

2 tablespoons fish sauce

½ teaspoon honey

1 clove garlic, crushed

2 tablespoons chopped fresh cilantro

1 tablespoon chopped fresh mint

Italian Vinaigrette

6 tablespoons extra-virgin olive oil

¼ cup apple cider vinegar

¼ teaspoon dried oregano leaves

¼ teaspoon dried rosemary

¼ teaspoon dried marjoram leaves

¼ teaspoon dried thyme leaves

¼ teaspoon dried savory

1 clove garlic, crushed

Pinch of salt

PREP TIME: 5 to 10 minutes

SERVINGS: 2 to 8

SPECIAL EQUIPMENT

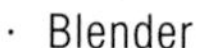

- Blender

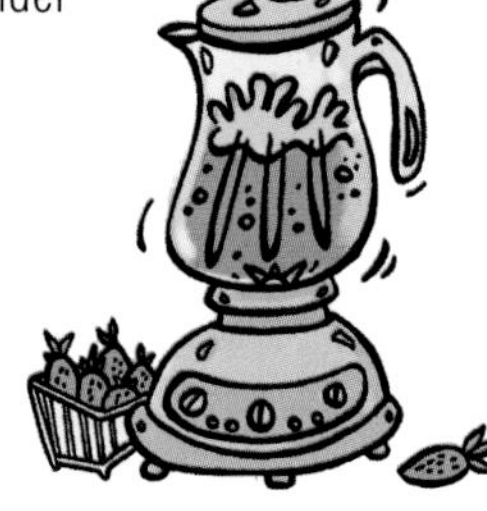

1. Combine all the ingredients in a blender. (If making the Basic Vinaigrette, simply combine the ingredients in a jar and shake before serving.)
2. Blend until fully combined.
3. Store in the fridge and warm to room temperature before serving (just take it out of the fridge about 30 minutes before mealtime). Creamy Balsamic Dressing and Thai Salad Dressing will keep in the fridge for 3 to 4 days. The other dressings will keep for about a month.

FODMAP ALERT *Replace the garlic with green garlic or garlic scapes (green part only) or omit. Do not make the Creamy Balsamic Dressing. Instead of honey in the Thai Salad Dressing, use ¼ teaspoon evaporated cane juice.*

NUTRITION FACTS	
Serving Size	19.6 g
Recipe Yields	157 g
Calories	**70.5**
Fats	**7.32 g**
MUFA	5.32 g
Omega-3	0.06 g
Omega-6	0.72 g
Saturated Fat	1.01 g
Carbohydrates	**1.12 g**
Fiber	0.13 g
Starch	0.23 g
Fructose	0.3 g
Glucose	0.3 g
Sucrose	0.01 g
Protein	**0.12 g**
Alanine	0 g
Arginine	0 g
Aspartic acid	0.01 g
Cystine	0 g
Glutamic acid	0.01 g
Glycine	0 g
Histidine	0 g
Isoleucine	0 g
Leucine	0 g
Lysine	0 g
Methionine	0 g
Phenylalanine	0 g
Proline	0 g
Serine	0 g
Threonine	0 g
Tryptophan	0 g
Tyrosine	0 g
Valine	0 g
Vitamins	
Vitamin B1	0 mg
Vitamin B12	0 mcg
Vitamin B2	0 mg
Vitamin B3	0.05 mg
Vitamin B5	0.02 mg
Vitamin B6	0.01 mg
Choline	0.53 mg
Folate	1.99 mcg
Vitamin A	0.49 mcg
Vitamin C	1.07 mg
Vitamin D	0 IU
Vitamin E	1.06 mg
Vitamin K	5.09 mcg
Minerals	
Calcium	3.92 mg
Copper	0.01 mg
Iron	0.2 mg
Magnesium	2.95 mg
Manganese	0.03 mg
Phosphorus	2.54 mg
Potassium	20.8 mg
Selenium	0.14 mcg
Sodium	83.1 mg
Zinc	0.02 mg

nutrition content estimated using the USDA database. values are based on an average of all variations.

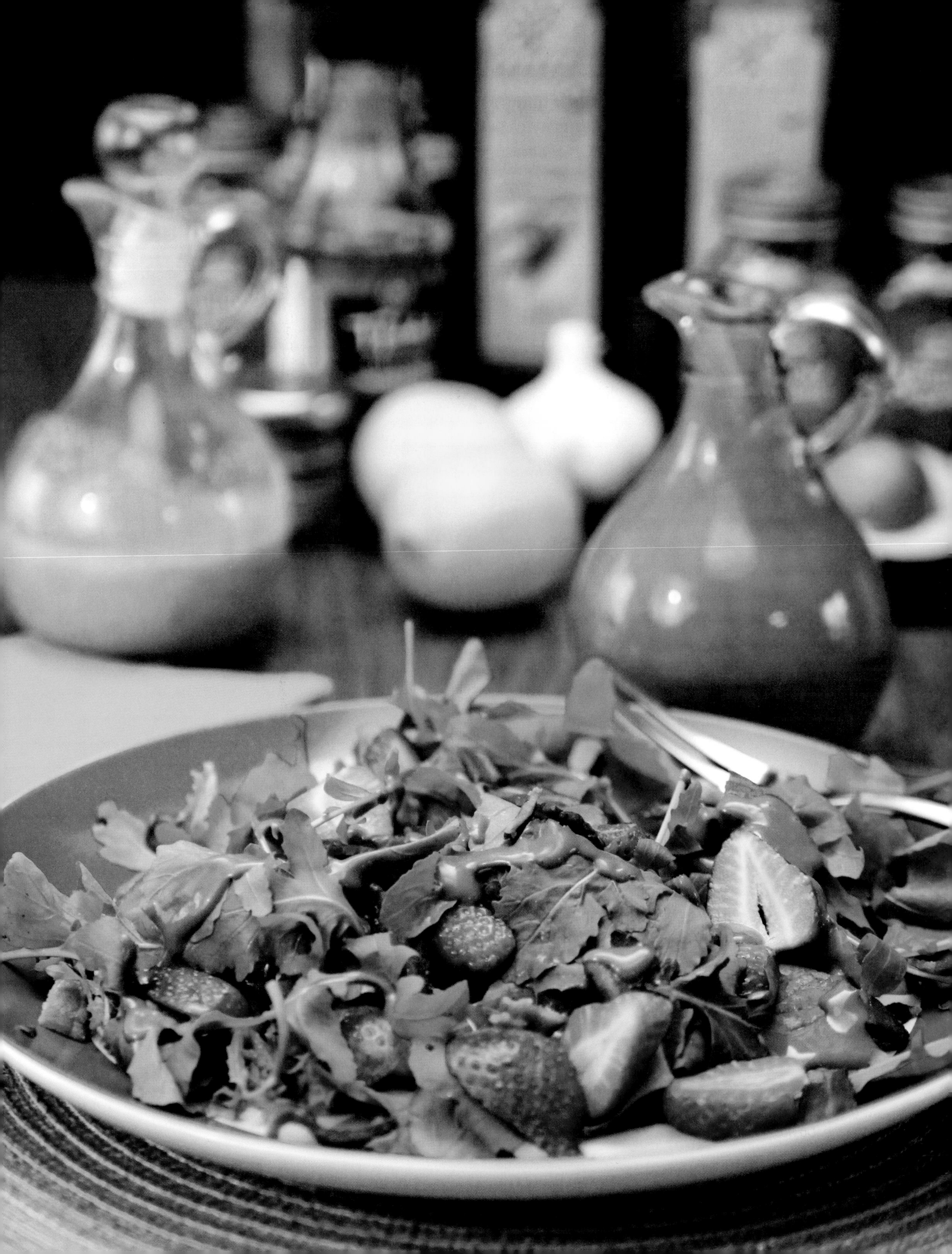

Chapter 5
Breakfast Foods

breakfast [brek.fəst]: *A meal eaten in the morning, the first of the day.*

Nowhere in the definition of breakfast does it say "scrambled eggs and toast" or "toaster waffles with blueberry syrup" or "steel-cut oats with brown sugar and cream." There is no need to redefine what breakfast means, because the definition is already pretty accurate. Breakfast is whatever you eat for your first meal of the day. Although you may have to adjust your preconceived notions of which foods make good breakfast options.

Any food that is good for your body can be a breakfast food. Leftovers make a fantastically quick and simple breakfast and typically provide a better balance of animal- and plant-based foods than what many of us are used to eating for breakfast. Soups and stews can be extremely satisfying meals to wake up to, and they are easy to digest and rich in glycine. For busy weekday mornings, it's nice to have something quick to prepare, and anything that simply requires reheating (or can be eaten cold) fits the bill.

If you really want to have "normal" breakfast foods, there are some great options. Bacon, sausage (provided it's made with Paleo Approach–friendly seasonings), and kippers are traditional breakfast proteins that can still be enjoyed. Berries or grapefruit make an excellent and familiar addition, maybe with some coconut milk yogurt. Sauerkraut is a delicious accompaniment to sausage. Throw in some leftover salad, veggie sticks, and/or steamed or braised vegetables and you have a wonderfully balanced meal, albeit one that may be starting to look unfamiliar again.

While this chapter focuses on reproductions of more familiar breakfast foods, I urge you to be creative and start thinking of breakfast as just another opportunity to nourish your body with health-promoting foods.

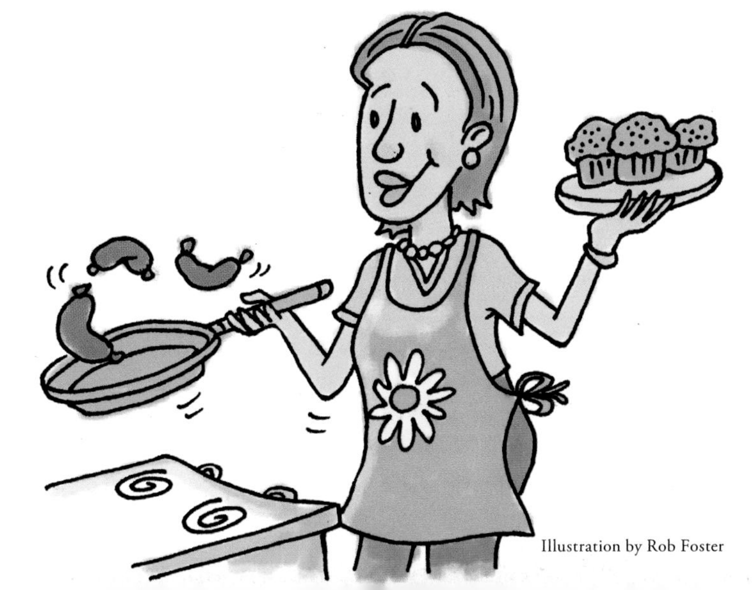

Illustration by Rob Foster

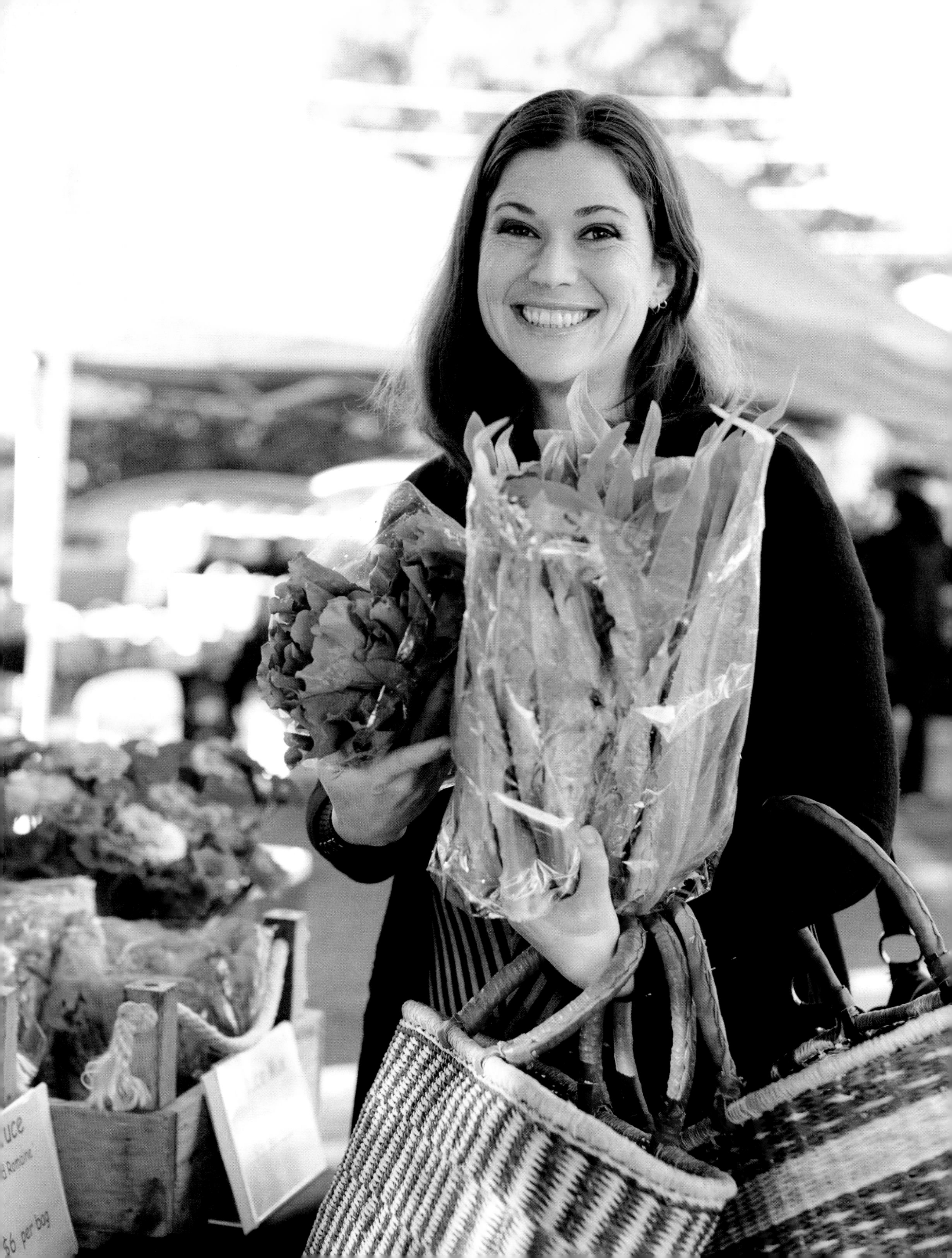
$6 per bag

Homemade Sausage (9 Variations)

Sausage is a great source of protein. It is also an excellent opportunity to camouflage organ meat and start your day with a terrifically nutrient-dense meal. And of course, sausage is delicious at any time of the day!

It can be challenging to source premade sausage made with high-quality meat and exclusively Paleo Approach–friendly seasonings. Fortunately, sausage is very easy to make at home. Sausage is just spiced ground meat, after all.

With a little planning, you can make two or three different types of sausage at once to give you a month or even two months of easy breakfasts with a choice of flavors in the morning—all for a 1- to 4-hour time commitment.

To keep you feeling as if you're not missing a thing, you will find below a variety of traditional and regional sausage styles. As you become a practiced sausage maker, you'll learn how a small tweak in spices can make a big difference in the taste of the finished product, and you'll soon come up with your own variations. My favorite is Farmer's Sausage made with 2 pounds ground beef heart, 2 pounds ground bison liver, and 2 pounds ground pork. Delicious!

Sausage usually works better with dried spices, because grinding dried spices before adding them to the meat makes it much easier to get uniform seasoning. However, some spices just don't have any flavor after being dried (including basil and parsley, which are used in the recipes below). If you are using fresh spices, make sure to chop them very, very finely, which helps distribute the flavor more thoroughly. You may substitute fresh herbs wherever you see dried herbs if you prefer. As a general rule, 1 teaspoon dried herbs is equivalent to 1 tablespoon fresh.

When making sausage, typically the fattier the meat used, the better the sausage tastes. Aim for a 30- to 40-percent fat content (or 60- to 70-percent lean). Depending on where you source your meat, this might mean adding a little fat (or using it straight out of the package). If you are buying your meat from a butcher, you can ask them to grind some fat trimmings to add to ground meat (typically done at no extra charge or for a nominal fee). If you are grinding your own meat, you can use the fattiest cuts to make sausage and even add extra fat (which you might have on hand if you bought half a pig or cow, for example). If getting a little extra fat into your ground meat to make sausage just isn't practical, don't worry about it. The sausages will be more reminiscent of spiced hamburgers, but they'll still be good.

Sausage really is best when stuffed into casings, because the casings help retain fat and moisture throughout cooking. Most home meat grinders come with sausage stuffer attachments, and natural hog casings are fairly inexpensive. A meat grinder is a worthwhile investment if you think that you might enjoy sausage frequently. The sausage can then be parboiled and frozen for quick breakfasts all week long (or more!).

Don't fret if stuffing sausage into casings is too much work or too daunting of a task for you. There's no rule that says sausage has to be stuffed into casings. You can try it loose (add some veggies to make a scramble or some grated root vegetables to make a hash!) or form it into patties. These can be precooked by baking or pan-frying and then frozen for quick breakfasts all week long (or more!).

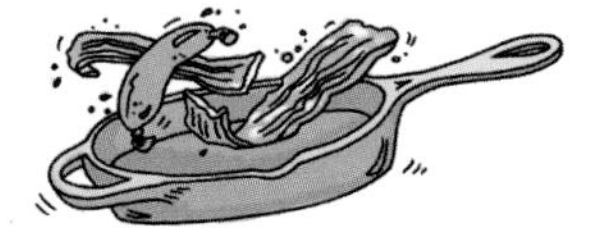

NUTRITION FACTS	
Serving Size	119 g
Recipe Yields	2273 g
Calories	**306**
Fats	**20.1 g**
MUFA	8.9 g
Omega-3	0.1 g
Omega-6	1.51 g
Saturated Fat	7.5 g
Carbohydrates	**0.86 g**
Fiber	0.17 g
Starch	0.14 g
Fructose	0.21 g
Glucose	0.11 g
Sucrose	0.11 g
Protein	**28.6 g**
Alanine	1.58 g
Arginine	1.67 g
Aspartic acid	2.42 g
Cystine	0.31 g
Glutamic acid	4.04 g
Glycine	1.42 g
Histidine	0.96 g
Isoleucine	1.23 g
Leucine	2.1 g
Lysine	2.32 g
Methionine	0.68 g
Phenylalanine	1.06 g
Proline	1.15 g
Serine	1.08 g
Threonine	1.15 g
Tryptophan	0.28 g
Tyrosine	0.89 g
Valine	1.39 g
Vitamins	
Vitamin B1	0.48 mg
Vitamin B12	2.01 mcg
Vitamin B2	0.33 mg
Vitamin B3	5.62 mg
Vitamin B5	0.8 mg
Vitamin B6	0.41 mg
Choline	106 mg
Folate	9.18 mcg
Vitamin A	2.85 mcg
Vitamin C	1.1 mg
Vitamin D	13.5 IU
Vitamin E	0.32 mg
Vitamin K	7.71 mcg
Minerals	
Calcium	30.3 mg
Copper	0.11 mg
Iron	3.02 mg
Magnesium	27.7 mg
Manganese	0.04 mg
Phosphorus	258 mg
Potassium	442 mg
Selenium	33.8 mcg
Sodium	222 mg
Zinc	4.15 mg

nutrition content estimated using the USDA database. values are based on an average of all variations.

INGREDIENTS:

Natural hog casings if you are stuffing your sausage

English Bangers

1 teaspoon ground mace

½ teaspoon dried thyme leaves

½ teaspoon dried marjoram leaves

5 teaspoons dried rubbed sage

1 tablespoon plus 1 teaspoon salt

5 pounds ground pork

Breakfast Sausage

1 tablespoon dried rubbed sage

½ teaspoon ground ginger

1½ teaspoons ground mace

1½ teaspoons dried thyme leaves

1 tablespoon salt

5 pounds ground pork

Irish Sausage

1 tablespoon dried thyme leaves

2 teaspoons dried rosemary

1 tablespoon dried marjoram leaves

1 tablespoon dried oregano leaves

1 tablespoon salt

5 pounds ground pork

8 cloves garlic, crushed

Farmer's Sausage (Pork and Beef)

2 teaspoons ground mace

1 teaspoon ground cloves

1½ teaspoons dried rubbed sage

1 tablespoon plus 1 teaspoon salt

3 pounds ground pork

3 pounds ground beef

Sweet Italian Sausage

¼ teaspoon dried oregano

¼ teaspoon dried rosemary

1 tablespoon dried tarragon

1 teaspoon salt

5 pounds ground pork

6 or 7 cloves garlic, crushed

1 teaspoon minced fresh basil

¼ cup minced fresh parsley

Beef Sausage

1½ teaspoons dried rubbed sage

1 tablespoon salt

4 pounds ground beef or ground chuck (70% to 75% lean)

3 tablespoons minced fresh parsley

Lamb Sausage

1 teaspoon dried tarragon

1½ teaspoons salt

4 pounds ground lamb

2 teaspoons minced fresh basil

1 tablespoon pomegranate molasses

Beef Heart Sausage

½ teaspoon dried thyme leaves

½ teaspoon dried savory

2½ teaspoons salt

3 pounds ground beef heart

1 pound ground pork

1 pound ground pork fat or additional ground pork

½ cup dry red wine

PREP TIME: 20 to 40 minutes if making patties and baking or frying, 1 to 2 hours if stuffing into casings and parboiling, plus 24 hours marinating time

COOK TIME: 20 minutes

SERVINGS: 8 to 20 servings

INGREDIENTS:

Natural hog casings if you are stuffing your sausage

Apple Chicken Sausage:

1 medium onion, very finely chopped

1 to 2 tablespoons cooking fat

2 large Granny Smith apples, peeled and diced

2 teaspoons dried rubbed sage

1 teaspoon dried thyme leaves

½ teaspoon dried rosemary

½ teaspoon dried marjoram leaves

1½ teaspoons salt

4 pounds ground chicken or turkey (or substitute pork)

¼ cup minced fresh parsley

FOR THE EIGHT SAUSAGE VARIATIONS ABOVE:

1. Combine the dried spices in a spice grinder and grind until they are a fine powder. You can also do this in a mortar and pestle, clean coffee grinder, mini blender, or mini food processor.
2. Place the dried herbs, salt, ground meat, and any other ingredients in a large mixing bowl.
3. Use your hands to thoroughly incorporate the spices into the meat. Alternatively, mix the ingredients in the bowl of a stand mixer on low speed for 3 to 4 minutes.
4. Cover with plastic wrap and refrigerate overnight or up to 24 hours.

APPLE CHICKEN SAUSAGE:

1. In a skillet, sauté the onion in the cooking fat over medium-high heat for 8 to 10 minutes, until soft and starting to caramelize. Add the apples and sauté for 5 additional minutes. Let cool before adding to the ground meat. To complete, follow the instructions for first eight sausage variations above.

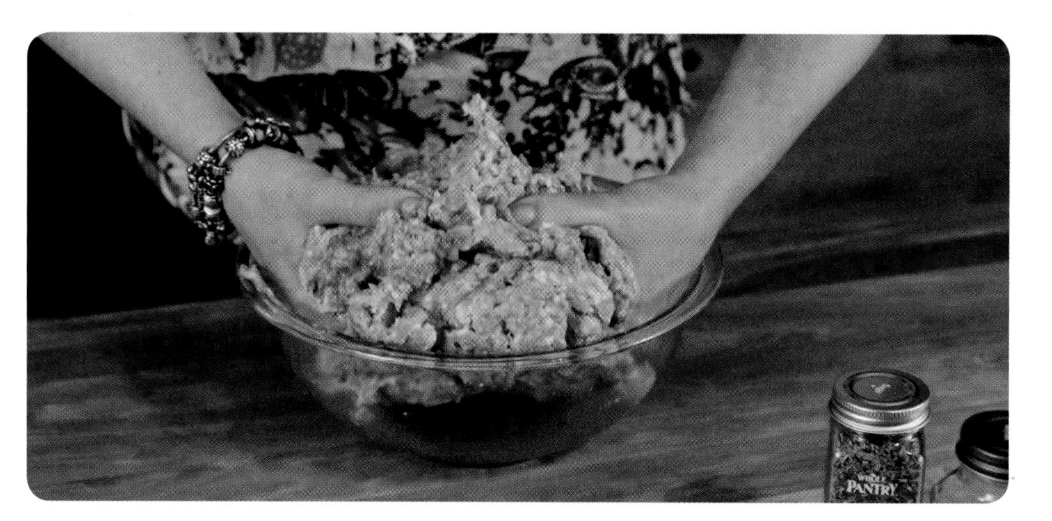

SPECIAL EQUIPMENT

- Meat grinder or food processor (if grinding your own meat)
- Spice grinder
- Sausage stuffer (if stuffing into casings)
- Very large stockpot and oil/candy thermometer for parboiling (if stuffing into casings)

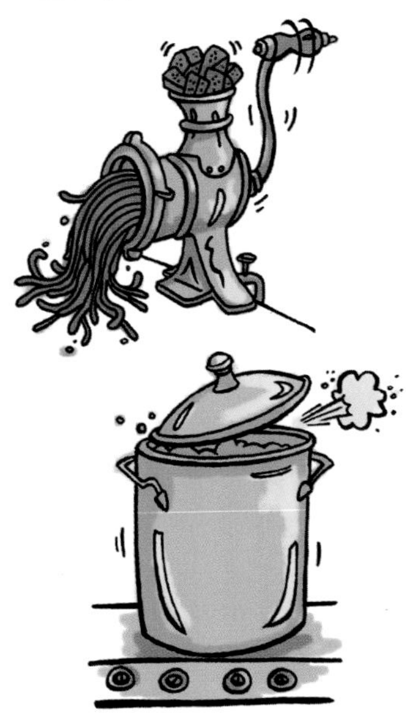

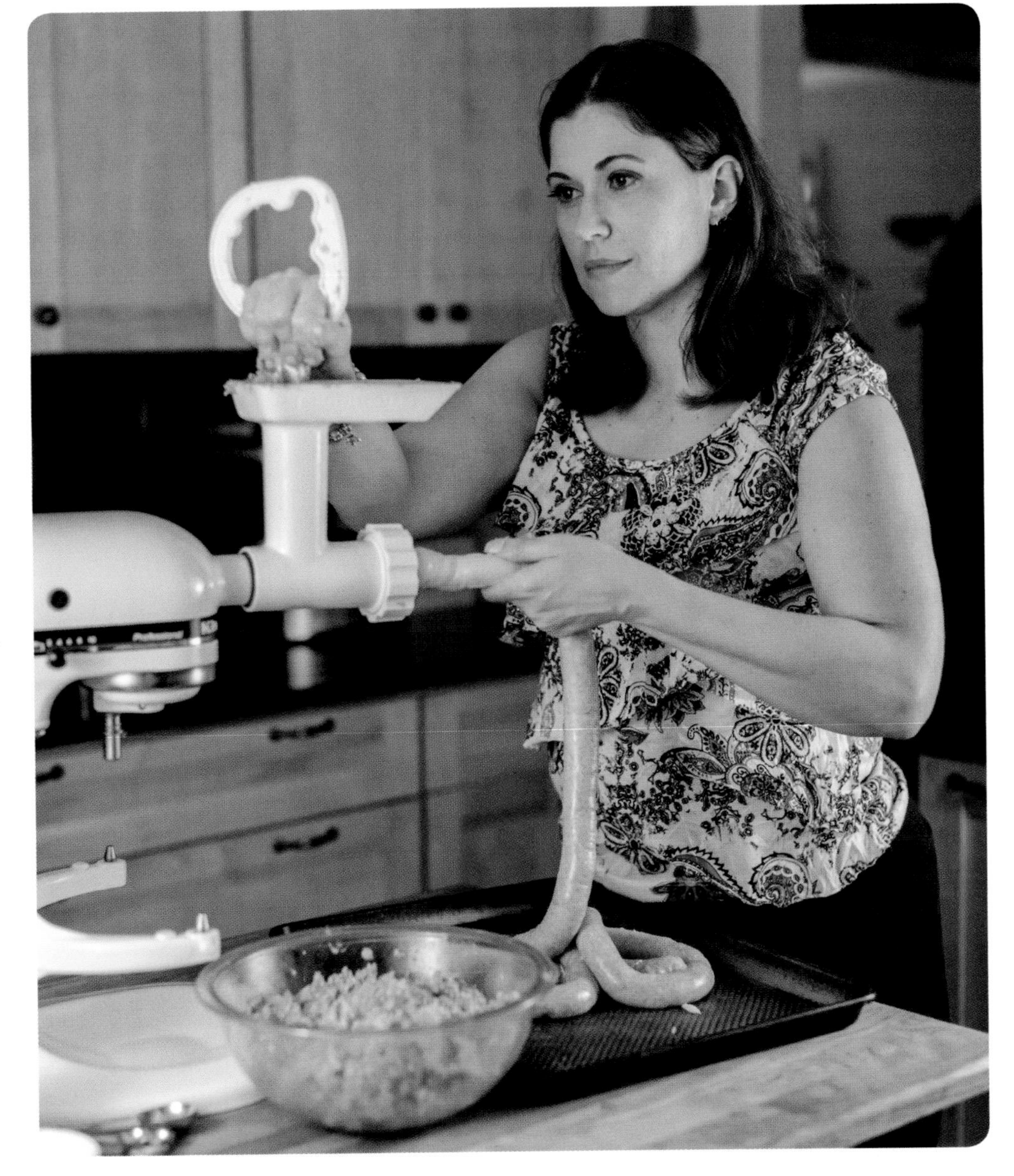

TO STUFF INTO CASINGS:

1. Follow the directions on the packaging for your natural hog casings (typically rinsing and then soaking them in warm water for 30 minutes).
2. Attach the sausage stuffer attachment to the meat grinder per the manufacturer's instructions. Alternatively, you can use a manual sausage stuffer (a contraption that is vaguely reminiscent of a water pump) or even a jerky gun or pastry bag without a tip attached.
3. Grease the funnel end of your sausage stuffer attachment with lard, palm shortening, or coconut oil. Feed the sausage casing onto the funnel until the entire casing is scrunched/folded up on the funnel, leaving only 3 to 4 inches over the end (to tie a knot when you're done—but leave it untied for now so you don't get air bubbles in your sausage).
4. Turn on your meat grinder per the manufacturer's instructions (typically on low speed for stuffing sausages). Feed your sausage mix through the feeding spout, pressing down with the tamping tool or a wooden pestle. If you are using a manual sausage stuffer, fill the feeding tube with the sausage mix and then press down on the handle to push the sausage mix into the casing.

FODMAP ALERT *Apple Chicken sausage cannot be made low-FODMAP. For other variations, replace the garlic with green garlic or garlic scapes (green part only) or omit.*

TIPS:

Sausage is an outstanding opportunity to hide organ meat. Try replacing up to a third of the ground meat with ground liver (you can run it through a meat grinder or process it in a food processor to grind it yourself, or ask your butcher to do it for you) and up to another third of the ground meat with ground heart meat. Bison, lamb, and chicken liver are the easiest to "hide." Ground heart meat tastes very much like the muscle meat of whatever animal it comes from (for example, ground beef heart tastes like ground beef). The only limitation to using it in sausage is that it can be a little too lean, necessitating the addition of extra fat to maintain an ideal fat-to-lean ratio.

Miss the umami flavor of the black or red pepper found in many sausages? Substitute truffle salt for the salt in any sausage recipe (look for a brand that uses unrefined sea salt as its base). For a little heat, try adding 1 teaspoon or more wasabi powder.

5. As the sausage mix fills the casing, it will gradually inflate, ease away from the funnel, and coil in ropelike fashion. Make sure that the casing is filling completely, but do not overstuff your sausage, or the casing may burst when you cook it. If you want kinks in your sausage to make links, simply pause and twist a few times to create a kink.
6. Fill the casing to within 3 to 4 inches of the other end. Tie a knot in both ends and set aside.
7. Repeat until all of your sausage mix has been stuffed into casings.
8. To parboil your sausage, attach an oil/candy thermometer to the side of a large stockpot. Fill the pot half to three-quarters full with water (you can add a teaspoon of salt to make it heat faster). Bring the water up to 165°F, just shy of a simmer. Place the sausages in the pot (do not overfill; you may have to do this in batches depending on how big your pot is). Keep the temperature as close to 165°F as you can.
9. Poach the sausages until the internal temperature reaches 150°F (15 to 20 minutes, depending on the size of the sausages).
10. Remove from the pot and set aside. If freezing, refrigerate the sausage until cold and then slice into single servings before freezing. Freeze on a baking sheet, then move to a resealable freezer bag or container.
11. Fry in a skillet over medium heat for 5 to 10 minutes (longer if frying frozen) and enjoy! You can also freeze after pan-frying if you want to be able to reheat your sausages from frozen in the microwave for a very quick breakfast.

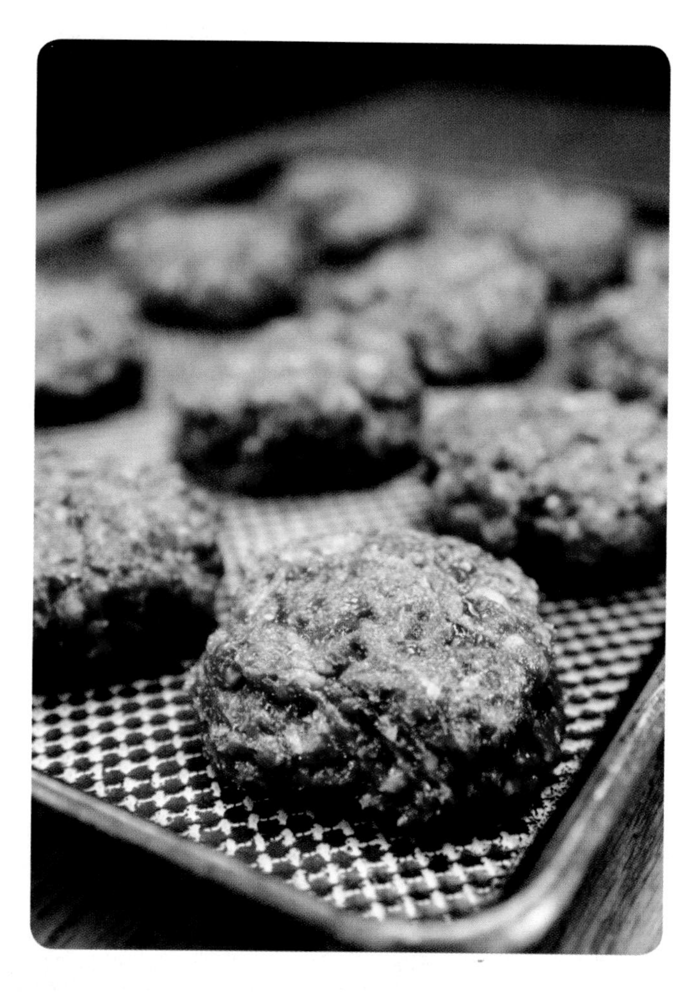

TO FORM INTO PATTIES:

1. Preheat the oven to 400°F.
2. Form 4- to 8-ounce patties with your hands, just as you would make hamburger patties. Place on a rimmed baking sheet, spacing them about 1 inch apart (how big you make the patties will depend on how big a serving size you are aiming for). You may need 2 baking sheets, depending on how thick you make your patties.
3. Bake for 15 to 25 minutes (depending on thickness), until the internal temperature reaches a minimum of 160°F for beef, lamb, and pork sausage and 165°F for chicken and turkey sausage. Alternatively, you can fry the patties in a skillet or on a griddle over medium-high heat.
4. If freezing, freeze on a baking sheet, then move to a resealable freezer bag or container. You can reheat frozen patties in the microwave or fry them in a skillet.

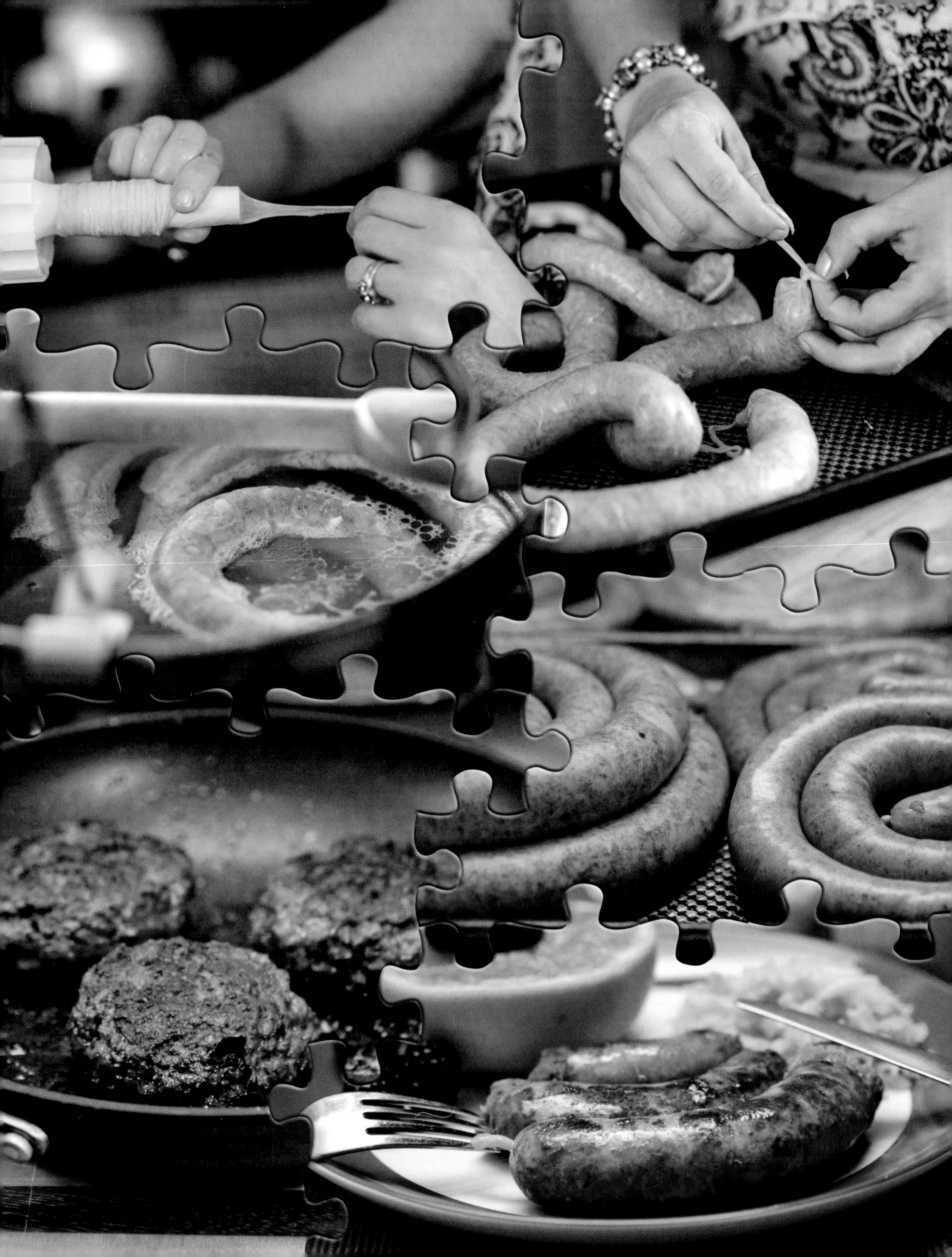

Bacon Fruit Cups

This recipe is for those days when you want to dress up your bacon, perhaps because your in-laws are coming for Sunday brunch. You can even make these cups ahead and refrigerate them. Before serving, remove from the fridge and let come to room temperature.

While the Bacon Bowl does this job efficiently, you don't need this kitchen gadget to make awesome bacon cups.

PREP TIME: 15 minutes
COOK TIME: 45 minutes to 1 hour
SERVINGS: 2

INGREDIENTS:

12 thick slices bacon

Berries, melon cubes or balls, or fruit of choice

SPECIAL EQUIPMENT

- 2 (3- to 4-inch) metal sieves or strainers with no plastic components

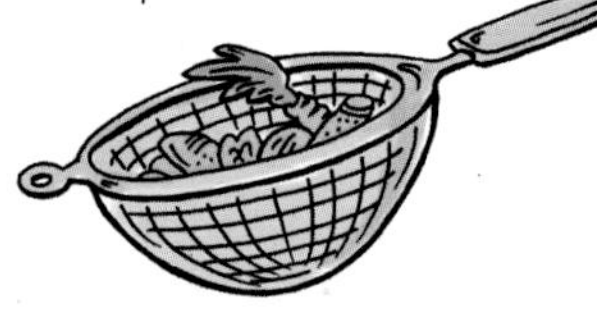

1. Preheat the oven to 375°F. Place 2 (3- to 4-inch) metal sieves upside down in a baking dish.
2. Take 6 slices of bacon and weave 3 slices horizontal and 3 slices vertical in a simple over-under-over, under-over-under, over-under-over pattern. (Now you're ready to try baskets!) Push the slices of bacon tightly together.
3. Carefully transfer your woven bacon to drape over the top of an upside-down metal sieve. The bacon will want to come unwoven at the corners, so tuck those ends underneath each other to complete your bowl shape.
4. Repeat for the second bacon cup.
5. Bake for 30 minutes, until the bacon is starting to crisp and looks browned.
6. Remove from the oven. Drain the excess bacon fat. Carefully remove each bacon cup from the sieve using tongs. Using tongs or oven mitts, turn the sieves over. Place the bacon cups right-side-up in the sieves.
7. Place the bacon cups back in the oven and cook for an additional 15 to 25 minutes, until the cups are completely crisp.
8. Serve warm or cooled, filled with berries, melon cubes or balls, or any other fruit you enjoy with bacon.

TIPS:

The cooking time will vary based on how thick and how fatty the bacon is. Keep a close eye on it once you get close to the end of the cooking time. You want the bacon to cook until fully crisp (or else the bowls won't hold their shape), but you don't want it to burn, either.

Some bacon, especially bacon cured with a lot of sugar or natural sweeteners like maple syrup, just doesn't crisp well; it is likely to burn before it goes crisp, even when cooked at a lower temperature. Save it for recipes like Bacon-Braised Brussels Sprouts (page 321) or Bacon-Apple Chicken Burgers with Maple-Cranberry Sauce (page 222).

If you don't have a metal sieve that will work as a "mold," try making your own out of several sheets of thick foil balled together. You could also try a small ovenproof bowl. These solid mold options will require a slightly longer cooking time.

VARIATIONS:

Instead of fruit, use bacon bowls to serve a side salad or vegetable.

NUTRITION FACTS	
Serving Size	130 g
Recipe Yields	260 g
Calories	**293**
Fats	**21.2 g**
MUFA	9.28 g
Omega-3	0.15 g
Omega-6	2.13 g
Saturated Fat	6.92 g
Carbohydrates	**7.1 g**
Fiber	1.19 g
Starch	0.03 g
Fructose	1.76 g
Glucose	1.44 g
Sucrose	1.93 g
Protein	**18 g**
Alanine	1.16 g
Arginine	1.15 g
Aspartic acid	1.75 g
Cystine	0.2 g
Glutamic acid	2.68 g
Glycine	1.24 g
Histidine	0.66 g
Isoleucine	0.83 g
Leucine	1.38 g
Lysine	1.46 g
Methionine	0.39 g
Phenylalanine	0.71 g
Proline	0.97 g
Serine	0.69 g
Threonine	0.69 g
Tryptophan	0.15 g
Tyrosine	0.56 g
Valine	0.94 g
Vitamins	
Vitamin B1	0.2 mg
Vitamin B12	0.56 mcg
Vitamin B2	0.14 mg
Vitamin B3	5.61 mg
Vitamin B5	0.6 mg
Vitamin B6	0.2 mg
Choline	63.3 mg
Folate	19.3 mcg
Vitamin A	73.3 mcg
Vitamin C	39.1 mg
Vitamin D	0 IU
Vitamin E	0.3 mg
Vitamin K	1.96 mcg
Minerals	
Calcium	15.1 mg
Copper	0.12 mg
Iron	0.98 mg
Magnesium	24.8 mg
Manganese	0.19 mg
Phosphorus	262 mg
Potassium	432 mg
Selenium	29 mcg
Sodium	1072 mg
Zinc	1.76 mg

nutrition content estimated using the USDA database. values vary based on iongredient selection.

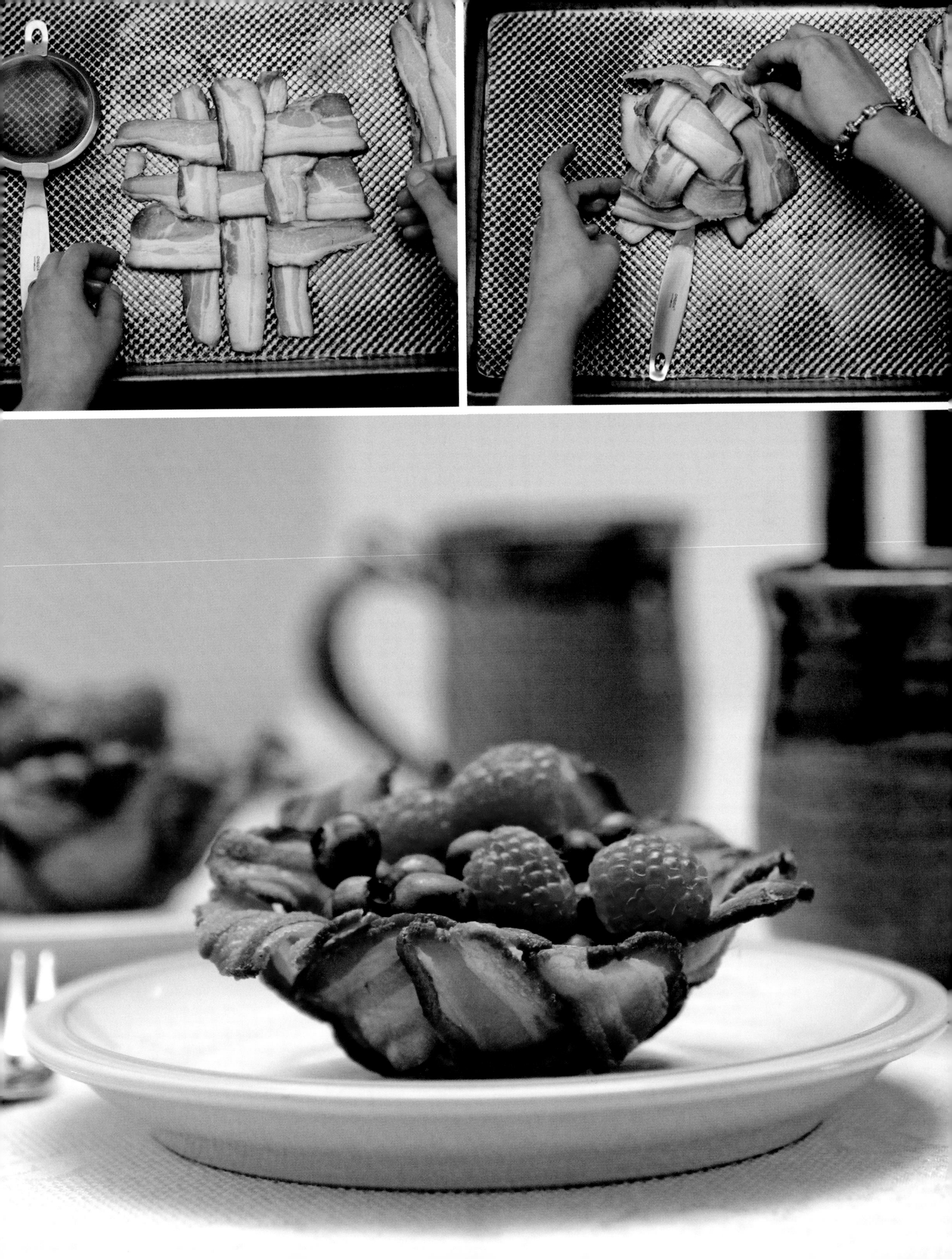

Taro Hash

Taro is a delicious root vegetable and, when presteamed before frying or roasting, loses its mucilaginous texture. This hash is sure to become a breakfast favorite!

PREP TIME: 15 minutes
COOK TIME: 30 to 40 minutes
SERVINGS: 3 to 4

INGREDIENTS:

1 pound taro roots

4 thick slices bacon, chopped

1 clove garlic, crushed

2 tablespoons chopped green onion or chives

FODMAP ALERT *Replace the garlic with green garlic or garlic scapes (green part only) or omit. If using green onion, use the green part only.*

SPECIAL EQUIPMENT

- Steamer pot

1. Place the whole taro roots in a steamer insert with 1 inch of water in the saucepot underneath. Bring to a boil and steam for 10 to 15 minutes, until the taro is soft enough to pierce easily with a knife (but is not mushy). Remove the steamer insert from the pot and allow the taro to cool enough to handle.
2. Place the chopped bacon in a skillet, then turn on the heat to medium-high. Sauté the bacon, stirring occasionally, until browned, 7 to 8 minutes.
3. Meanwhile, peel the dark brown skin off the steamed taro (it should come off easily). Cut the taro into ¼-inch dice.
4. Add the taro to the skillet with the bacon. Continue to sauté, gently stirring occasionally, until the taro has browned, 10 to 15 minutes. Add the garlic and green onion and cook for 2 to 3 minutes more. Serve.

TIPS:

You can steam the taro root ahead of time to make this dish quicker to prepare in the morning.

VARIATIONS:

Use your favorite sausage mix (page 132) instead of bacon.

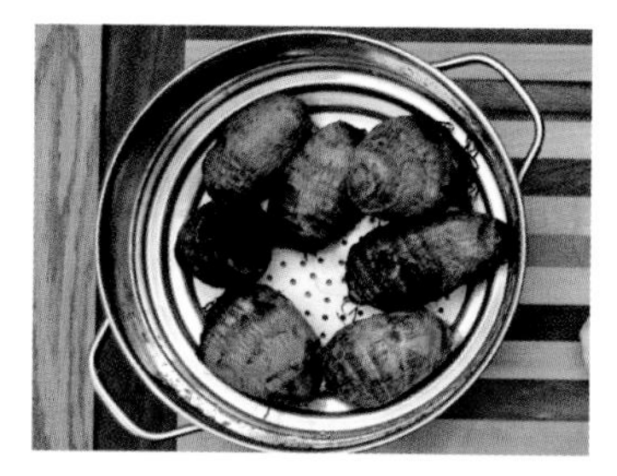

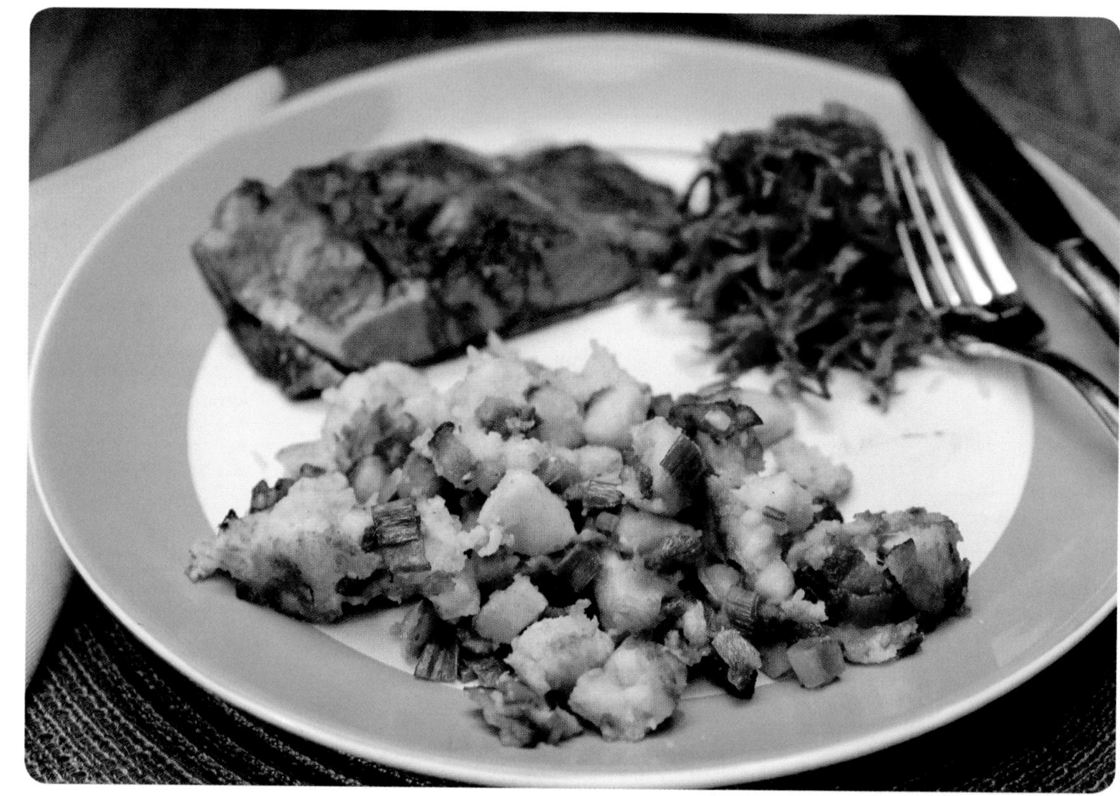

NUTRITION FACTS	
Serving Size	125 g
Recipe Yields	501 g
Calories	**207**
Fats	**3.65 g**
MUFA	1.56 g
Omega-3	0.03 g
Omega-6	0.39 g
Saturated Fat	1.18 g
Carbohydrates	**39.8 g**
Fiber	5.85 g
Starch	33.1 g
Fructose	0.08 g
Glucose	0.06 g
Sucrose	<0.01 g
Protein	**3.56 g**
Alanine	0.21 g
Arginine	0.23 g
Aspartic acid	0.35 g
Cystine	0.05 g
Glutamic acid	0.5 g
Glycine	0.23 g
Histidine	0.12 g
Isoleucine	0.16 g
Leucine	0.27 g
Lysine	0.27 g
Methionine	0.07 g
Phenylalanine	0.15 g
Proline	0.18 g
Serine	0.15 g
Threonine	0.14 g
Tryptophan	0.03 g
Tyrosine	0.11 g
Valine	0.19 g
Vitamins	
Vitamin B1	0.15 mg
Vitamin B12	0.09 mcg
Vitamin B2	0.05 mg
Vitamin B3	1.45 mg
Vitamin B5	0.47 mg
Vitamin B6	0.41 mg
Choline	34.1 mg
Folate	22.6 mcg
Vitamin A	11.4 mcg
Vitamin C	6.31 mg
Vitamin D	0 IU
Vitamin E	3.36 mg
Vitamin K	6.07 mcg
Minerals	
Calcium	24.1 mg
Copper	0.25 mg
Iron	0.97 mg
Magnesium	37.1 mg
Manganese	0.53 mg
Phosphorus	129 mg
Potassium	600 mg
Selenium	5.92 mcg
Sodium	195 mg
Zinc	0.59 mg

nutrition content estimated using the USDA database.

Plantain and Apple Fritters

These fritters taste like little apple pie pancakes. They are tasty warm or chilled and are great combined with pork sausage or bacon (or both!). For an extra decadent breakfast, you can add a spoonful of Coconut Whipped Topping (page 116).

PREP TIME: 5 to 10 minutes
COOK TIME: 17 to 20 minutes
SERVINGS: 8

INGREDIENTS:

2 ripe plantains, peeled

1 small apple, peeled, cored, and grated

½ teaspoon ground cinnamon

2 to 4 tablespoons coconut oil

FODMAP ALERT
This recipe cannot be made low-FODMAP.

1. Mash the plantains in a bowl with a fork or a wire potato masher (the fritters taste better if you leave some lumps and don't overmash). Add the grated apple and cinnamon and mix to combine.
2. Heat 1 to 2 tablespoons of the coconut oil in a skillet over medium heat. Drop heaping spoonfuls of the plantain batter into the pan and flatten with the back of a spoon. The fritters should be 2 to 3 inches in diameter, or about the same size as your spatula; otherwise, they can be tricky to flip. Depending on the size of your skillet, you may have to cook the fritters in batches.
3. Cook for 10 to 12 minutes, until golden brown on the bottom. Add a little extra coconut oil if the fritters absorb it all. If they are browning too fast, turn down the heat.
4. Carefully flip the fritters and cook for 7 to 8 minutes on the other side. Again, add a little extra coconut oil if the fritters absorb it all. Enjoy!

TIPS:

Ripe plantains should be covered in black spots, if not almost completely black. The blacker the peel, the better!

If cooking in batches, you can keep the finished fritters warm on a baking dish in a 200°F oven.

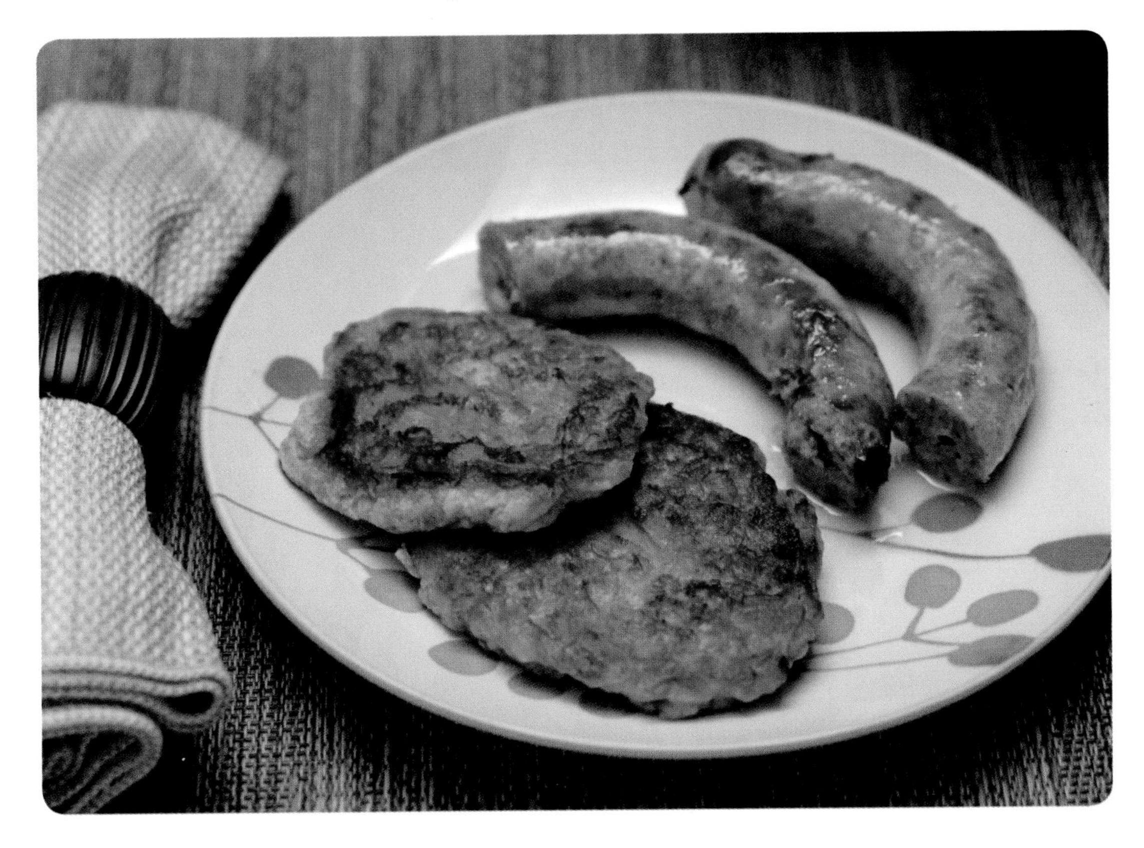

NUTRITION FACTS	
Serving Size	65 g
Recipe Yields	519 g
Calories	**92.3**
Fats	**3.59 g**
MUFA	0.21 g
Omega-3	0.01 g
Omega-6	0.09 g
Saturated Fat	3.01 g
Carbohydrates	**16.5 g**
Fiber	1.33 g
Starch	6.8 g
Fructose	1 g
Glucose	0.54 g
Sucrose	0.14 g
Protein	**0.63 g**
Alanine	0.03 g
Arginine	0.05 g
Aspartic acid	0.06 g
Cystine	<0.01 g
Glutamic acid	0.06 g
Glycine	0.02 g
Histidine	0.03 g
Isoleucine	0.02 g
Leucine	0.03 g
Lysine	0.03 g
Methionine	<0.01 g
Phenylalanine	0.02 g
Proline	0.02 g
Serine	0.02 g
Threonine	0.02 g
Tryptophan	<0.01 g
Tyrosine	0.01 g
Valine	0.02 g
Vitamins	
Vitamin B1	0.03 mg
Vitamin B12	0 mcg
Vitamin B2	0.03 mg
Vitamin B3	0.32 mg
Vitamin B5	0.13 mg
Vitamin B6	0.14 mg
Choline	6.64 mg
Folate	9.86 mcg
Vitamin A	25.4 mcg
Vitamin C	8.91 mg
Vitamin D	0 IU
Vitamin E	0.08 mg
Vitamin K	0.48 mcg
Minerals	
Calcium	3.8 mg
Copper	0.04 mg
Iron	0.3 mg
Magnesium	17.3 mg
Manganese	0.03 mg
Phosphorus	17.2 mg
Potassium	239 mg
Selenium	0.68 mcg
Sodium	1.81 mg
Zinc	0.07 mg

nutrition content estimated using the USDA database.

Carrot-Raisin Muffins

These muffins pack a carbohydrate punch and should be reserved for an occasional treat.

PREP TIME: 20 minutes
COOK TIME: 40 minutes
YIELD: 8 muffins

INGREDIENTS:

- Lard or palm shortening, for greasing the pan (if not using liners)
- 1½ cups puréed green plantains (2 medium)
- ½ cup lard
- 2 tablespoons muscovado sugar or evaporated cane juice
- 1 teaspoon ground cinnamon
- ½ teaspoon salt
- 1 teaspoon baking soda
- ½ cup Pumpkin Flour (page 121)
- 1½ cups grated carrots
- ½ cup raisins

1. Preheat the oven to 350°F. Grease 8 muffin cups with lard or palm shortening, or use silicone or paper muffin liners.
2. Combine the plantains, lard, sugar, cinnamon, and salt in a food processor and process until a smooth puree is formed, 3 to 5 minutes.
3. Add the baking soda and pumpkin flour and pulse to combine. Remove the blade from the food processor and fold in the grated carrots and raisins.
4. Spoon the batter into the prepared muffin cups, filling them nearly to the top. Smooth out the tops with the back of a spoon.
5. Bake for 40 minutes, until the muffins are lightly browned on top and a toothpick inserted into the middle comes out clean. Remove from the pan by either gently inverting the pan over a cooling rack or by gently lifting each muffin out of the pan with a knife or narrow spatula inserted along the side.
6. Enjoy warm or allow to cool. Store leftovers in an airtight container in the fridge for up to 5 days, or freeze for up to 6 months. (To freeze, place on a baking sheet in the freezer until frozen, then move to a freezer bag or container.)

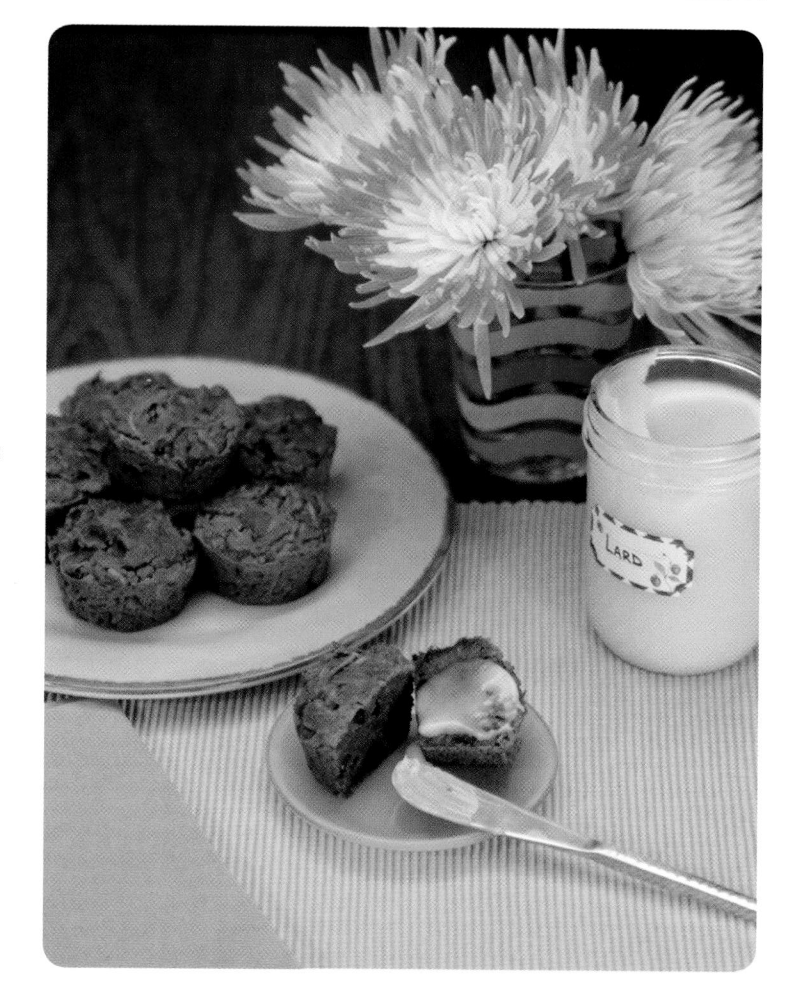

SPECIAL EQUIPMENT

- Food processor

TIPS:

These muffins are delicious spread with lard! Like all baked goods using plantains or plantain flour, they go stale quickly. Store in a resealable plastic bag with as much air pushed out as possible. Or, better yet, freeze any muffins you don't plan to eat the same day you bake them (freeze on a baking sheet and then move to a freezer-safe container once frozen).

VARIATIONS:

Substitute other dried fruit for the raisins, such as dried cranberries, chopped dried apricots, dried cherries, chopped dates, or even chopped prunes.

Parsnip-Carrot Muffins. *Substitute grated parsnip for half of the grated carrots and substitute chopped dates for the raisins. The parsnip gives these muffins a lovely nutty sweetness!*

NUTRITION FACTS

Serving Size	106 g
Recipe Yields	847 g
Calories	**268**
Fats	**13.2 g**
MUFA	5.8 g
Omega-3	0.14 g
Omega-6	1.35 g
Saturated Fat	5.1 g
Carbohydrates	**37.9 g**
Fiber	5.38 g
Starch	7.15 g
Fructose	2.81 g
Glucose	2.64 g
Sucrose	3.93 g
Protein	**1.92 g**
Alanine	0.06 g
Arginine	0.11 g
Aspartic acid	0.1 g
Cystine	0.03 g
Glutamic acid	0.14 g
Glycine	0.04 g
Histidine	0.04 g
Isoleucine	0.04 g
Leucine	0.06 g
Lysine	0.06 g
Methionine	0.01 g
Phenylalanine	0.04 g
Proline	0.06 g
Serine	0.04 g
Threonine	0.06 g
Tryptophan	0.01 g
Tyrosine	0.02 g
Valine	0.04 g
Vitamins	
Vitamin B1	0.23 mg
Vitamin B12	0 mcg
Vitamin B2	0.23 mg
Vitamin B3	1.72 mg
Vitamin B5	0.75 mg
Vitamin B6	0.36 mg
Choline	30.7 mg
Folate	44.3 mcg
Vitamin A	197 mcg
Vitamin C	26.6 mg
Vitamin D	13.1 IU
Vitamin E	2.36 mg
Vitamin K	5.53 mcg
Minerals	
Calcium	56.3 mg
Copper	0.26 mg
Iron	2.41 mg
Magnesium	44.7 mg
Manganese	0.3 mg
Phosphorus	115 mg
Potassium	1001 mg
Selenium	1.37 mcg
Sodium	242 mg
Zinc	0.72 mg

nutrition content estimated using the USDA database.

Superfood Smoothie

There are pros and cons to smoothies. One of the major pros is that they are a quick and easy way for most of us to get a nutrient-dense meal first thing in the morning. This smoothie takes advantage of banana to mask the flavors of some other great nutrient-dense foods. If you're going to add a lot of superfood add-ons, you may want to use a whole banana. Ripe bananas will be sweeter, whereas green bananas will give you more starch (including resistant starch).

PREP TIME: 5 minutes
COOK TIME: none
YIELD: 1 (12-ounce) serving

INGREDIENTS:

- ½ banana
- ¼ avocado
- 1 cup vegetable juice (homemade or store-bought) or water, chilled
- 2 to 3 cups fresh leafy greens (spinach, kale, lettuce, baby collards, etc.)
- 1 teaspoon to 2 tablespoons superfood add-ons: sea vegetables, desiccated liver or other organs, cubes of frozen liver or other organ meat, nutritional yeast (make sure it's gluten-free), coconut milk kefir or yogurt, high-quality extra-virgin olive oil, fermented cod liver oil, freeze-dried acai powder, kombucha, or bone broth or soft bones left over from making broth (optional)
- 1 to 2 tablespoons protein powder (beef isolate, beef plasma isolate, gelatin, collagen, insect powder/flour, or a mix)

1. Place all the ingredients except the protein powder in a blender and blend on high for 1 to 2 minutes, until smooth. Add the protein powder and pulse to incorporate.

TIPS:

Leftover sweet potato can be added to increase the starchy carbohydrate content.

A high-powered blender will create a smoother consistency and is definitely a worthwhile investment if you'll be making smoothies often.

Look for vegetable juice that doesn't contain any fruit ingredients (except maybe lemon). If making homemade vegetable juice, celery, cucumber, and leafy greens are great options.

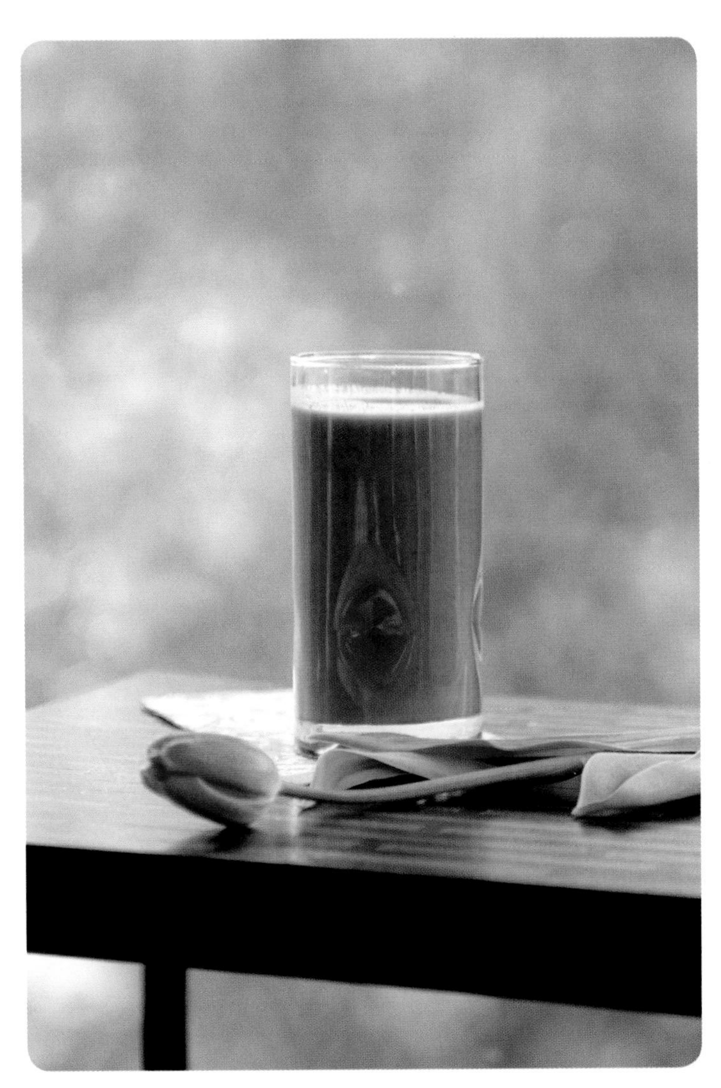

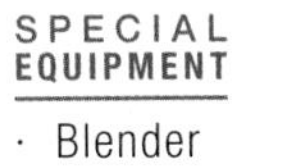

FODMAP ALERT *Omit the avocado, or substitute a drizzle of extra-virgin olive oil.*

SPECIAL EQUIPMENT

- Blender

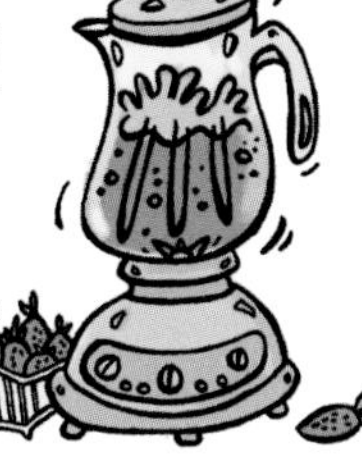

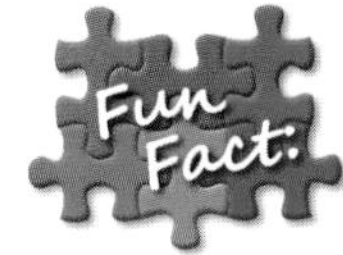

Citrus fruits aren't the only good sources of vitamin C. Leafy greens like spinach, as well as herbs like cilantro and chives, have lots, too!

NUTRITION FACTS	
Serving Size	462 g
Recipe Yields	462 g
Calories	**257**
Fats	**9.11 g**
MUFA	5.14 g
Omega-3	0.24 g
Omega-6	1.14 g
Saturated Fat	1.48 g
Carbohydrates	**35.9 g**
Fiber	9.91 g
Starch	5.64 g
Fructose	7.56 g
Glucose	6.3 g
Sucrose	1.95 g
Protein	**14.9 g**
Alanine	0.9 g
Arginine	0.82 g
Aspartic acid	1.01 g
Cystine	0.08 g
Glutamic acid	1.42 g
Glycine	1.65 g
Histidine	0.23 g
Isoleucine	0.4 g
Leucine	0.67 g
Lysine	0.63 g
Methionine	0.15 g
Phenylalanine	0.44 g
Proline	1.19 g
Serine	0.48 g
Threonine	0.38 g
Tryptophan	0.08 g
Tyrosine	0.24 g
Valine	0.51 g
Vitamins	
Vitamin B1	0.27 mg
Vitamin B12	5.06 mcg
Vitamin B2	0.6 mg
Vitamin B3	4.72 mg
Vitamin B5	1.89 mg
Vitamin B6	0.96 mg
Choline	65.8 mg
Folate	263 mcg
Vitamin A	1161 mcg
Vitamin C	166 mg
Vitamin D	1.32 IU
Vitamin E	2.96 mg
Vitamin K	641 mcg
Minerals	
Calcium	170 mg
Copper	2.29 mg
Iron	3.87 mg
Magnesium	115 mg
Manganese	1.23 mg
Phosphorus	187 mg
Potassium	1434 mg
Selenium	13 mcg
Sodium	550 mg
Zinc	1.96 mg

nutrition content estimated using the USDA database. values vary based on iongredient selection.

Breakfast Brew

If you are missing your morning cup of coffee, this herbal tea actually mimics the flavor very well. To make it feel even more like coffee, it is brewed in a French coffee press! This recipe scales up well if you want to make a whole pot. Serve black or with Coconut Cream (page 116).

PREP TIME: 2 minutes
COOK TIME: 3 to 5 minutes
YIELD: 1 (10-ounce) serving if using a 12-ounce coffee press, or 3 (10-ounce) servings if using a 34-ounce coffee press

INGREDIENTS:

For a 12-Ounce Coffee Press:

¾ teaspoon roasted dandelion root

1¼ teaspoons roasted chicory root

½ teaspoon carob powder

10 ounces boiling water

For a 34-Ounce Coffee Press:

2½ teaspoons roasted dandelion root

1 tablespoon plus 1 teaspoon roasted chicory root

2 teaspoons carob powder

3¾ cups boiling water

1. Combine the dandelion root, chicory root, and carob powder in the bottom of a coffee press.
2. Pour the boiling water over the ingredients in the coffee press.
3. Steep for 3 to 5 minutes. Press down the filter and enjoy!

TIPS:

If finding loose dandelion root is a bit of a challenge, ¾ teaspoon of roasted dandelion root is equivalent to a teabag. Use 3 teabags' worth of roasted dandelion root if you are making a pot.

If you don't have a coffee press, you can steep the herbs in a teapot or Pyrex measuring cup and pour through a mesh strainer into your cup.

SPECIAL EQUIPMENT

- 12-ounce or 34-ounce coffee press

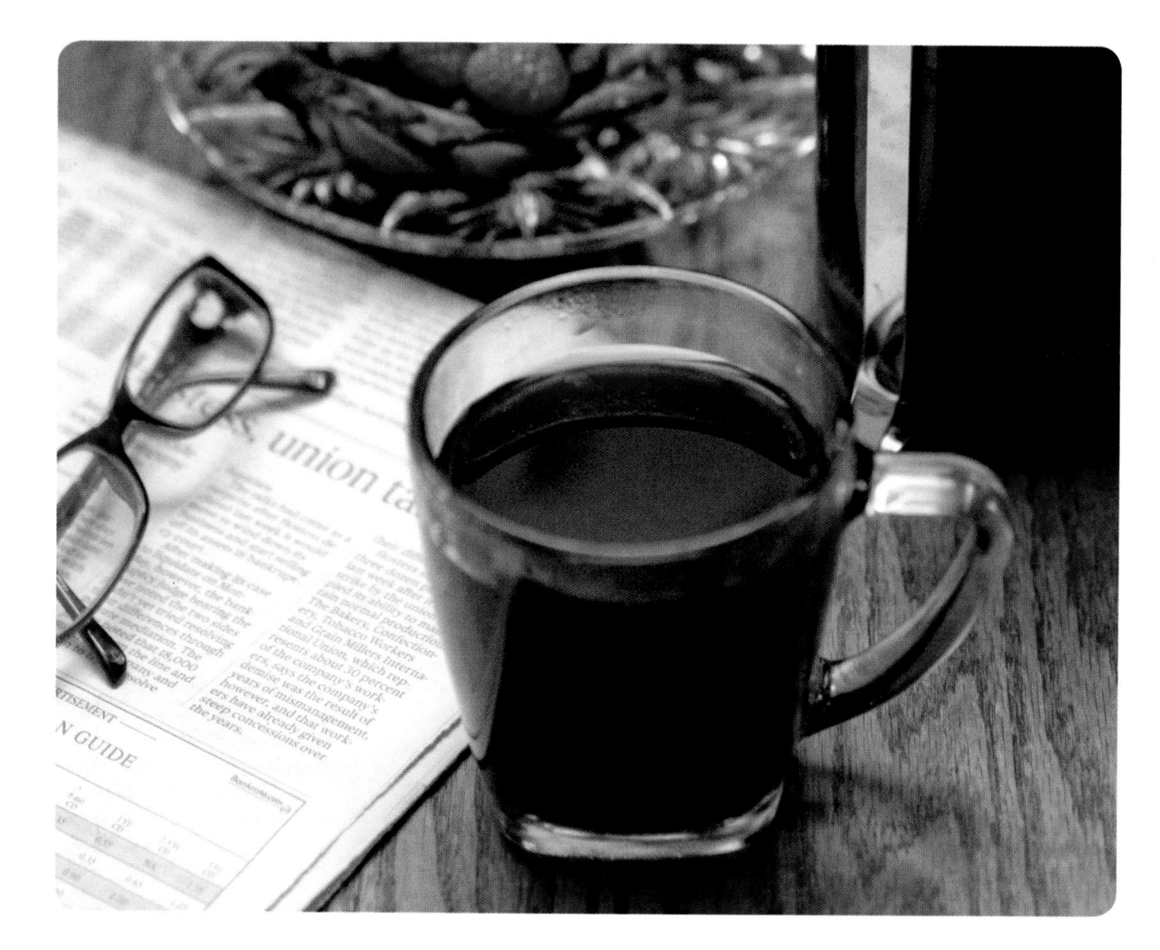

NUTRITION FACTS

Serving Size	310 g
Recipe Yields	310 g
Calories	**12.5**
Fats	**0.02 g**
MUFA	<0.01 g
Omega-3	<0.01 g
Omega-6	<0.01 g
Saturated Fat	<0.01 g
Carbohydrates	**2.91 g**
Fiber	0.45 g
Starch	0.81 g
Fructose	0 g
Glucose	0 g
Sucrose	0 g
Protein	**0.28 g**
Alanine	0 g
Arginine	0 g
Aspartic acid	0 g
Cystine	0 g
Glutamic acid	0 g
Glycine	0 g
Histidine	0 g
Isoleucine	0 g
Leucine	0 g
Lysine	0 g
Methionine	0 g
Phenylalanine	0 g
Proline	0 g
Serine	0 g
Threonine	0 g
Tryptophan	0 g
Tyrosine	0 g
Valine	0 g
Vitamins	
Vitamin B1	<0.01 mg
Vitamin B12	0 mcg
Vitamin B2	<0.01 mg
Vitamin B3	0.03 mg
Vitamin B5	0.02 mg
Vitamin B6	0.02 mg
Choline	0.41 mg
Folate	1.63 mcg
Vitamin A	5.6 mcg
Vitamin C	0.6 mg
Vitamin D	0 IU
Vitamin E	0.04 mg
Vitamin K	9.03 mcg
Minerals	
Calcium	4.81 mg
Copper	<0.01 mg
Iron	0.08 mg
Magnesium	1.75 mg
Manganese	0.02 mg
Phosphorus	4.44 mg
Potassium	21.6 mg
Selenium	0.05 mcg
Sodium	4.58 mg
Zinc	0.02 mg

nutrition content estimated using the USDA database.

Cinnamon Broiled Grapefruit

Cooking citrus fruit in this way may seem unusual, but broiling transforms grapefruit into a warm comfort food. It's also a fun way to "spice up" grapefruit for Sunday brunch!

PREP TIME: 5 to 10 minutes
COOK TIME: 4 to 6 minutes
SERVINGS: 2

INGREDIENTS:

1 grapefruit
¼ teaspoon ground cinnamon

SPECIAL EQUIPMENT

- Grapefruit knife

1. Position a rack in your oven so that the grapefruit will be about 6 inches from the top element. Preheat the broiler on high for 10 minutes while you prepare the grapefruit.
2. Cut the grapefruit in half. Use a grapefruit knife or paring knife to cut around each segment. Place the grapefruit halves cut side up on a roasting pan.
3. Sprinkle the top of the grapefruit with the cinnamon.
4. Broil for 5 to 6 minutes, until the grapefruit starts to bubble and brown on the top.

VARIATIONS:

Add ¼ teaspoon ground ginger or 1 teaspoon grated fresh ginger for a little added ginger "punch." You can also experiment with seasonings. A pinch of cloves, ground mace, ground bay leaf, and even a dash of salt can be added. You can also broil your grapefruit without any spices at all!

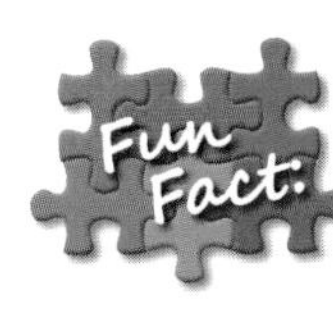

Pink and red grapefruit are typically sweeter than white grapefruit, but any type will work for this recipe.

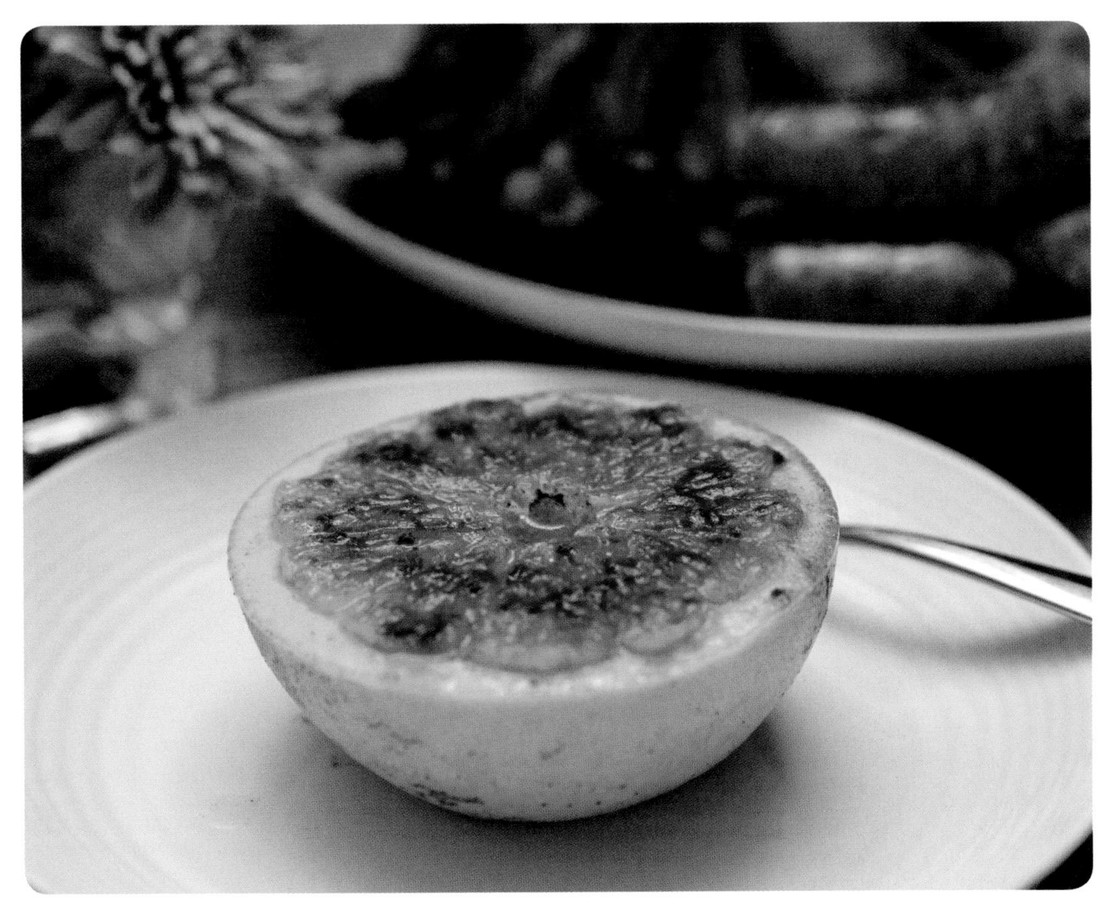

NUTRITION FACTS

Serving Size	119 g
Recipe Yields	237 g
Calories	**38.6**
Fats	**0.12 g**
MUFA	0.02 g
Omega-3	<0.01 g
Omega-6	0.02 g
Saturated Fat	0.02 g
Carbohydrates	**9.94 g**
Fiber	0.17 g
Starch	0.08 g
Fructose	<0.01 g
Glucose	<0.01 g
Sucrose	<0.01 g
Protein	**0.76 g**
Alanine	0.02 g
Arginine	0.08 g
Aspartic acid	0.13 g
Cystine	<0.01 g
Glutamic acid	0.19 g
Glycine	0.01 g
Histidine	<0.01 g
Isoleucine	<0.01 g
Leucine	0.02 g
Lysine	0.02 g
Methionine	<0.01 g
Phenylalanine	0.05 g
Proline	0.06 g
Serine	0.03 g
Threonine	0.01 g
Tryptophan	<0.01 g
Tyrosine	<0.01 g
Valine	0.01 g
Vitamins	
Vitamin B1	0.05 mg
Vitamin B12	0 mcg
Vitamin B2	0.02 mg
Vitamin B3	0.24 mg
Vitamin B5	0.34 mg
Vitamin B6	0.05 mg
Choline	0.04 mg
Folate	10.7 mcg
Vitamin A	0.05 mcg
Vitamin C	43.7 mg
Vitamin D	0 IU
Vitamin E	<0.01 mg
Vitamin K	0.1 mcg
Minerals	
Calcium	21 mg
Copper	0.07 mg
Iron	0.09 mg
Magnesium	10.8 mg
Manganese	0.07 mg
Phosphorus	8.48 mg
Potassium	179 mg
Selenium	0.01 mcg
Sodium	0.03 mg
Zinc	0.09 mg

nutrition content estimated using the USDA database.

Banana "Nut" Pancakes

These pancakes have a secret high-protein ingredient that makes them a great breakfast choice. Yes, cricket flour. Cricket flour has a wonderful nutty flavor and it's finely ground, so you can pretend you aren't eating what you're actually eating. And even though they know what's in these pancakes, my kids beg me to make them!

PREP TIME: 5 minutes
COOK TIME: 15 minutes
SERVINGS: 1 to 2

INGREDIENTS:

- 1 small green banana (about ¼ cup mashed)
- ¼ cup cricket flour or powder
- 1 tablespoon Sweet Potato Flour or Plantain Flour (page 121)
- 1 tablespoon arrowroot powder
- 1 teaspoon coconut flour
- ¼ cup homemade Coconut Milk (page 116) or canned full-fat coconut milk
- 1 tablespoon avocado oil
- ½ teaspoon vanilla extract or ⅛ teaspoon vanilla powder
- ¼ teaspoon baking soda
- Pinch of salt
- Coconut oil, for frying
- Fresh fruit and Coconut Milk Yogurt (page 118) or Coconut Whipped Topping (page 116), for serving

1. Combine all the ingredients in a blender and blend until smooth.
2. Heat a large skillet over medium heat. Melt 1 to 2 teaspoons of coconut oil in the hot skillet.
3. Pour the batter into the skillet to make small pancakes (2 to 3 inches in diameter). Depending on the size of your skillet, you may need to make several batches.
4. Cook for 5 to 6 minutes on the first side, until starting to dry around the edges. Flip.
5. Cook for 3 to 4 minutes on the other side.
6. Serve plain or with fresh fruit and coconut milk yogurt or coconut cream!

VARIATIONS:

Try adding chopped unsweetened banana chips to the batter for a little nutlike crunch.

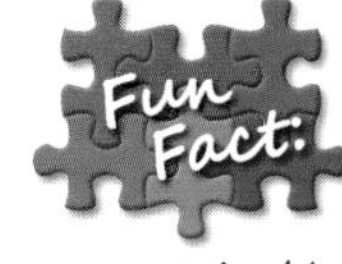

Insects are a fundamental part of the diet in many parts of the world. Crickets provide a sustainable and environmentally responsible complete protein while being rich in vitamins and minerals!

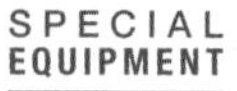

SPECIAL EQUIPMENT

- Blender

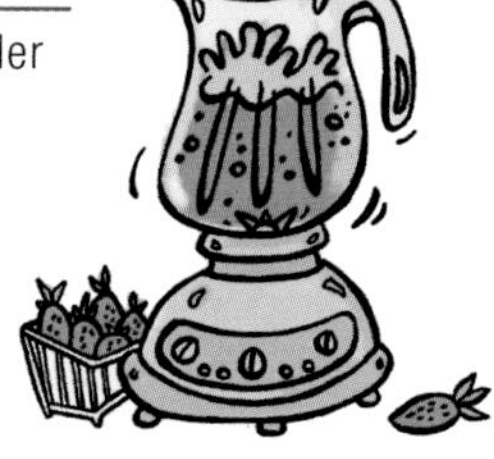

NUTRITION FACTS	
Serving Size	124 g
Recipe Yields	248 g
Calories	**240**
Fats	**13.9 g**
MUFA	5.08 g
Omega-3	0.08 g
Omega-6	0.95 g
Saturated Fat	6.36 g
Carbohydrates	**29.3 g**
Fiber	3.01 g
Starch	3.44 g
Fructose	2.49 g
Glucose	2.56 g
Sucrose	1.45 g
Protein	**12.1 g**
Alanine	0.06 g
Arginine	0.12 g
Aspartic acid	0.16 g
Cystine	0.02 g
Glutamic acid	0.23 g
Glycine	0.05 g
Histidine	0.06 g
Isoleucine	0.04 g
Leucine	0.09 g
Lysine	0.06 g
Methionine	0.02 g
Phenylalanine	0.06 g
Proline	0.04 g
Serine	0.06 g
Threonine	0.04 g
Tryptophan	0.01 g
Tyrosine	0.03 g
Valine	0.07 g
Vitamins	
Vitamin B1	0.03 mg
Vitamin B12	0.4 mcg
Vitamin B2	0.05 mg
Vitamin B3	0.64 mg
Vitamin B5	0.29 mg
Vitamin B6	0.22 mg
Choline	8.41 mg
Folate	15.1 mcg
Vitamin A	78.1 mcg
Vitamin C	6.24 mg
Vitamin D	0 IU
Vitamin E	0.96 mg
Vitamin K	6.66 mcg
Minerals	
Calcium	29.5 mg
Copper	0.12 mg
Iron	1.8 mg
Magnesium	29.2 mg
Manganese	0.43 mg
Phosphorus	43 mg
Potassium	283 mg
Selenium	0.52 mcg
Sodium	240 mg
Zinc	0.27 mg

nutrition content estimated using the USDA database.

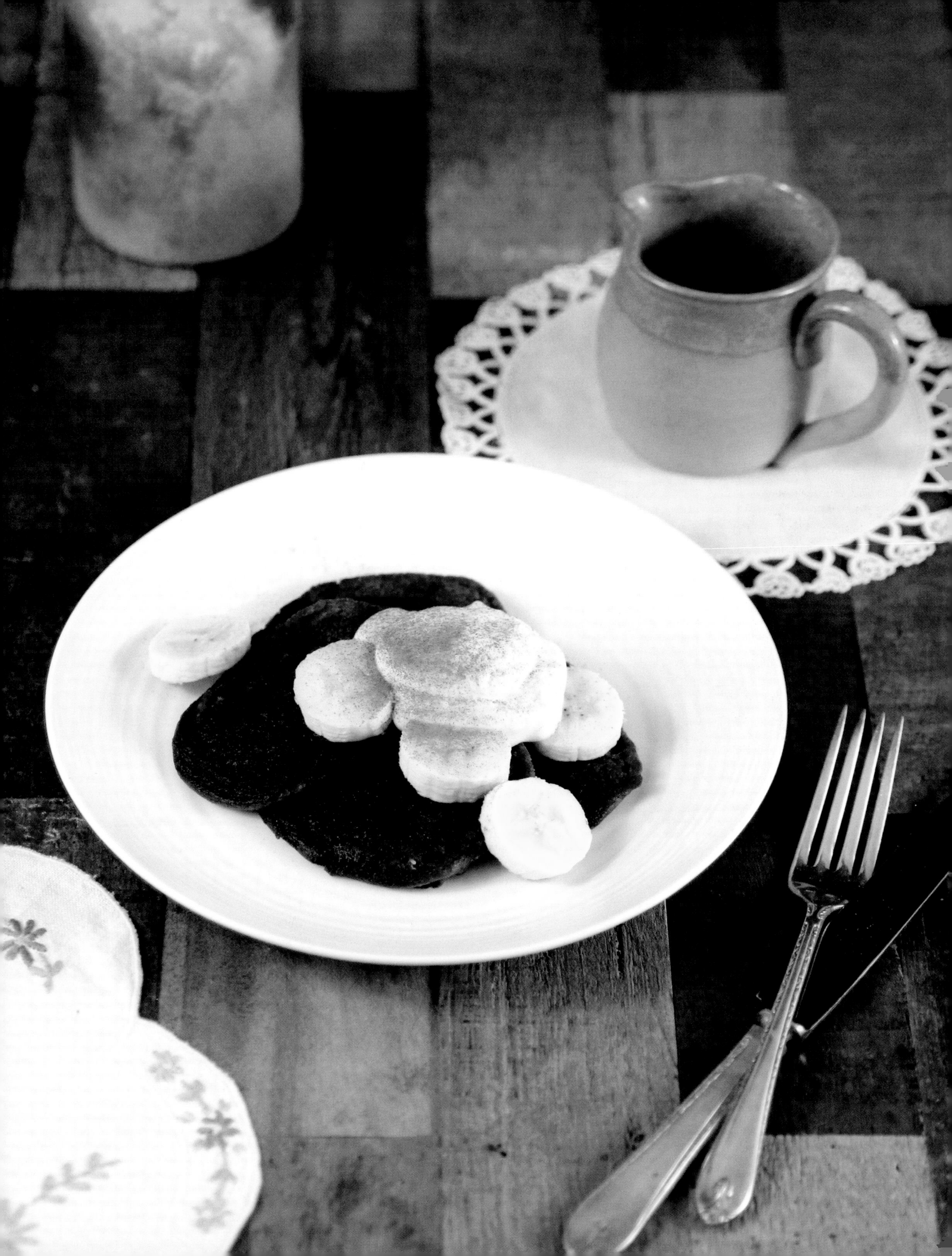

Chapter 6
Appetizers, Salads, and Snacks

The recipes in this chapter can be used as a snack on their own, an appetizer or canapé for a party, or a delightful accompaniment to a meal. Look to this chapter for lunch ideas and for what to make for your next Super Bowl party!

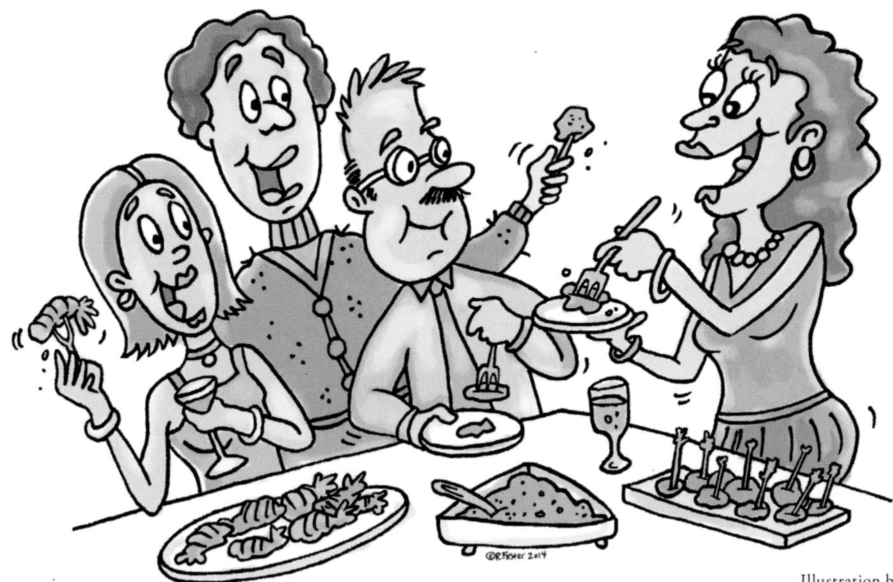

Illustration by Rob Foster

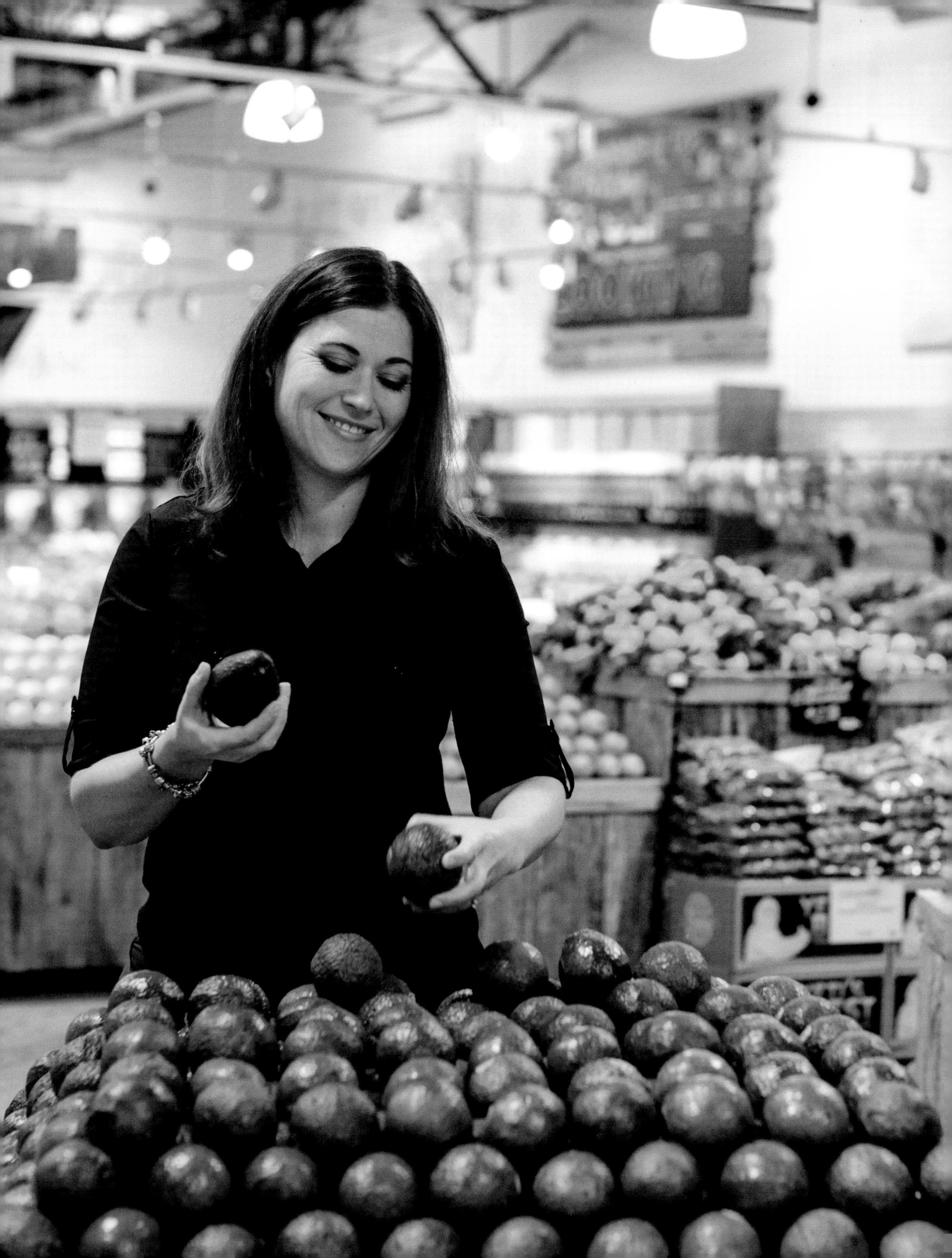

Plantain Crackers

Green plantains have a very neutral and starchy flavor and make the perfect nutrient-dense base for these delicious, crunchy crackers.

PREP TIME: 10 to 15 minutes
COOK TIME: 60 to 80 minutes
SERVINGS: 6 to 10

INGREDIENTS:

2 large or 3 medium green plantains
½ cup coconut oil, melted
½ teaspoon salt, to taste

SPECIAL EQUIPMENT

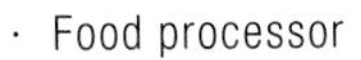

· Food processor

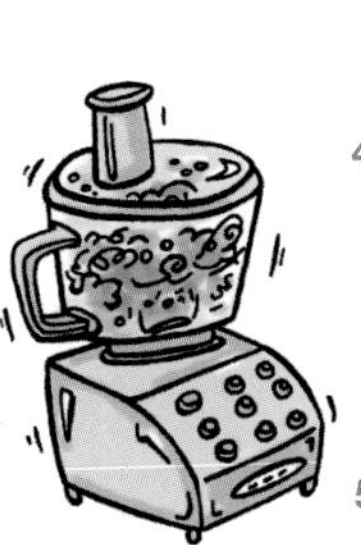

1. Preheat the oven to 300°F. Line a 13-by-18-inch rimmed baking sheet with parchment paper or a silicone liner. Make sure that the parchment goes right up to each edge of the pan.
2. Peel the plantains and place in a food processor with the coconut oil and salt. Process until a completely smooth puree forms, 3 to 5 minutes, turning off the processor and scraping down the sides at least once. (You should have about 2 cups of puree.)
3. Pour the batter (it should look like hummus) onto the prepared baking sheet. Use a rubber spatula to smooth it out and cover the entire sheet uniformly. The batter should be about ⅛ inch thick.
4. Bake for 10 minutes. Remove from the oven and score the batter with a pastry wheel, pizza cutter, or pastry scraper. You can make whatever size crackers you like. The crackers will pull away from each other slightly while cooking and will shrink up a bit, but not much.
5. Return the pan to the oven and bake for 50 to 70 minutes, until the crackers are dark brown.
6. Remove from the oven and let cool slightly in the pan. Move to a cooling rack (you will probably be moving fairly big pieces of several crackers stuck together). Once completely cool, you can break apart any crackers that are stuck together.
7. Store in an airtight container at room temperature. Enjoy!

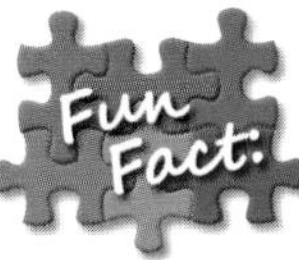

Plantains are a member of the banana family (which is why they look so similar to bananas and are often found in the same area in stores). They go by different names in different regions, so if you can't find them, look for "raw bananas" or "cooking bananas."

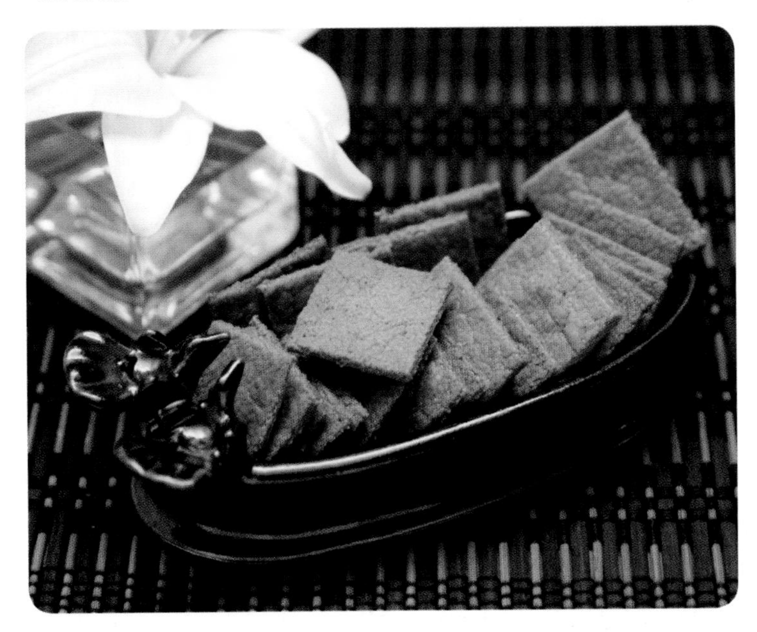

TIPS:

You can buy several green plantains, purée in a food processor, and then freeze for use in recipes such as this or in desserts that use puréed plantain.

VARIATIONS:

You can substitute other cooking fats for the coconut oil. Lard, palm shortening, and avocado oil are all good options.

Herb Crackers. Add 2 to 3 tablespoons of your favorite seasoning mix to make herb crackers. Try 2 tablespoons herbes de Provence (page 108); or 3 tablespoons nutritional yeast with 1 teaspoon garlic powder; or 1 teaspoon garlic powder with 2 tablespoons dried rosemary.

Dessert Crackers. Using partially or fully ripe plantains yields a sweeter, more dessert-like cracker (delicious crumbled on top of yogurt and fruit). You can also omit the salt and add cinnamon or other sweet spices to make these feel like cookies. Because of the naturally higher water content of ripe plantains, they will take up to 30 minutes longer to crisp up in the oven.

NUTRITION FACTS	
Serving Size	47 g
Recipe Yields	470 g
Calories	**138**
Fats	**11 g**
MUFA	0.64 g
Omega-3	<0.01 g
Omega-6	0.21 g
Saturated Fat	9.48 g
Carbohydrates	**11.4 g**
Fiber	0.82 g
Starch	5.22 g
Fructose	0 g
Glucose	0 g
Sucrose	0 g
Protein	**0.47 g**
Alanine	0.02 g
Arginine	0.04 g
Aspartic acid	0.04 g
Cystine	<0.01 g
Glutamic acid	0.04 g
Glycine	0.02 g
Histidine	0.02 g
Isoleucine	0.01 g
Leucine	0.02 g
Lysine	0.02 g
Methionine	<0.01 g
Phenylalanine	0.02 g
Proline	0.02 g
Serine	0.01 g
Threonine	0.01 g
Tryptophan	<0.01 g
Tyrosine	0.01 g
Valine	0.02 g
Vitamins	
Vitamin B1	0.02 mg
Vitamin B12	0 mcg
Vitamin B2	0.02 mg
Vitamin B3	0.25 mg
Vitamin B5	0.09 mg
Vitamin B6	0.11 mg
Choline	4.87 mg
Folate	7.88 mcg
Vitamin A	20.1 mcg
Vitamin C	6.59 mg
Vitamin D	0 IU
Vitamin E	0.06 mg
Vitamin K	0.31 mcg
Minerals	
Calcium	1.66 mg
Copper	0.03 mg
Iron	0.52 mg
Magnesium	13.3 mg
Manganese	0 mg
Phosphorus	12.2 mg
Potassium	180 mg
Selenium	0.54 mcg
Sodium	52.8 mg
Zinc	0.05 mg

nutrition content estimated using the USDA database.

Ahi Tuna Ceviche

Ceviche is essentially a raw fish salsa in which the acidity of the lime juice "cooks" the fish. Cucumber is a delicious alternative to the corn chips that are typically served with this dish.

PREP TIME: 30 minutes
COOK TIME: 1 hour marinating time
SERVINGS: 4 to 6

INGREDIENTS:

¾ pounds sushi-grade ahi tuna, sliced into very thin strips

½ red onion, thinly sliced

⅔ cup fresh lime juice

1 teaspoon finely grated lime zest

¼ teaspoon salt

2 to 3 cucumbers

½ cup chopped fresh cilantro

1 large avocado, peeled, pitted, and cubed (optional)

1. Combine the tuna, onion, lime juice and zest, and salt. Cover and refrigerate for 1 hour, stirring every 15 to 20 minutes.
2. Slice the cucumbers on the bias for serving, or make cucumber cups by cutting the cucumbers into 1½-inch-thick rounds and then using a melon baller to scoop out the middle to form a "cup."
3. Stir the cilantro and avocado, if using, into the tuna mixture and spoon onto cucumber slices or into cucumber cups to serve.

TIPS:

Ahi tuna is much easier to slice when it is still mostly frozen. Thaw for 2 to 3 hours in the refrigerator, then slice with a sharp knife.

VARIATIONS:

Instead of cucumber, serve in lettuce leaves or serve with Plantain Crackers (page 149), Sweet Potato Chips (page 168), or Dehydrator Plantain Chips (page 170). You can also serve as a salad over a bed of mixed greens.

Substitute any fish you like for the ahi tuna, but buy sushi quality.

Shrimp and Mango Ceviche. Use shrimp instead of ahi tuna (buy sushi quality) and add 1 peeled, seeded, and diced mango.

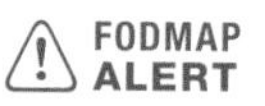

FODMAP ALERT

This recipe cannot be made low-FODMAP.

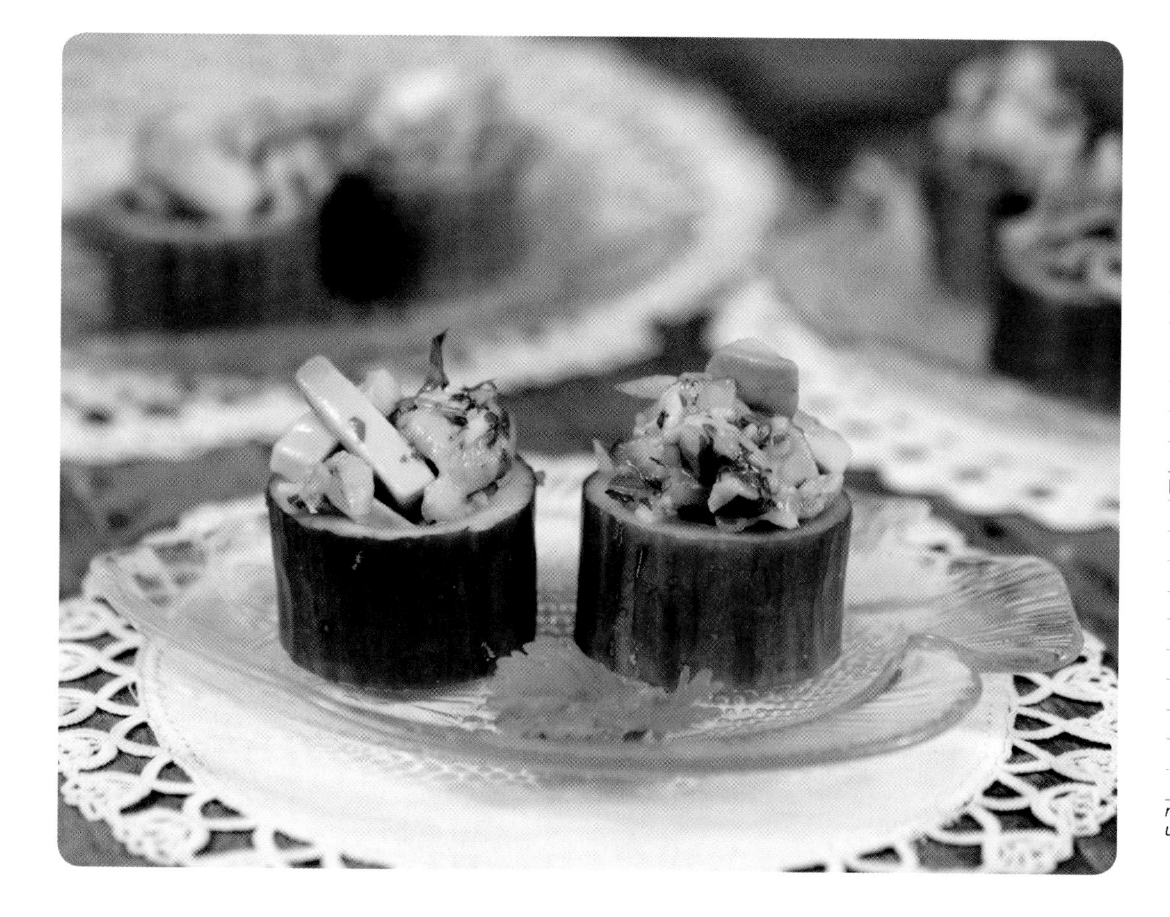

NUTRITION FACTS	
Serving Size	212 g
Recipe Yields	1274 g
Calories	**141**
Fats	**5.77 g**
MUFA	2.88 g
Omega-3	0.19 g
Omega-6	0.82 g
Saturated Fat	1.14 g
Carbohydrates	**8.62 g**
Fiber	3.64 g
Starch	2.07 g
Fructose	0.91 g
Glucose	1.86 g
Sucrose	0.22 g
Protein	**15 g**
Alanine	0.89 g
Arginine	0.88 g
Aspartic acid	1.55 g
Cystine	0.16 g
Glutamic acid	2.32 g
Glycine	0.72 g
Histidine	0.42 g
Isoleucine	0.67 g
Leucine	1.18 g
Lysine	1.31 g
Methionine	0.42 g
Phenylalanine	0.6 g
Proline	0.54 g
Serine	0.63 g
Threonine	0.63 g
Tryptophan	0.17 g
Tyrosine	0.48 g
Valine	0.76 g
Vitamins	
Vitamin B1	0.29 mg
Vitamin B12	0.29 mcg
Vitamin B2	0.08 mg
Vitamin B3	5.98 mg
Vitamin B5	1.11 mg
Vitamin B6	0.61 mg
Choline	42.7 mg
Folate	33.5 mcg
Vitamin A	21.4 mcg
Vitamin C	21 mg
Vitamin D	62.3 IU
Vitamin E	1.74 mg
Vitamin K	9.2 mcg
Minerals	
Calcium	31.2 mg
Copper	0.26 mg
Iron	0.97 mg
Magnesium	51.9 mg
Manganese	0.13 mg
Phosphorus	150 mg
Potassium	574 mg
Selenium	20.8 mcg
Sodium	67.5 mg
Zinc	0.65 mg

nutrition content estimated using the USDA database.

Lox Canapé

Lox is salmon that has been cured with a mild brine and then cold smoked. It has a very different texture and flavor than hot smoked salmon, which is typically cured with salt and sugar before being hot smoked.

This canapé works wonderfully at a party, as an hors d'oeuvre, or as a meal with salad on the side.

PREP TIME: 15 minutes
COOK TIME: none
SERVINGS: 1 to 16

INGREDIENTS:

- 1 clove garlic
- 12 to 16 Plantain Crackers (page 149)
- 4 ounces lox, sliced
- 2 tablespoons thinly sliced red onion
- 2 teaspoons capers

FODMAP ALERT *Omit the garlic and use green onion or chives instead of red onion.*

1. Cut the garlic clove in half. Rub the cut side over the surface of each cracker.
2. Lay slices of lox over each cracker (depending on the size of your crackers, you may or may not have to slice the lox to fit).
3. Add a couple of slices of onion and a few capers on top of each piece of lox. Enjoy!

VARIATIONS:

Sliced cucumber works very well in place of crackers (skip the garlic).

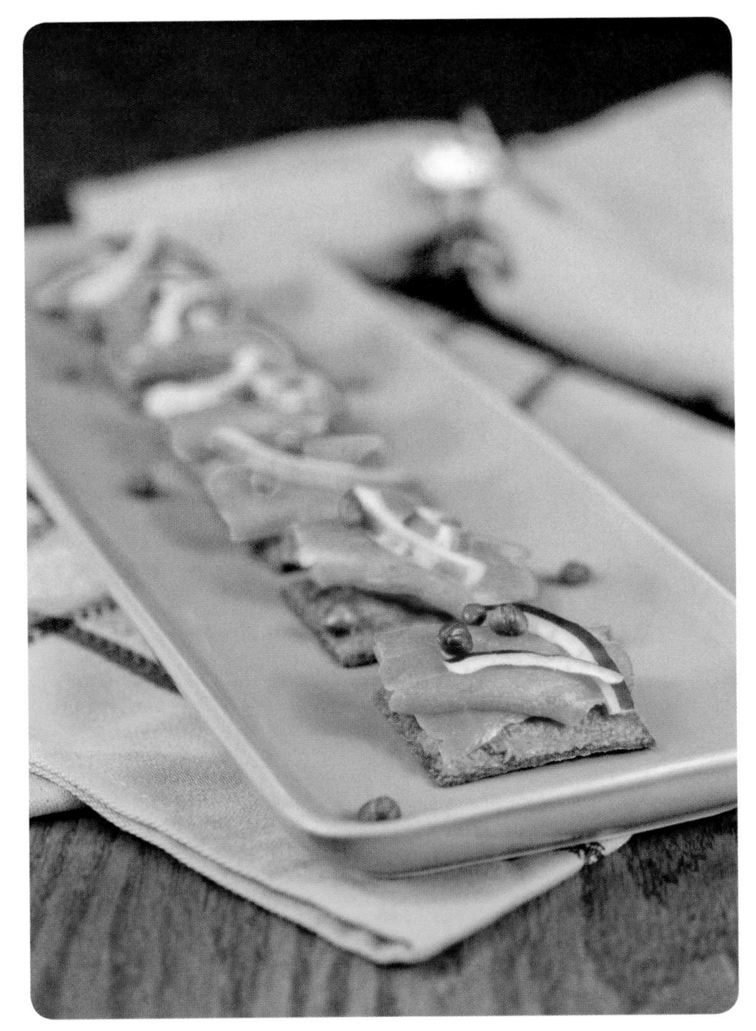

NUTRITION FACTS	
Serving Size	31 g
Recipe Yields	495 g
Calories	**73.9**
Fats	**5.5 g**
MUFA	0.45 g
Omega-3	0.04 g
Omega-6	0.13 g
Saturated Fat	4.52 g
Carbohydrates	**5.56 g**
Fiber	0.42 g
Starch	2.56 g
Fructose	0.02 g
Glucose	0.02 g
Sucrose	0.01 g
Protein	**1.55 g**
Alanine	0.09 g
Arginine	0.1 g
Aspartic acid	0.15 g
Cystine	0.02 g
Glutamic acid	0.22 g
Glycine	0.07 g
Histidine	0.05 g
Isoleucine	0.07 g
Leucine	0.12 g
Lysine	0.13 g
Methionine	0.04 g
Phenylalanine	0.06 g
Proline	0.05 g
Serine	0.06 g
Threonine	0.06 g
Tryptophan	0.02 g
Tyrosine	0.05 g
Valine	0.08 g
Vitamins	
Vitamin B1	0.01 mg
Vitamin B12	0.23 mcg
Vitamin B2	0.02 mg
Vitamin B3	0.46 mg
Vitamin B5	0.11 mg
Vitamin B6	0.07 mg
Choline	2.43 mg
Folate	4.17 mcg
Vitamin A	11.3 mcg
Vitamin C	3.26 mg
Vitamin D	0 IU
Vitamin E	0.03 mg
Vitamin K	0.24 mcg
Minerals	
Calcium	2.33 mg
Copper	0.03 mg
Iron	0.32 mg
Magnesium	7.8 mg
Manganese	<0.01 mg
Phosphorus	18.1 mg
Potassium	100 mg
Selenium	3 mcg
Sodium	177 mg
Zinc	0.05 mg

nutrition content estimated using the USDA database.

Bacon and Bison Liver Pâté with Fresh Fig Jam

While the flavor of bison liver is fantastic, you can make this pâté with any type of liver. Lamb liver and chicken liver are particularly good options, but calf's liver also works very well.

This recipe makes a delightful soft spreadable pâté, perfect to serve on Plantain Crackers. To make it extra special, serve it with a touch of fresh fig jam.

PREP TIME: 10 to 15 minutes
COOK TIME: 30 minutes
SERVINGS: 6 to 16

INGREDIENTS:

Fresh Fig Jam (optional):

- 1 pound fresh figs
- ½ cup water
- 1 tablespoon fresh lemon juice

Pâté:

- 8 ounces bacon, chopped
- 1 small onion, finely chopped
- 2 cloves garlic, sliced
- 1 tablespoon chopped fresh sage (10 to 12 leaves)
- 1 sprig fresh rosemary
- 4 or 5 sprigs fresh thyme
- ⅛ teaspoon ground mace
- 1 bay leaf
- 1 pound liver, sliced
- ⅓ cup cognac, dry sherry, or Bone Broth (beef, page 110)
- ¼ teaspoon salt
- ½ cup bacon fat or lard
- 1 teaspoon truffle oil (optional)
- 1 recipe Plantain Crackers (page 149), for serving

FODMAP ALERT *Replace the garlic with green garlic or garlic scapes (green part only) or omit. Replace the onion with green onion or leek (green part only) or chives or omit. Skip the Fresh Fig Jam.*

SPECIAL EQUIPMENT

- Blender or food processor

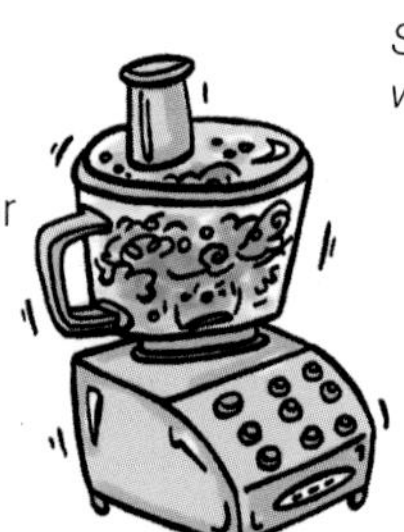

FRESH FIG JAM:

1. Remove the stems from the figs and roughly chop the figs.
2. Combine the figs, water, and lemon juice in a small saucepot. Bring to a boil over high heat, then reduce the heat to maintain a simmer.
3. Simmer for 20 to 25 minutes, until the figs are thoroughly cooked and soft. Mash with a fork for a lumpier jam, or purée with an immersion blender for a smooth jam. Store in the refrigerator for up to a month or in the freezer for long-term storage.

PÂTÉ:

1. Cook the bacon, onion, garlic, sage, rosemary, thyme, mace, and bay leaf in a large skillet over medium-high heat until the bacon is fully cooked and the onions are soft and caramelized, about 15 minutes.
2. Add the liver and cognac to the pan and cook at a rapid simmer until you can't smell alcohol in the steam, 6 to 10 minutes.
3. Remove from the heat. Remove and discard the bay leaf and stems of rosemary and thyme. Add the salt and the bacon fat.
4. Pour the hot liver mixture into a blender or food processor and process until smooth. Add the truffle oil, if using, and pulse until fully combined.
5. Pour into a serving dish such as a loaf pan or a pair of 10- to 14-ounce ramekins. Cover with wax paper or parchment paper, applying it directly to the surface to prevent oxidation (you'll still get some, which is okay, but covering with paper helps your pâté stay a nice pink color).
6. Refrigerate overnight or up to a few days before eating. Serve with fig jam, if desired, and Plantain Crackers.

TIPS:

Look for truffle oil made with extra-virgin olive oil with no artificial flavors.

VARIATIONS:

Sliced cucumber and celery also make great vessels for this pâté if you want to skip the Plantain Crackers.

NUTRITION FACTS

Serving Size	125 g
Recipe Yields	2005 g
Calories	**299**
Fats	**21 g**
MUFA	6.33 g
Omega-3	0.11 g
Omega-6	1.63 g
Saturated Fat	11.3 g
Carbohydrates	**14.9 g**
Fiber	1.49 g
Starch	3.57 g
Fructose	0.07 g
Glucose	0.1 g
Sucrose	0.05 g
Protein	**13.9 g**
Alanine	0.81 g
Arginine	0.85 g
Aspartic acid	1.32 g
Cystine	0.21 g
Glutamic acid	1.84 g
Glycine	0.83 g
Histidine	0.46 g
Isoleucine	0.64 g
Leucine	1.17 g
Lysine	1.08 g
Methionine	0.33 g
Phenylalanine	0.65 g
Proline	0.68 g
Serine	0.57 g
Threonine	0.56 g
Tryptophan	0.15 g
Tyrosine	0.49 g
Valine	0.79 g
Vitamins	
Vitamin B1	0.14 mg
Vitamin B12	20.1 mcg
Vitamin B2	1.03 mg
Vitamin B3	6.78 mg
Vitamin B5	2.31 mg
Vitamin B6	0.44 mg
Choline	145 mg
Folate	80 mcg
Vitamin A	2687 mcg
Vitamin C	6.39 mg
Vitamin D	20.4 IU
Vitamin E	0.3 mg
Vitamin K	3.56 mcg
Minerals	
Calcium	18.6 mg
Copper	4.11 mg
Iron	2.68 mg
Magnesium	24.6 mg
Manganese	0.16 mg
Phosphorus	227 mg
Potassium	368 mg
Selenium	19.1 mcg
Sodium	401 mg
Zinc	2.08 mg

nutrition content estimated using the USDA database.

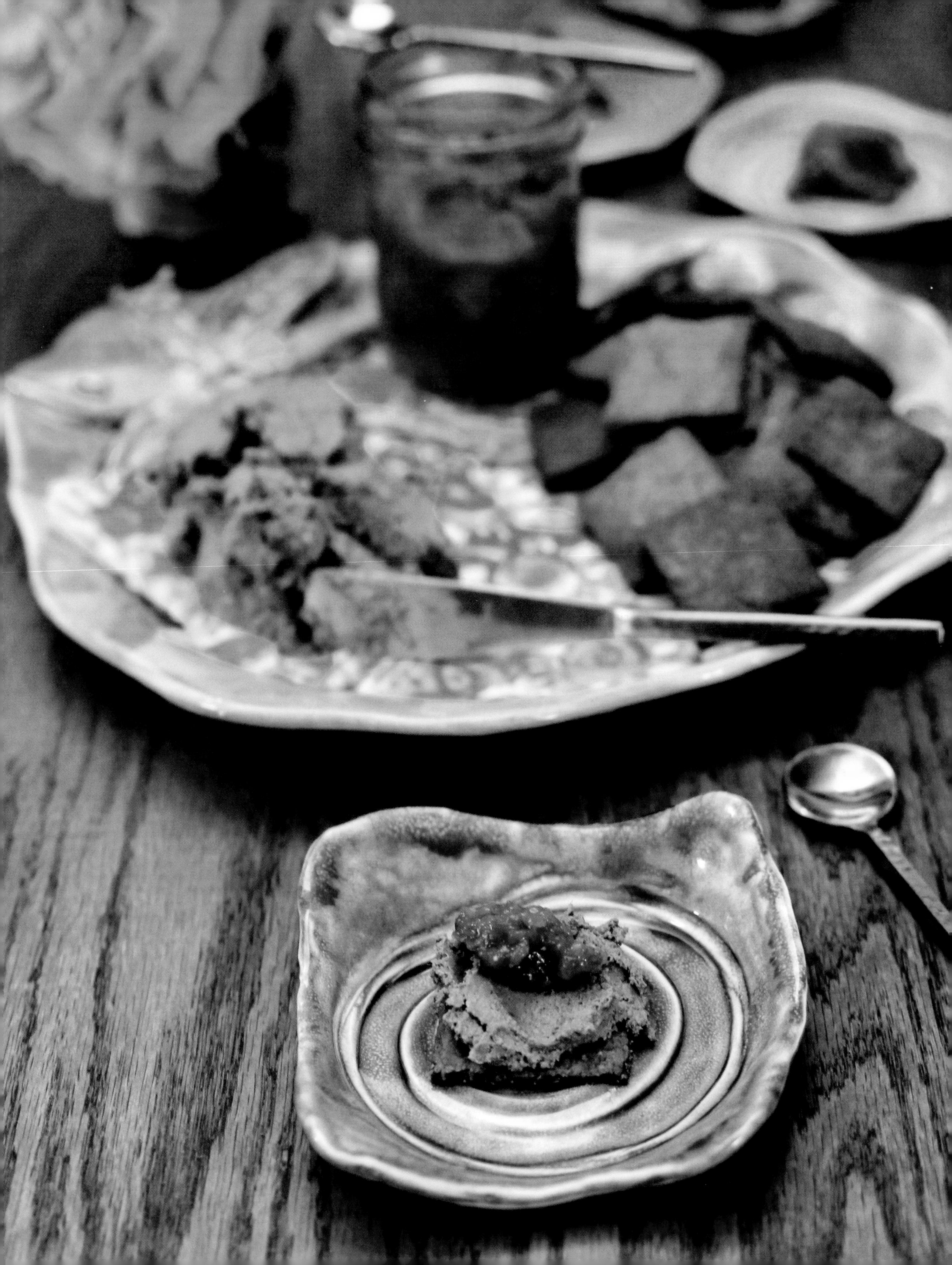

Shrimp and Avocado Skewers

These shrimp skewers are a delicious appetizer and can be made ahead of time.

PREP TIME: 20 to 30 minutes, plus at least 3 hours marinating time
COOK TIME: none
YIELD: 25 to 30

INGREDIENTS:

- 2 tablespoons extra-virgin olive oil
- 2 tablespoons fresh lime juice
- 1 teaspoon finely grated lime zest
- ⅓ cup chopped fresh cilantro
- Pinch of salt
- ½ pound small shrimp (51 to 60 per pound), cooked
- 2 medium avocados, peeled, pitted, and cut into large chunks

1. In a small bowl, combine the olive oil, lime juice and zest, cilantro, and salt. Pour over the shrimp and refrigerate for at least 3 hours and up to overnight.
2. To serve, skewer 1 shrimp and 1 chunk of avocado with a toothpick (they hold together better if you skewer one end of the shrimp, then the avocado, then the other end of the shrimp). Repeat with the rest of your shrimp. (You can also add several shrimp and chunks of avocado to a skewer, kabob style.)
3. Drizzle a little of the marinade over the skewers. Serve!

TIPS:

Want to keep this simple? Dump it in a bowl and eat it with a fork!

VARIATIONS:

Shrimp and Avocado Salad. You can easily turn this dish into a salad by pouring the marinated shrimp, avocado, and leftover marinade onto some mixed greens. Serves 2.

FODMAP ALERT

This recipe cannot be made low-FODMAP.

SPECIAL EQUIPMENT

- Toothpicks or skewers

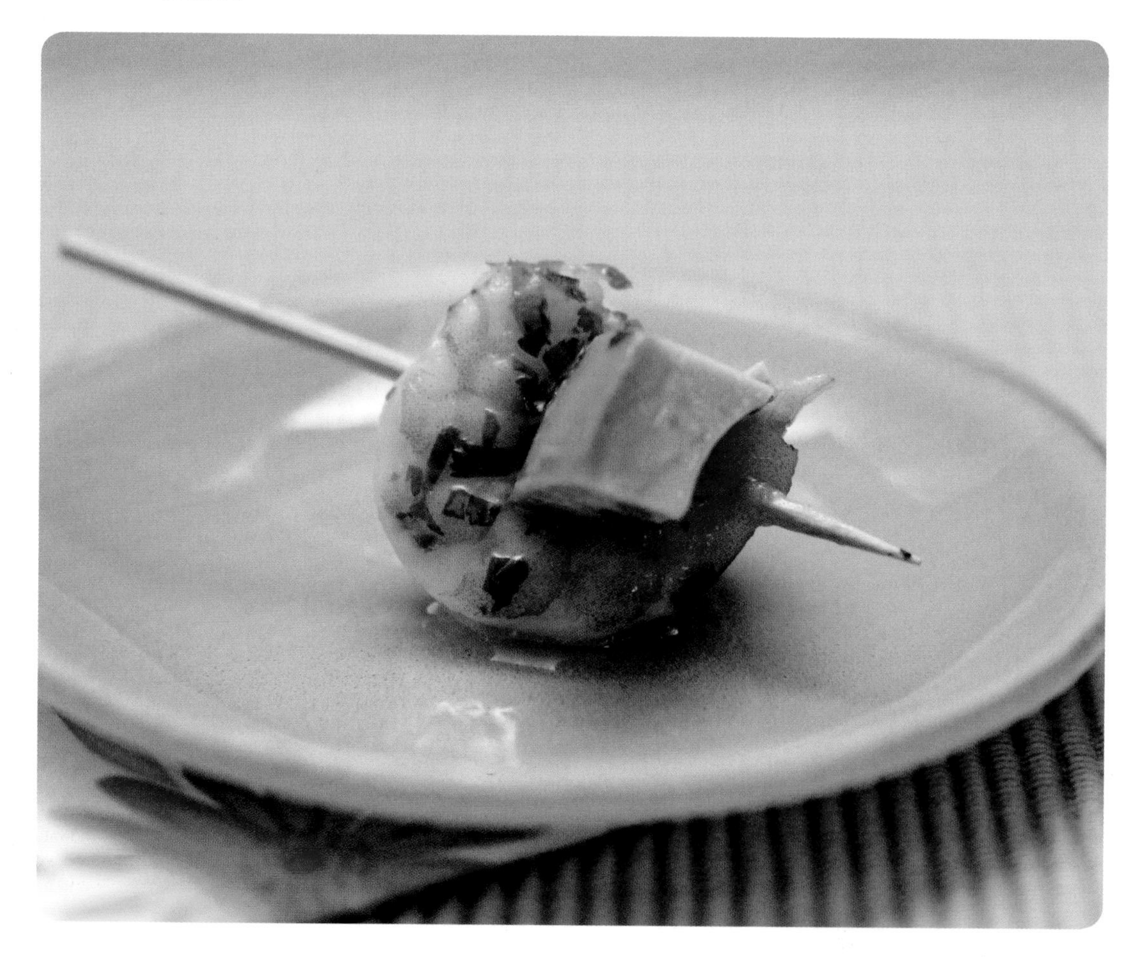

NUTRITION FACTS	
Serving Size	60 g
Recipe Yields	900 g
Calories	**81.2**
Fats	**6.14 g**
MUFA	3.59 g
Omega-3	0.13 g
Omega-6	0.83 g
Saturated Fat	1.09 g
Carbohydrates	**3.51 g**
Fiber	2.3 g
Starch	0.13 g
Fructose	0.11 g
Glucose	0.89 g
Sucrose	<0.01 g
Protein	**3.99 g**
Alanine	0.22 g
Arginine	0.31 g
Aspartic acid	0.43 g
Cystine	0.05 g
Glutamic acid	0.66 g
Glycine	0.23 g
Histidine	0.08 g
Isoleucine	0.19 g
Leucine	0.31 g
Lysine	0.33 g
Methionine	0.1 g
Phenylalanine	0.17 g
Proline	0.15 g
Serine	0.17 g
Threonine	0.16 g
Tryptophan	0.05 g
Tyrosine	0.12 g
Valine	0.19 g
Vitamins	
Vitamin B1	0.01 mg
Vitamin B12	0.18 mcg
Vitamin B2	0.03 mg
Vitamin B3	0.67 mg
Vitamin B5	0.39 mg
Vitamin B6	0.05 mg
Choline	12.4 mg
Folate	15.8 mcg
Vitamin A	12.2 mcg
Vitamin C	8.23 mg
Vitamin D	0.6 IU
Vitamin E	1.52 mg
Vitamin K	2.13 mcg
Minerals	
Calcium	12.7 mg
Copper	0.17 mg
Iron	0.5 mg
Magnesium	15.6 mg
Manganese	0.05 mg
Phosphorus	47.7 mg
Potassium	175 mg
Selenium	5.75 mcg
Sodium	32 mg
Zinc	0.33 mg

nutrition content estimated using the USDA database.

Bacon-Wrapped Scallops

There's a reason why bacon-wrapped scallops are a classic appetizer: it's hard to imagine a better pairing. You can skewer these on shish kabob skewers or use sturdy toothpicks.

PREP TIME: 20 to 30 minutes
COOK TIME: 20 to 35 minutes
YIELD: 15

INGREDIENTS:

1 pound sea scallops (about 15 large)

10 to 15 slices bacon

1. Preheat the oven to 375°F. Line a rimmed baking sheet with parchment paper, aluminum foil, or a silicone liner.
2. Cut the bacon slices long enough to wrap around each scallop with about a ¾-inch overlap—likely about three-quarters of the length of your bacon slices. You may even use a whole slice of bacon if your scallops are particularly large.
3. Wrap each scallop in a slice of bacon, skewering through the bacon overlap to the other side to hold in place (you can also use 2 shorter pieces of bacon and overlap on both ends).
4. Arrange the scallops on the prepared baking sheet so that the bottom of each scallop is on the sheet and the bacon is perpendicular to the sheet. Bake until the bacon is browned and fully cooked (20 to 35 minutes, depending on the thickness of your bacon).

TIPS:

Thinly sliced bacon will take less time to cook than thick-cut bacon. It's best to use thinly sliced bacon if your scallops are on the small side.

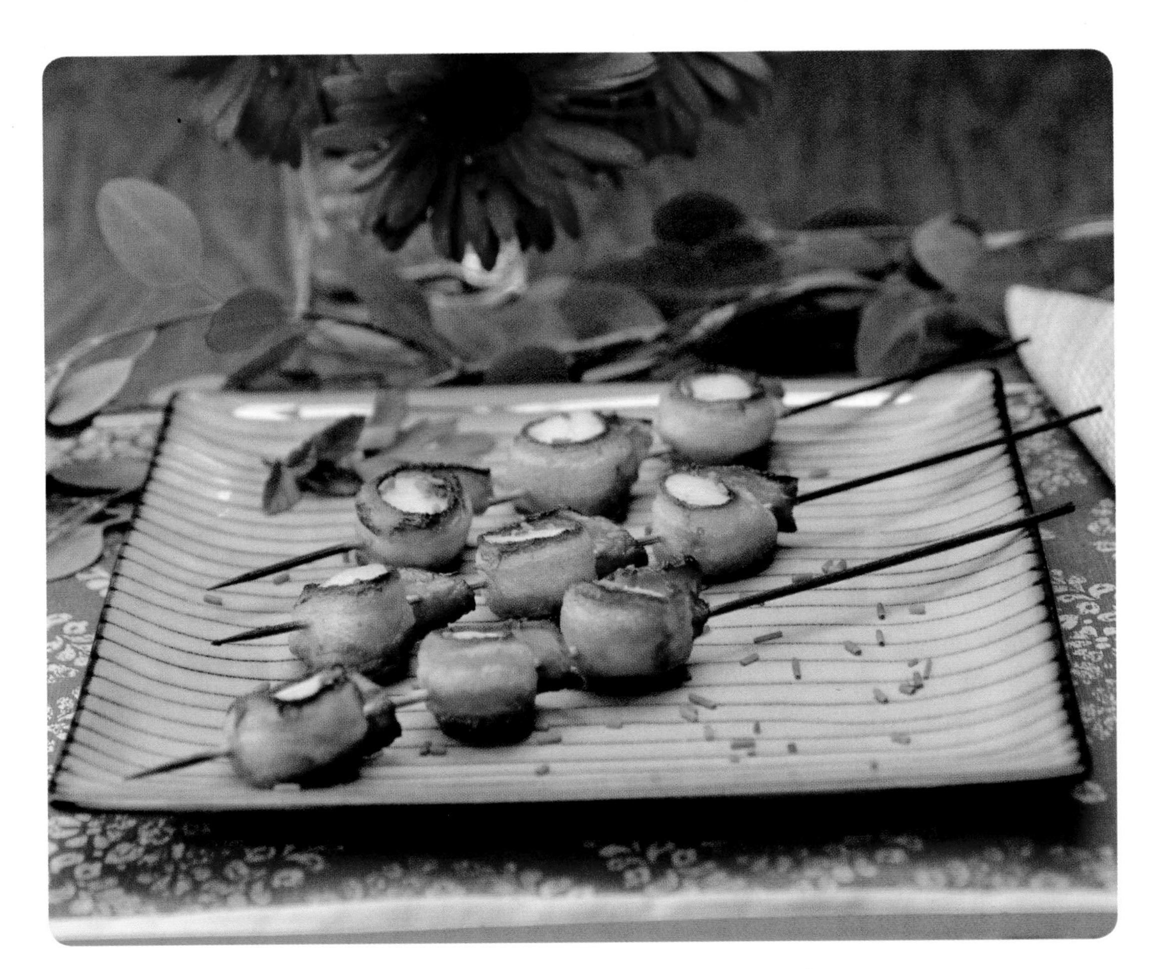

NUTRITION FACTS

Serving Size	67 g
Recipe Yields	535 g
Calories	**94.9**
Fats	**4.67 g**
MUFA	1.96 g
Omega-3	0.08 g
Omega-6	0.44 g
Saturated Fat	1.51 g
Carbohydrates	**1.94 g**
Fiber	0 g
Starch	1.23 g
Fructose	0 g
Glucose	0 g
Sucrose	0 g
Protein	**10.5 g**
Alanine	0.54 g
Arginine	0.6 g
Aspartic acid	0.87 g
Cystine	0.11 g
Glutamic acid	1.33 g
Glycine	0.84 g
Histidine	0.24 g
Isoleucine	0.4 g
Leucine	0.69 g
Lysine	0.72 g
Methionine	0.24 g
Phenylalanine	0.34 g
Proline	0.36 g
Serine	0.34 g
Threonine	0.35 g
Tryptophan	0.09 g
Tyrosine	0.28 g
Valine	0.41 g
Vitamins	
Vitamin B1	0.04 mg
Vitamin B12	0.92 mcg
Vitamin B2	0.03 mg
Vitamin B3	1.48 mg
Vitamin B5	0.23 mg
Vitamin B6	0.07 mg
Choline	49.1 mg
Folate	9.3 mcg
Vitamin A	1.69 mcg
Vitamin C	0 mg
Vitamin D	0.57 IU
Vitamin E	0.03 mg
Vitamin K	0.01 mcg
Minerals	
Calcium	4.43 mg
Copper	0.03 mg
Iron	0.37 mg
Magnesium	15.6 mg
Manganese	0.01 mg
Phosphorus	241 mg
Potassium	171 mg
Selenium	13.3 mcg
Sodium	445 mg
Zinc	0.86 mg

nutrition content estimated using the USDA database.

Har Gow–Inspired Shrimp Balls

Har gow was my favorite dim sum dish growing up. You can enjoy these har gow–inspired shrimp balls as a snack or an appetizer, or add some vegetables to make it a meal. These also make a wonderful breakfast protein!

PREP TIME: 20 minutes
COOK TIME: 10 minutes
YIELD: 16 to 20

INGREDIENTS:

- 1 pound raw shrimp, shelled
- 1 teaspoon fish sauce
- 1½ teaspoons coconut oil, melted
- 1 tablespoon arrowroot powder
- ⅛ teaspoon salt
- ⅓ cup finely chopped bamboo shoots

1. Preheat the oven to 350°F. Line a baking sheet with parchment paper, aluminum foil, or a silicone liner.
2. Place the shrimp, fish sauce, coconut oil, arrowroot powder, and salt in a food processor. Process until the shrimp is finely ground.
3. Add the chopped bamboo shoots and pulse once or twice to incorporate.
4. Wet your hands with cold water and form the mixture into 1 to 1½-inch balls. If the mixture starts to stick to your hands, wet them again. Arrange the shrimp balls on the prepared baking sheet.
5. Bake for 10 minutes, until fully cooked and pink throughout. Enjoy!

SPECIAL EQUIPMENT

- Food processor

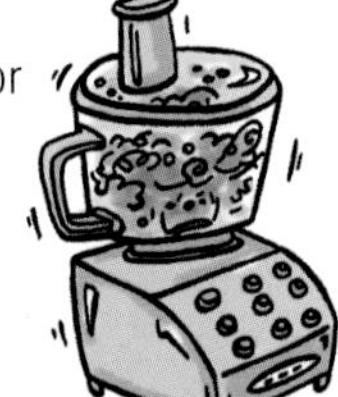

TIPS:

Large shrimp are typically deveined when you buy them, and small shrimp are not. You don't have to devein shrimp, but some people find the vein (which is actually the shrimp's intestinal tract) to be a little bitter.

While a food processor is great for grinding shrimp, the texture of very finely hand-chopped bamboo shoots actually works much better in these shrimp balls.

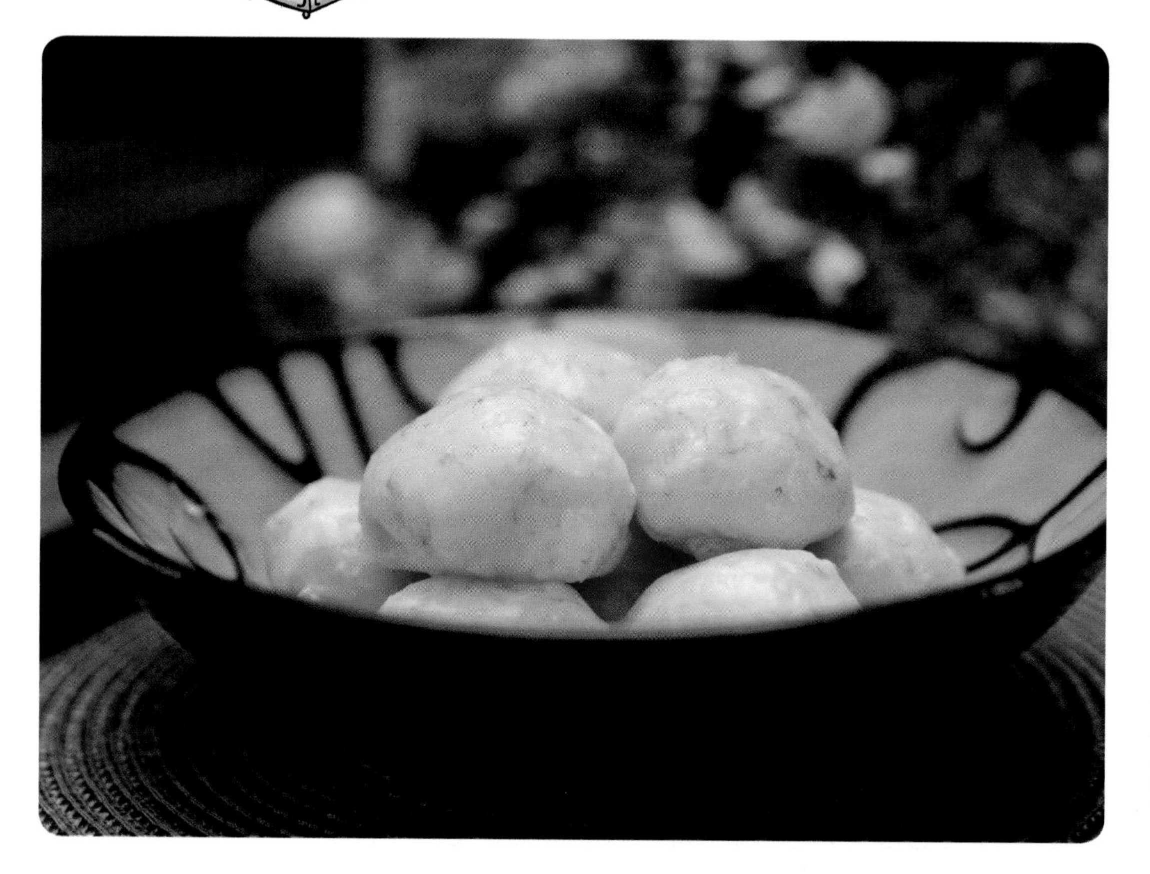

NUTRITION FACTS

Serving Size	130 g
Recipe Yields	519 g
Calories	**145**
Fats	**3.7 g**
MUFA	0.39 g
Omega-3	0.61 g
Omega-6	0.16 g
Saturated Fat	1.85 g
Carbohydrates	**3.2 g**
Fiber	0.22 g
Starch	0 g
Fructose	0 g
Glucose	0 g
Sucrose	0 g
Protein	**23.4 g**
Alanine	1.32 g
Arginine	2.02 g
Aspartic acid	2.42 g
Cystine	0.26 g
Glutamic acid	3.96 g
Glycine	1.4 g
Histidine	0.47 g
Isoleucine	1.13 g
Leucine	1.84 g
Lysine	2.02 g
Methionine	0.65 g
Phenylalanine	0.98 g
Proline	0.78 g
Serine	0.92 g
Threonine	0.94 g
Tryptophan	0.32 g
Tyrosine	0.77 g
Valine	1.09 g
Vitamins	
Vitamin B1	0.03 mg
Vitamin B12	1.33 mcg
Vitamin B2	0.04 mg
Vitamin B3	2.95 mg
Vitamin B5	0.1 mg
Vitamin B6	0.14 mg
Choline	92.2 mg
Folate	10.2 mcg
Vitamin A	61.6 mcg
Vitamin C	2.4 mg
Vitamin D	4.55 IU
Vitamin E	1.32 mg
Vitamin K	<0.01mcg
Minerals	
Calcium	61 mg
Copper	0.31 mg
Iron	2.98 mg
Magnesium	45.1 mg
Manganese	0.08 mg
Phosphorus	236 mg
Potassium	224 mg
Selenium	43.4 mcg
Sodium	319 mg
Zinc	1.34 mg

nutrition content estimated using the USDA database.

Pot Sticker Meatballs

These pot sticker–inspired meatballs make a wonderful snack or appetizer on their own, can be enjoyed as a dim sum–style breakfast, or can easily be turned into a meal with the addition of a salad or some veggie sticks on the side.

PREP TIME: 15 to 20 minutes
COOK TIME: 12 minutes
YIELD: 20 to 24

INGREDIENTS:

- 1 pound ground pork
- 2 cups very finely chopped Napa cabbage (about 7 ounces)
- ¼ cup very finely chopped green onion (about 2 large)
- 1 tablespoon peeled and grated fresh ginger
- 1 teaspoon coconut aminos
- 1 teaspoon coconut water vinegar
- 1 teaspoon fish sauce
- ¼ teaspoon salt, to taste
- 2 tablespoons arrowroot powder

1. Preheat the oven to 400°F. Line a rimmed baking sheet with parchment paper, aluminum foil, or a silicone liner.
2. Combine all the ingredients in a bowl and mix thoroughly. Form into 1-inch balls with your hands and arrange on the prepared baking sheet.
3. Bake for 12 minutes, until fully cooked. Enjoy!

TIPS:

You can save time by using a food processor to chop the cabbage and green onions. Give them a rough chop first to measure the right amounts, then pulse in the food processor until finely chopped.

FODMAP ALERT

This recipe cannot be made low-FODMAP.

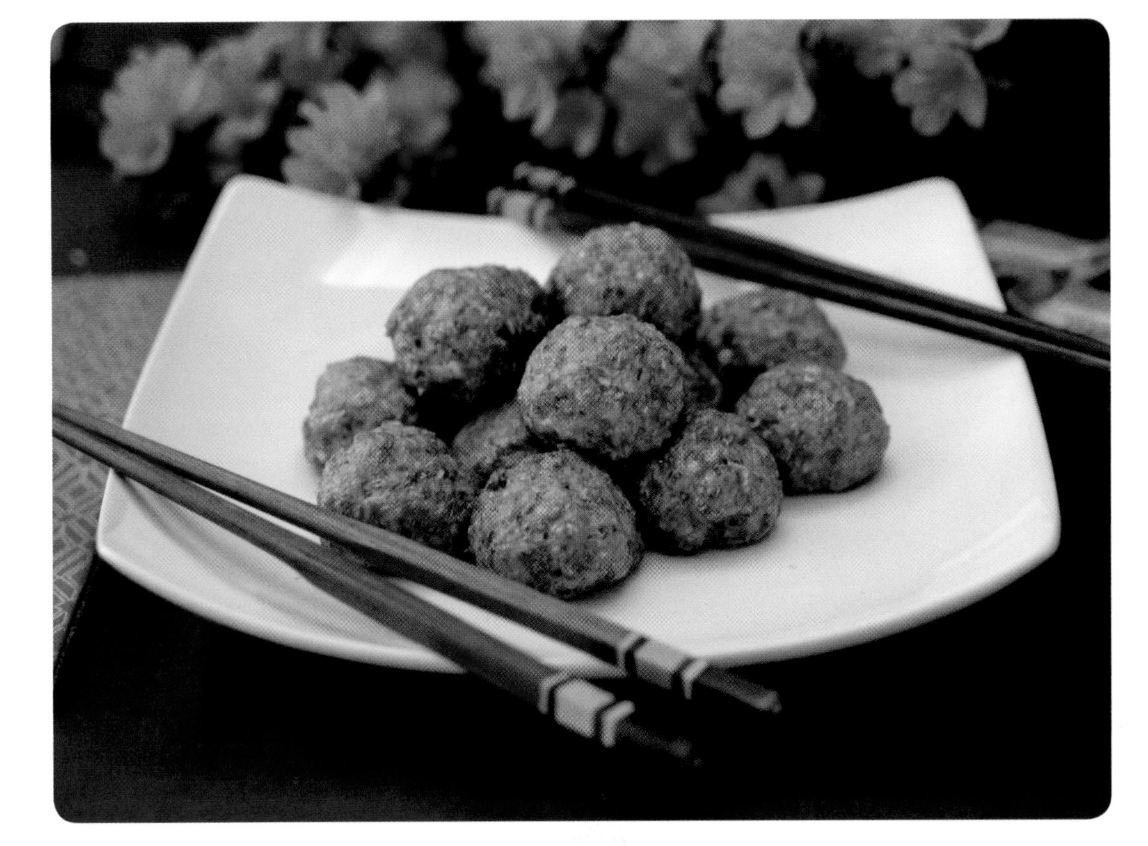

NUTRITION FACTS	
Serving Size	27 g
Recipe Yields	651 g
Calories	**60.4**
Fats	**3.92 g**
MUFA	1.74 g
Omega-3	0.01 g
Omega-6	0.31 g
Saturated Fat	1.46 g
Carbohydrates	**1.06 g**
Fiber	0.18 g
Starch	0.04 g
Fructose	0.1 g
Glucose	0.11 g
Sucrose	<0.01 g
Protein	**4.93 g**
Alanine	0.28 g
Arginine	0.31 g
Aspartic acid	0.46 g
Cystine	0.06 g
Glutamic acid	0.77 g
Glycine	0.23 g
Histidine	0.19 g
Isoleucine	0.23 g
Leucine	0.39 g
Lysine	0.44 g
Methionine	0.13 g
Phenylalanine	0.19 g
Proline	0.2 g
Serine	0.2 g
Threonine	0.22 g
Tryptophan	0.06 g
Tyrosine	0.17 g
Valine	0.26 g
Vitamins	
Vitamin B1	0.14 mg
Vitamin B12	0.1 mcg
Vitamin B2	0.04 mg
Vitamin B3	0.82 mg
Vitamin B5	0.11 mg
Vitamin B6	0.08 mg
Choline	17.4 mg
Folate	4 mcg
Vitamin A	2.15 mcg
Vitamin C	2.37 mg
Vitamin D	3.95 IU
Vitamin E	0.05 mg
Vitamin K	5.57 mcg
Minerals	
Calcium	7.13 mg
Copper	0.01 mg
Iron	0.34 mg
Magnesium	5.88 mg
Manganese	0.01 mg
Phosphorus	44.3 mg
Potassium	81.4 mg
Selenium	6.71 mcg
Sodium	49.8 mg
Zinc	0.62 mg

nutrition content estimated using the USDA database.

Crab-Stuffed Mushroom Caps

Avocado takes the place of mayonnaise in this traditional appetizer.

PREP TIME: 20 to 30 minutes
COOK TIME: 20 to 35 minutes
YIELD: 12

INGREDIENTS:

- 12 ounces large stuffing mushrooms
- 8 ounces precooked or canned crab meat (about 2 [6-ounce] cans)
- 1 small avocado, peeled, pitted, and diced
- 1 green onion, minced
- 2 tablespoons fresh lemon juice
- ¼ teaspoon salt
- ⅓ cup minced fresh parsley
- 1 clove garlic, crushed

FODMAP ALERT

This recipe cannot be made low-FODMAP.

1. Preheat the oven to 400°F.
2. Pull the stems out of the mushroom caps and use a knife or melon baller to gently widen the "hole" for the stuffing. Place in a baking dish or on a rimmed baking sheet.
3. Combine the remaining ingredients in a bowl. Mash with a fork until completely combined. Spoon into the prepared mushrooms caps (it's okay if they're a little overstuffed).
4. Bake for 20 to 25 minutes, until lightly browned on top and bubbling. Serve warm.

VARIATIONS:

Try sprinkling a little nutritional yeast mixed with crushed Plantain Chips (page 170) or Plantain Crackers (page 149) on the top before baking to emulate the traditional Parmesan and bread crumble on crab-stuffed mushroom caps.

Shrimp-Stuffed Mushroom Caps. Replace the crab meat with finely chopped precooked shrimp.

Lobster-Stuffed Mushroom Caps. Replace the crab meat with finely diced precooked lobster meat.

NUTRITION FACTS	
Serving Size	77 g
Recipe Yields	770 g
Calories	**51.2**
Fats	**2.41 g**
MUFA	1.38 g
Omega-3	0.06 g
Omega-6	0.29 g
Saturated Fat	0.36 g
Carbohydrates	**3 g**
Fiber	1.47 g
Starch	0.3 g
Fructose	0.24 g
Glucose	0.75 g
Sucrose	0.02 g
Protein	**5.14 g**
Alanine	0.28 g
Arginine	0.44 g
Aspartic acid	0.5 g
Cystine	0.05 g
Glutamic acid	0.75 g
Glycine	0.29 g
Histidine	0.12 g
Isoleucine	0.22 g
Leucine	0.36 g
Lysine	0.38 g
Methionine	0.12 g
Phenylalanine	0.2 g
Proline	0.2 g
Serine	0.2 g
Threonine	0.21 g
Tryptophan	0.07 g
Tyrosine	0.16 g
Valine	0.23 g
Vitamins	
Vitamin B1	0.04 mg
Vitamin B12	0.77 mcg
Vitamin B2	0.09 mg
Vitamin B3	2.45 mg
Vitamin B5	0.83 mg
Vitamin B6	0.13 mg
Choline	28 mg
Folate	37.2 mcg
Vitamin A	11.9 mcg
Vitamin C	6.02 mg
Vitamin D	3.4 IU
Vitamin E	0.71 mg
Vitamin K	37.3 mcg
Minerals	
Calcium	27.8 mg
Copper	0.31 mg
Iron	0.59 mg
Magnesium	13.6 mg
Manganese	0.07 mg
Phosphorus	99.3 mg
Potassium	270 mg
Selenium	16.2 mcg
Sodium	121 mg
Zinc	1.17 mg

nutrition content estimated using the USDA database.

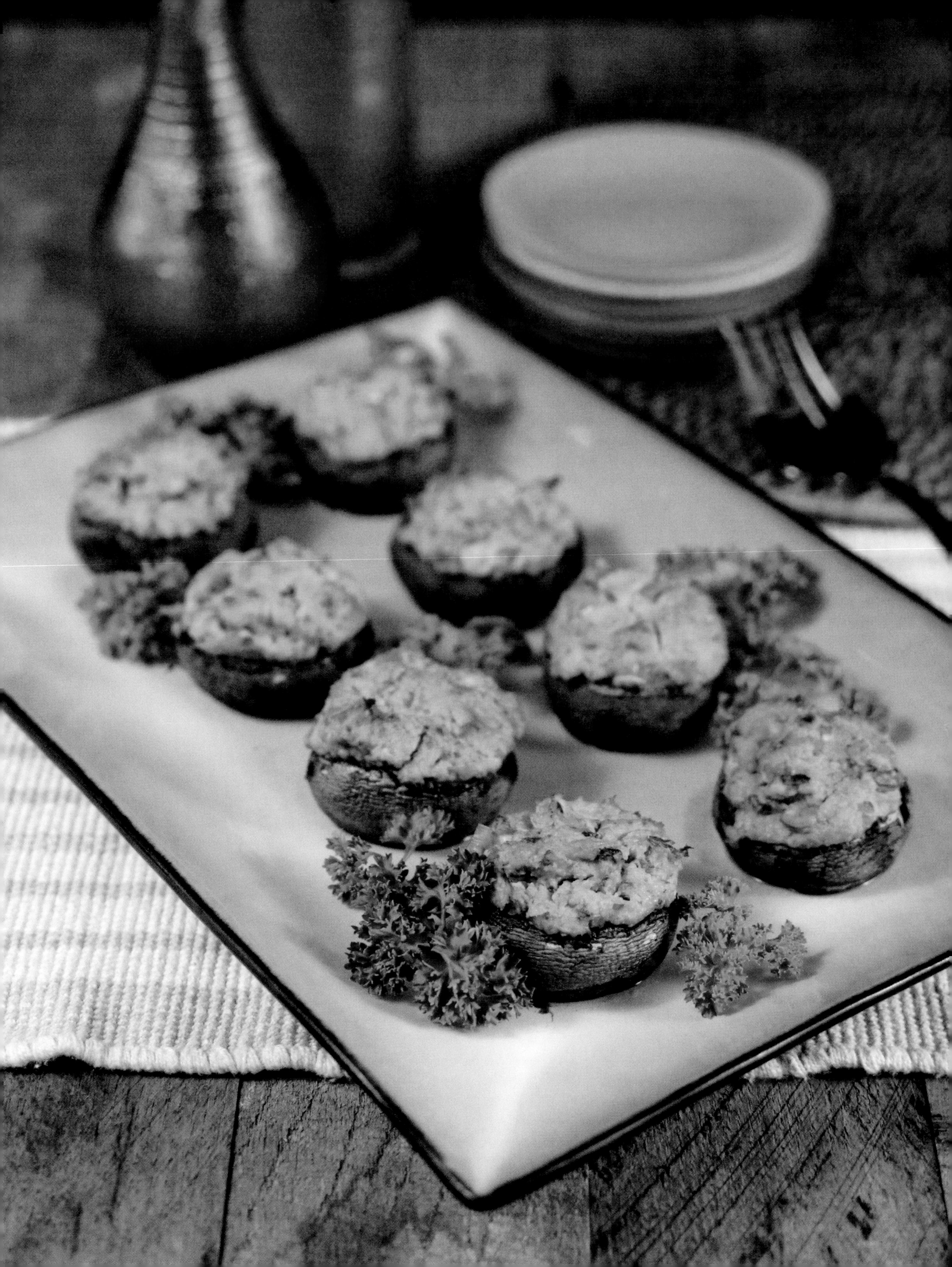

Garden Salad

If you are used to a garden salad containing lettuce, cucumber, tomatoes, and sweet peppers, you may feel like salad is pointless now that nightshades are out of your diet. However, there is a vast array of wonderful salad vegetables that you can still enjoy, yielding endless variations. Dozens of different leafy greens can be used alone or in combination for the base of your salad. Similarly, dozens of different vegetables can be added for color, flavor, and texture. Vegetables can be added raw or cooked and chilled (a great use for leftover roasted or grilled vegetables).

This is more of a collection of ideas than an actual recipe, including leafy greens, vegetable and fruit additions, items to add a little fat or protein, herbs that work well in salads, and items to give a little extra crunch. Keep in mind that many of the listed suggestions encompass dozens of varieties. For example, there are many, many varieties of lettuce, kale, spinach, radishes, and turnips, all of which are delicious in salads. A collection of different salad dressing recipes are included on page 126.

PREP TIME: 5 to 10 minutes

COOK TIME: usually none

SERVINGS: variable

1. Combine your favorites from the lists below, select a Salad Dressing (page 126), and enjoy!

INGREDIENTS:

Leafy Greens:
- Arugula
- Baby collards
- Beet greens
- Broccoli leaves
- Cabbage
- Carrot greens
- Celery leaves
- Chard
- Endive
- Kale
- Kohlrabi greens
- Lettuce
- Mizuna
- Mustard greens
- Pea leaves
- Radicchio
- Radish tops
- Sorrel
- Spinach
- Sweet potato leaves
- Turnip greens
- Watercress

Salad Veggie Extras:
- Asparagus (raw, broiled, grilled)
- Beets (raw, roasted, steamed)
- Broccoli florets (raw or steamed)
- Broccoli slaw
- Carrots (sliced, shredded)
- Celery root
- Cucumber
- Fennel (leaves or root)
- Jicama
- Kelp noodles
- Kohlrabi
- Microgreens
- Mushrooms
- Onions (green, red, spring, shallots, etc.)
- Radish sprouts
- Radishes
- Sea vegetables
- Seaweed
- Sunflower sprouts
- Turnips
- Wakame noodles
- Zucchini and other summer squash

Salad Herb Extras:
- Basil
- Chervil
- Chives
- Cilantro
- Dill
- Fennel
- Mint
- Oregano
- Parsley
- Tarragon

Salad Fat and Protein Extras:
- Avocado
- Bacon Bits (page 120)
- Fish (cooked shrimp, salmon, tuna, scallops, canned fish, etc.)
- Olives
- Meat or poultry (sliced steak, cold chicken, cold sausage, etc.)
- Toasted Coconut (see Tips)

Salad Fruit Extras:
- Apple
- Apricot
- Asian pear
- Berries
- Citrus segments
- Fresh figs
- Grapes, halved
- Mango
- Melon
- Pear
- Pomegranate seeds
- Dried fruit in moderation

Extra Crunch:
- Bacon Bits (page 120)
- Crunchy veggies (jicama, celery root, radishes, turnips, etc.)
- Crunchy fruit (apple, Asian pear)
- Kelp noodles
- Toasted Coconut (see Tips)
- Unsweetened banana chips (see Tips)
- Plantain Chips (homemade, page 170; or store-bought)
- Plantain Crackers (page 149)

TIPS:

When purchasing unsweetened banana chips or plantain chips, be sure to read the ingredients label to verify that no sugar or preservatives have been added and that they are cooked in a healthy fat.

Toasted Coconut. Preheat the oven to 325°F. Spread unsweetened coconut flakes on a rimmed baking sheet. Bake for 5 to 10 minutes, until fragrant and turning golden brown.

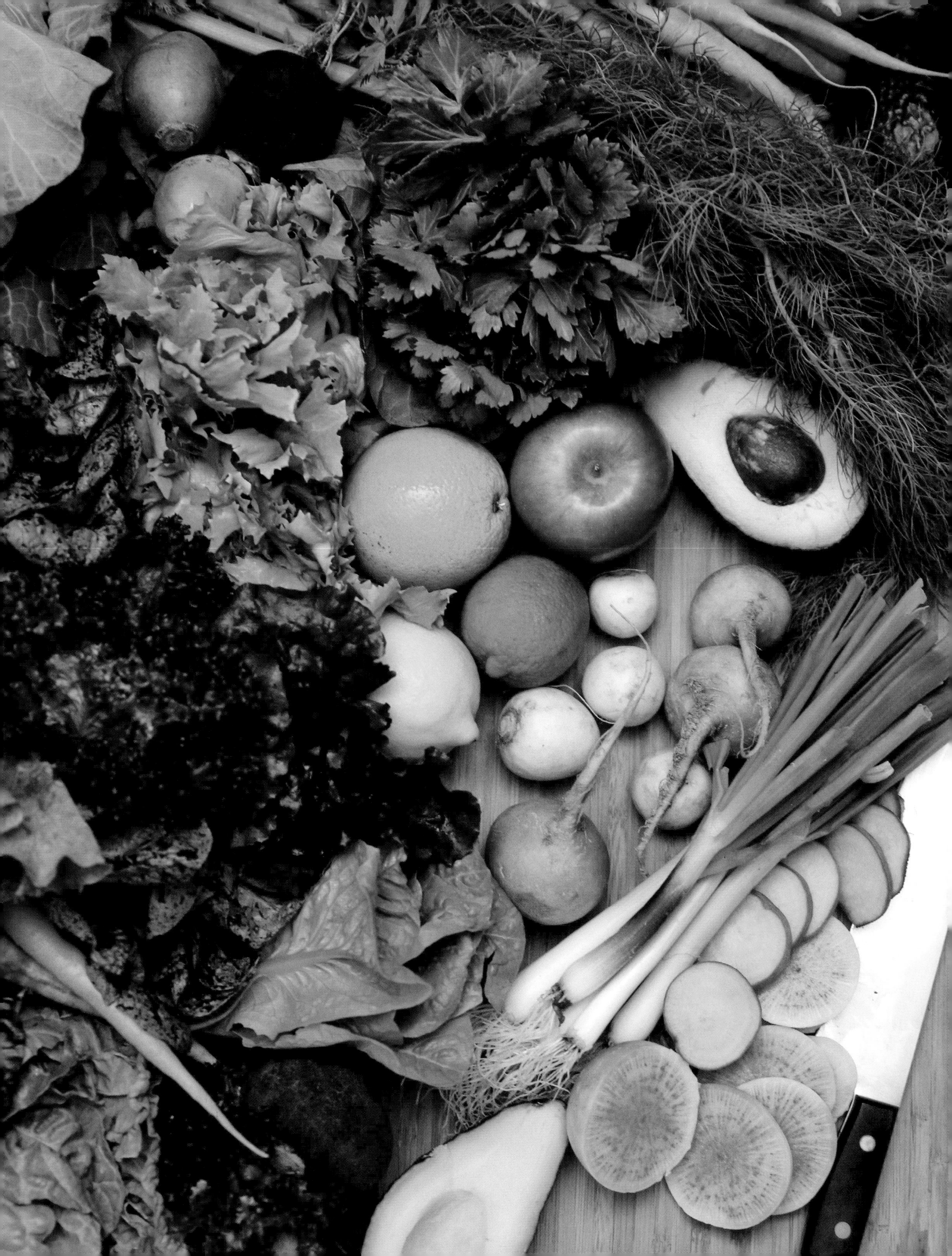

Radish Salad

There are many, many different varieties of radish, and all of them are delicious in this simple salad! Watermelon radishes are probably my favorite, both for their beautiful color and for the combination of their sweeter red inside and extra peppery green outside.

PREP TIME: 15 minutes
COOK TIME: none
SERVINGS: 3 to 5

INGREDIENTS:

- 1 tablespoon white wine vinegar
- 1 teaspoon honey
- 2 tablespoons extra-virgin olive oil
- ⅛ teaspoon salt
- 1½ pounds radishes (about 3 bunches), very thinly sliced
- 1 tablespoon chopped fresh oregano
- 1 tablespoon chopped fresh mint
- 1 tablespoon chopped fresh tarragon leaves

1. In a small bowl, thoroughly combine the vinegar, honey, olive oil, and salt.
2. Sprinkle over the thinly sliced radishes and toss with the herbs.
3. Serve!

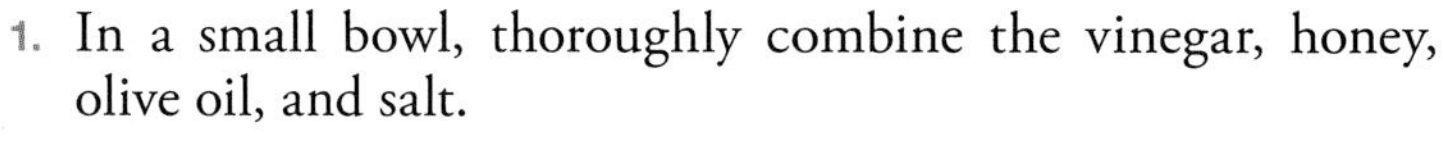

TIPS:
A mandoline slicer makes the job of slicing the radishes much faster, but isn't essential.

VARIATIONS:
Turnip Salad. This recipe can also be made with turnips instead of radishes. Japanese turnips (aka Hakurei turnips) are especially nice for this variation.

FODMAP ALERT *Leave out the honey or substitute ½ teaspoon evaporated cane juice.*

SPECIAL EQUIPMENT
- Mandoline slicer (optional)

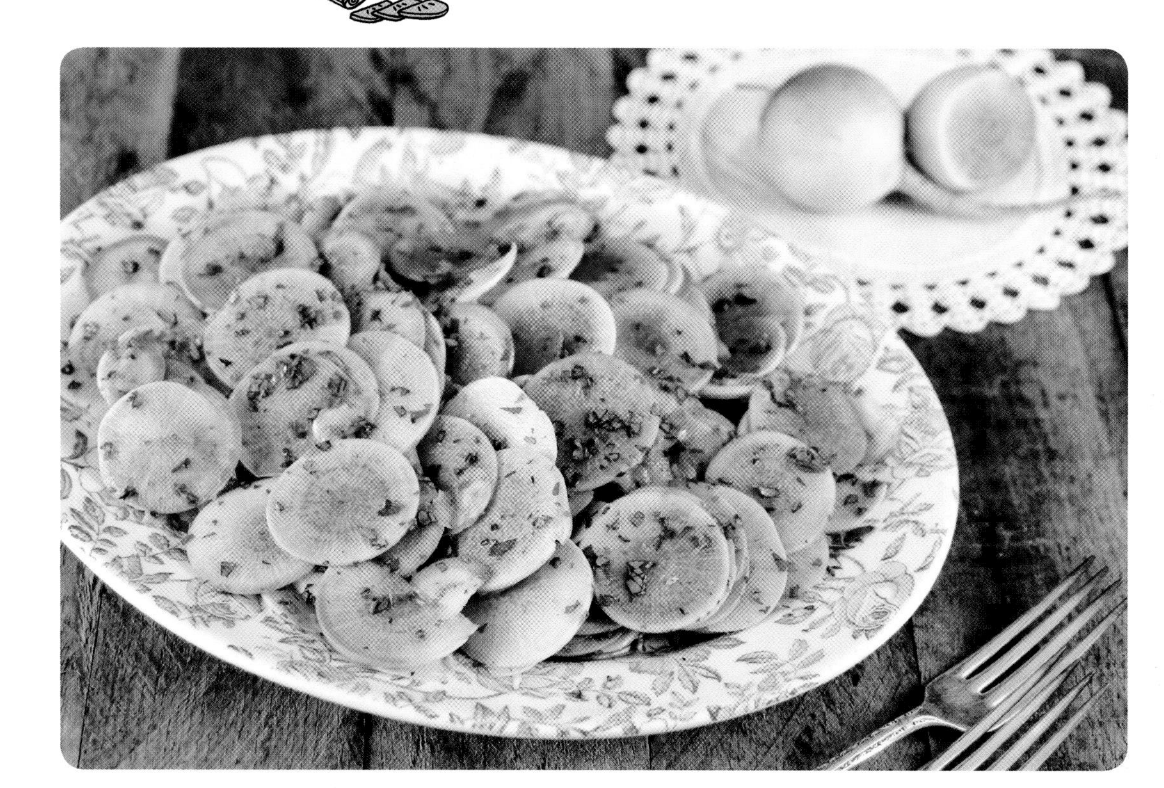

NUTRITION FACTS

Serving Size	146 g
Recipe Yields	730 g
Calories	**74.3**
Fats	**5.54 g**
MUFA	3.96 g
Omega-3	0.08 g
Omega-6	0.55 g
Saturated Fat	0.79 g
Carbohydrates	**5.78 g**
Fiber	2.18 g
Starch	<0.01 g
Fructose	1.53 g
Glucose	1.92 g
Sucrose	0.15 g
Protein	**0.93 g**
Alanine	0.04 g
Arginine	0.05 g
Aspartic acid	0.09 g
Cystine	0.01 g
Glutamic acid	0.21 g
Glycine	0.04 g
Histidine	0.02 g
Isoleucine	0.03 g
Leucine	0.04 g
Lysine	0.05 g
Methionine	0.01 g
Phenylalanine	0.05 g
Proline	0.03 g
Serine	0.04 g
Threonine	0.03 g
Tryptophan	0.01 g
Tyrosine	0.01 g
Valine	0.05 g
Vitamins	
Vitamin B1	0.02 mg
Vitamin B12	0 mcg
Vitamin B2	0.05 mg
Vitamin B3	0.35 mg
Vitamin B5	0.23 mg
Vitamin B6	0.1 mg
Choline	8.89 mg
Folate	34.1 mcg
Vitamin A	0 mcg
Vitamin C	20.2 mg
Vitamin D	0 IU
Vitamin E	0.77 mg
Vitamin K	5.02 mcg
Minerals	
Calcium	34.6 mg
Copper	0.07 mg
Iron	0.66 mg
Magnesium	13.8 mg
Manganese	0.1 mg
Phosphorus	27.5 mg
Potassium	320 mg
Selenium	0.83 mcg
Sodium	79.2 mg
Zinc	0.38 mg

nutrition content estimated using the USDA database.

Sardine Salad

Sardines are one of the most nutrient-dense foods you can eat. While you warm up to eating them straight out of the can, try them in this delicious salad.

PREP TIME: 10 minutes
COOK TIME: none
SERVINGS: 2

INGREDIENTS:

- 2 tablespoons extra-virgin olive oil
- 1 teaspoon finely grated lemon zest
- Juice of 1 lemon
- 1 tablespoon capers
- 2 tablespoons chopped fresh parsley
- 1 tablespoon chopped fresh tarragon
- 2 stalks celery, finely diced
- 2 (4-ounce) cans sardines packed in olive oil, drained
- 6 to 10 cups arugula or mustard greens

1. In a bowl, mix together the olive oil, lemon zest and juice, capers, parsley, tarragon, and celery.
2. Toss the sardines with the dressing. Place the arugula on 2 serving plates and pour the sardine mixture over the top.

TIPS:

If you really don't like sardines straight out of the can, try frying them using the Pan-Fried Sardines recipe (page 252) before tossing them with the dressing.

VARIATIONS:

This salad is also delicious with an avocado cut into chunks.

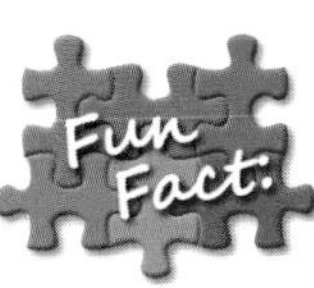

Sardines are an outstanding source of the heart-healthy nutrient Coenzyme Q10.

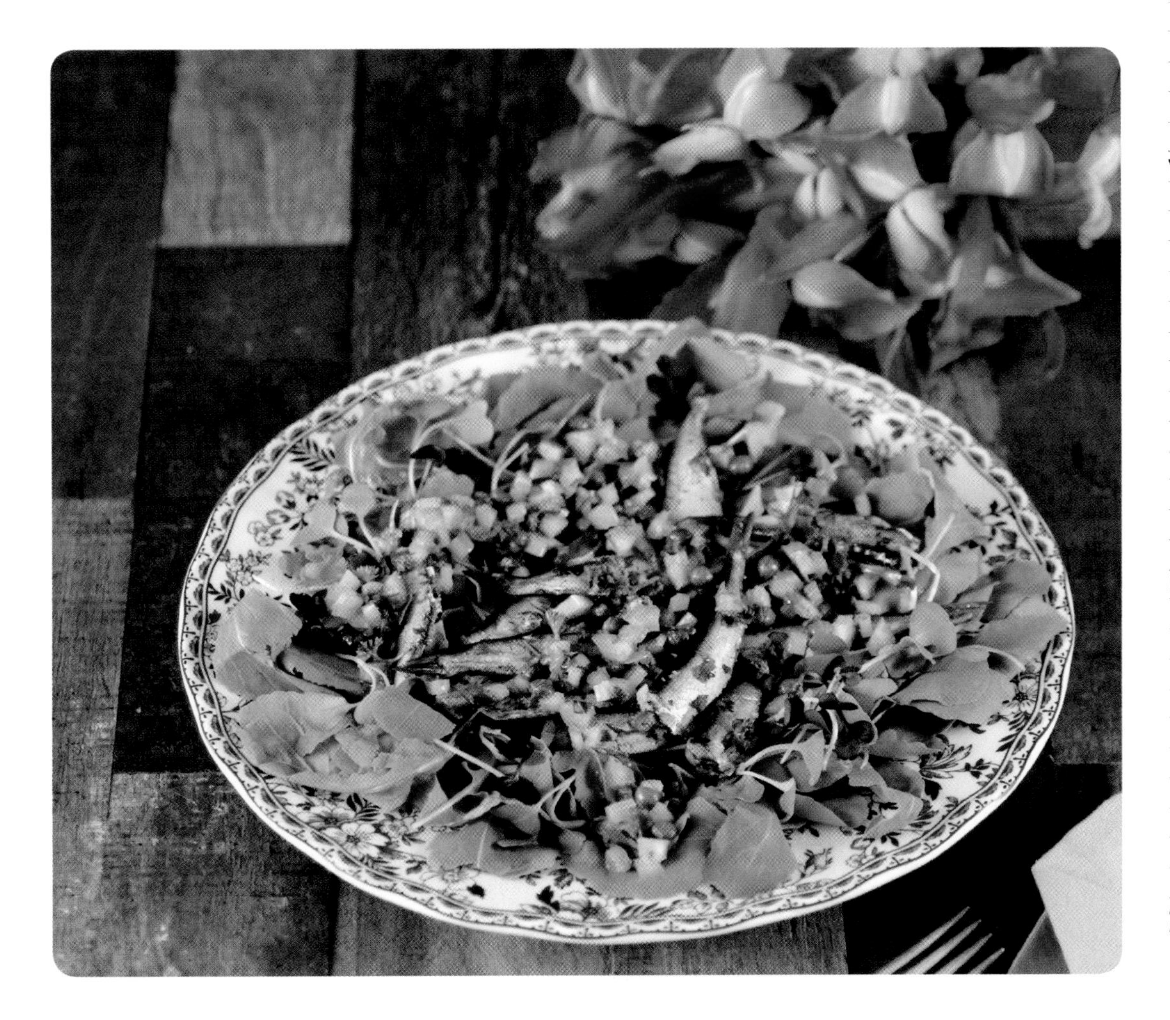

NUTRITION FACTS

Serving Size	261 g
Recipe Yields	521 g
Calories	**387**
Fats	**27.1 g**
MUFA	14.3 g
Omega-3	2.05 g
Omega-6	5.46 g
Saturated Fat	3.7 g
Carbohydrates	**6 g**
Fiber	2.09 g
Starch	1.08 g
Fructose	0.47 g
Glucose	0.47 g
Sucrose	0.15 g
Protein	**30.2 g**
Alanine	1.71 g
Arginine	1.69 g
Aspartic acid	2.92 g
Cystine	0.3 g
Glutamic acid	4.24 g
Glycine	1.36 g
Histidine	0.83 g
Isoleucine	1.3 g
Leucine	2.29 g
Lysine	2.58 g
Methionine	0.83 g
Phenylalanine	1.11 g
Proline	1 g
Serine	1.15 g
Threonine	1.24 g
Tryptophan	0.32 g
Tyrosine	0.95 g
Valine	1.46 g
Vitamins	
Vitamin B1	0.14 mg
Vitamin B12	10.1 mcg
Vitamin B2	0.36 mg
Vitamin B3	6.42 mg
Vitamin B5	1.14 mg
Vitamin B6	0.3 mg
Choline	99.1 mg
Folate	97.5 mcg
Vitamin A	134 mcg
Vitamin C	26.4 mg
Vitamin D	219 IU
Vitamin E	4.73 mg
Vitamin K	151 mcg
Minerals	
Calcium	563 mg
Copper	0.3 mg
Iron	4.91 mg
Magnesium	84.2 mg
Manganese	0.43 mg
Phosphorus	603 mg
Potassium	846 mg
Selenium	60.2 mcg
Sodium	751 mg
Zinc	1.91 mg

nutrition content estimated using the USDA database.

Cran-Apple Coleslaw

This simple slaw is inspired by my mom's recipe. The secret is to slice the cabbage as thinly as possible. This slaw makes a delicious accompaniment to almost any dish and is always a hit at barbecues and potlucks.

PREP TIME: 10 minutes
COOK TIME: none
SERVINGS: 4 to 6

INGREDIENTS:

- 1 pound red cabbage, cored
- 2 tablespoons extra-virgin olive oil
- 1½ teaspoons coconut water vinegar or white wine vinegar
- ⅛ teaspoon salt
- 1 apple, peeled, cored, and diced
- ½ cup fresh cranberries (or thawed frozen)

FODMAP ALERT

This recipe cannot be made low-FODMAP.

SPECIAL EQUIPMENT

- Mandoline slicer or food processor

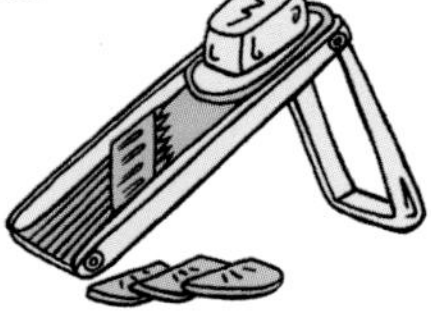

1. Use a mandoline slicer or food processor to slice the cabbage very finely, ideally 1⁄16 inch thick (see Tips). Place in a serving bowl.
2. Combine the olive oil, vinegar, and salt in a small bowl. Pour over the cabbage and toss to coat.
3. Add the apple and cranberries, toss to combine, and serve. This coleslaw will keep well for up to 4 days in the fridge.

TIPS:

If you don't have a mandoline slicer or food processor to slice the cabbage, you can slice it with a knife, sprinkle it with 2 tablespoons salt, and let it sit in a colander in the sink for 1 hour. Rinse the salt off thoroughly, dry with paper towels or in a salad spinner, then follow steps 2 and 3.

VARIATIONS:

This coleslaw is delicious with dried cranberries instead of fresh. Also try substituting Asian pear for the apple.

Carrot-Raisin Coleslaw. Replace the red cabbage with a half-and-half mix of green cabbage and grated carrot and toss with ¾ cup raisins instead of the apple and cranberries. Also add a generous pinch of cinnamon, 1 teaspoon finely grated orange zest, and ½ red onion, very finely sliced.

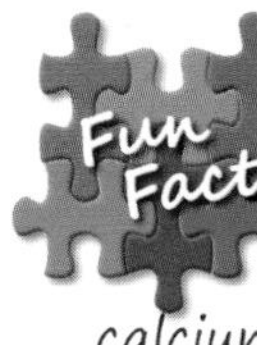

In addition to fiber, vitamin B_1, vitamin B_5, vitamin B_6, vitamin K, folate, manganese, iron, magnesium, phosphorous, calcium, and potassium, cabbage is high in phytonutrients such as thiocyanates, lutein, zeaxanthin, isothiocyanates, and sulforaphane. Red cabbage is additionally rich in anthocyanin polyphenols, which are potent antioxidants with diverse health benefits.

NUTRITION FACTS	
Serving Size	120 g
Recipe Yields	721 g
Calories	**83**
Fats	**4.68 g**
MUFA	3.29 g
Omega-3	0.07 g
Omega-6	0.48 g
Saturated Fat	0.65 g
Carbohydrates	**10.8 g**
Fiber	2.7 g
Starch	1.4 g
Fructose	2.96 g
Glucose	2.32 g
Sucrose	1.09 g
Protein	**1.19 g**
Alanine	0.04 g
Arginine	0.07 g
Aspartic acid	0.14 g
Cystine	<0.01 g
Glutamic acid	0.27 g
Glycine	0.03 g
Histidine	0.02 g
Isoleucine	0.03 g
Leucine	0.04 g
Lysine	0.04 g
Methionine	0.01 g
Phenylalanine	0.03 g
Proline	0.05 g
Serine	0.05 g
Threonine	0.03 g
Tryptophan	<0.01 g
Tyrosine	0.02 g
Valine	0.04 g
Vitamins	
Vitamin B1	0.05 mg
Vitamin B12	0 mcg
Vitamin B2	0.06 mg
Vitamin B3	0.35 mg
Vitamin B5	0.15 mg
Vitamin B6	0.17 mg
Choline	14.4 mg
Folate	14.6 mcg
Vitamin A	43.4 mcg
Vitamin C	45.6 mg
Vitamin D	0 IU
Vitamin E	0.88 mg
Vitamin K	32.6 mcg
Minerals	
Calcium	36.7 mg
Copper	0.03 mg
Iron	0.69 mg
Magnesium	14.2 mg
Manganese	0.22 mg
Phosphorus	27.2 mg
Potassium	223.5 mg
Selenium	0.46 mcg
Sodium	69.7 mg
Zinc	0.19 mg

nutrition content estimated using the USDA database.

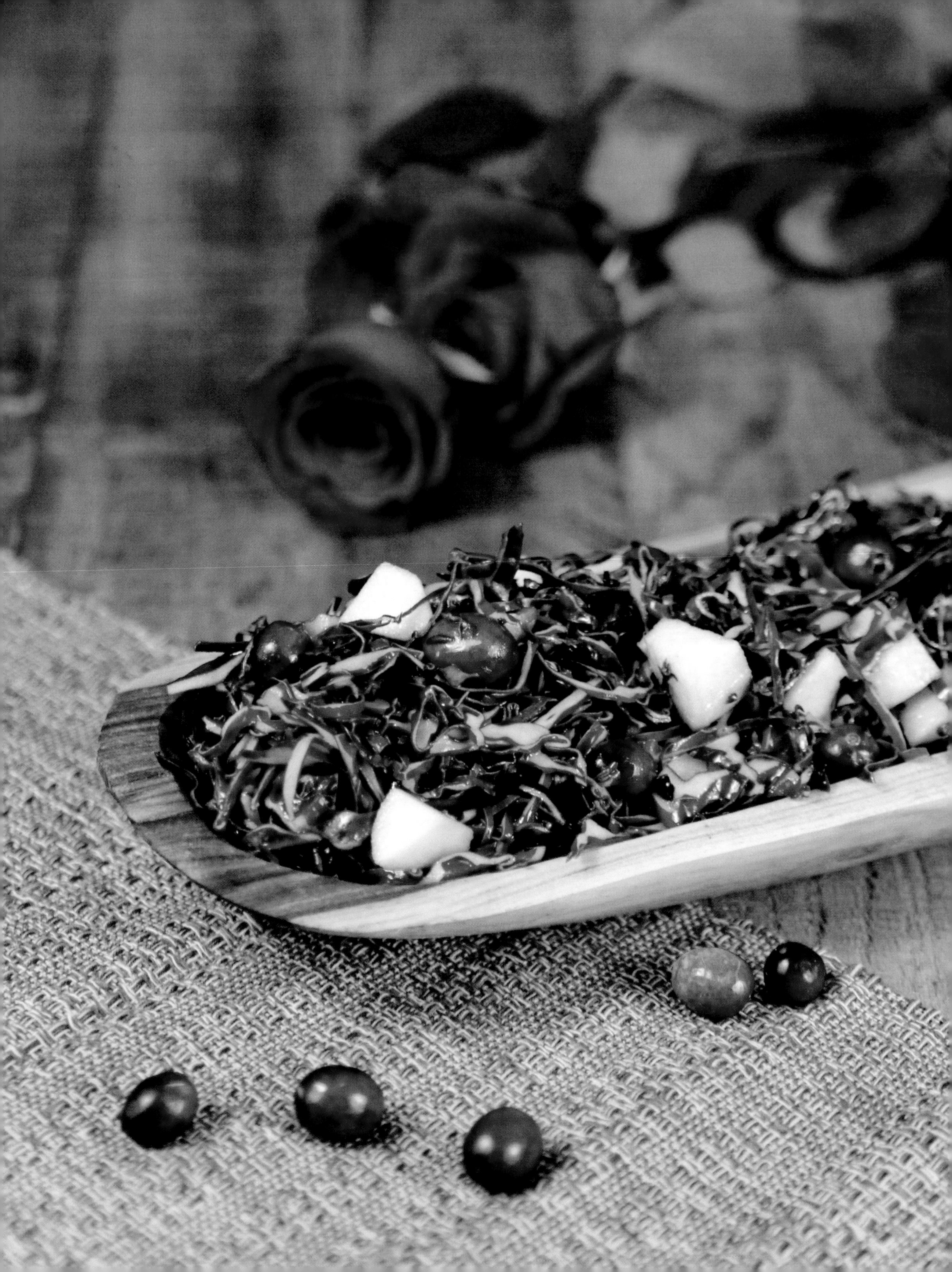

Kale Chips

Kale chips are one of the easiest and most delicious ways to dramatically increase your vegetable intake. They have an addictive quality, and leftovers will likely be a rare occurrence.

There are many varieties of kale, most of which make excellent kale chips. Varieties with very flat leaves don't work as well, but as long as there is some curl in the leaves, they will crisp up nicely in the oven. More tender-leaved varieties take less time to crisp up in the oven. Thicker leaves take more time.

PREP TIME: 10 minutes
COOK TIME: 40 to 60 minutes
SERVINGS: 2 to 4

INGREDIENTS:

1 bunch kale, tough stems removed, torn into 1 to 1½-inch pieces (approximately 8 loosely packed cups)

2 tablespoons coconut oil, melted

¼ teaspoon salt

1. Preheat the oven to 275°F.
2. Wash and thoroughly dry the kale, using a salad spinner, tea towels, or paper towels to remove all the water. Place in a plastic container or large bowl.
3. Pour the coconut oil over the kale. Mix with your hands to thoroughly coat each leaf (if you put it in a container with a lid, you can also close the lid and shake the container vigorously to coat).
4. Spread out on a large baking sheet. Sprinkle with the salt.
5. Bake for 40 to 60 minutes, depending on the variety of kale you are using, until crispy. Enjoy!

TIPS:

If you have leftover kale chips that get a little soggy, just pop them back into a 275°F oven for 5 minutes.

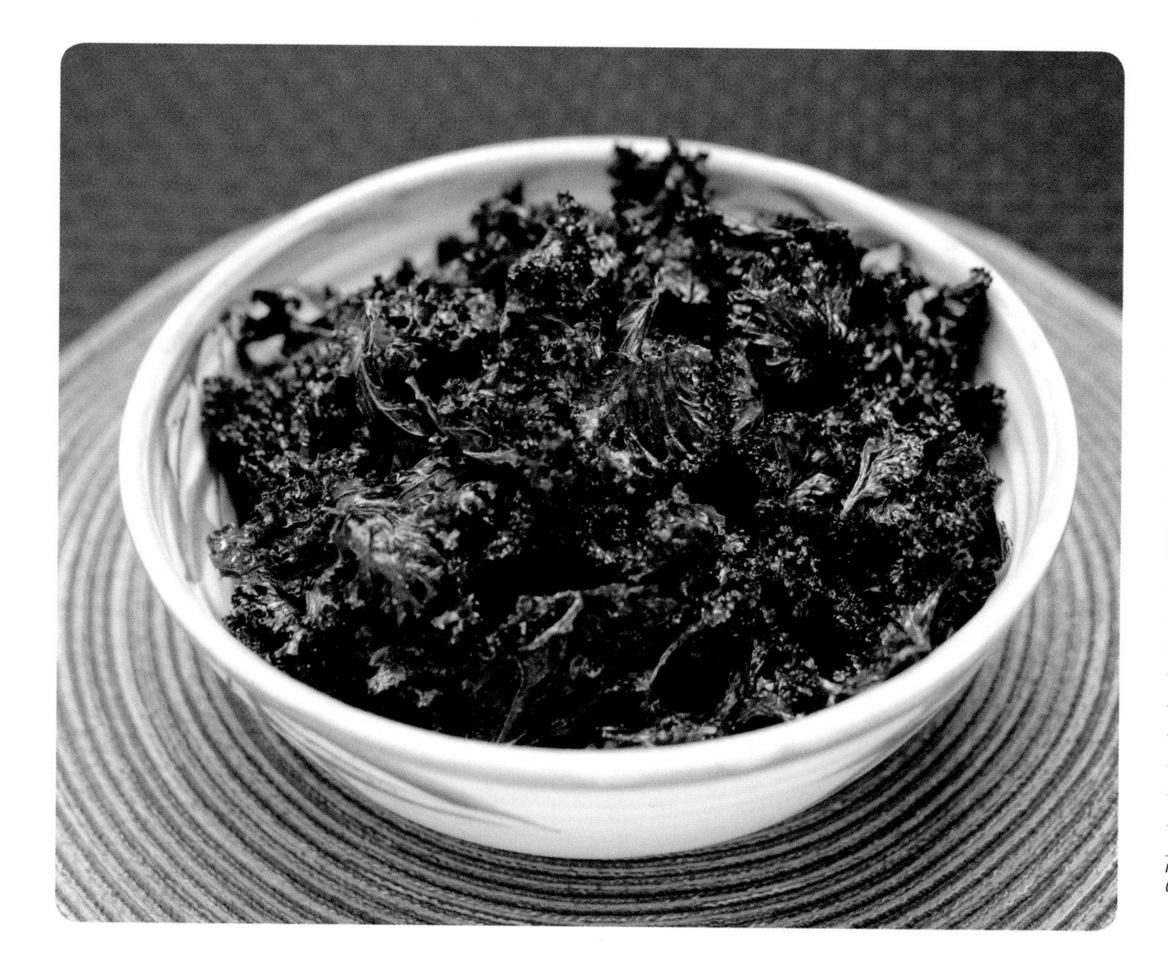

NUTRITION FACTS	
Serving Size	141 g
Recipe Yields	565 g
Calories	**124**
Fats	**8.04 g**
MUFA	0.46 g
Omega-3	0.24 g
Omega-6	0.31 g
Saturated Fat	6 g
Carbohydrates	**11.7 g**
Fiber	4.82 g
Starch	3.87 g
Fructose	0 g
Glucose	0 g
Sucrose	0 g
Protein	**5.73 g**
Alanine	0 g
Arginine	0 g
Aspartic acid	0 g
Cystine	0 g
Glutamic acid	0 g
Glycine	0 g
Histidine	0 g
Isoleucine	0 g
Leucine	0 g
Lysine	0 g
Methionine	0 g
Phenylalanine	0 g
Proline	0 g
Serine	0 g
Threonine	0 g
Tryptophan	0 g
Tyrosine	0 g
Valine	0 g
Vitamins	
Vitamin B1	0.15 mg
Vitamin B12	0 mcg
Vitamin B2	0.17 mg
Vitamin B3	1.34 mg
Vitamin B5	0.12 mg
Vitamin B6	0.36 mg
Choline	1.09 mg
Folate	189 mcg
Vitamin A	669 mcg
Vitamin C	161 mg
Vitamin D	0 IU
Vitamin E	2.07 mg
Vitamin K	943 mcg
Minerals	
Calcium	202 mg
Copper	2.01 mg
Iron	2.35 mg
Magnesium	62.9 mg
Manganese	0.88 mg
Phosphorus	123 mg
Potassium	659 mg
Selenium	1.2 mcg
Sodium	115 mg
Zinc	0.75 mg

nutrition content estimated using the USDA database.

Pork Rinds

I learned how to make light and airy pork rinds from Beyond Bacon *by Stacy Toth and Matthew McCarry. Matt and Stacy's version just can't be beat, so this recipe is adapted with permission from their Curried Cracklin's recipe.*

The toughest thing about making pork rinds is cutting the pork skins into small pieces. Fortunately, this is something that your butcher can do for you. If you are doing it yourself, try using sharp kitchen scissors instead of a knife.

PREP TIME: 20 minutes
COOK TIME: 7 to 24 hours
SERVINGS: 6 to 12

INGREDIENTS:

2 pounds pork skins, cut into small pieces or strips

2 to 4 teaspoons salt

Lard and palm shortening, for deep-frying

SPECIAL EQUIPMENT

- Dehydrator
- Countertop deep-fryer or heavy-bottomed pot with an oil thermometer

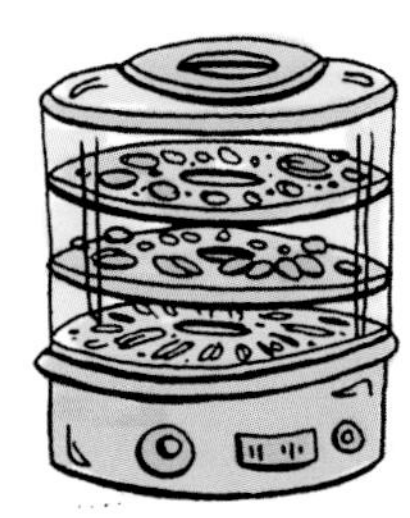

1. Bring a stockpot full of water to a boil on the stovetop. Add the pork skins and simmer for 10 minutes.
2. Remove the skins from the water and place on a kitchen towel or paper towels to drain. Cover with additional paper towels and press to remove any excess water.
3. Arrange the pork skins on the racks of a dehydrator. Dehydrate for 6 to 24 hours, depending on your dehydrator, until the skins are rock-hard little bricks.
4. When ready, heat a mixture of half lard and half palm shortening to 375°F in a countertop deep-fryer or heavy-bottomed pot over medium to medium-high heat with a deep-fry thermometer attached to the side. Add enough fat to fill the deep-fryer to the fill line or to have about 2 inches of fat in the pot.
5. Fry the pork skins in batches, being careful not to overcrowd, until puffed up, light, and airy (7 to 10 minutes, depending on the size of the pieces). They will float and more than double in size, so put in fewer than you think will fit and err on the side of frying more batches.
6. Remove from the deep-fryer and drain on a towel or paper towels. Sprinkle liberally with salt while still warm.

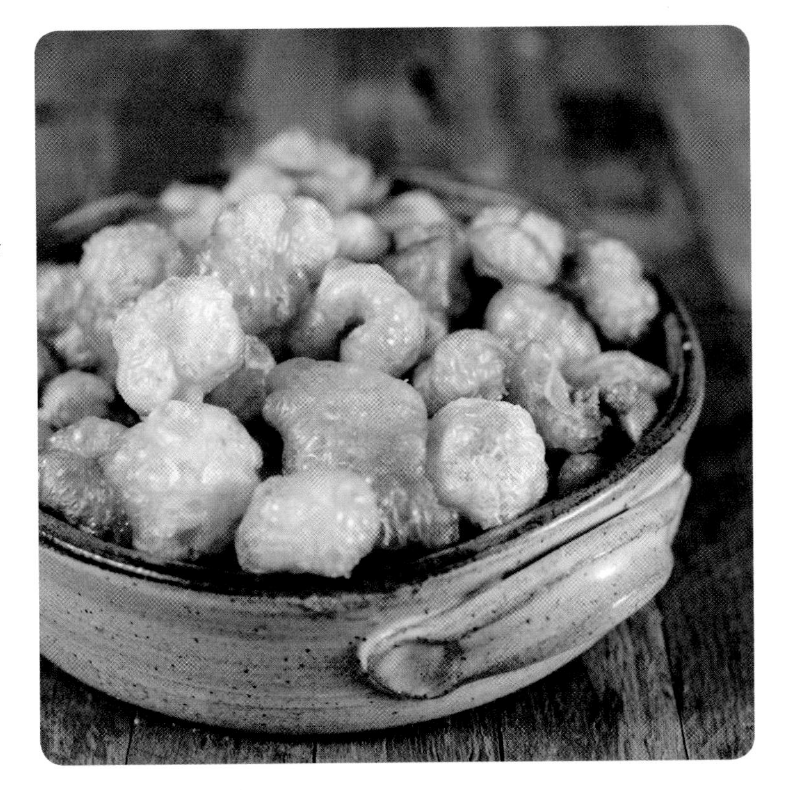

TIPS:

If you don't own a dehydrator, you can also dehydrate the pork skins in your oven at the lowest temperature setting. If the skins have a good lining of fat, it can be hard to gauge whether they are dehydrated enough to fry. If they aren't puffing up in the fryer for you, they need to be dehydrated longer.

The use of palm shortening allows for higher-temperature deep-frying without exceeding the smoke point.

NUTRITION FACTS	
Serving Size	79 g
Recipe Yields	945 g
Calories	**432**
Fats	**25.9 g**
MUFA	12.2 g
Omega-3	0.22 g
Omega-6	2.76 g
Saturated Fat	9.46 g
Carbohydrates	**0 g**
Fiber	0 g
Starch	0 g
Fructose	0 g
Glucose	0 g
Sucrose	0 g
Protein	**46.5 g**
Alanine	4.41 g
Arginine	3.67 g
Aspartic acid	3.39 g
Cystine	0.4 g
Glutamic acid	5.78 g
Glycine	9.04 g
Histidine	0.55 g
Isoleucine	1.05 g
Leucine	2.52 g
Lysine	2.11 g
Methionine	0.36 g
Phenylalanine	1.47 g
Proline	5.51 g
Serine	1.97 g
Threonine	1.38 g
Tryptophan	0.09 g
Tyrosine	0.91 g
Valine	1.84 g
Vitamins	
Vitamin B1	0.08 mg
Vitamin B12	0.49 mcg
Vitamin B2	0.21 mg
Vitamin B3	1.18 mg
Vitamin B5	0.33 mg
Vitamin B6	0.02 mg
Choline	126 mg
Folate	0 mcg
Vitamin A	9.1 mcg
Vitamin C	0.38 mg
Vitamin D	2.18 IU
Vitamin E	0.41 mg
Vitamin K	0 mcg
Minerals	
Calcium	23.7 mg
Copper	0.07 mg
Iron	0.67 mg
Magnesium	8.43 mg
Manganese	0.05 mg
Phosphorus	64.5 mg
Potassium	96.3 mg
Selenium	31.1 mcg
Sodium	1770 mg
Zinc	0.43 mg

nutrition content estimated using the USDA database.

Sweet Potato Chips

These sweet potato chips have a wonderful salty crunch with a hint of sweetness. They are fantastic fried in lard, but can be made in any high-smoke-point cooking fat.

PREP TIME: 20 minutes, plus 1 to 2 hours salting time
COOK TIME: 1 hour
SERVINGS: 2 to 6

INGREDIENTS:

1 to 2 sweet potatoes

1 to 1½ tablespoons salt

4 to 8 cups high-smoke-point cooking fat (enough to have about 2 inches of oil in a pot or to fill a countertop deep-fryer)

FODMAP ALERT *Stick with Root Vegetable Chips and Fried Plantain Chips.*

SPECIAL EQUIPMENT

- Countertop deep-fryer or deep, wide-bottomed pot with an oil thermometer
- Deep-fry basket or wire skimmer
- Mandoline slicer or food processor

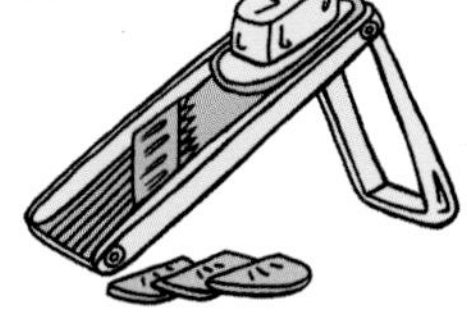

1. Slice the sweet potatoes as thinly as possible, ideally 1/16 inch thick. A mandoline slicer or food processor makes this task much easier. The thinner they are, the more evenly and quickly they will crisp up when fried.
2. Place the sweet potato slices in a bowl and toss with 2 to 3 teaspoons of the salt. Place in a colander in your kitchen sink and let drain for 1 to 2 hours (or more).
3. Rinse the excess salt off the sweet potato slices and pat dry with clean tea towels or paper towels. It's important that the slices be completely dry before you put them in the oil. Any excess water on them will cause the oil to bubble aggressively.
4. Meanwhile, heat the cooking fat in a countertop deep-fryer or a fairly deep, wide-bottomed pot over medium heat with a deep-fry thermometer attached to the side. Aim to get the oil to 350°F to 365°F if using lard, or 370°F to 375°F if using tallow or palm shortening. Line a baking sheet with newsprint or paper towels to put your sweet potato chips on after they are fried.
5. Add a generous handful of sweet potato slices to the oil, but do not overcrowd. Watch them. When they start to curl slightly and brown a little, they are done. Using a deep-fry basket or a wire skimmer, transfer the chips onto the prepared baking sheet. Sprinkle with salt and let cool before eating. Repeat with the remaining sweet potato slices, working in batches. If you aren't sure whether they done, remove the chips from the oil and let them cool a little (but don't sprinkle with salt yet) to see if they are entirely crisp. If they aren't, you can put them back in the oil to continue cooking. Depending on how big and thick your sweet potato slices are and how hot your oil is, frying may take as little as 2 to 3 minutes or as long as 6 to 7 minutes. Once you've done a few batches, you'll have a better idea of how long they take to cook and what they look like when perfectly crisp.

TIPS:

Store any leftovers in an airtight container at room temperature. If the chips were fully crisp, they will keep for about a week.

VARIATIONS:

You can use many varieties of sweet potato to make these chips.

Root Vegetable Chips. *You can also make chips out of other starchy root vegetables, such as beets, parsnips, carrots, and taro root. If you want to experiment with different combinations of root vegetables, keep them separate until after you have deep-fried them, since different vegetables take different lengths of time to crisp up.*

Fried Plantain Chips. *You can also make chips out of green plantains. Slice as thinly as possible and skip steps 2 and 3. These are particularly good when fried in lard or coconut oil (but don't heat extra-virgin coconut oil above 350°F.)*

NUTRITION FACTS	
Serving Size	24 g
Recipe Yields	144 g
Calories	**36.4**
Fats	**2.17 g**
MUFA	0.96 g
Omega-3	0.02 g
Omega-6	0.23 g
Saturated Fat	0.84 g
Carbohydrates	**3.94 g**
Fiber	0.63 g
Starch	1.34 g
Fructose	0.1 g
Glucose	0.11 g
Sucrose	0.43 g
Protein	**0.38 g**
Alanine	0.02 g
Arginine	0.01 g
Aspartic acid	0.09 g
Cystine	<0.01 g
Glutamic acid	0.04 g
Glycine	0.02 g
Histidine	<0.01 g
Isoleucine	0.01 g
Leucine	0.02 g
Lysine	0.02 g
Methionine	<0.01 g
Phenylalanine	0.02 g
Proline	0.01 g
Serine	0.02 g
Threonine	0.02 g
Tryptophan	<0.01 g
Tyrosine	<0.01 g
Valine	0.02 g
Vitamins	
Vitamin B1	0.02 mg
Vitamin B12	0 mcg
Vitamin B2	0.02 mg
Vitamin B3	0.28 mg
Vitamin B5	0.17 mg
Vitamin B6	0.05 mg
Choline	3.56 mg
Folate	1.14 mcg
Vitamin A	183 mcg
Vitamin C	3.73 mg
Vitamin D	2.18 IU
Vitamin E	0.15 mg
Vitamin K	0.44 mcg
Minerals	
Calcium	13 mg
Copper	0.03 mg
Iron	3.1 mg
Magnesium	5.14 mg
Manganese	0.09 mg
Phosphorus	10.3 mg
Potassium	108 mg
Selenium	0.04 mcg
Sodium	514 mg
Zinc	0.06 mg

nutrition content estimated using the USDA database.

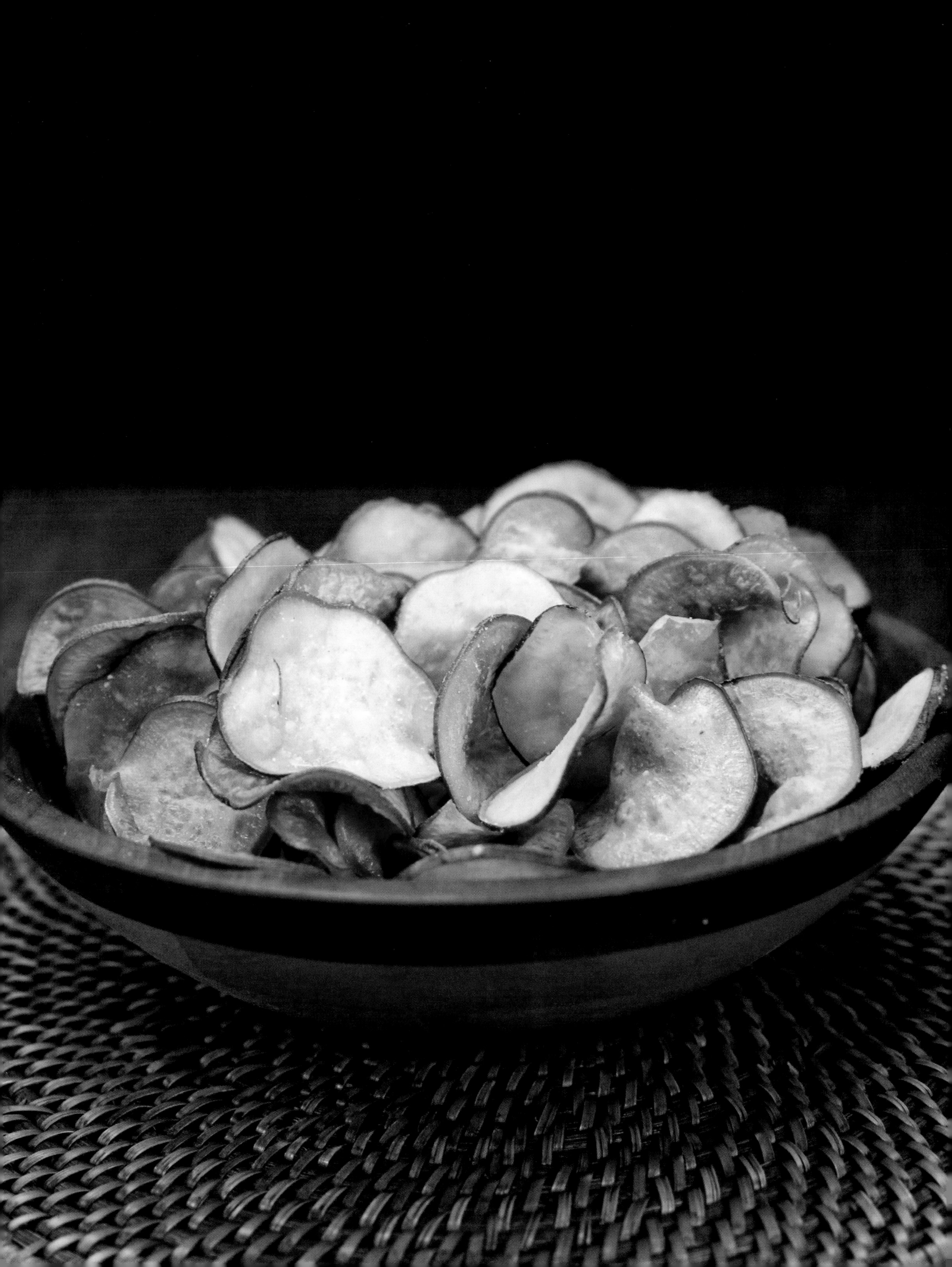

Dehydrator Plantain Chips

Plantain chips can be deep-fried (see page 168) or baked in the oven, but making them in a dehydrator has two great advantages. First, it preserves the resistant starch, meaning that these plantain chips won't have as big an impact on your blood sugar, and they're great food for probiotic bacteria in your gut. Second, they're really easy to make and don't require dealing with hot oil!

PREP TIME: 10 minutes
COOK TIME: 6 to 12 hours
SERVINGS: 8 to 12

INGREDIENTS:

- 4 green plantains, peeled and very thinly sliced
- 3 tablespoons melted coconut oil
- 1 teaspoon salt, to taste

1. Gently toss the sliced plantains with the coconut oil and salt.
2. Lay the slices on the racks of a dehydrator. Dehydrate for 6 to 12 hours, until crunchy.

VARIATIONS:

You can easily substitute avocado oil, olive oil, lard, or red palm oil for the coconut oil.

Sweet and Salty Plantain Chips. Replace the coconut oil with red palm oil and add 1 teaspoon ground cinnamon. Try using half-ripe plantains (yellow peel) for even sweeter chips.

SPECIAL EQUIPMENT

- Dehydrator

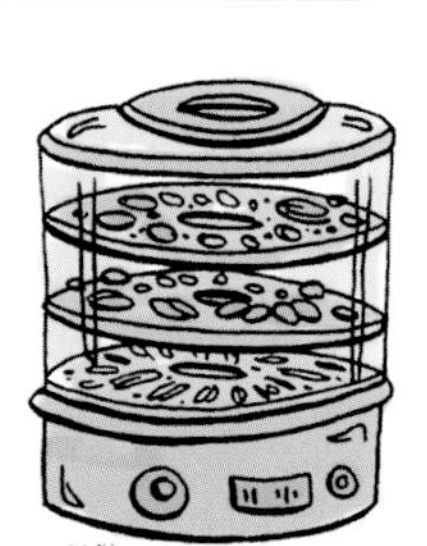

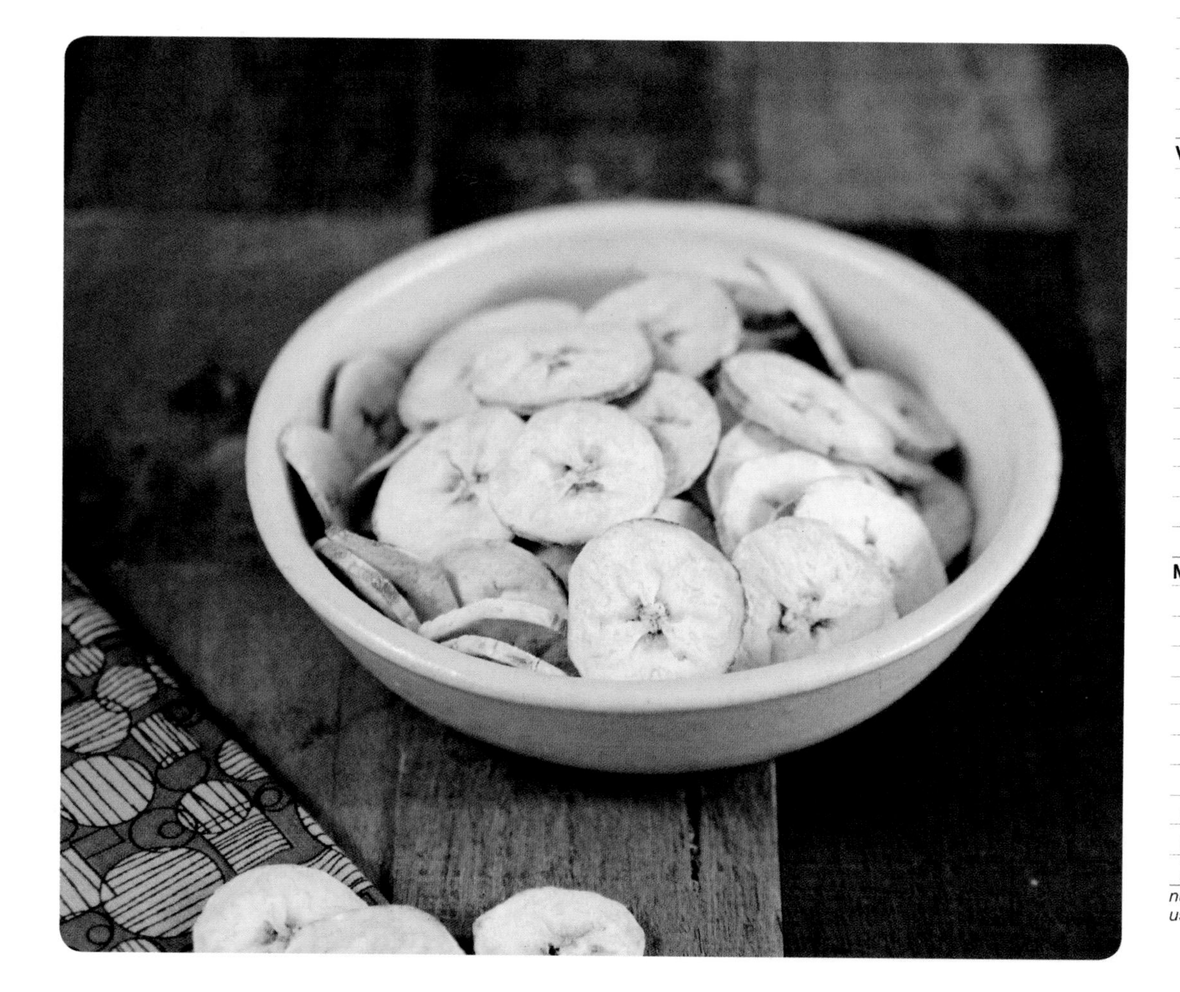

NUTRITION FACTS	
Serving Size	64 g
Recipe Yields	763 g
Calories	**103**
Fats	**3.65 g**
MUFA	0.22 g
Omega-3	0.02 g
Omega-6	0.09 g
Saturated Fat	3.05 g
Carbohydrates	**19.2 g**
Fiber	1.38 g
Starch	8.76 g
Fructose	0 g
Glucose	0 g
Sucrose	0 g
Protein	**0.78 g**
Alanine	0.03 g
Arginine	0.06 g
Aspartic acid	0.06 g
Cystine	0.01 g
Glutamic acid	0.07 g
Glycine	0.03 g
Histidine	0.04 g
Isoleucine	0.02 g
Leucine	0.04 g
Lysine	0.04 g
Methionine	0.01 g
Phenylalanine	0.03 g
Proline	0.03 g
Serine	0.02 g
Threonine	0.02 g
Tryptophan	<0.01 g
Tyrosine	0.02 g
Valine	0.03 g
Vitamins	
Vitamin B1	0.03 mg
Vitamin B12	0 mcg
Vitamin B2	0.03 mg
Vitamin B3	0.41 mg
Vitamin B5	0.16 mg
Vitamin B6	0.18 mg
Choline	8.12 mg
Folate	13.2 mcg
Vitamin A	33.6 mcg
Vitamin C	11.1 mg
Vitamin D	0 IU
Vitamin E	0.09 mg
Vitamin K	0.44 mcg
Minerals	
Calcium	2.25 mg
Copper	0.05 mg
Iron	0.36 mg
Magnesium	22.3 mg
Manganese	0 mg
Phosphorus	20.4 mg
Potassium	300 mg
Selenium	0.9 mcg
Sodium	199 mg
Zinc	0.09 mg

nutrition content estimated using the USDA database.

Guacamole

This classic guacamole makes a great dip for vegetables or a perfect side for burgers or grilled chicken.

PREP TIME: 10 minutes
COOK TIME: none
SERVINGS: 2 to 4

INGREDIENTS:

- 2 medium ripe avocados
- 2 tablespoons fresh lime juice (1 to 2 limes)
- ¼ teaspoon truffle salt or pink or gray salt
- ⅓ cup chopped fresh cilantro
- 2 tablespoons finely diced red onion (optional)

1. Cut the avocados in half, remove the pits, and scoop the flesh into a bowl. Mash with a fork to the desired consistency (I like mine a little lumpy).
2. Add the remaining ingredients and stir to combine. Serve!

TIPS:

Great dipping vegetables include carrots, celery, broccoli, mushrooms, jicama, radishes, kohlrabi, Belgian endive, asparagus spears, and sliced raw beet, turnip, and rutabaga. Other great dipping options are Dehydrator Plantain Chips (page 170), Sweet Potato Chips (page 168), and Plantain Crackers (page 149).

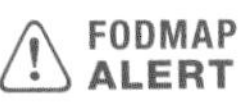

FODMAP ALERT

This recipe cannot be made low-FODMAP.

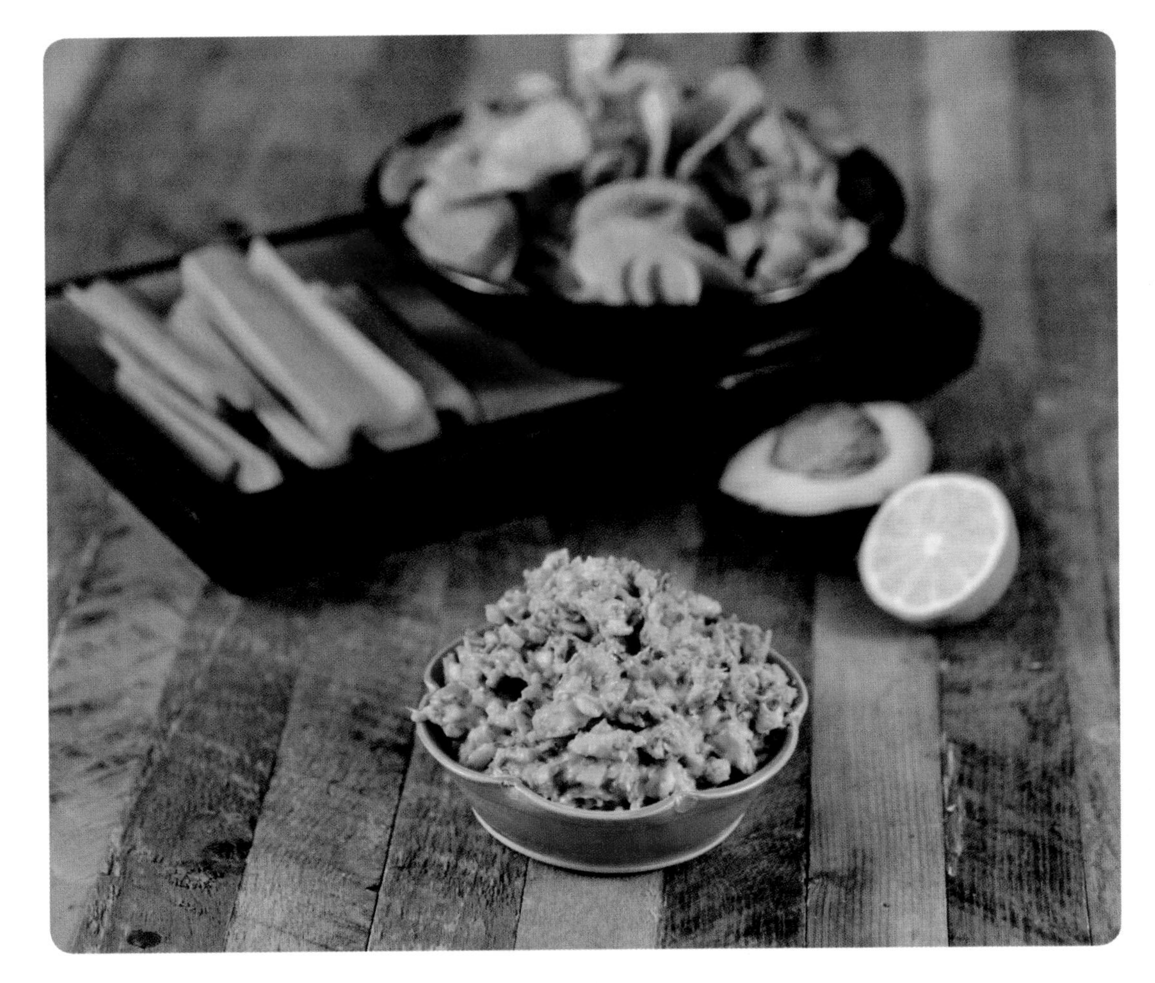

NUTRITION FACTS	
Serving Size	167 g
Recipe Yields	669 g
Calories	**187**
Fats	**15.3 g**
MUFA	8.37 g
Omega-3	0.15 g
Omega-6	2.4 g
Saturated Fat	2.98 g
Carbohydrates	**13.1 g**
Fiber	8.65 g
Starch	0.49 g
Fructose	0.5 g
Glucose	3.46 g
Sucrose	0.1 g
Protein	**3.51 g**
Alanine	0.19 g
Arginine	0.16 g
Aspartic acid	0.41 g
Cystine	0.05 g
Glutamic acid	0.51 g
Glycine	0.18 g
Histidine	0.08 g
Isoleucine	0.14 g
Leucine	0.25 g
Lysine	0.23 g
Methionine	0.06 g
Phenylalanine	0.17 g
Proline	0.17 g
Serine	0.2 g
Threonine	0.13 g
Tryptophan	0.04 g
Tyrosine	0.08 g
Valine	0.18 g
Vitamins	
Vitamin B1	0.04 mg
Vitamin B12	0 mcg
Vitamin B2	0.09 mg
Vitamin B3	1.05 mg
Vitamin B5	1.44 mg
Vitamin B6	0.13 mg
Choline	0.92 mg
Folate	55.8 mcg
Vitamin A	15 mcg
Vitamin C	29.5 mg
Vitamin D	0 IU
Vitamin E	4.08 mg
Vitamin K	3.94 mcg
Minerals	
Calcium	19.2 mg
Copper	0.48 mg
Iron	0.67 mg
Magnesium	37.9 mg
Manganese	0.16 mg
Phosphorus	64.1 mg
Potassium	559 mg
Selenium	0.05 mcg
Sodium	68 mg
Zinc	0.63 mg

nutrition content estimated using the USDA database.

Veggies and Dip

There are endless variations for delicious dip that you can make with Paleo Approach–friendly ingredients. Either avocado combined with some of your favorite salad dressing or coconut yogurt or kefir combined with your favorite spice blend (or the seasoning ingredients of your favorite salad dressing, minus the liquid ingredients) makes a fantastic base for your favorite herbs and spices.

PREP TIME: 10 to 15 minutes
COOK TIME: none
SERVINGS: 4 to 10

INGREDIENTS:

Avocado Dip:

¼ cup Salad Dressing of your choice (page 126)

1 large avocado, peeled and pitted

Your favorite veggies, for dipping

Yogurt Dip:

1 tablespoon Handy-Dandy Spice Blends of your choice (page 108) or salad dressing seasonings of your choice (page 126)

½ cup Coconut Milk Yogurt (page 118) or kefir

Your favorite veggies, for dipping

1. Combine the ingredients in a small blender or food processor. Process until smooth or until the desired consistency is reached. Enjoy with veggies for dipping!

TIPS:

Great dipping vegetables include carrots, celery, broccoli, mushrooms, jicama, radishes, kohlrabi, Belgian endive, asparagus spears, beet, turnips, and rutabaga. Other good dipping options are Dehydrator Plantain Chips (page 170), Sweet Potato Chips (page 168), and Plantain Crackers (page 149).

FODMAP ALERT *Do not make the Avocado Dip. If you do not tolerate Coconut Milk Yogurt, you can try using mashed low-FODMAP vegetables thinned with broth as a base.*

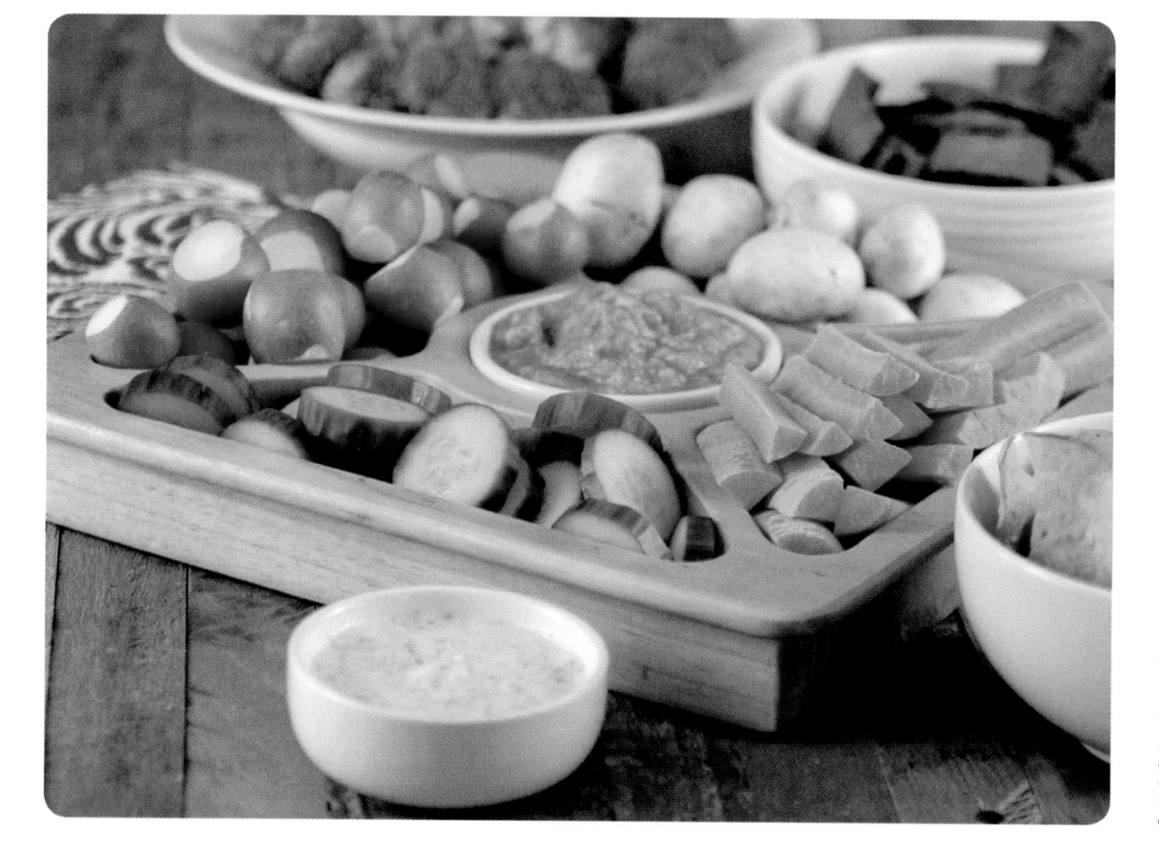

NUTRITION FACTS	
Serving Size	17 g
Recipe Yields	172 g
Calories	**46.1**
Fats	**4.62 g**
MUFA	1.19 g
Omega-3	0.14 g
Omega-6	1.09 g
Saturated Fat	1.93 g
Carbohydrates	**1.35 g**
Fiber	0.66 g
Starch	0.04 g
Fructose	0.1 g
Glucose	0.09 g
Sucrose	0.09 g
Protein	**0.37 g**
Alanine	0.02 g
Arginine	0.04 g
Aspartic acid	0.04 g
Cystine	0.01 g
Glutamic acid	0.07 g
Glycine	0.03 g
Histidine	0.01 g
Isoleucine	0.02 g
Leucine	0.03 g
Lysine	0.02 g
Methionine	0.01 g
Phenylalanine	0.02 g
Proline	0.02 g
Serine	0.02 g
Threonine	0.01 g
Tryptophan	0 g
Tyrosine	0.01 g
Valine	0.02 g
Vitamins	
Vitamin B1	0.01 mg
Vitamin B12	0 mcg
Vitamin B2	0.01 mg
Vitamin B3	0.2 mg
Vitamin B5	0.12 mg
Vitamin B6	0.03 mg
Choline	1.7 mg
Folate	7.66 mcg
Vitamin A	0.78 mcg
Vitamin C	0.86 mg
Vitamin D	0 IU
Vitamin E	0.31mg
Vitamin K	6.7 mcg
Minerals	
Calcium	4.46 mg
Copper	0.03 mg
Iron	0.24 mg
Magnesium	5.15 mg
Manganese	0.09 mg
Phosphorus	11.3 mg
Potassium	55.7 mg
Selenium	1.37 mcg
Sodium	42.2 mg
Zinc	0.11 mg

nutrition content estimated using the USDA database. values are based on an average of all variations.

Prosciutto-Wrapped Melon

Sometimes you just can't beat the classics, although you can definitely experiment with different types of melon for this recipe!

PREP TIME: 20 to 30 minutes
COOK TIME: none
SERVINGS: 4 to 10

INGREDIENTS:

- ½ pound very thinly sliced prosciutto
- ½ small cantaloupe, cut into 1-inch cubes
- ½ small honeydew melon, cut into 1-inch cubes
- 2 to 3 dozen seedless grapes
- Balsamic vinegar (optional)

1. Cut each slice of prosciutto in half lengthwise.
2. Wrap a piece of prosciutto tightly around each chunk of melon and top with a grape. Skewer with a toothpick to hold it together, and arrange on a serving platter.
3. If desired, drizzle a single drop of balsamic vinegar over each piece just before serving (you may want to use an eyedropper!).

VARIATIONS:

Watermelon, canary melon, papaya, mango, pineapple, and strawberries are all great options in lieu of honeydew and cantaloupe.

Lox-Wrapped Melon. Cold-smoked salmon is a delicious alternative to prosciutto, and is particularly good with watermelon. Skip the grapes and the balsamic vinegar.

FODMAP ALERT

Omit the grapes.

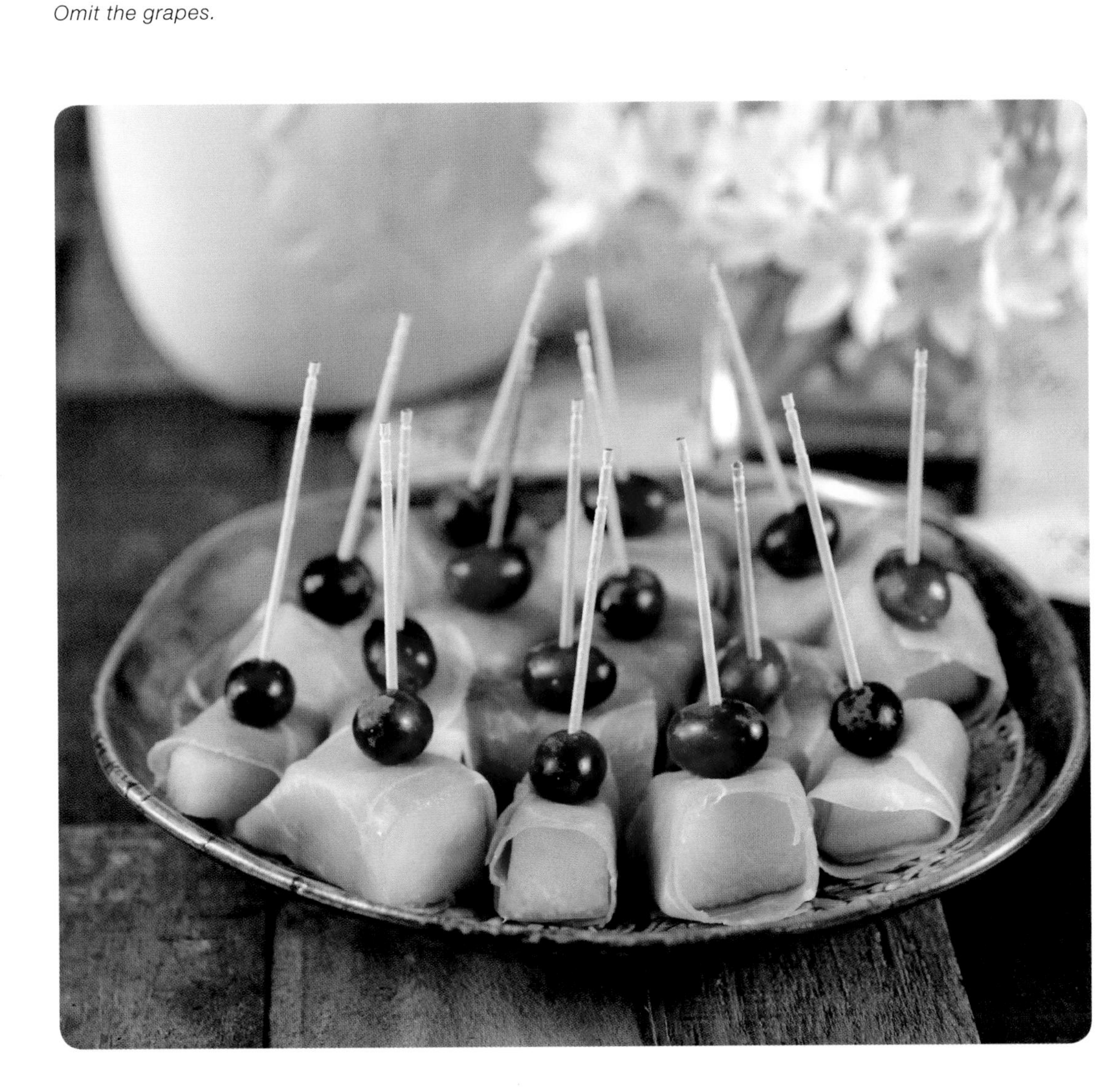

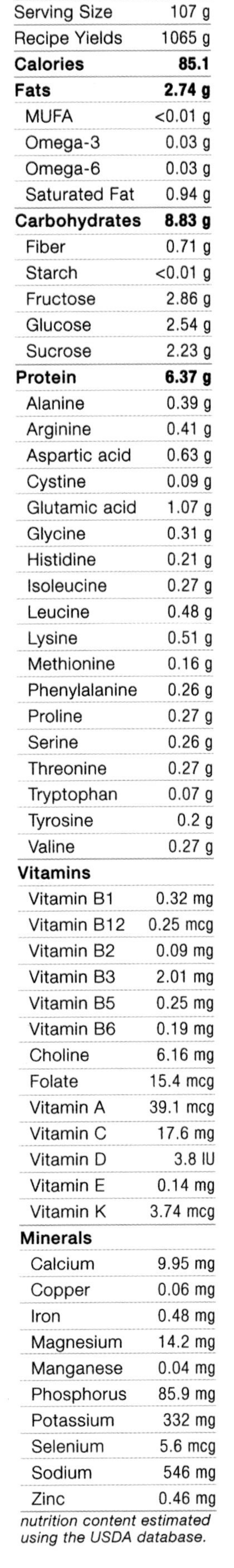

NUTRITION FACTS	
Serving Size	107 g
Recipe Yields	1065 g
Calories	**85.1**
Fats	**2.74 g**
MUFA	<0.01 g
Omega-3	0.03 g
Omega-6	0.03 g
Saturated Fat	0.94 g
Carbohydrates	**8.83 g**
Fiber	0.71 g
Starch	<0.01 g
Fructose	2.86 g
Glucose	2.54 g
Sucrose	2.23 g
Protein	**6.37 g**
Alanine	0.39 g
Arginine	0.41 g
Aspartic acid	0.63 g
Cystine	0.09 g
Glutamic acid	1.07 g
Glycine	0.31 g
Histidine	0.21 g
Isoleucine	0.27 g
Leucine	0.48 g
Lysine	0.51 g
Methionine	0.16 g
Phenylalanine	0.26 g
Proline	0.27 g
Serine	0.26 g
Threonine	0.27 g
Tryptophan	0.07 g
Tyrosine	0.2 g
Valine	0.27 g
Vitamins	
Vitamin B1	0.32 mg
Vitamin B12	0.25 mcg
Vitamin B2	0.09 mg
Vitamin B3	2.01 mg
Vitamin B5	0.25 mg
Vitamin B6	0.19 mg
Choline	6.16 mg
Folate	15.4 mcg
Vitamin A	39.1 mcg
Vitamin C	17.6 mg
Vitamin D	3.8 IU
Vitamin E	0.14 mg
Vitamin K	3.74 mcg
Minerals	
Calcium	9.95 mg
Copper	0.06 mg
Iron	0.48 mg
Magnesium	14.2 mg
Manganese	0.04 mg
Phosphorus	85.9 mg
Potassium	332 mg
Selenium	5.6 mcg
Sodium	546 mg
Zinc	0.46 mg

nutrition content estimated using the USDA database.

Smoked Salmon and Roe Endive Boats

Hot-smoked salmon is typically cured in salt and sugar before being smoked. Similar to other cures, very little of the sugar and salt remain in the finished product. However, check the ingredients before buying.

PREP TIME: 20 to 30 minutes
COOK TIME: none
SERVINGS: 4 to 10

INGREDIENTS:

- 4 ounces smoked salmon
- ½ cup Coconut Milk Yogurt (page 118)
- 2 green onions, finely chopped
- ¾ teaspoon chopped fresh dill, plus more for garnish, if desired
- 1½ teaspoons fresh lemon juice
- 1¾ ounces salmon caviar (see Tips)
- 2 heads Belgian endive

FODMAP ALERT *Use only the green parts of the green onions. If you do not tolerate Coconut Milk Yogurt, do not make this recipe.*

1. Using a fork, break apart the smoked salmon in a small bowl.
2. Add the yogurt, green onions, dill, and lemon juice and stir to fully combine. Fold in the caviar.
3. Separate the endive leaves (this can be done easily by progressively slicing thin slices off the bottom of the head of endive and removing the leaves as they are cut off).
4. Spoon the salmon mixture onto the base of each leaf and arrange on a serving platter. Garnish with additional chopped fresh dill, if desired. Enjoy!

TIPS:

Salmon caviar, also called salmon roe, is likely the easiest type of caviar to find without problematic added ingredients such as preservatives and food dyes (it is also one of the most affordable types of caviar). However, check the label before buying.

VARIATIONS:

You can use smoked trout in place of the smoked salmon. Lox can also be used for a very different flavor. Other types of caviar can be used as well.

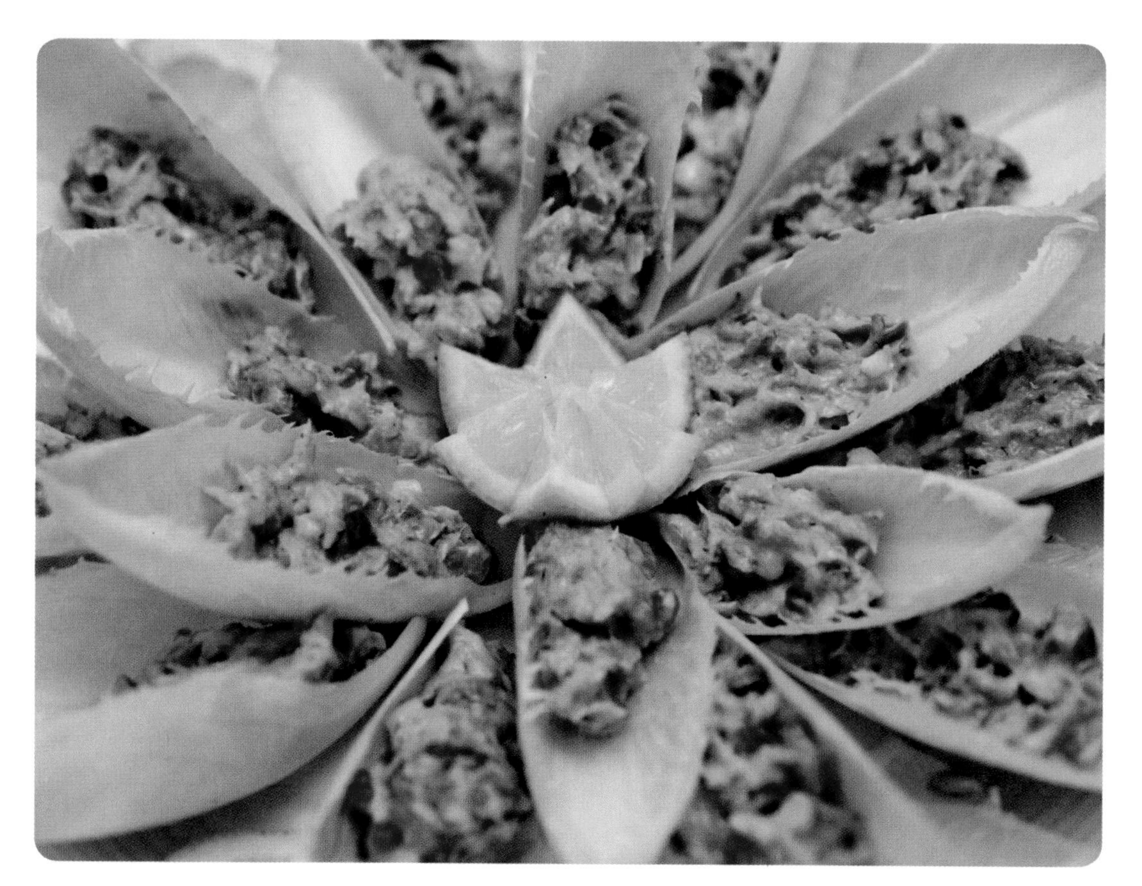

NUTRITION FACTS

Serving Size	139 g
Recipe Yields	1393 g
Calories	**79**
Fats	**4.91 g**
MUFA	0.61 g
Omega-3	0.41 g
Omega-6	0.2 g
Saturated Fat	3.32 g
Carbohydrates	**5.13 g**
Fiber	3.58 g
Starch	0.23 g
Fructose	0.33 g
Glucose	0.27 g
Sucrose	0.02 g
Protein	**5.05 g**
Alanine	0.3 g
Arginine	0.33 g
Aspartic acid	0.5 g
Cystine	0.06 g
Glutamic acid	0.74 g
Glycine	0.23 g
Histidine	0.12 g
Isoleucine	0.23 g
Leucine	0.4 g
Lysine	0.36 g
Methionine	0.11 g
Phenylalanine	0.21 g
Proline	0.22 g
Serine	0.25 g
Threonine	0.22 g
Tryptophan	0.05 g
Tyrosine	0.17 g
Valine	0.26 g
Vitamins	
Vitamin B1	0.1 mg
Vitamin B12	1.36 mcg
Vitamin B2	0.12 mg
Vitamin B3	1.08 mg
Vitamin B5	1.23 mg
Vitamin B6	0.08 mg
Choline	53.1 mg
Folate	153 mcg
Vitamin A	138 mcg
Vitamin C	8.32 mg
Vitamin D	11 IU
Vitamin E	0.73 mg
Vitamin K	244 mcg
Minerals	
Calcium	73.8 mg
Copper	0.17 mg
Iron	1.82 mg
Magnesium	38.4 mg
Manganese	0.57 mg
Phosphorus	80.3 mg
Potassium	398 mg
Selenium	8.04 mcg
Sodium	189 mg
Zinc	1 mg

nutrition content estimated using the USDA database.

Smoked Salmon and Mango Salsa Nori Wraps

These nori wraps make an excellent snack or lunch food. The recipe can easily be doubled or tripled.

PREP TIME: 15 minutes
COOK TIME: none
SERVINGS: 1 to 2

INGREDIENTS:

- 3 tablespoons peeled, pitted, and finely diced avocado
- 1 tablespoon finely diced red onion
- 2 tablespoons finely diced mango
- ¼ cup finely diced cucumber (peel if desired)
- 2 (8-by-8-inch) nori sheets
- 2 to 3 ounces lox
- ½ cup sunflower sprouts or radish sprouts

1. In a bowl, mix together the avocado, red onion, mango, and cucumber.
2. Lay the nori sheets out on a cutting board. Divide the lox among the sheets, laying it over one-quarter of each sheet and leaving the rest of the sheet empty for wrapping. Top the lox with the mango salsa and sunflower sprouts. Wrap each nori sheet around the filling, forming a cone or burrito shape. Wet the edge of the nori sheet with a little cold water to make it stick. Enjoy!

VARIATIONS:

Want to give these wraps some kick? Add a little wasabi! Look for wasabi powder. Simply mix wasabi powder with a little hot water to the desired thickness, and let sit for 5 minutes before spreading on your nori wraps.

Shrimp Salad Nori Wraps. A delicious alternative to lox and mango salsa is to fill the nori sheets with cooked small shrimp mixed with a tablespoon or two of Coconut Milk Yogurt (page 118) and shredded lettuce.

FODMAP ALERT

This recipe cannot be made low-FODMAP.

NUTRITION FACTS	
Serving Size	149 g
Recipe Yields	75 g
Calories	**56.6**
Fats	**2.23 g**
MUFA	1.1 g
Omega-3	0.23 g
Omega-6	0.26 g
Saturated Fat	0.46 g
Carbohydrates	**3.48 g**
Fiber	0.64 g
Starch	0.11 g
Fructose	0.68 g
Glucose	0.45 g
Sucrose	0.79 g
Protein	**6.06 g**
Alanine	0.35 g
Arginine	0.34 g
Aspartic acid	0.58 g
Cystine	0.06 g
Glutamic acid	0.86 g
Glycine	0.27 g
Histidine	0.16 g
Isoleucine	0.26 g
Leucine	0.45 g
Lysine	0.5 g
Methionine	0.16 g
Phenylalanine	0.22 g
Proline	0.2 g
Serine	0.23 g
Threonine	0.25 g
Tryptophan	0.06 g
Tyrosine	0.19 g
Valine	0.29 g
Vitamins	
Vitamin B1	0.03 mg
Vitamin B12	0.93 mcg
Vitamin B2	0.07 mg
Vitamin B3	1.83 mg
Vitamin B5	0.46 mg
Vitamin B6	0.15 mg
Choline	31 mg
Folate	23.8 mcg
Vitamin A	22.7 mcg
Vitamin C	8.85 mg
Vitamin D	96.9 IU
Vitamin E	0.37 mg
Vitamin K	3.73 mcg
Minerals	
Calcium	15.1 mg
Copper	0.11 mg
Iron	0.46 mg
Magnesium	14.1 mg
Manganese	0.09 mg
Phosphorus	67.9 mg
Potassium	136 mg
Selenium	11.1 mcg
Sodium	573 mg
Zinc	0.25 mg

nutrition content estimated using the USDA database.

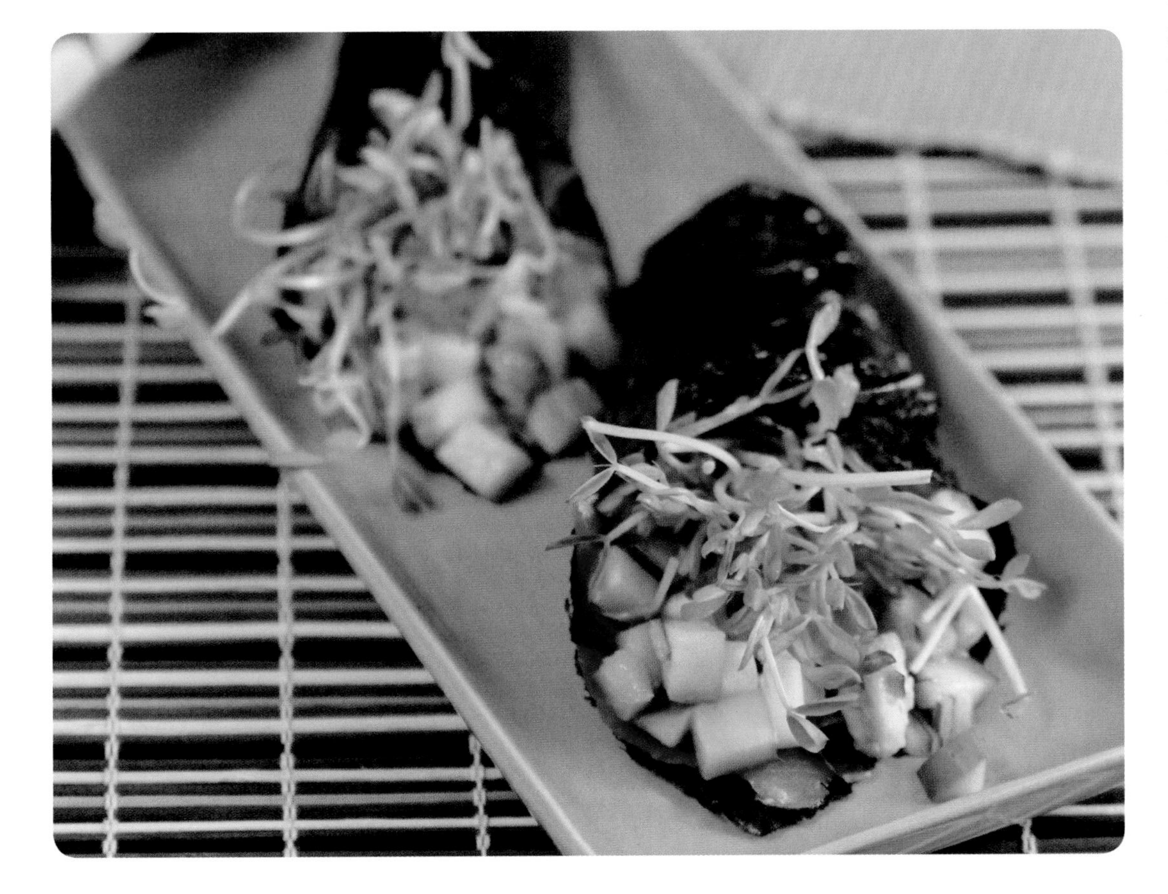

Vietnamese-Style Fresh "Spring Rolls"

These Vietnamese-style spring rolls have a fantastic flavor. You can mix the filling in advance, but it's best to assemble the rolls right before eating them.

PREP TIME: 30 minutes
COOK TIME: none
SERCINGS: 4 to 8

INGREDIENTS:

- 2 teaspoons fish sauce
- 1 tablespoon fresh lime juice
- 1 small clove garlic, crushed
- 1 teaspoon honey
- 1 carrot, grated
- ½ cup thinly sliced lettuce
- ½ cup sunflower sprouts or radish sprouts
- 1 tablespoon chopped fresh Thai basil leaves
- 3 tablespoons chopped fresh mint
- 3 tablespoons chopped fresh cilantro
- 2 ounces kelp noodles
- 8 coconut wraps
- 8 large cooked shrimp
- 4 ounces leftover pork, thinly sliced
- 8 large slices cucumber

FODMAP ALERT *Replace the garlic with green garlic or garlic scapes (green part only) or omit. Skip the honey or replace with evaporated cane juice. Use one of the alternatives for coconut wraps suggested in the variations.*

1. In a small bowl, mix together the fish sauce, lime juice, garlic, and honey.
2. In another bowl, mix the grated carrot, lettuce, sunflower sprouts, Thai basil, mint, and cilantro. Pour the fish sauce mixture over the vegetables and toss to thoroughly combine.
3. To assemble the spring rolls, place a few tablespoons of the kelp noodles in the middle of a coconut wrap. Layer a shrimp and a couple slices of pork over the top. Top with a spoonful of the grated carrot mixture and a cucumber slice.
4. Fold the coconut wrap around the filling. Repeat until all 8 spring rolls are made.

TIPS:

Kelp noodles and coconut wraps can be found in many specialty and ethnic grocery stores or ordered online.

Love the sauce? Double the batch in step 1 and use the rest as a dipping sauce!

VARIATIONS:

Don't want to wrap in coconut wraps? Nori wraps, lettuce leaves, tender collard leaves, and Swiss chard leaves are all great wrapping options.

NUTRITION FACTS	
Serving Size	67 g
Recipe Yields	533 g
Calories	**98.7**
Fats	**3.22 g**
MUFA	0.22 g
Omega-3	0.04 g
Omega-6	0.1 g
Saturated Fat	2.74 g
Carbohydrates	**10.5 g**
Fiber	0.45 g
Starch	0.49 g
Fructose	0.49 g
Glucose	0.43 g
Sucrose	0.35 g
Protein	**5.49 g**
Alanine	0.33 g
Arginine	0.4 g
Aspartic acid	0.55 g
Cystine	0.07 g
Glutamic acid	0.9 g
Glycine	0.26 g
Histidine	0.2 g
Isoleucine	0.26 g
Leucine	0.46 g
Lysine	0.5 g
Methionine	0.15 g
Phenylalanine	0.23 g
Proline	0.23 g
Serine	0.23 g
Threonine	0.24 g
Tryptophan	0.06 g
Tyrosine	0.2 g
Valine	0.28 g
Vitamins	
Vitamin B1	0.18 mg
Vitamin B12	0.19 mcg
Vitamin B2	0.07 mg
Vitamin B3	1.84 mg
Vitamin B5	0.25 mg
Vitamin B6	0.16 mg
Choline	22.7 mg
Folate	11.8 mcg
Vitamin A	86.7 mcg
Vitamin C	7.33 mg
Vitamin D	1.66 IU
Vitamin E	0.22 mg
Vitamin K	7.7 mcg
Minerals	
Calcium	65.7 mg
Copper	0.05 mg
Iron	1.11 mg
Magnesium	21.3 mg
Manganese	0.1 mg
Phosphorus	106 mg
Potassium	249 mg
Selenium	8.67 mcg
Sodium	434 mg
Zinc	0.52 mg

nutrition content estimated using the USDA database.

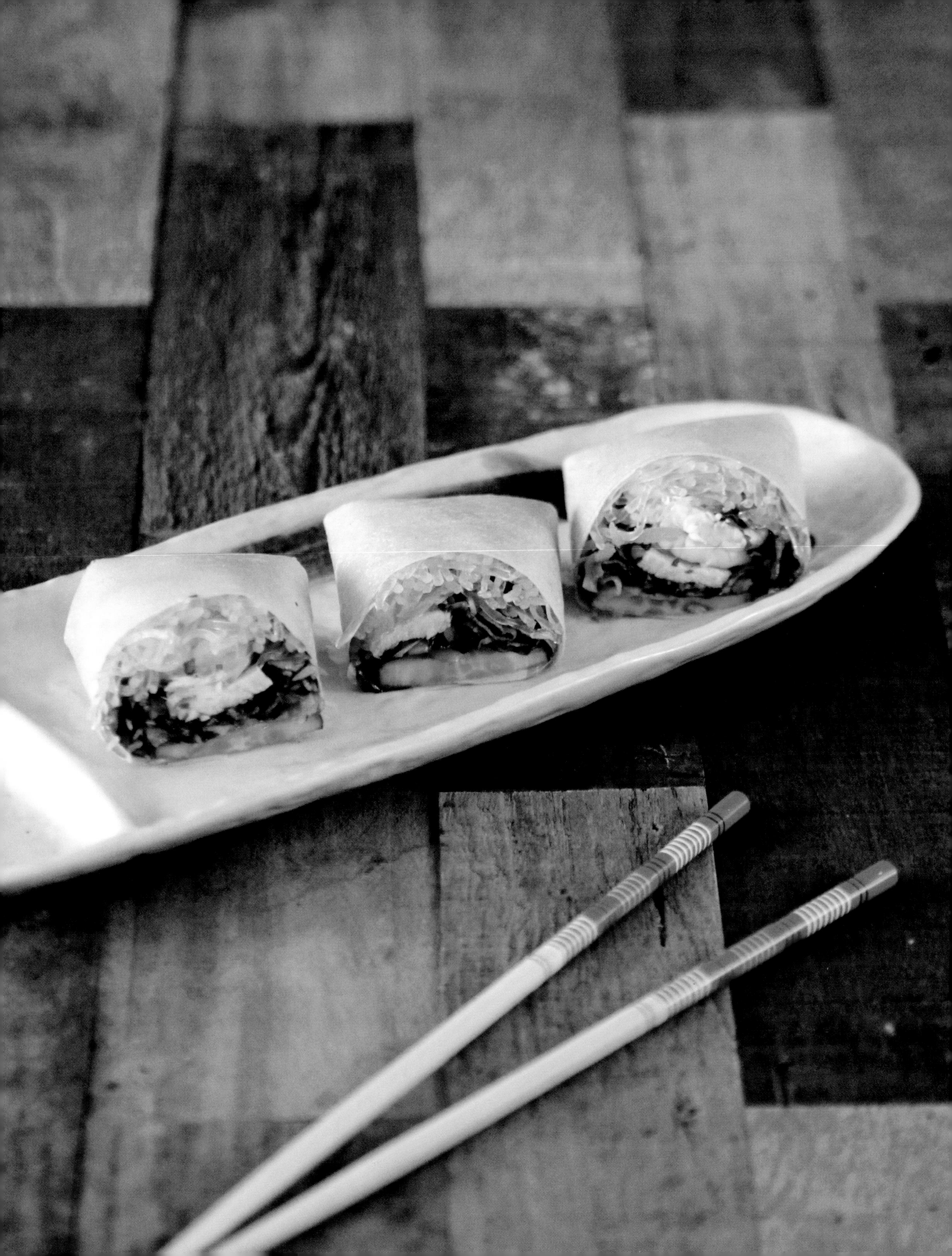

Sweet-and-Sour Beef Heart Jerky

It's pretty typical that Paleo Approach–friendly jerky involves very simple seasoning, often just salt. But that doesn't mean you're doomed to boring jerky for the rest of your life! In fact, jerky is quite easy to make at home, and there are many wonderful ways to enjoy it!

PREP TIME: 30 minutes, plus up to 24 hours marinating time
COOK TIME: 4 to 6 hours
SERVINGS: 4 to 8

INGREDIENTS:

- 3 large Medjool dates
- ¼ cup boiling water
- 2 teaspoons coconut oil
- 2 shallots, thinly sliced
- 2 tablespoons tamarind paste
- 1 tablespoon fish sauce
- 1 pound beef heart, sliced ¼ inch thick

1. Pit the dates and place in a small heatproof bowl or measuring cup. Pour the boiling water over them and soak for at least 20 minutes.
2. Meanwhile, heat the coconut oil in a skillet over medium-high heat. Add the shallots and sauté, stirring frequently, until caramelized, 5 to 8 minutes.
3. Place the shallots, dates and their soaking water, tamarind paste, and fish sauce in a blender and blend until smooth.
4. Coat the beef heart slices with the marinade, cover, and place in the refrigerator. Marinate overnight and up to 24 hours.
5. Place the beef heart slices on a dehydrator tray, discarding the excess marinade. Dehydrate for 4 to 6 hours, until chewy.
6. Store in the refrigerator for up to 2 weeks or freeze.

FODMAP ALERT *Because the dates are used in a marinade, most people with FODMAP intolerance will probably be okay with this jerky. An alternative is to use 1 to 2 tablespoons evaporated cane juice dissolved in 2 to 3 tablespoons water.*

SPECIAL EQUIPMENT

- Blender
- Dehydrator

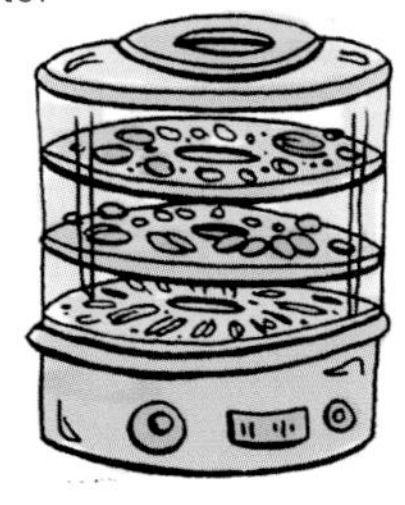

VARIATIONS:

You can use any thinly sliced meat in place of the beef heart in this recipe.

You can also dehydrate the marinated meat in your oven on the lowest temperature or in a smoker.

Sweet-and-Sour Pork. Use the marinade as a sweet-and-sour sauce for an Asian-inspired dish! Stir-fry pieces of pork or chicken with onion wedges, sliced carrot, and pineapple chunks, add the sauce to coat, and serve over Cauliflower Rice (page 298).

Teriyaki Beef Jerky. Use Teriyaki Marinade (page 250) instead of the sweet-and-sour marinade to marinate the beef heart slices.

Barbecue Beef Jerky. Use Barbecue Sauce (page 124) instead of the sweet-and-sour marinade to marinate the beef heart slices.

NUTRITION FACTS	
Serving Size	82 g
Recipe Yields	657 g
Calories	**136**
Fats	**3.84 g**
MUFA	0.64 g
Omega-3	0.01 g
Omega-6	0.56 g
Saturated Fat	1.78 g
Carbohydrates	**8.7 g**
Fiber	0.82 g
Starch	0.46 g
Fructose	2.87 g
Glucose	3.03 g
Sucrose	0.13 g
Protein	**16.6 g**
Alanine	1.03 g
Arginine	1.1 g
Aspartic acid	1.54 g
Cystine	0.22 g
Glutamic acid	2.64 g
Glycine	0.87 g
Histidine	0.46 g
Isoleucine	0.73 g
Leucine	1.46 g
Lysine	1.37 g
Methionine	0.42 g
Phenylalanine	0.75 g
Proline	0.79 g
Serine	0.77 g
Threonine	0.78 g
Tryptophan	0.18 g
Tyrosine	0.6 g
Valine	0.87 g
Vitamins	
Vitamin B1	0.07 mg
Vitamin B12	6.13 mcg
Vitamin B2	0.7 mg
Vitamin B3	4.02 mg
Vitamin B5	0.99 mg
Vitamin B6	0.18 mg
Choline	131 mg
Folate	6.86 mcg
Vitamin A	0.76 mcg
Vitamin C	0.38 mg
Vitamin D	1.7 IU
Vitamin E	0.17 mg
Vitamin K	0.61 mcg
Minerals	
Calcium	12.5 mg
Copper	0.36 mg
Iron	3.81 mg
Magnesium	23.3 mg
Manganese	0.06 mg
Phosphorus	154 mg
Potassium	217 mg
Selenium	22.3 mcg
Sodium	211 mg
Zinc	1.69 mg

nutrition content estimated using the USDA database.

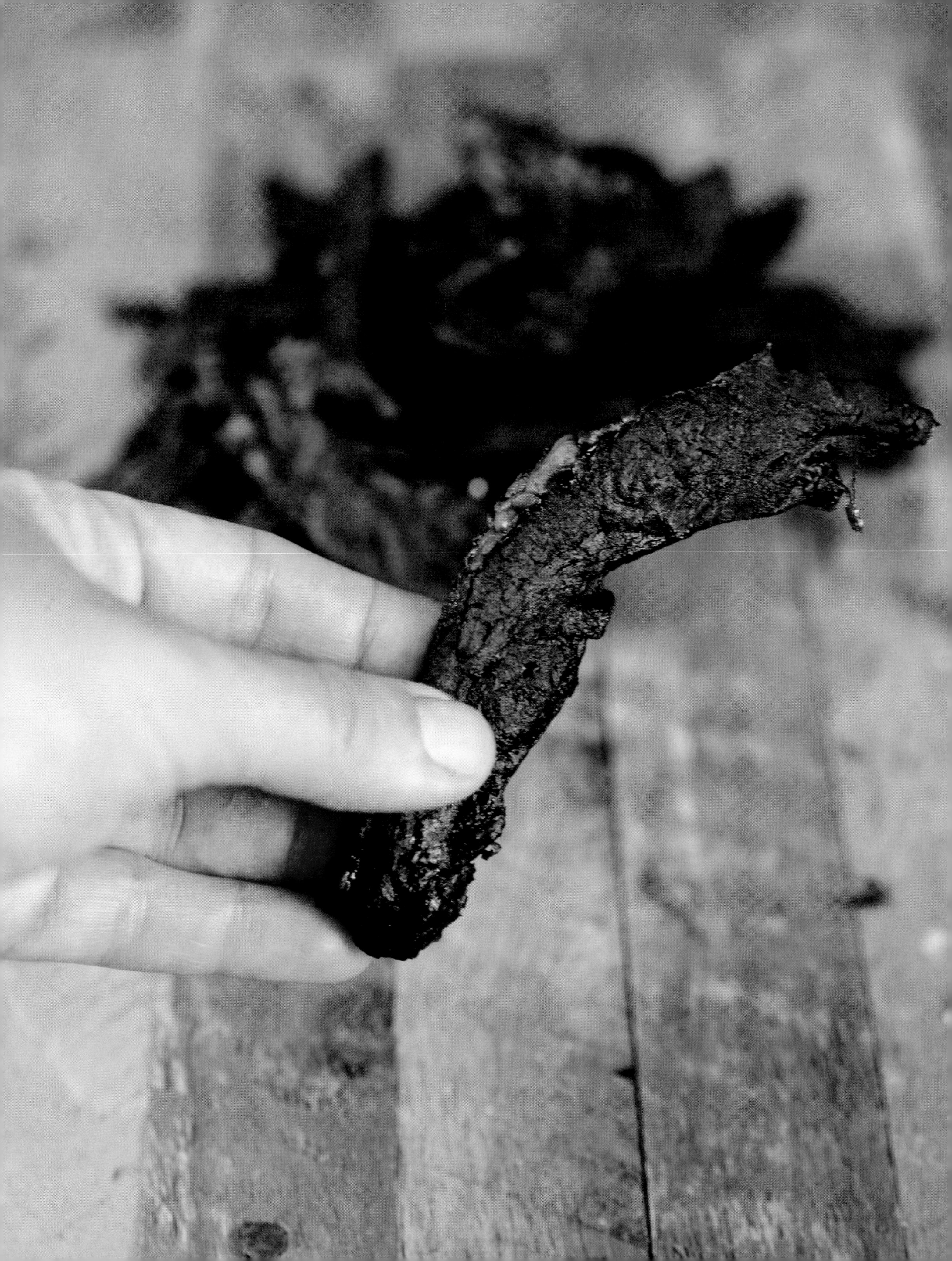

Chapter 7

Soups and Stews

Soups and stews are wonderfully convenient meals to have in your freezer and can be very comforting on a cold winter day. They even make great breakfasts. This chapter includes a range of different flavors and textures, from super simple to sublimely elegant, to give you some great options for your next "soup day."

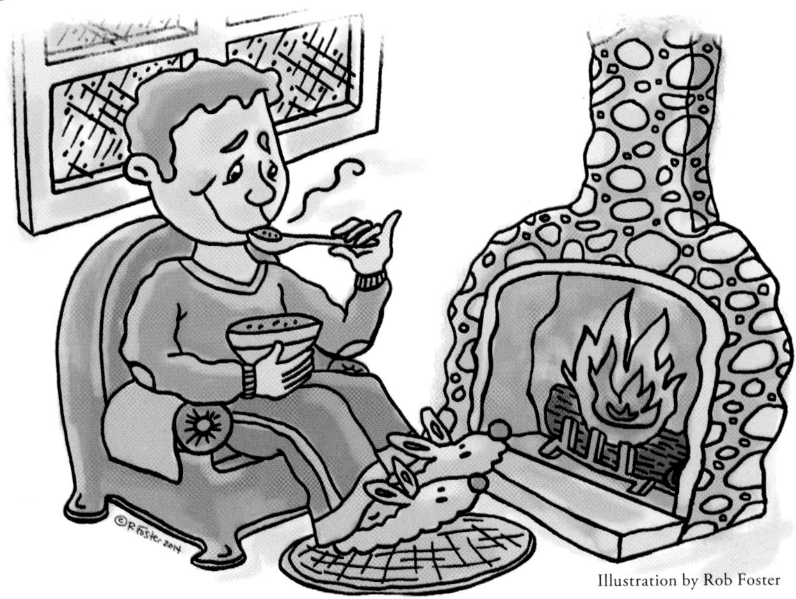

Illustration by Rob Foster

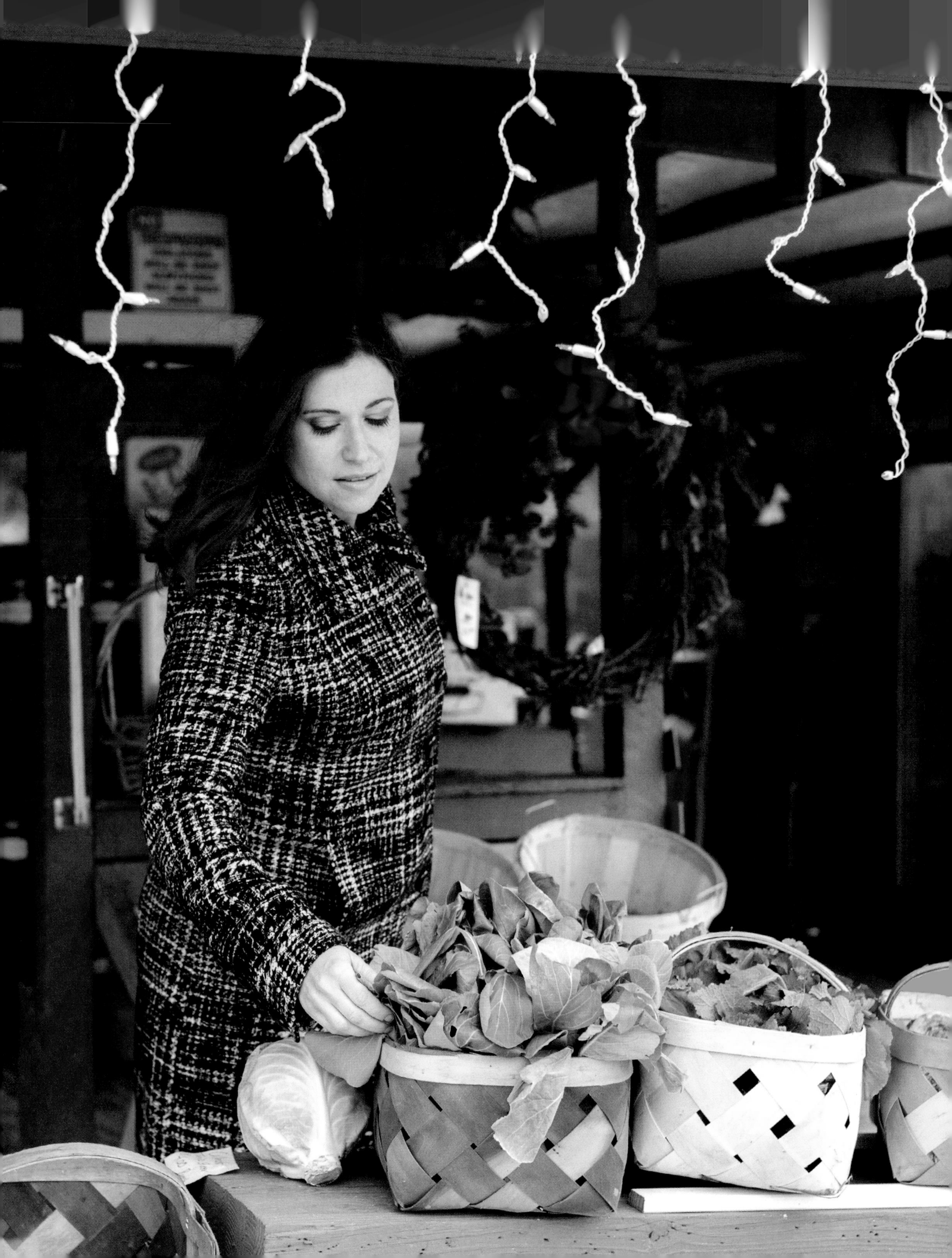

"Cream" of Broccoli Soup

This simple soup can be enjoyed warm or chilled. Serve it with chunks of leftover chicken, steak, or crab to make it a complete meal.

PREP TIME: 5 to 10 minutes
COOK TIME: 12 to 15 minutes
SERVINGS: 3 to 5

INGREDIENTS:

- 2 pounds broccoli
- 2 small avocados
- 4 cups Bone Broth (chicken, page 110)
- ¼ teaspoon ground mace
- Salt, to taste

1. Wash and cut the broccoli into florets. Slice the stems (peel them if they are tough). Peel and pit the avocados and cut the flesh into medium-sized chunks.
2. Bring the bone broth to a simmer in a saucepot over medium-high heat.
3. Add the broccoli and cook for 7 to 8 minutes, until dark green and tender.
4. Reduce the heat to low. Add the mace and avocado to the pot. Cook for 3 to 4 more minutes, until the avocado has warmed.
5. Purée with an immersion blender (or in a blender or food processor). Taste and add salt, if desired. Enjoy!

FODMAP ALERT

This recipe cannot be made low-FODMAP.

SPECIAL EQUIPMENT

- Immersion blender, blender, or food processor

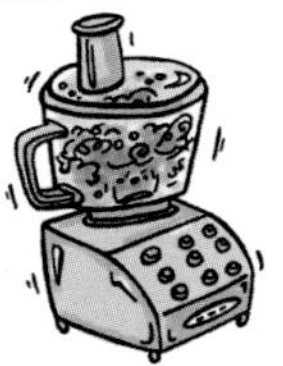

VARIATIONS:

You can replace the broccoli with cauliflower, broccoflower, or any mix of fresh vegetables you like.

Cream of Asparagus Soup. Replace the broccoli with asparagus, omit the mace, and add 1 cup Coconut Cream (page 116).

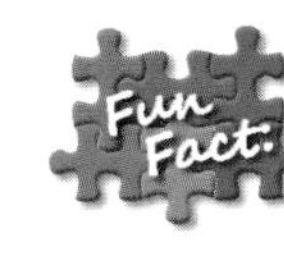

Dairy isn't the only source of calcium! A serving of broccoli has the same amount as a serving of cottage cheese.

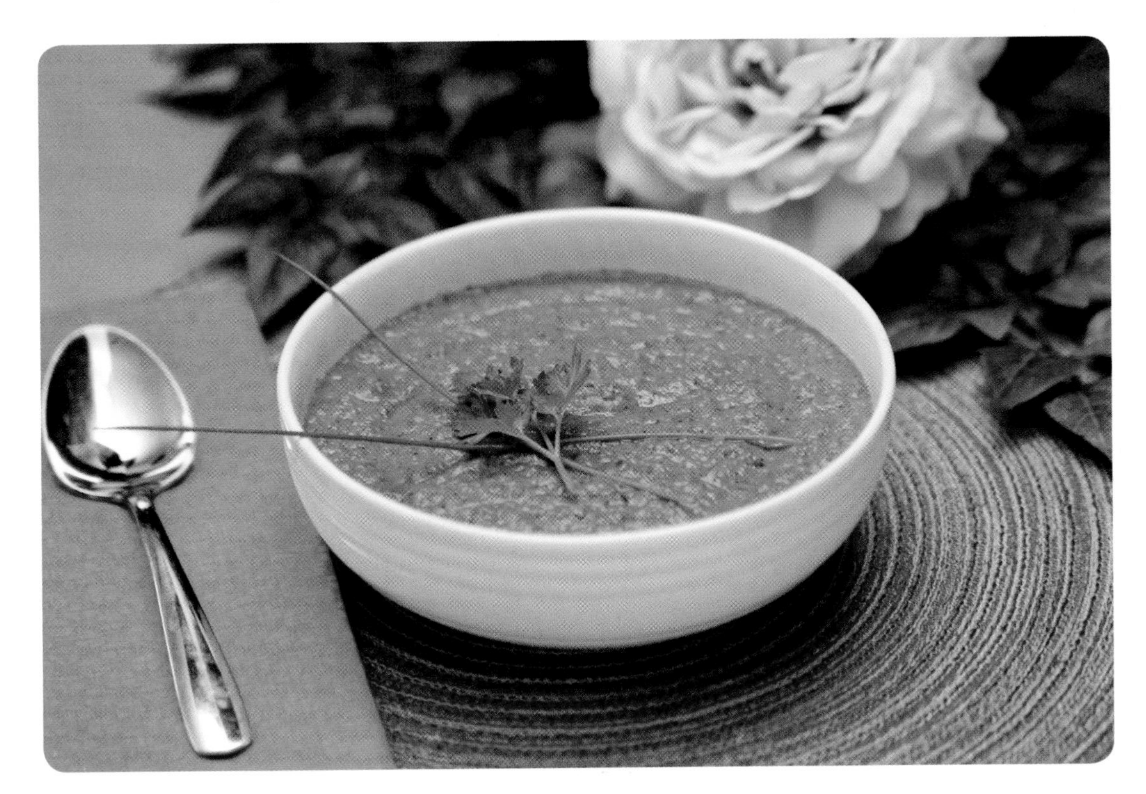

NUTRITION FACTS	
Serving Size	502 g
Recipe Yields	2512 g
Calories	**220**
Fats	**13.3 g**
MUFA	6.76 g
Omega-3	0.15 g
Omega-6	1.97 g
Saturated Fat	2.49 g
Carbohydrates	**22.5 g**
Fiber	11.5 g
Starch	4.24 g
Fructose	1.54 g
Glucose	3.52 g
Sucrose	0.18 g
Protein	**9.1 g**
Alanine	0.34 g
Arginine	0.47 g
Aspartic acid	0.91 g
Cystine	0.09 g
Glutamic acid	1.37 g
Glycine	0.3 g
Histidine	0.17 g
Isoleucine	0.26 g
Leucine	0.43 g
Lysine	0.42 g
Methionine	0.12 g
Phenylalanine	0.34 g
Proline	0.33 g
Serine	0.37 g
Threonine	0.26 g
Tryptophan	0.09 g
Tyrosine	0.16 g
Valine	0.37 g
Vitamins	
Vitamin B1	0.2 mg
Vitamin B12	0.04 mcg
Vitamin B2	0.39 mg
Vitamin B3	2.41 mg
Vitamin B5	2.17 mg
Vitamin B6	0.41 mg
Choline	35.9 mg
Folate	157 mcg
Vitamin A	64.7 mcg
Vitamin C	183 mg
Vitamin D	0 IU
Vitamin E	4.73 mg
Vitamin K	184 mcg
Minerals	
Calcium	106 mg
Copper	0.5 mg
Iron	1.83 mg
Magnesium	69.4 mg
Manganese	0.53 mg
Phosphorus	176 mg
Potassium	1036 mg
Selenium	5.33 mcg
Sodium	826 mg
Zinc	1.37 mg

nutrition content estimated using the USDA database.

"Wonton" Soup

The only thing missing from this wonton soup is the wonton wrappers—and the flavor is so wonderful, you won't even miss them!

PREP TIME: 30 minutes
COOK TIME: 12 to 20 minutes
SERVINGS: 4 to 8

INGREDIENTS:

- 3 dried or fresh shiitake mushrooms
- 1 (5-ounce) can sliced bamboo shoots, drained and rinsed
- 1 (5-ounce) can sliced water chestnuts, drained and rinsed
- 1 pound raw shrimp, shelled
- 1 pound ground pork
- 1 teaspoon fish sauce
- 1 teaspoon coconut water vinegar
- ¼ teaspoon salt, plus more to taste
- 1 tablespoon arrowroot powder
- 8 to 10 cups Bone Broth (chicken or pork, page 110)
- 1 (2-inch-long) piece fresh ginger, peeled and sliced
- ¾ cup thinly sliced carrots
- 6 to 8 ounces baby bok choy
- 4 ounces oyster mushrooms
- ½ cup chopped green onions

1. Preheat the oven to 400°F. Line a rimmed baking sheet with parchment paper, aluminum foil, or a silicone liner.
2. If using dried shiitake mushrooms, soak in hot water for 30 minutes. Drain and rinse, then thinly slice the caps and stems. If using fresh shiitake, thinly slice the caps and stems.
3. Finely chop ¼ cup of the bamboo shoots and ¼ cup of the water chestnuts.
4. Place the shrimp in a food processor and process until a chunky paste forms. Combine with the ground pork, chopped bamboo shoots, chopped water chestnuts, fish sauce, coconut water vinegar, salt, and arrowroot powder in a mixing bowl. Mix by hand to combine.
5. Wet your hands so that the meat mixture won't stick to them. Using your hands, form into 1-inch meatballs and arrange on the prepared baking sheet. Bake for 12 minutes. Remove from the oven and set aside.
6. Meanwhile, combine the broth and ginger in a saucepot and bring to a boil over high heat. Reduce the heat to maintain a simmer and simmer for 5 to 8 minutes, until the ginger is soft. Remove the ginger slices. If the broth is underseasoned, add salt to taste.
7. Add the carrots, baby bok choy, remaining water chestnuts, remaining bamboo shoots, oyster mushrooms, and shiitake mushrooms. Simmer for 6 to 8 minutes, until the vegetables are cooked to your liking.
8. Add the meatballs and green onions to the soup. Taste and add additional salt, if desired. Serve.

VARIATIONS:

Seafood (especially squid and shrimp) and leftover barbecue pork are great additions to wonton soup. Kai-lan is a wonderful vegetable to add. Regular bok choy or sui choy can substitute for the baby bok choy. You can also add or substitute different kinds of mushrooms, such as forest or wood ear mushrooms.

FODMAP ALERT *Omit the mushrooms and use only the green part of the green onion.*

SPECIAL EQUIPMENT

- Food processor

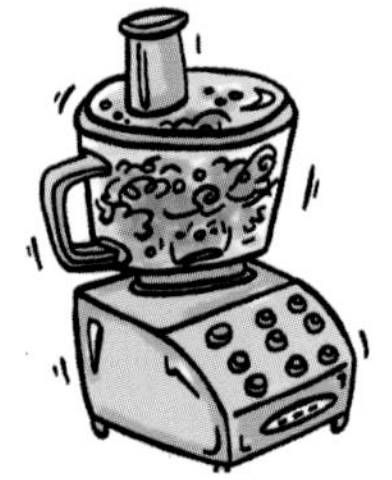

NUTRITION FACTS

Serving Size	463 g
Recipe Yields	3700 g
Calories	**237**
Fats	**6.98 g**
MUFA	2.57 g
Omega-3	0.34 g
Omega-6	0.51 g
Saturated Fat	2.19 g
Carbohydrates	**11.8 g**
Fiber	2.02 g
Starch	3.93 g
Fructose	0.18 g
Glucose	0.49 g
Sucrose	0.42 g
Protein	**31.1 g**
Alanine	1.69 g
Arginine	2.09 g
Aspartic acid	2.86 g
Cystine	0.36 g
Glutamic acid	4.8 g
Glycine	1.52 g
Histidine	0.91 g
Isoleucine	1.38 g
Leucine	2.3 g
Lysine	2.54 g
Methionine	0.77 g
Phenylalanine	1.19 g
Proline	1.08 g
Serine	1.18 g
Threonine	1.28 g
Tryptophan	0.38 g
Tyrosine	0.98 g
Valine	1.5 g
Vitamins	
Vitamin B1	0.51 mg
Vitamin B12	1.02mcg
Vitamin B2	0.45 mg
Vitamin B3	6.05 mg
Vitamin B5	0.89 mg
Vitamin B6	0.47 mg
Choline	121 mg
Folate	34.9 mcg
Vitamin A	184 mcg
Vitamin C	13.4 mg
Vitamin D	25.3 IU
Vitamin E	1.28 mg
Vitamin K	18.2 mcg
Minerals	
Calcium	84 mg
Copper	0.37 mg
Iron	2.91 mg
Magnesium	52.2 mg
Manganese	0.27 mg
Phosphorus	285 mg
Potassium	681 mg
Selenium	51.2 mcg
Sodium	1158 mg
Zinc	2.69 mg

nutrition content estimated using the USDA database.

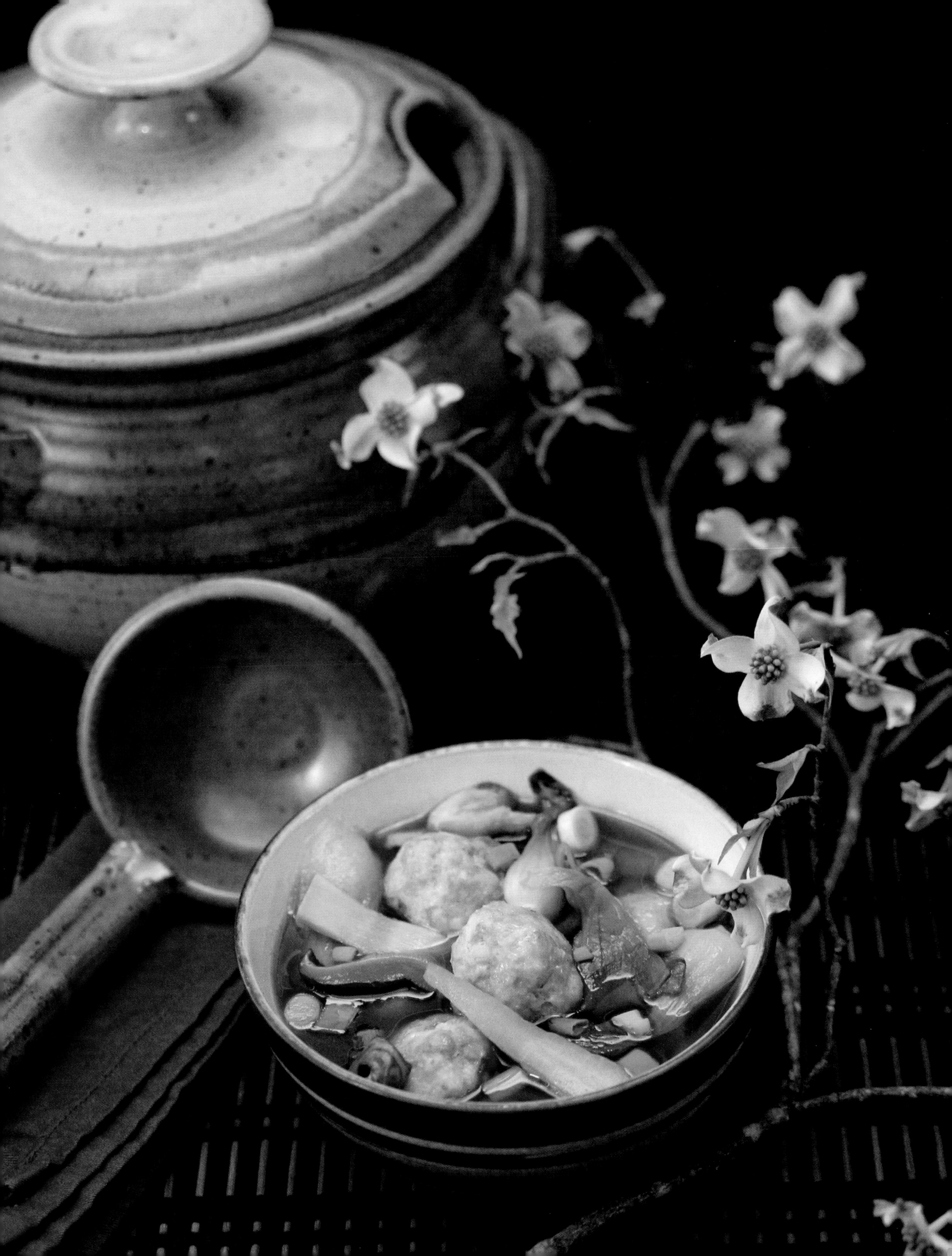

Lobster Bisque

A real lobster bisque takes time to prepare, but the flavor is so glorious that it is absolutely worth every minute. In this version, umeboshi paste and tamarind paste take the place of the more traditional tomato paste.

PREP TIME: 45 minutes
COOK TIME: 4 hours
SERVINGS: 4 to 6

INGREDIENTS:

- 3 pounds whole raw lobsters (two 1½-pounders or three 1-pounders)
- ⅓ cup tamarind paste
- ⅓ cup umeboshi paste
- 1 large onion, coarsely chopped
- 3 to 4 stalks celery (including leaves), coarsely chopped
- 2 large carrots, coarsely chopped
- 1 sprig fresh thyme
- 3 sprigs fresh flat-leaf parsley, chopped, plus extra for garnish
- ¼ teaspoon saffron
- 3 to 3⅓ cups homemade Coconut Milk (page 116) or 2 (13½-ounce) cans full-fat coconut milk
- 1 cup dry sherry, white wine, cognac, apple cider, or Bone Broth (chicken or fish, page 110)
- ¼ cup kuzu starch or arrowroot powder
- ¼ cup cold water
- Salt, to taste

1. Fill a large stockpot with water and bring to a boil. There should be enough water to cover the lobsters completely when immersed. Place the live lobsters headfirst in the boiling water (keeping the elastic bands on their pinchers, which you can remove later) to minimize splashing. Bring the water back to a boil, then reduce the heat to maintain a simmer.
2. Simmer for 20 minutes. Remove the lobsters from the pot using tongs (also remove the rubber bands if they fell off the claws during cooking) and keep the stock in the pot.
3. Once the lobsters have cooled enough to handle, remove the tail and claw meat and refrigerate until ready to serve. Return the shells and the bodies, including the roe and tomalley, to the pot. Add the tamarind paste and umeboshi paste. Simmer uncovered on low heat for 2 hours, stirring occasionally.
4. Strain out and discard all the shells. The easiest way to do so is to pour the stock through a sieve into another stockpot.
5. Add the onion, celery, carrots, thyme, parsley, and saffron to the strained stock. Simmer for 1 hour.
6. Blend the soup with an immersion blender or in batches in a countertop blender. (Be careful not to burn yourself!)
7. Add the coconut milk and sherry. Simmer on low heat for another 20 minutes.
8. Mix the kuzu starch with the cold water and slowly add to the bisque while whisking continuously. Simmer on low heat for another 20 minutes. Taste and add salt, if desired.
9. To serve, place pieces of the reserved lobster meat in bowls and pour the bisque over the top. Garnish with flat-leaf parsley.

FODMAP ALERT

This recipe cannot be made low-FODMAP.

VARIATIONS:

You may have more bisque than lobster meat to serve it with. That's okay! The bisque is also delicious with salmon or shrimp, or just plain!

NUTRITION FACTS	
Serving Size	477 g
Recipe Yields	2864 g
Calories	**557**
Fats	**26.2 g**
MUFA	1.64 g
Omega-3	0.58 g
Omega-6	0.47 g
Saturated Fat	21.9 g
Carbohydrates	**26.6 g**
Fiber	2.24 g
Starch	1.16 g
Fructose	0.72 g
Glucose	0.95 g
Sucrose	1 g
Protein	**46.5 g**
Alanine	2.44 g
Arginine	4.4 g
Aspartic acid	4.49 g
Cystine	0.54 g
Glutamic acid	7.03 g
Glycine	3 g
Histidine	1.14 g
Isoleucine	2 g
Leucine	3.32 g
Lysine	3.39 g
Methionine	1.13 g
Phenylalanine	1.91 g
Proline	2.04 g
Serine	1.8 g
Threonine	1.84 g
Tryptophan	0.6 g
Tyrosine	1.61 g
Valine	2.1 g
Vitamins	
Vitamin B1	0.17 mg
Vitamin B12	3.24 mcg
Vitamin B2	0.1 mg
Vitamin B3	5.51 mg
Vitamin B5	4.13 mg
Vitamin B6	0.39 mg
Choline	201 mg
Folate	59.8 mcg
Vitamin A	180 mcg
Vitamin C	6.65 mg
Vitamin D	2.27 IU
Vitamin E	2.48 mg
Vitamin K	18 mcg
Minerals	
Calcium	276 mg
Copper	3.83 mg
Iron	5.13 mg
Magnesium	173 mg
Manganese	1.18 mg
Phosphorus	566 mg
Potassium	1058 mg
Selenium	166 mcg
Sodium	1457 mg
Zinc	9.99 mg

nutrition content estimated using the USDA database.

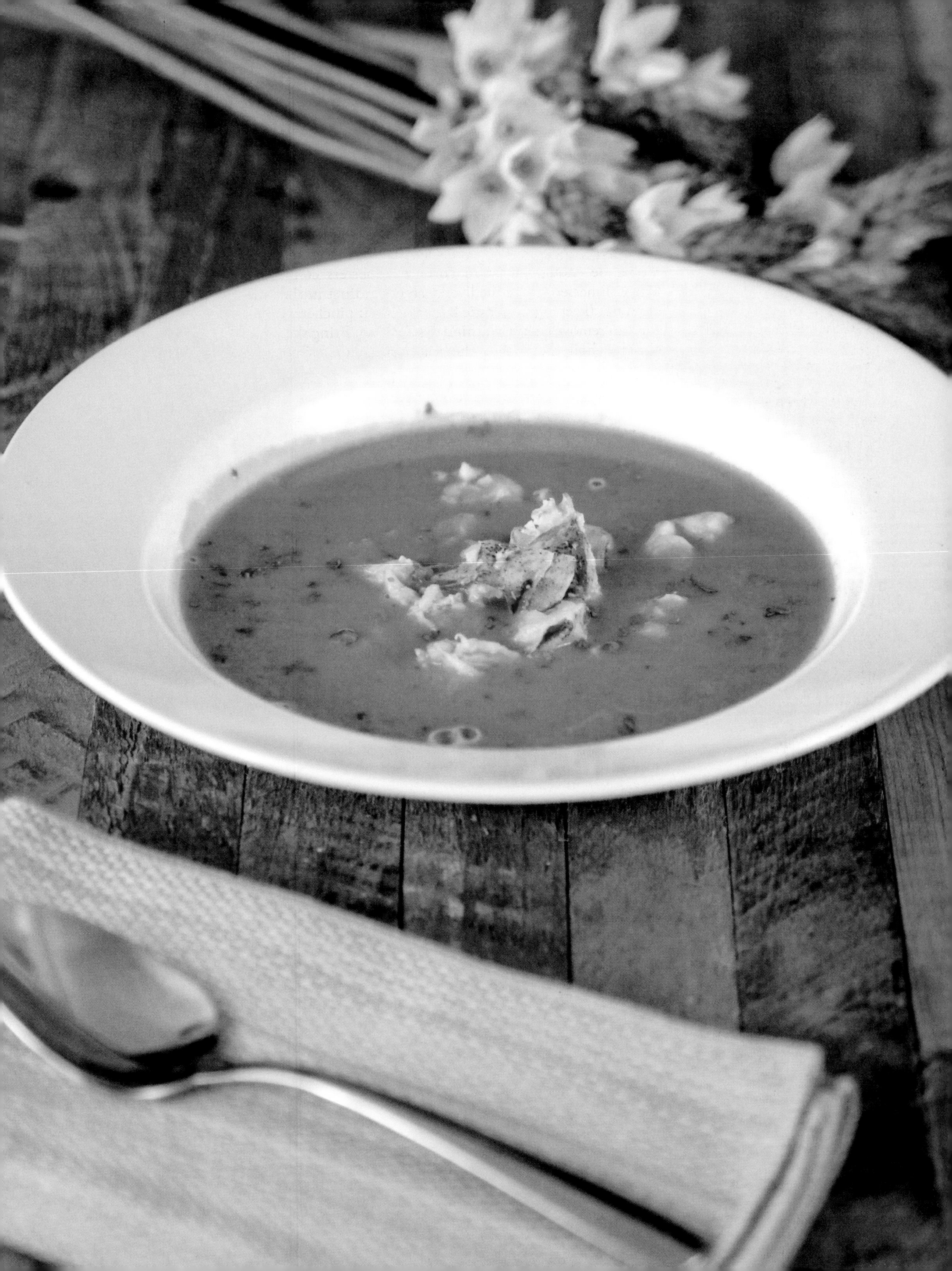

Garden Green Vichyssoise

Vichyssoise is a rich and creamy potato and leek soup (traditionally made with only the white part of the leek) that is usually served chilled. This potatoless green version is full of flavor, with the richness of avocado and the refreshing flavor of cilantro. Perfect for a hot summer's day!

PREP TIME: 20 minutes
COOK TIME: 30 to 35 minutes, plus 4 hours chilling time
SERVINGS: 6 to 8

INGREDIENTS:

- 4 cups Bone Broth (chicken, page 110)
- 1 head cauliflower, cored and cut into florets
- 3 leeks (green and white parts), chopped
- 2 cups packed fresh spinach (about 4 ounces)
- ½ teaspoon salt, plus more to taste
- ¼ cup lard, avocado oil, or olive oil
- 3 to 4 avocados, peeled, pitted, and finely chopped, for serving
- 6 to 8 tablespoons chopped fresh cilantro, for serving
- 6 to 8 tablespoons Coconut Milk Yogurt (page 118), for serving (optional)

1. Combine the broth, cauliflower, and leeks in a large pot. Cover and bring to a boil over high heat, then reduce the heat to maintain a simmer. Simmer for 25 to 30 minutes, until the vegetables are soft.
2. Add the spinach and simmer for 3 to 4 minutes, until the spinach has wilted. Remove from the heat and let cool.
3. Add the lard. Purée the soup with an immersion blender, or pour into a blender and process until smooth. Season with salt to taste.
4. Refrigerate the soup until cold, about 4 hours.
5. To serve, add half a chopped avocado and 1 tablespoon fresh cilantro to each bowl. Serve with a dollop of Coconut Milk Yogurt, if desired. Enjoy!

VARIATIONS:

You can also make this as a rich and comforting hot soup. Skip the avocado and cilantro and serve with crab meat, fresh parsley, and a drizzle of olive oil.

Because this soup embraces the color green, you can substitute broccoli or broccoflower for the cauliflower.

FODMAP ALERT

This recipe cannot be made low-FODMAP.

SPECIAL EQUIPMENT

- Blender or immersion blender

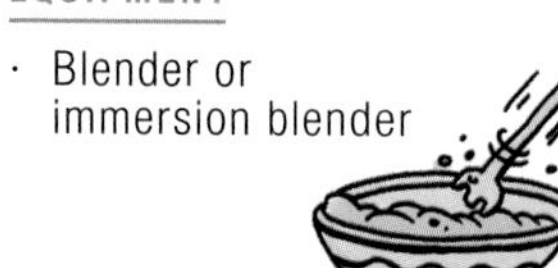

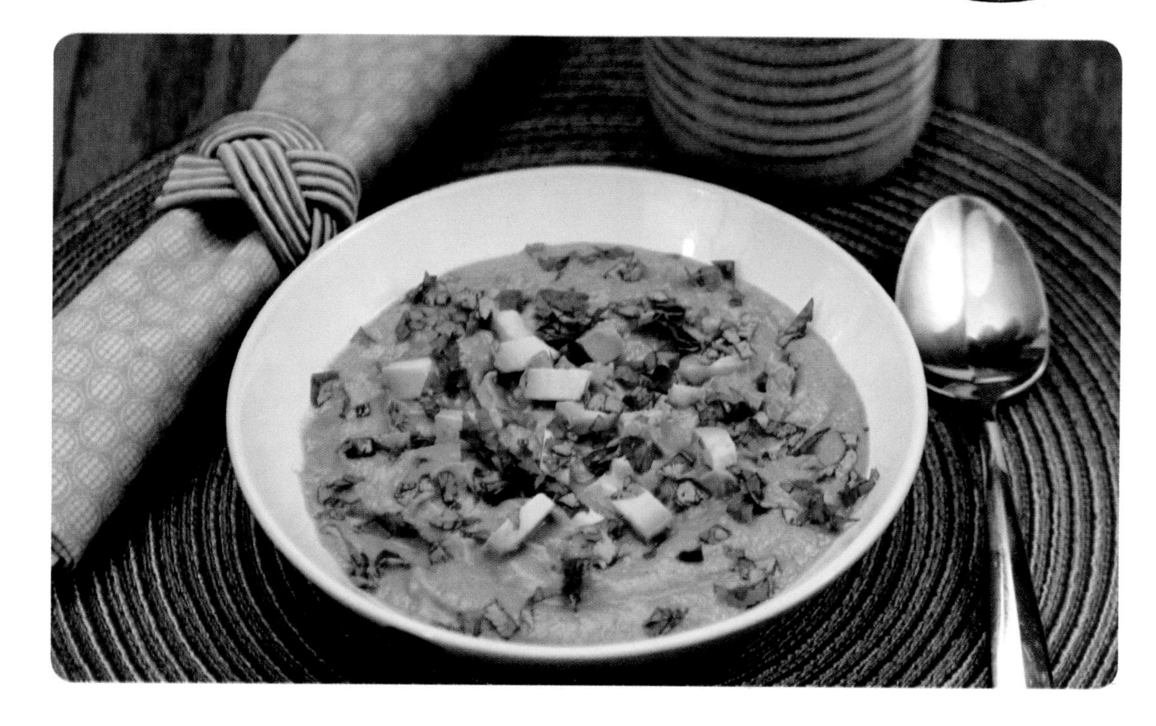

NUTRITION FACTS

Serving Size	360 g
Recipe Yields	2883 g
Calories	**242**
Fats	**18.5 g**
MUFA	9.2 g
Omega-3	0.22 g
Omega-6	2.49 g
Saturated Fat	4.82 g
Carbohydrates	**18.1 g**
Fiber	8.63 g
Starch	3.67 g
Fructose	1.01 g
Glucose	3.17 g
Sucrose	<0.01 g
Protein	**5.48 g**
Alanine	0.26 g
Arginine	0.21 g
Aspartic acid	0.5 g
Cystine	0.06 g
Glutamic acid	0.66 g
Glycine	0.22 g
Histidine	0.12 g
Isoleucine	0.19 g
Leucine	0.31 g
Lysine	0.37 g
Methionine	0.07 g
Phenylalanine	0.2 g
Proline	0.21 g
Serine	0.25 g
Threonine	0.18 g
Tryptophan	0.05 g
Tyrosine	0.12 g
Valine	0.26 g
Vitamins	
Vitamin B1	0.11 mg
Vitamin B12	0.02 mcg
Vitamin B2	0.2 mg
Vitamin B3	1.61 mg
Vitamin B5	1.61 mg
Vitamin B6	0.32 mg
Choline	41.7 mg
Folate	118 mcg
Vitamin A	73.3 mcg
Vitamin C	61.5 mg
Vitamin D	6.53 IU
Vitamin E	3.65 mg
Vitamin K	65.6 mcg
Minerals	
Calcium	60.8 mg
Copper	0.45 mg
Iron	1.88 mg
Magnesium	55 mg
Manganese	0.47 mg
Phosphorus	98.5 mg
Potassium	750 mg
Selenium	1.37 mcg
Sodium	563 mg
Zinc	0.83 mg

nutrition content estimated using the USDA database.

Carrot-Ginger Soup

This is one of those throw-everything-into-a-pot-and-purée-later soups, which I love because there is so little prep work.

PREP TIME: 5 to 10 minutes
COOK TIME: 40 minutes
SERVINGS: 3 to 4

INGREDIENTS:

- 6 cups Bone Broth (chicken, page 110)
- ¼ medium onion, roughly chopped
- 1 pound carrots, roughly chopped
- 1 thumb fresh ginger, peeled and sliced
- 1 (3-inch-long) piece fresh turmeric root, peeled and chopped
- Salt, to taste

FODMAP ALERT

Omit the onion.

SPECIAL EQUIPMENT

- Blender or immersion blender

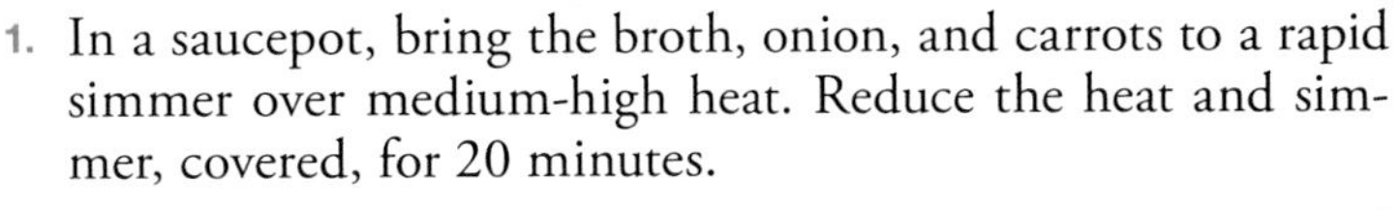

1. In a saucepot, bring the broth, onion, and carrots to a rapid simmer over medium-high heat. Reduce the heat and simmer, covered, for 20 minutes.
2. Add the ginger and turmeric and continue to simmer until the carrots are extremely soft, 15 to 20 additional minutes.
3. Blend the soup with an immersion blender until it is a smooth puree (you can also use a countertop model, being careful not to burn yourself). Serve!

TIPS:

If you can't find fresh turmeric root, you can use 2 teaspoons ground turmeric.

VARIATIONS:

Add ½ cup Coconut Cream (page 116) at the end to make a creamier soup.

Serve with a dollop of Coconut Milk Yogurt (page 118) and Bacon Bits (page 120).

This soup is also good chilled.

Winter Squash Soup. This soup is also very nice when made with butternut squash or pumpkin in place of the carrots.

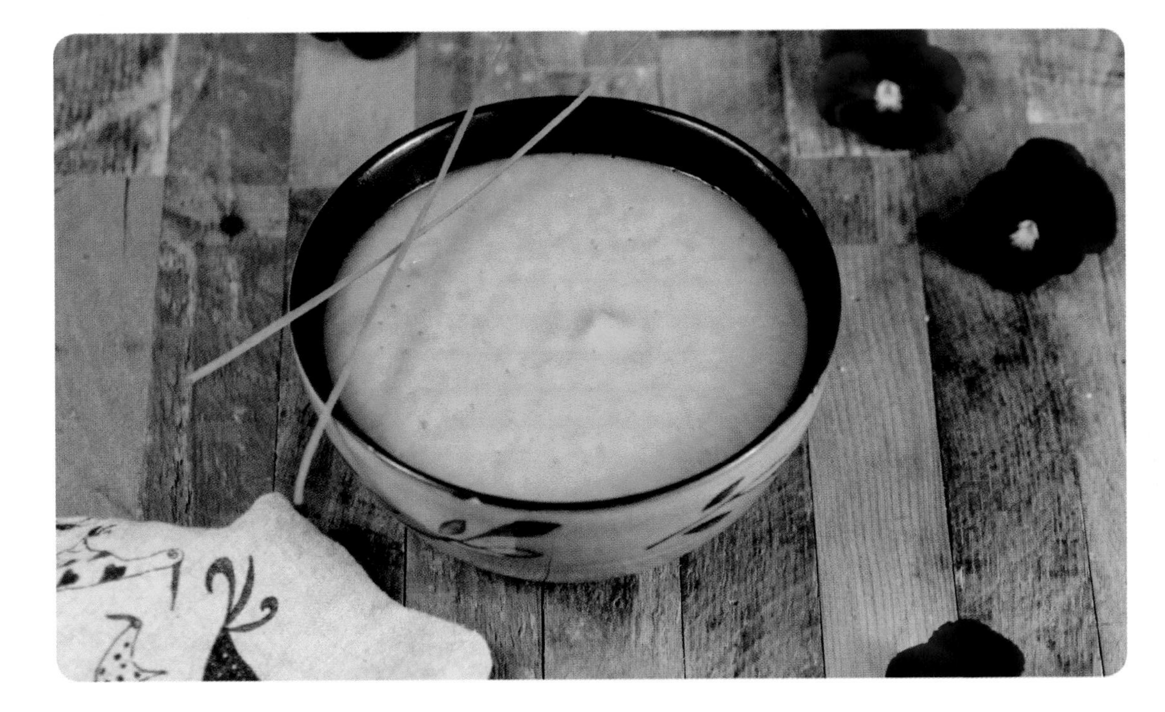

NUTRITION FACTS

Serving Size	484 g
Recipe Yields	1936 g
Calories	**111**
Fats	**2.52 g**
MUFA	1.02 g
Omega-3	0.05 g
Omega-6	0.56 g
Saturated Fat	0.71 g
Carbohydrates	**16.7 g**
Fiber	3.47 g
Starch	2.51 g
Fructose	0.72 g
Glucose	0.81 g
Sucrose	4.15 g
Protein	**8.43 g**
Alanine	0.13 g
Arginine	0.11 g
Aspartic acid	0.23 g
Cystine	0.09 g
Glutamic acid	0.44 g
Glycine	0.06 g
Histidine	0.05 g
Isoleucine	0.09 g
Leucine	0.12 g
Lysine	0.12 g
Methionine	0.02 g
Phenylalanine	0.07 g
Proline	0.06 g
Serine	0.06 g
Threonine	0.22 g
Tryptophan	0.01 g
Tyrosine	0.05 g
Valine	0.08 g
Vitamins	
Vitamin B1	0.08 mg
Vitamin B12	0.36 mcg
Vitamin B2	0.18 mg
Vitamin B3	6.11 mg
Vitamin B5	0.33 mg
Vitamin B6	0.21 mg
Choline	22.7 mg
Folate	23.4 mcg
Vitamin A	947 mcg
Vitamin C	7.5 mg
Vitamin D	0 IU
Vitamin E	0.78 mg
Vitamin K	15.1 mcg
Minerals	
Calcium	55 mg
Copper	0.25 mg
Iron	1.36 mg
Magnesium	20.3 mg
Manganese	0.22 mg
Phosphorus	152 mg
Potassium	709 mg
Selenium	0.19 mcg
Sodium	223 mg
Zinc	0.68 mg

nutrition content estimated using the USDA database.

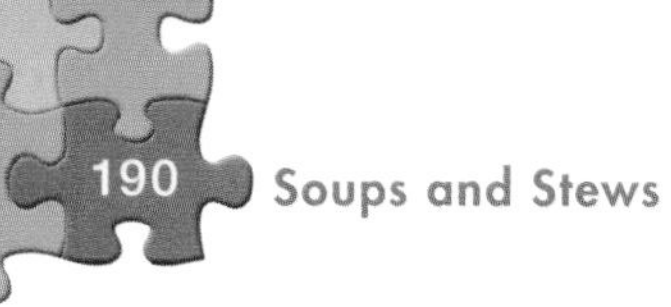

Seafood and Leek Soup

Somewhere between cioppino and potato leek soup, this soup is full of flavor and remarkably satisfying.

PREP TIME: 15 minutes
COOK TIME: 20 minutes
SERVINGS: 4

INGREDIENTS:

- 6 cups Bone Broth (fish, page 110)
- 2 pounds leeks, sliced (about 8 cups)
- 1 pound turnips, peeled and cubed
- 1 medium carrot, diced
- 12 to 14 ounces salmon fillets, cut into large chunks
- 1 pound mixed shellfish
- 2 cloves garlic, sliced
- 3 tablespoons chopped fresh oregano leaves
- 2 tablespoons chopped fresh parsley
- Salt, to taste

1. Bring the broth to a simmer in a stockpot over medium-high heat. Add the leeks, turnips, and carrot and simmer for 10 minutes.
2. Add the salmon chunks, shellfish, and garlic. Simmer for 10 more minutes, until the salmon and shellfish are fully cooked and opaque throughout. Stir in the oregano and parsley. Taste and add salt, if desired. Serve.

VARIATIONS:

You can use any mix of shellfish you like in this recipe and replace the salmon with your favorite oily fish or whitefish. You can also use chicken Bone Broth (page 110) in place of fish Bone Broth. Substitute rutabaga or radishes for the turnips.

If you have access to ramps, you can substitute ramps for the leeks.

FODMAP ALERT *Replace the garlic with green garlic or garlic scapes (green part only) or omit. Use only the green tops of the leeks.*

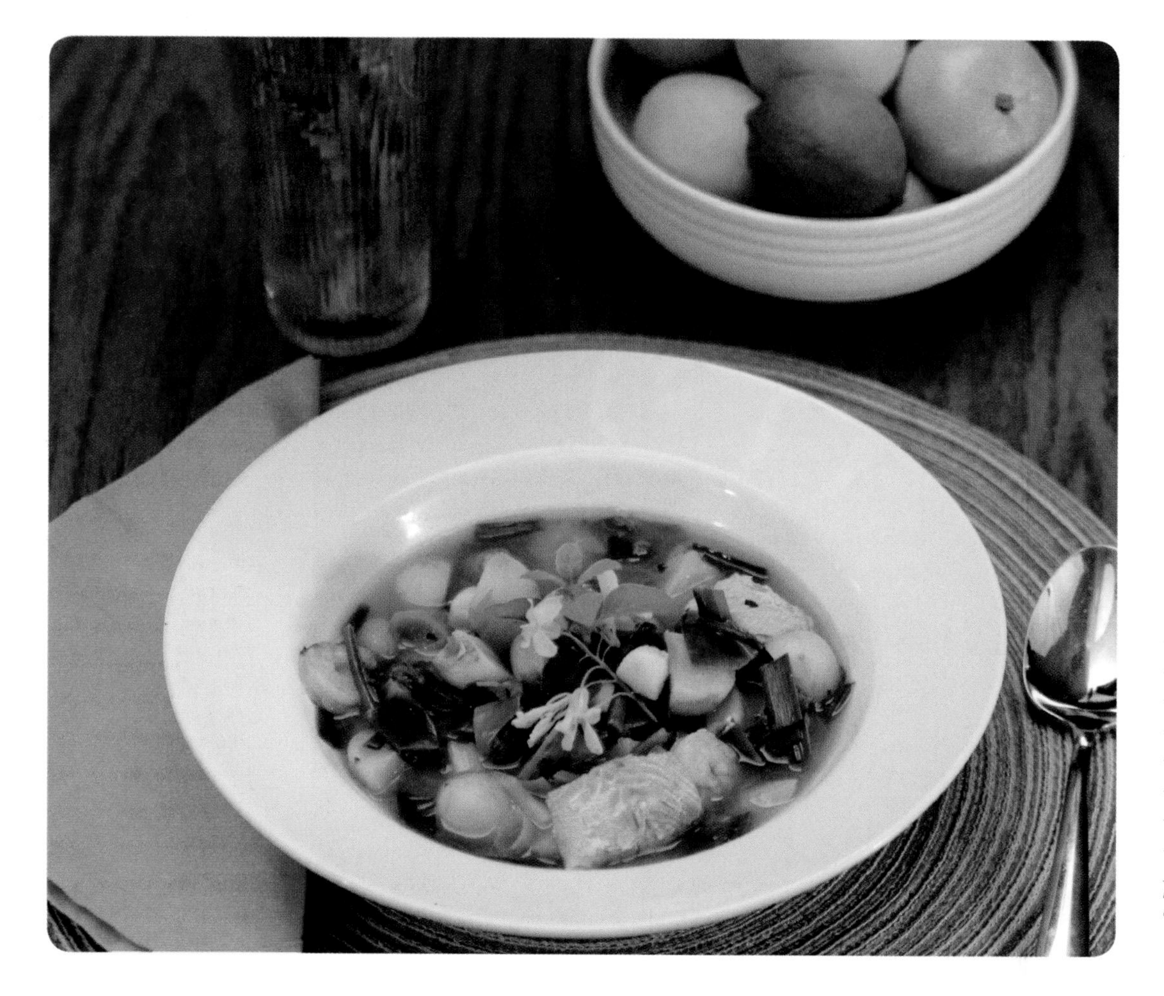

NUTRITION FACTS	
Serving Size	922 g
Recipe Yields	3687 g
Calories	**485**
Fats	**9.56 g**
MUFA	2.1 g
Omega-3	2.31 g
Omega-6	0.43 g
Saturated Fat	1.83 g
Carbohydrates	**43.5 g**
Fiber	7.75 g
Starch	20.3 g
Fructose	0.07 g
Glucose	0.09 g
Sucrose	0.33 g
Protein	**55.9 g**
Alanine	2.87 g
Arginine	3.55 g
Aspartic acid	5.44 g
Cystine	0.49 g
Glutamic acid	7.59 g
Glycine	2.88 g
Histidine	1.1 g
Isoleucine	2.26 g
Leucine	3.71 g
Lysine	4.04 g
Methionine	1.3 g
Phenylalanine	2 g
Proline	1.87 g
Serine	2.08 g
Threonine	2.22 g
Tryptophan	0.59 g
Tyrosine	1.64 g
Valine	2.39 g
Vitamins	
Vitamin B1	0.29 mg
Vitamin B12	5.71 mcg
Vitamin B2	0.37 mg
Vitamin B3	17.5 mg
Vitamin B5	1.68 mg
Vitamin B6	1.41 mg
Choline	256 mg
Folate	193 mcg
Vitamin A	397 mcg
Vitamin C	46.1 mg
Vitamin D	449 IU
Vitamin E	4.86 mg
Vitamin K	155 mcg
Minerals	
Calcium	392 mg
Copper	0.85 mg
Iron	9.86 mg
Magnesium	155 mg
Manganese	1.4 mg
Phosphorus	728 mg
Potassium	1579 mg
Selenium	80.5 mcg
Sodium	1481 mg
Zinc	2.55 mg

nutrition content estimated using the USDA database.

Oxtail and Pearl Onion Soup

This recipe is inspired by French onion soup, but it gets added flavor from the use of oxtail and skips the traditional bread and cheese.

PREP TIME: 15 to 20 minutes
COOK TIME: 4 hours
SERVINGS: 2 to 3

INGREDIENTS:

1 pound oxtail

5 to 6 cups water or Bone Broth (beef, page 110)

10 ounces white pearl onions

1 tablespoon melted tallow or avocado oil

Salt, to taste

FODMAP ALERT *Omit the onions and use a variety of other vegetables instead. Carrots and turnips are particularly good!*

1. Add the oxtail and enough water or broth to cover to a saucepot. Bring to a boil, then reduce the heat to maintain a simmer. Simmer covered for at least 3 to 4 hours, until the meat is falling off the bone. Check periodically and top up with more liquid if necessary to keep the oxtail bones covered.
2. Meanwhile, preheat the oven to 425°F.
3. Peel the onions and toss with the tallow. Place on a rimmed baking sheet and roast for 30 minutes, stirring at both the 20-minute mark and the 25-minute mark.
4. Remove the bones and meat from the saucepot using a slotted spoon or sieve. Save the bones for making bone broth (there's a lot of goodness left in them!). Give the meat a rough chop and add it back to the broth. Add the onions to the broth. Taste the broth and season with salt, if desired.

TIPS:

This soup doubles or triples easily and freezes very well.

VARIATIONS:

You can use regular onions for this soup, cut into half moons and sautéed with fat in a skillet until caramelized.

This soup is also delicious with chunks of roasted turnip, parsnip, plantain, or sweet potato added. Mushrooms are another great addition.

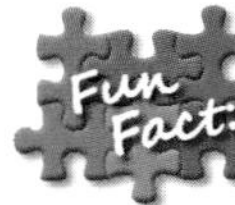

The smaller the onion, the greater its concentration of phytonutrients. Two small onions offer more nutrients than one large onion.

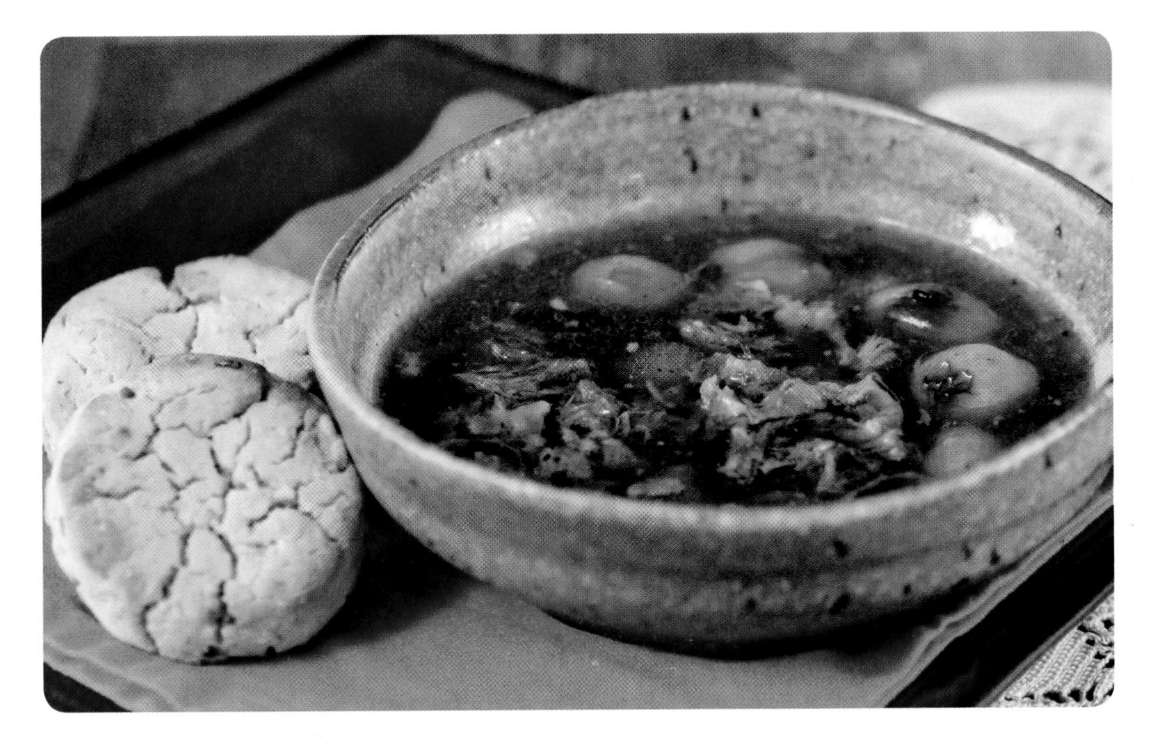

NUTRITION FACTS

Serving Size	650 g
Recipe Yields	1951 g
Calories	**523**
Fats	**30 g**
MUFA	14.1 g
Omega-3	0.29 g
Omega-6	1.74 g
Saturated Fat	10.3 g
Carbohydrates	**14.4 g**
Fiber	1.32 g
Starch	0 g
Fructose	1.36 g
Glucose	2.07 g
Sucrose	1.04 g
Protein	**49.7 g**
Alanine	2.46 g
Arginine	2.75 g
Aspartic acid	3.7 g
Cystine	0.54 g
Glutamic acid	6.19 g
Glycine	2.48 g
Histidine	1.29 g
Isoleucine	1.86 g
Leucine	3.22 g
Lysine	3.43 g
Methionine	1.05 g
Phenylalanine	1.61 g
Proline	1.94 g
Serine	1.61 g
Threonine	1.62 g
Tryptophan	0.28 g
Tyrosine	1.3 g
Valine	2.01 g
Vitamins	
Vitamin B1	0.16 mg
Vitamin B12	2.49 mcg
Vitamin B2	0.35 mg
Vitamin B3	16.2 mg
Vitamin B5	0.9 mg
Vitamin B6	1.05 mg
Choline	173 mg
Folate	26.3 mcg
Vitamin A	0.08 mcg
Vitamin C	4.91 mg
Vitamin D	42.3 IU
Vitamin E	1.26 mg
Vitamin K	7.04 mcg
Minerals	
Calcium	70.1 mg
Copper	0.38 mg
Iron	3.53 mg
Magnesium	49.2 mg
Manganese	0.16 mg
Phosphorus	475 mg
Potassium	1014 mg
Selenium	44.1 mcg
Sodium	257 mg
Zinc	7.93 mg

nutrition content estimated using the USDA database.

Beef Heart Borscht

Borscht is a richly flavored soup packed with nutrient-dense foods. It is traditionally served with sour cream, but coconut milk yogurt makes a delightful accompaniment to this comforting meal.

PREP TIME: 15 minutes
COOK TIME: 1 hour
SERVINGS: 3 to 4

INGREDIENTS:

- 2 to 3 tablespoons tallow or other cooking fat
- 1 pound beef heart, trimmed and cut into small pieces
- 1 medium onion, quartered and sliced
- 3 large beets
- 3 medium carrots
- 2 stalks celery
- 4 cups Bone Broth (beef, page 110)
- 2 cups thinly sliced cabbage
- ½ cup chopped fresh dill
- 1 tablespoon fresh lemon juice
- 2 tablespoons balsamic vinegar
- ½ teaspoon salt, plus more to taste
- ½ cup Coconut Milk Yogurt (page 118)

FODMAP ALERT

This recipe cannot be made low-FODMAP.

1. Heat 2 tablespoons of the tallow in a large saucepan or stockpot over medium-high heat. Add the beef heart and brown, 3 to 4 minutes.
2. Add the onion, beets, carrots, and celery. Add a little more tallow if they are sticking to the pan. Cook until the onion is starting to caramelize, 8 to 10 minutes.
3. Add the broth. Reduce the heat to a simmer and cover. Simmer for 30 minutes.
4. Add the cabbage and stir. Cover and simmer for 15 more minutes.
5. Add the dill, lemon juice, vinegar, and salt. Cook for 1 to 2 minutes. Taste and add more salt, if desired. Serve with coconut milk yogurt.

VARIATIONS:

You don't have to use beef heart for this stew; use beef if you prefer.

NUTRITION FACTS	
Serving Size	594 g
Recipe Yields	2376 g
Calories	**394**
Fats	**18.8 g**
MUFA	4.35 g
Omega-3	0.07 g
Omega-6	1.22 g
Saturated Fat	10.6 g
Carbohydrates	**18.2 g**
Fiber	4.59 g
Starch	1.77 g
Fructose	2.47 g
Glucose	2.99 g
Sucrose	1.25 g
Protein	**38.2 g**
Alanine	0.15 g
Arginine	0.25 g
Aspartic acid	0.32 g
Cystine	0.05 g
Glutamic acid	0.74 g
Glycine	0.13 g
Histidine	0.06 g
Isoleucine	0.1 g
Leucine	0.15 g
Lysine	0.14 g
Methionine	0.04 g
Phenylalanine	0.11 g
Proline	0.13 g
Serine	0.13 g
Threonine	0.13 g
Tryptophan	0.03 g
Tyrosine	0.07 g
Valine	0.13 g
Vitamins	
Vitamin B1	0.22 mg
Vitamin B12	12.4 mcg
Vitamin B2	1.51 mg
Vitamin B3	10.3 mg
Vitamin B5	2.28 mg
Vitamin B6	0.53 mg
Choline	298 mg
Folate	85.9 mcg
Vitamin A	307 mcg
Vitamin C	37.1 mg
Vitamin D	5.19 IU
Vitamin E	1.09 mg
Vitamin K	94.1 mcg
Minerals	
Calcium	97.2 mg
Copper	0.78 mg
Iron	9.64 mg
Magnesium	68.5 mg
Manganese	0.71 mg
Phosphorus	410 mg
Potassium	909 mg
Selenium	48.8 mcg
Sodium	1168 mg
Zinc	3.87 mg

nutrition content estimated using the USDA database.

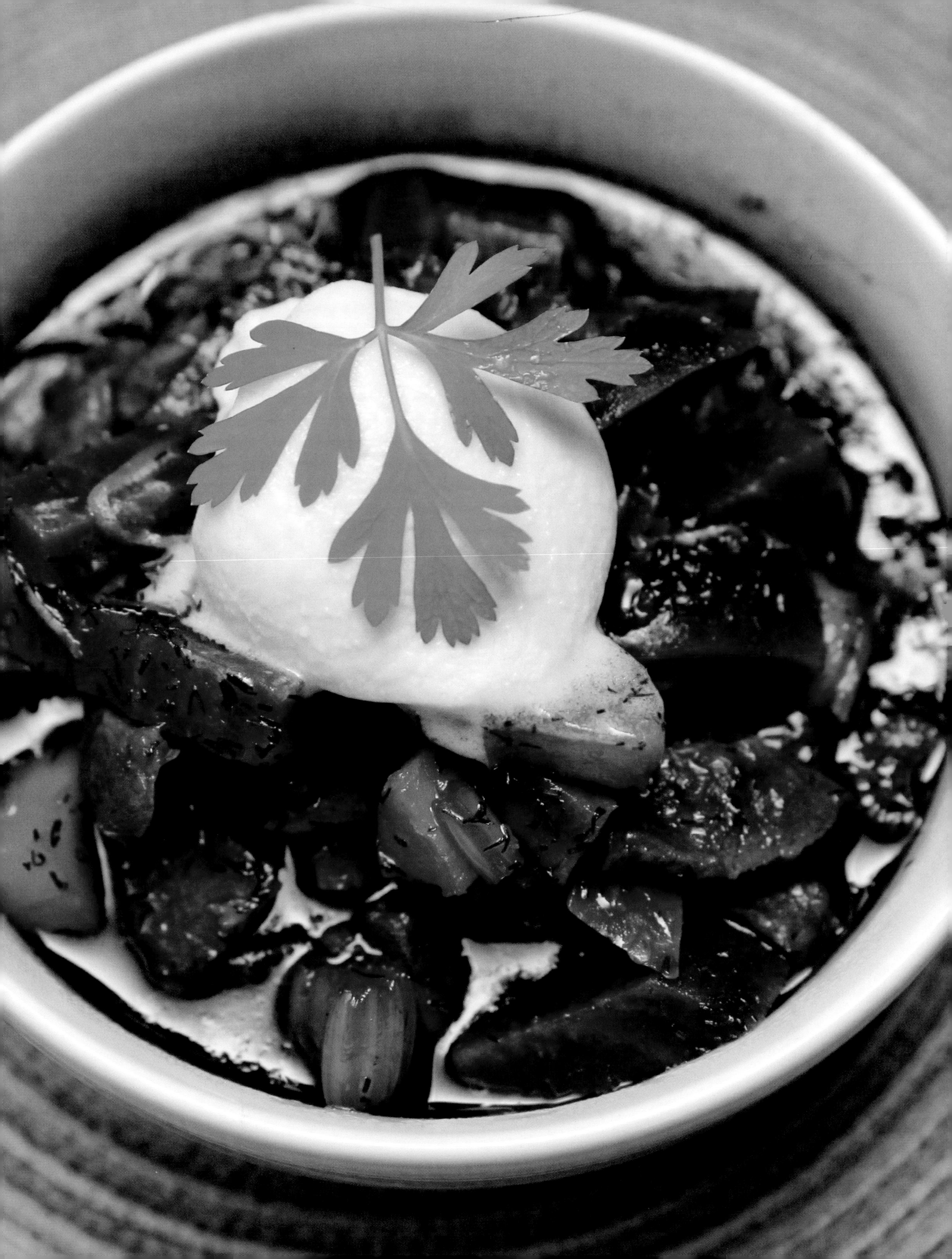

Vegetable Soup with Chicken Sausage

This simple vegetable soup has tons of flavor on its own but becomes even more wonderful when you add some Apple Chicken Sausage to it. You can slice parboiled sausage or a precooked sausage patty. If you're making sausage just for this soup, double or triple the soup recipe, and shape your sausage into meatballs instead of patties before baking.

PREP TIME: 10 minutes
COOK TIME: 20 minutes
SERVINGS: 3 to 4

INGREDIENTS:

- 4 cups Bone Broth (chicken or pork, page 110)
- 1 cup sliced leeks
- 1½ cups sliced carrots
- ½ cup diced turnip
- ½ cup diced kohlrabi
- 1½ cups chopped carrot greens
- ¼ to ½ recipe Apple Chicken Sausage (page 132; optional)
- ¼ teaspoon salt, plus more to taste

FODMAP ALERT *Use only the green parts of the leeks. Substitute a different variety of sausage, or use leftover chicken, pork, or beef instead.*

1. Bring the broth, leeks, carrots, turnip, and kohlrabi to a simmer in a large saucepan over medium-high heat. Cook until the vegetables are cooked al dente, about 15 minutes (depending on how large your vegetable pieces are).
2. Add the carrot greens and precooked sausage, if using, and cook for 3 to 4 more minutes. Season with salt to taste.

VARIATIONS:

You can really play with different vegetables in this soup. You can use all turnip or all kohlrabi or use rutabaga or radishes instead. Celery and onion are welcome additions. You can add fresh spinach instead of or in addition to carrot greens. Chopped fresh parsley adds a lovely flavor to this soup (add it with or instead of the carrot greens).

Another option is to add diced leftover roasted chicken, pork, beef, or lamb instead of sausage.

Italian Wedding Soup. Make meatballs with the Sweet Italian Sausage meat mixture (page 132) and bake at 400°F for 15 minutes. Use these instead of Apple Chicken Sausage. Replace the carrot greens with parsley. Season with truffle salt instead of regular salt.

Chicken Noodle Soup. Omit the carrot greens and sausage. Boil sweet potato noodles in water for 5 minutes. Drain and add to the soup. Also add cubes of leftover chicken.

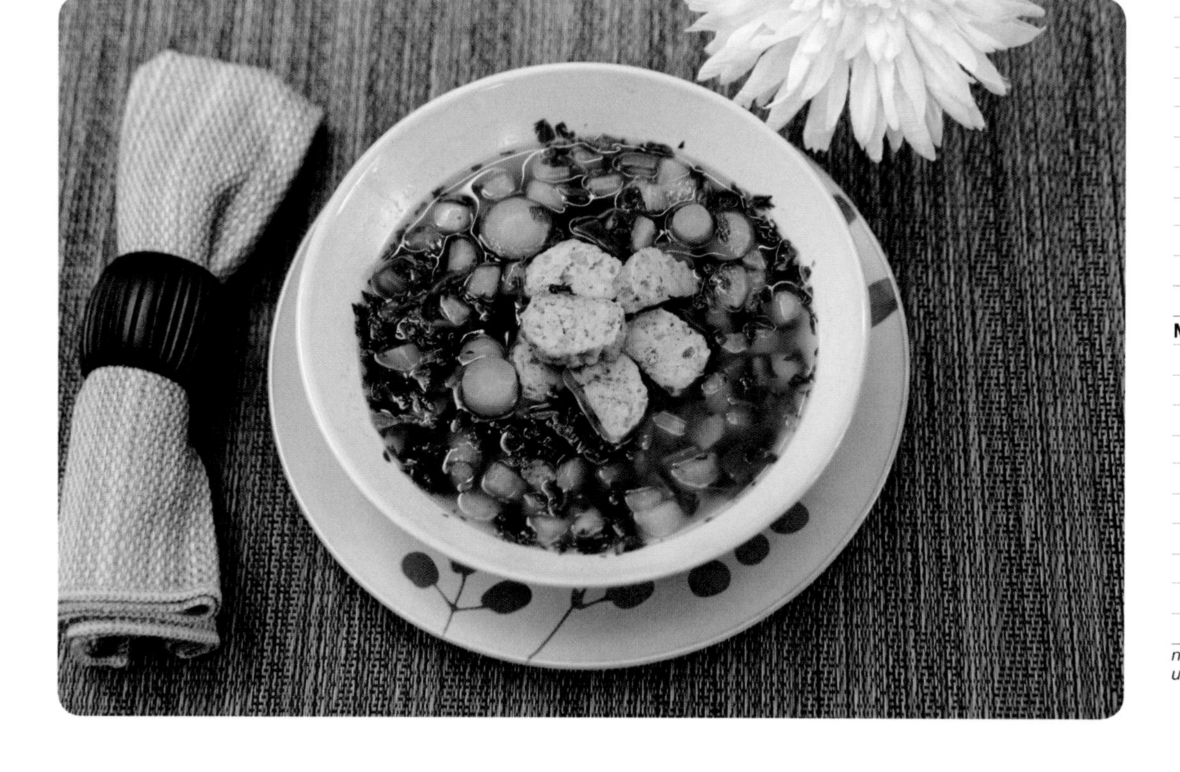

NUTRITION FACTS	
Serving Size	544 g
Recipe Yields	2177 g
Calories	**300**
Fats	**14.1 g**
MUFA	5.96 g
Omega-3	0.21 g
Omega-6	2.26 g
Saturated Fat	3.94 g
Carbohydrates	**16.4 g**
Fiber	4.16 g
Starch	2.82 g
Fructose	2 g
Glucose	1.15 g
Sucrose	2.22 g
Protein	**29.7 g**
Alanine	1.6 g
Arginine	1.82 g
Aspartic acid	2.62 g
Cystine	0.34 g
Glutamic acid	4.24 g
Glycine	1.33 g
Histidine	0.84 g
Isoleucine	1.29 g
Leucine	2.18 g
Lysine	2.39 g
Methionine	0.7 g
Phenylalanine	1.11 g
Proline	1.06 g
Serine	1.17 g
Threonine	1.24 g
Tryptophan	0.24 g
Tyrosine	0.96 g
Valine	1.33 g
Vitamins	
Vitamin B1	0.27 mg
Vitamin B12	0.63 mcg
Vitamin B2	0.56 mg
Vitamin B3	9.35 mg
Vitamin B5	1.82 mg
Vitamin B6	0.85 mg
Choline	80.9 mg
Folate	64.7 mcg
Vitamin A	634 mcg
Vitamin C	31.9 mg
Vitamin D	0.82 IU
Vitamin E	2.05 mg
Vitamin K	87.9 mcg
Minerals	
Calcium	105 mg
Copper	0.25 mg
Iron	3.26 mg
Magnesium	59 mg
Manganese	0.38 mg
Phosphorus	326 mg
Potassium	1190 mg
Selenium	18.2 mcg
Sodium	1222 mg
Zinc	2.66 mg

nutrition content estimated using the USDA database.

Asian-Inspired Noodle Soup

This simple soup is a great way to get some seaweed into your diet. Try this basic version, which is similar to a Japanese dashi, or get creative with any number of add-ons!

PREP TIME: 5 minutes
COOK TIME: 25 minutes
SERVINGS: 4

INGREDIENTS:

- 4 to 5 cups water
- 2 (4-inch) pieces kombu
- 1 cup loosely packed bonito flakes
- 2 tablespoons coconut aminos (optional)
- 1 tablespoon coconut water vinegar (optional)
- 6 ounces sweet potato noodles (dangmyeon)
- 7 ounces wakame noodles

FODMAP ALERT *Skip the sweet potato noodles and replace with a low-FODMAP alternative like kelp noodles.*

1. Combine the water, kombu, and bonito flakes in a stockpot or saucepot. Bring to a boil over high heat, then reduce the heat to maintain a simmer for 20 minutes.
2. Strain and discard the kombu and bonito flakes. Add the coconut aminos and coconut water vinegar, if using.
3. Meanwhile, bring a pot of water to a boil. Add the sweet potato noodles and simmer uncovered for 5 minutes. Drain.
4. Rinse the wakame noodles.
5. Add the wakame noodles and sweet potato noodles to the soup and serve.

TIPS:

You can find the ingredients for this dish in many specialty and ethnic grocery stores or order them online.

Wakame noodles tend to lose their texture if heated for too long. If you don't plan to eat all of this soup immediately, add some wakame noodles directly to your bowl before serving and keep the rest in the fridge until you're ready for more soup.

VARIATIONS:

Instead of sweet potato noodles and wakame noodles, try kelp noodles, spiral-cut veggies, or broccoli slaw. Any seafood and/or leftover meat plus wild mushrooms (shiitake, oyster mushrooms, forest mushrooms, etc.), baby bok choy, sui choy, broccoli rabe, arame, and/or wakame are great additions to this soup.

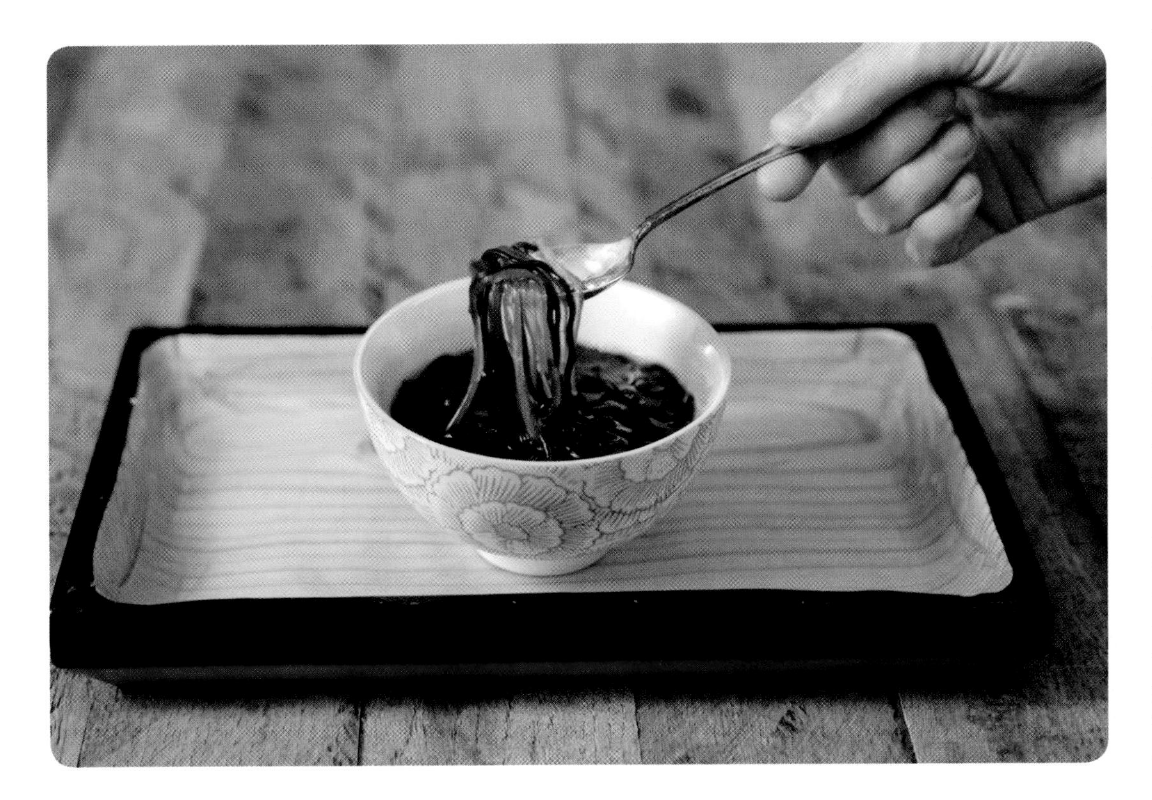

NUTRITION FACTS	
Serving Size	337 g
Recipe Yields	1349 g
Calories	**71**
Fats	**0.37 g**
MUFA	0.03 g
Omega-3	0.09 g
Omega-6	0.02 g
Saturated Fat	0.08 g
Carbohydrates	**13.6 g**
Fiber	1.59 g
Starch	5.76 g
Fructose	0.3 g
Glucose	0.65 g
Sucrose	1.07 g
Protein	**4.25 g**
Alanine	0.11 g
Arginine	0.07 g
Aspartic acid	0.26 g
Cystine	0.03 g
Glutamic acid	0.18 g
Glycine	0.09 g
Histidine	0.02 g
Isoleucine	0.07 g
Leucine	0.17 g
Lysine	0.09 g
Methionine	0.04 g
Phenylalanine	0.1 g
Proline	0.07 g
Serine	0.08 g
Threonine	0.12 g
Tryptophan	0.03 g
Tyrosine	0.04 g
Valine	0.14 g
Vitamins	
Vitamin B1	0.07 mg
Vitamin B12	0 mcg
Vitamin B2	0.15 mg
Vitamin B3	1.05 mg
Vitamin B5	0.72 mg
Vitamin B6	0.09 mg
Choline	12.8 mg
Folate	111 mcg
Vitamin A	311 mcg
Vitamin C	2.66 mg
Vitamin D	0 IU
Vitamin E	0.65 mg
Vitamin K	6.69 mcg
Minerals	
Calcium	103 mg
Copper	0.24 mg
Iron	1.48 mg
Magnesium	72.1 mg
Manganese	0.81 mg
Phosphorus	61.8 mg
Potassium	198 mg
Selenium	0.64 mcg
Sodium	485 mg
Zinc	0.4 mg

nutrition content estimated using the USDA database.

New England Clam Chowder

All the thick creaminess of this soup comes from green plantain and coconut cream. You'll be amazed that no dairy, potato, or flour is used to achieve one of the thickest, creamiest, most delicious clam chowders you will ever eat!

PREP TIME: 20 minutes
COOK TIME: 35 minutes
SERVINGS: 6

INGREDIENTS:

- 4 thick slices bacon, chopped
- 1 onion, diced
- 2 to 3 stalks celery, thinly sliced
- 1 large carrot, diced
- 1 large turnip, cut into ¾-inch cubes
- 3 cups Bone Broth (chicken, pork, or fish, page 110)
- 3 (5- to 6-ounce) cans clams, drained
- 1 green plantain, peeled and grated
- 2 bay leaves
- Leaves from 4 to 5 sprigs fresh thyme
- 2 cups Coconut Cream (page 116)
- 3 tablespoons chopped fresh parsley
- Salt or truffle salt, to taste

FODMAP ALERT *Omit the onion or replace with leek (green part only). While coconut cream is not as high in fructans as whole coconut products, it may cause a problem for some people.*

1. Add the chopped bacon to a medium stockpot, then turn on the heat to medium-high. Cook, stirring occasionally, until the bacon is crisp.
2. Add the onion, celery, carrot, and turnip to the pot. Cook until fragrant, stirring occasionally, about 5 minutes.
3. Add the broth, clams, grated plantain, bay leaves, and thyme. Bring to a boil, then reduce the heat to maintain a simmer for 20 minutes. Stir occasionally.
4. Add the coconut cream and parsley. Taste and season with salt or truffle salt, if desired. Cook for 1 to 2 more minutes and serve.

VARIATIONS:

Add 1 to 2 tablespoons peeled and grated fresh horseradish for some bite.

Try adding copious amounts of smoked salmon or chunks of any fish you like.

Add 1 to 2 sliced green onions and some chopped fresh dill or tarragon with or instead of the parsley.

Use smoked clams for an extra dimension of flavor.

NUTRITION FACTS	
Serving Size	386 g
Recipe Yields	2314 g
Calories	**343**
Fats	**22.6 g**
MUFA	1.98 g
Omega-3	0.13 g
Omega-6	0.52 g
Saturated Fat	17.9 g
Carbohydrates	**22.6 g**
Fiber	4 g
Starch	6.41 g
Fructose	0.36 g
Glucose	0.49 g
Sucrose	0.56 g
Protein	**16.1 g**
Alanine	0.89 g
Arginine	1.36 g
Aspartic acid	1.61 g
Cystine	0.2 g
Glutamic acid	2.47 g
Glycine	0.71 g
Histidine	0.36 g
Isoleucine	0.69 g
Leucine	1.19 g
Lysine	1.09 g
Methionine	0.39 g
Phenylalanine	0.6 g
Proline	0.57 g
Serine	0.69 g
Threonine	0.69 g
Tryptophan	0.2 g
Tyrosine	0.56 g
Valine	0.78 g
Vitamins	
Vitamin B1	0.12 mg
Vitamin B12	8.08 mcg
Vitamin B2	0.16 mg
Vitamin B3	2.23 mg
Vitamin B5	0.54 mg
Vitamin B6	0.22 mg
Choline	71.1 mg
Folate	41.3 mcg
Vitamin A	179 mcg
Vitamin C	20 mg
Vitamin D	0.71 IU
Vitamin E	0.84 mg
Vitamin K	37 mcg
Minerals	
Calcium	75.7 mg
Copper	0.35 mg
Iron	3.42 mg
Magnesium	66.9 mg
Manganese	0.94 mg
Phosphorus	285 mg
Potassium	612 mg
Selenium	31.2 mcg
Sodium	1082 mg
Zinc	1.4 mg

nutrition content estimated using the USDA database.

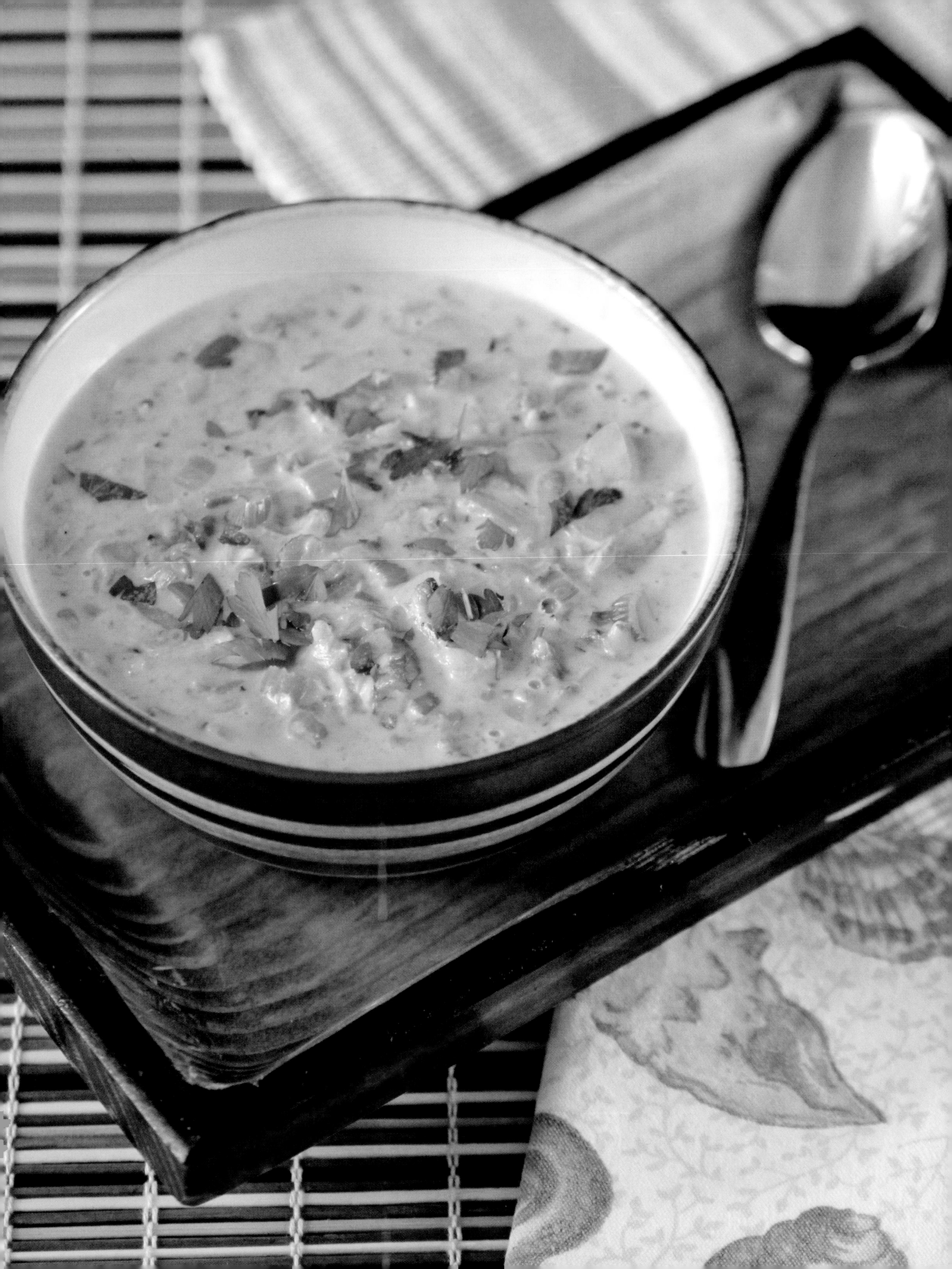

Beef Cheek and Daikon Radish Stew

One of the wonderful things about beef cheek is that it is so rich that it makes its own broth. When slowly simmered, this richly flavored meat melts in your mouth.

PREP TIME: 10 to 20 minutes
COOK TIME: 2 to 2¼ hours
SERVINGS: 5 to 8

INGREDIENTS:

- 2 tablespoons tallow
- 2 medium onions, cut into thick wedges
- 8 to 10 cloves garlic, sliced
- 4 medium carrots
- 4 stalks celery
- 2 pounds daikon radish, cut into 1-inch cubes (about 6 cups)
- 2½ pounds beef cheek, cut into 1-inch cubes
- 4 cups boiling water
- 4 or 5 sprigs fresh thyme
- 1 sprig fresh rosemary
- 1 bay leaf
- 1 tablespoon apple cider vinegar
- 1 teaspoon salt, or to taste
- ¼ cup arrowroot powder
- ⅓ cup cold water

FODMAP ALERT *Replace the garlic with green garlic or garlic scapes (green part only) or omit. Replace the onion with green onion or leek (green part only) or chives or omit.*

1. Heat the tallow in a large saucepot or stockpot over medium-high heat. Add the onions and cook until they start to caramelize, 7 to 10 minutes.
2. Add the garlic, carrots, celery, daikon, and cheek to the pot and pour the boiling water over the top. Add the thyme, rosemary, bay leaf, vinegar, and salt. Stir to combine.
3. Reduce the heat to a simmer. Cover and cook for 1½ to 2 hours, stirring very occasionally, until the meat is tender.
4. Mix the arrowroot powder with the cold water. Pour into the pot and stir to incorporate. Simmer uncovered for 4 to 5 more minutes, until the broth has thickened.

VARIATIONS:

This stew is also very good with some chopped kale or fresh spinach added toward the end of the cooking time (the last 7 to 8 minutes for kale or the last 2 to 3 minutes for spinach).

Basic Stew. *You can use beef, bison, lamb, or goat stew meat in place of cheek in this recipe to make a more basic stew. If using stew meat, replace the hot water with hot beef Bone Broth (page 110). Use turnips or rutabaga in place of daikon radish. Another option is to add chunks of peeled green plantain (either instead of or in addition to the daikon radish), but add it only for the last 20 to 25 minutes of cooking.*

NUTRITION FACTS	
Serving Size	468 g
Recipe Yields	3743 g
Calories	**432**
Fats	**25.4 g**
MUFA	12 g
Omega-3	0.12 g
Omega-6	0.68 g
Saturated Fat	10.5 g
Carbohydrates	**13.8 g**
Fiber	3.58 g
Starch	1.88 g
Fructose	0.57 g
Glucose	0.77 g
Sucrose	0.92 g
Protein	**35.5 g**
Alanine	2.32 g
Arginine	2.44 g
Aspartic acid	3.19 g
Cystine	0.35 g
Glutamic acid	5.31 g
Glycine	2.85 g
Histidine	1.08 g
Isoleucine	1.58 g
Leucine	2.72 g
Lysine	2.85 g
Methionine	0.84 g
Phenylalanine	1.41 g
Proline	2.06 g
Serine	1.47 g
Threonine	1.34 g
Tryptophan	0.13 g
Tyrosine	1.03 g
Valine	1.74 g
Vitamins	
Vitamin B1	0.11 mg
Vitamin B12	3.49 mcg
Vitamin B2	0.3 mg
Vitamin B3	6.16 mg
Vitamin B5	1.03 mg
Vitamin B6	0.61 mg
Choline	130 mg
Folate	44.8 mcg
Vitamin A	202 mcg
Vitamin C	22.8 mg
Vitamin D	0.9 IU
Vitamin E	1.02 mg
Vitamin K	14.9 mcg
Minerals	
Calcium	98.7 mg
Copper	0.26 mg
Iron	4.54 mg
Magnesium	43.5 mg
Manganese	0.23 mg
Phosphorus	288 mg
Potassium	835 mg
Selenium	28.8 mcg
Sodium	279 mg
Zinc	8.6 mg

nutrition content estimated using the USDA database.

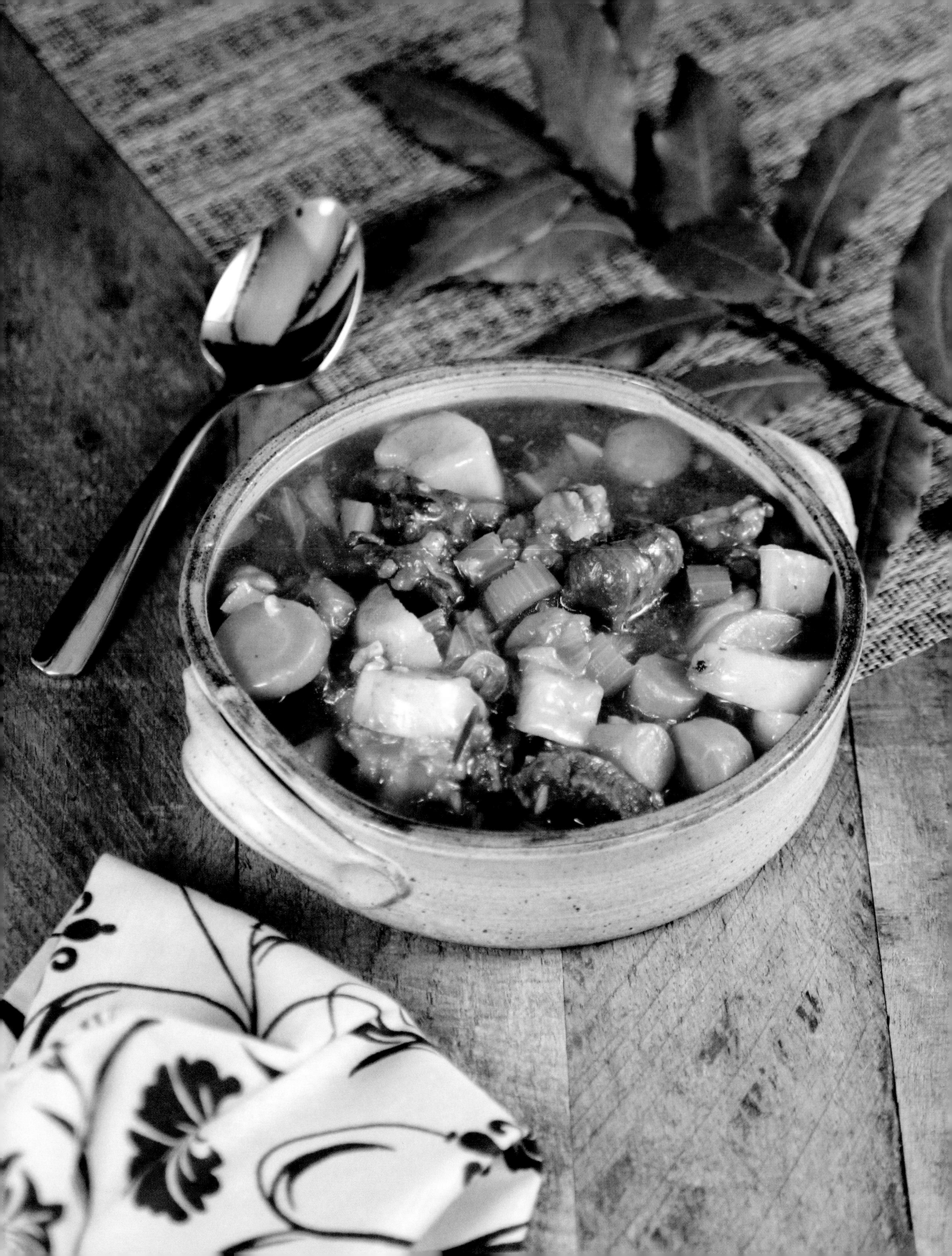

Rabbit and Wild Mushroom Stew

This rustic French-inspired stew uses traditional French techniques and a layering of flavors to achieve a truly remarkable result.

PREP TIME: 30 minutes
COOK TIME: 3 hours
SERVINGS: 4 to 8

INGREDIENTS:

- 2 heads garlic
- 1 tablespoon avocado oil
- 1 whole (2½- to 3-pound) rabbit, including giblets, cut into parts
- 3 to 4 tablespoons duck fat or lard
- 1 onion, diced
- 1 pound wild mushrooms
- 1½ teaspoons fresh thyme leaves (12 to 14 sprigs)
- 4 cups Bone Broth (chicken, page 110), divided
- 1 cup dry white wine, dry sherry, cognac, or broth
- 1 teaspoon salt, plus more to taste
- 3 tablespoons chopped fresh parsley
- 1½ teaspoons chopped fresh tarragon leaves

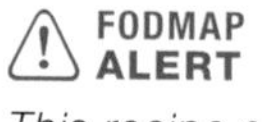

This recipe cannot be made low-FODMAP.

1. Preheat the oven to 375°F. Slice off the tops of the heads of garlic (but leave the heads whole) to expose the individual cloves. Drizzle with the avocado oil. Wrap loosely in aluminum foil and bake for 45 minutes to 1 hour. Let cool.
2. Once cool, squeeze the soft roasted garlic out of the peels and set aside.
3. Pat the rabbit dry. Reserve the liver (put it in the fridge for now). Heat 2 tablespoons of the duck fat in a medium stockpot over medium-high heat. Brown the rabbit pieces and giblets (other than the reserved liver) in batches for 3 to 4 minutes per side, adding more fat as needed to prevent the rabbit from sticking to the pan. Remove the browned pieces and set aside.
4. Add the onion to the stockpot and cook, stirring frequently, for 5 minutes. Add the mushrooms, roasted garlic, thyme, 3½ cups of the chicken broth (reserving ½ cup), wine, and browned rabbit pieces.
5. Bring to a boil, then reduce the heat to maintain a simmer for 1 hour and 30 minutes, stirring occasionally. Taste and add salt, if desired.
6. In a blender, purée the reserved liver with the reserved ½ cup of broth on high speed until completely smooth. Add the puréed liver, parsley, and tarragon to the stew. Stir and cook for 2 to 3 more minutes. Taste one final time and adjust the seasoning, if needed. Serve.

TIPS:

If the rabbit does not come with giblets, you can use 2 chicken livers to thicken the stew instead.

VARIATIONS:

Classically, crème fraîche would be added to this stew at the very end of cooking. If desired, you can add ¼ cup Coconut Milk Yogurt (page 118) right before serving.

This stew can also be made with a stewing hen or guinea fowl.

Roasted Garlic. Roasted garlic is a delicious accompaniment to just about any meat dish. Simply follow step 1 and serve warm out of the oven.

NUTRITION FACTS

Serving Size	376 g
Recipe Yields	3006 g
Calories	**356**
Fats	**12 g**
MUFA	4.78 g
Omega-3	0.27 g
Omega-6	1.58 g
Saturated Fat	3.63 g
Carbohydrates	**4.88 g**
Fiber	0.89 g
Starch	0.88 g
Fructose	0.27 g
Glucose	1.11 g
Sucrose	0.14 g
Protein	**49.7 g**
Alanine	2.94 g
Arginine	2.96 g
Aspartic acid	4.71 g
Cystine	0.6 g
Glutamic acid	7.75 g
Glycine	2.6 g
Histidine	1.35 g
Isoleucine	2.27 g
Leucine	3.73 g
Lysine	4.17 g
Methionine	1.19 g
Phenylalanine	1.98 g
Proline	2.34 g
Serine	2.13 g
Threonine	2.16 g
Tryptophan	0.64 g
Tyrosine	1.7 g
Valine	2.52 g
Vitamins	
Vitamin B1	0.11 mg
Vitamin B12	9.28 mcg
Vitamin B2	0.41 mg
Vitamin B3	11.5 mg
Vitamin B5	0.89 mg
Vitamin B6	0.59 mg
Choline	200 mg
Folate	26.5 mcg
Vitamin A	6.6 mcg
Vitamin C	4.64 mg
Vitamin D	8.87 IU
Vitamin E	0.68 mg
Vitamin K	25.7 mcg
Minerals	
Calcium	44.7 mg
Copper	0.46 mg
Iron	8.27 mg
Magnesium	56.2 mg
Manganese	0.12 mg
Phosphorus	406 mg
Potassium	750 mg
Selenium	27.6 mcg
Sodium	660 mg
Zinc	3.85 mg

nutrition content estimated using the USDA database.

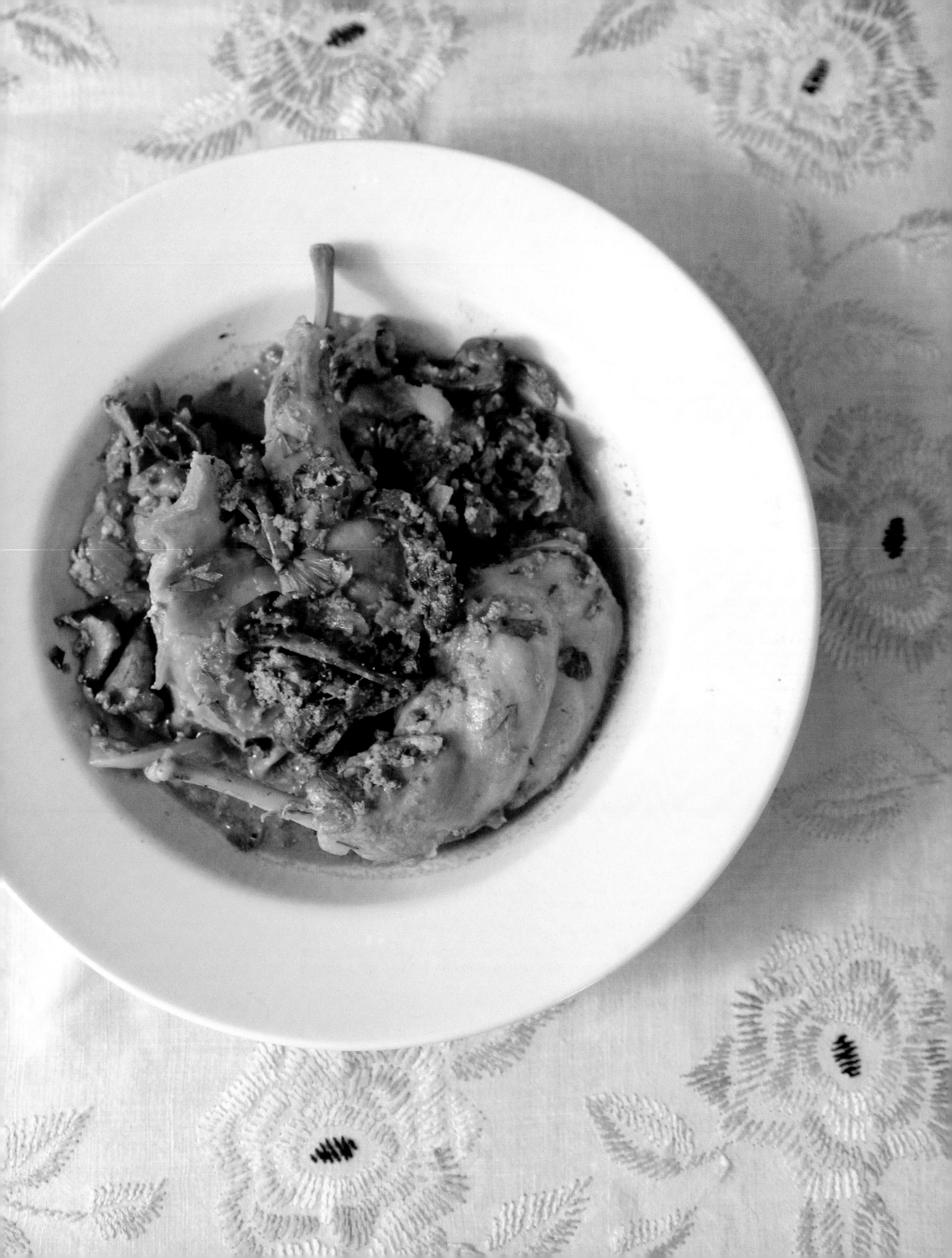

Chapter 8
Meat and Poultry

This chapter focuses on some of the most common cuts of meat, but also many larger roasts because of the convenience of having leftovers. You'll find that many of the recipes in this chapter yield a large number of servings or can easily be scaled up so that you can stock your freezer or feed a hungry horde.

Illustration by Rob Foster

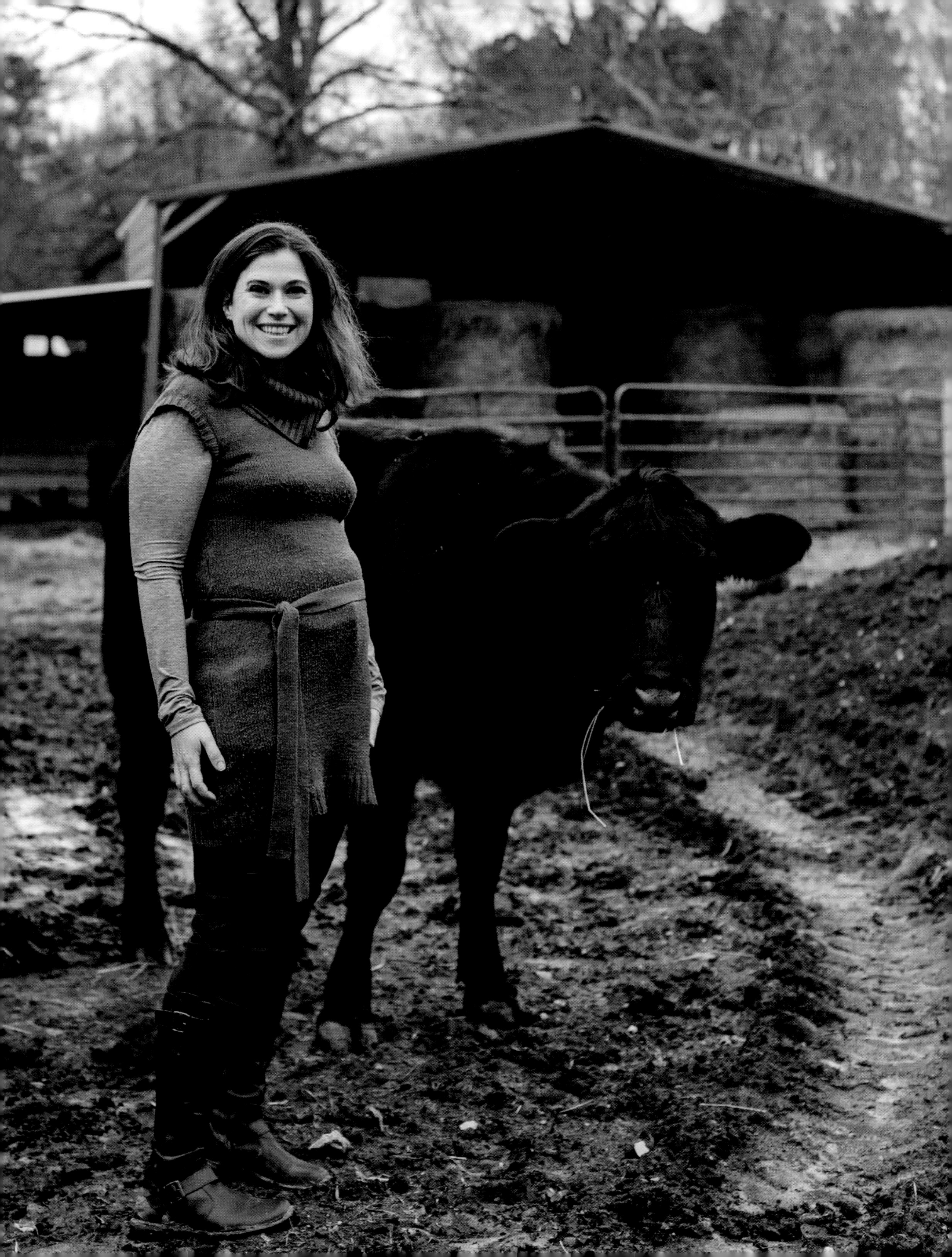

Garlic and Rosemary Roast Beef

Roast beef may seem like an intimidating dish to make, but it's actually very simple and quite forgiving, and it yields one of the most delicious meals imaginable with plenty of leftovers!

This cooking method is designed to give a perfectly rare, tender, and evenly cooked roast. You can cook it to medium-rare or medium simply by increasing the cooking time to reach a higher internal temperature (cook to 145°F for medium-rare, about 30 more minutes; or 160°F for medium, about 60 more minutes) or by following the cooking guide on page 77.

PREP TIME: 15 minutes
COOK TIME: 2 to 2½ hours
SERVINGS: 6 to 10

INGREDIENTS:

- 1 (3- to 4-pound) rib roast or top sirloin
- 5 cloves garlic
- ½ teaspoon salt
- 1 tablespoon chopped fresh rosemary
- 2 tablespoons tallow, lard, or coconut oil

FODMAP ALERT *Replace the garlic with green garlic or garlic scapes (green part only) or omit. (Yes, this is still tasty without the garlic.)*

SPECIAL EQUIPMENT

- Oven-safe meat thermometer

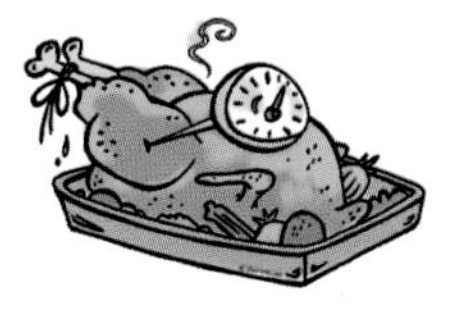

TIPS:

The most important aspect of having a delicious roast beef is to start with a tender cut of meat. Rib roasts are the most tender. Top sirloin roasts (also called center cut or top butt) are a good close second. Top round roasts are a little tougher but still work well. Rump roasts are better saved for pot roasts if you are buying grass-fed meat.

If you have a large roast, you can skip the pan-searing. Instead, preheat the oven to 500°F. Roast for 20 minutes, then reduce the oven temperature to 225°F for the remainder of the cooking time, about 20 to 30 minutes per pound.

1. Preheat the oven to 225°F.
2. Pat the roast dry with paper towels. Cut the garlic cloves lengthwise into thin slices. Take a sharp paring knife and insert the tip about 1 inch deep into the meat. Slide a slice of garlic along the blade into the cut and remove the knife (you may want to hold the garlic in place while you pull the knife out, but be careful!). Repeat with the remaining garlic slices, spacing them about 1 to 2 inches apart along the entire surface of the roast. Sprinkle the surface of the roast with the salt and rosemary.
3. Heat the tallow in a large skillet, Dutch oven, or saucepot (something with high sides that will contain the splatters when you brown the roast) over medium-high heat. Once hot, place the roast in the pan. Brown for 3 to 4 minutes on each side.
4. Place the roast on a roasting pan and insert an oven-safe meat thermometer. Roast in the oven until the internal temperature of the meat reaches 135°F, about 1½ to 2 hours.
5. Remove from the oven and let rest for 10 minutes before carving.

VARIATIONS:

Homemade Horseradish Sauce. *Horseradish sauce is a staple condiment for roast beef, and it's very easy to make at home. Simply combine 2 cups peeled and finely grated fresh horseradish root with ⅞ cup apple cider vinegar, 2 tablespoons lemon juice, and ¼ teaspoon salt. Store in a mason jar in the refrigerator for up to 2 months. For more heat, let the horseradish sit after grating for 30 minutes before mixing in the remaining ingredients.*

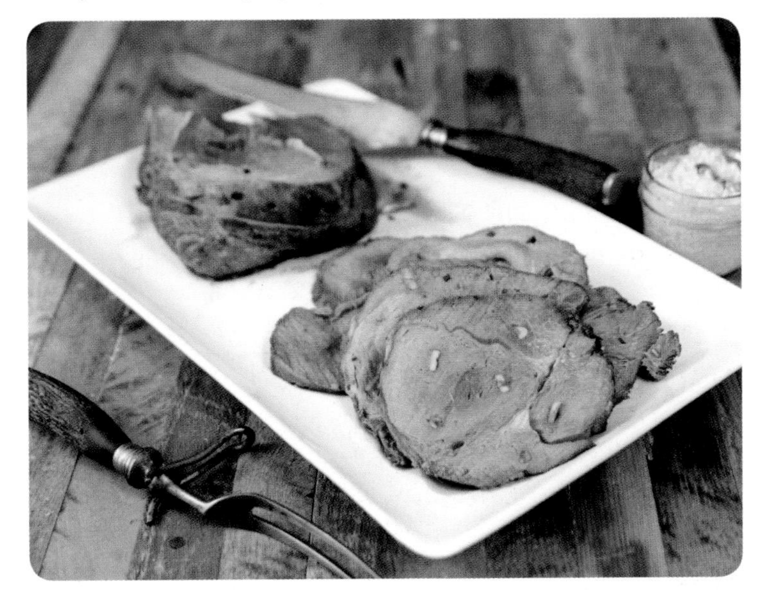

NUTRITION FACTS

Serving Size	141 g
Recipe Yields	1406 g
Calories	**209**
Fats	**8.86 g**
MUFA	3.6 g
Omega-3	0.05 g
Omega-6	0.3 g
Saturated Fat	3.61 g
Carbohydrates	**0.53 g**
Fiber	0.06 g
Starch	0.45 g
Fructose	0 g
Glucose	0 g
Sucrose	0 g
Protein	**29.9 g**
Alanine	1.81 g
Arginine	1.94 g
Aspartic acid	2.72 g
Cystine	0.39 g
Glutamic acid	4.49 g
Glycine	1.82 g
Histidine	0.95 g
Isoleucine	1.36 g
Leucine	2.38 g
Lysine	2.52 g
Methionine	0.78 g
Phenylalanine	1.18 g
Proline	1.42 g
Serine	1.18 g
Threonine	1.19 g
Tryptophan	0.2 g
Tyrosine	0.95 g
Valine	1.48 g
Vitamins	
Vitamin B1	0.09 mg
Vitamin B12	1.62 mcg
Vitamin B2	0.15 mg
Vitamin B3	10.1 mg
Vitamin B5	0.9 mg
Vitamin B6	0.84 mg
Choline	127 mg
Folate	17.9 mcg
Vitamin A	0.25 mcg
Vitamin C	0.51 mg
Vitamin D	3.44 IU
Vitamin E	0.52 mg
Vitamin K	1.79 mcg
Minerals	
Calcium	41.9 mg
Copper	0.1 mg
Iron	2.56 mg
Magnesium	31.8 mg
Manganese	0.05 mg
Phosphorus	281 mg
Potassium	474 mg
Selenium	34.9 mcg
Sodium	129 mg
Zinc	5.65 mg

nutrition content estimated using the USDA database.

Leg of Lamb with Mint Vinegar

Lamb is a tender and delicious meat, and mint is a classic companion. Buying a whole leg of lamb is also one of the most inexpensive ways to include grass-fed meat in your diet. This recipe is how my mom used to make it when I was little. It's still one of my favorite meals.

PREP TIME: 15 minutes
COOK TIME: 1 to 2½ hours
SERVINGS: 6 to 10

INGREDIENTS:

Lamb:

1 tablespoon minced fresh thyme

2 tablespoons minced fresh rosemary

¾ teaspoon salt

1 (4- to 6-pound) leg of lamb (bone-in or boneless)

Mint Vinegar:

⅓ cup minced fresh mint

⅔ cup coconut water vinegar or white wine vinegar

1. Preheat the oven to 325°F.
2. In a small food processor or with a mortar and pestle, combine the thyme, rosemary, and salt and process (or grind) to a paste.
3. Pat the lamb dry with paper towels and place on a roasting pan. Rub the herb paste over the entire surface of the lamb (this is easiest to do with your hands).
4. Insert an oven-safe meat thermometer into the lamb, place it in the oven, and bake for 15 minutes per pound for medium-rare (145°F), 20 minutes per pound for medium (160°F), or 25 minutes per pound for well-done (170°F).
5. While the lamb is cooking, make the mint vinegar: Combine the minced mint and coconut water vinegar in a bowl or measuring cup. Stir with a spoon, smushing the mint against the side of the bowl with the back of the spoon for a few minutes to thoroughly crush the mint. Let sit at room temperature for an hour before serving (or 2 hours or more in the fridge).
6. After removing the lamb from the oven, let it rest for 10 minutes before carving. Serve with mint vinegar drizzled over the top.

SPECIAL EQUIPMENT

- Food processor or mortar and pestle
- Oven-safe meat thermometer

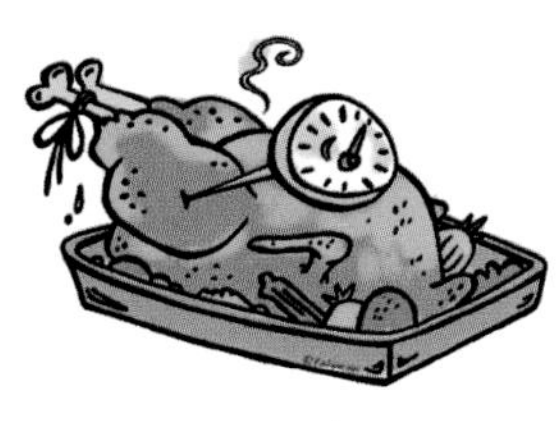

VARIATIONS:

This herb paste also works well with roast beef, bison, or emu.

NUTRITION FACTS	
Serving Size	206 g
Recipe Yields	2060 g
Calories	**370**
Fats	**16.3 g**
MUFA	7.68 g
Omega-3	0.18 g
Omega-6	1.07 g
Saturated Fat	6.9 g
Carbohydrates	**0.91 g**
Fiber	0.6 g
Starch	0 g
Fructose	0.05 g
Glucose	0.02 g
Sucrose	0 g
Protein	**54.3 g**
Alanine	3.1 g
Arginine	3.06 g
Aspartic acid	4.55 g
Cystine	0.62 g
Glutamic acid	7.48 g
Glycine	2.52 g
Histidine	1.63 g
Isoleucine	2.49 g
Leucine	4.01 g
Lysine	4.54 g
Methionine	1.32 g
Phenylalanine	2.1 g
Proline	2.16 g
Serine	1.92 g
Threonine	2.21 g
Tryptophan	0.6 g
Tyrosine	1.73 g
Valine	2.78 g
Vitamins	
Vitamin B1	0.21 mg
Vitamin B12	4.1 mcg
Vitamin B2	0.52 mg
Vitamin B3	11.9 mg
Vitamin B5	1.31 mg
Vitamin B6	0.29 mg
Choline	190 mg
Folate	39.3 mcg
Vitamin A	21.9 mcg
Vitamin C	1.46 mg
Vitamin D	3.63 IU
Vitamin E	0.33 mg
Vitamin K	6.53 mcg
Minerals	
Calcium	69.1 mg
Copper	0.24 mg
Iron	4.57 mg
Magnesium	53.4 mg
Manganese	0.18 mg
Phosphorus	380 mg
Potassium	718 mg
Selenium	54.6 mcg
Sodium	221 mg
Zinc	9.06 mg

nutrition content estimated using the USDA database.

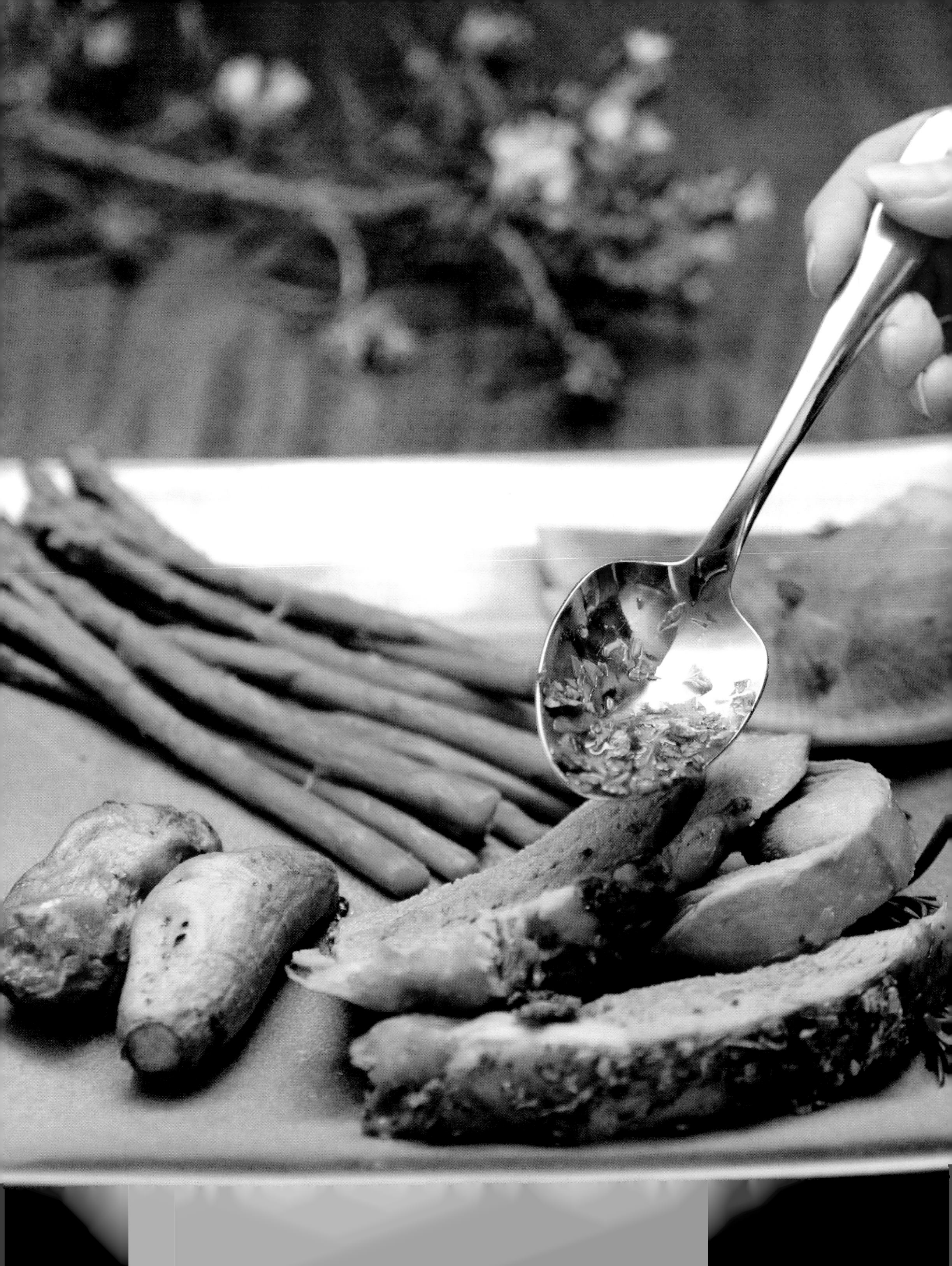

Tarragon Roasted Pork

Tarragon has a lovely aniselike flavor that pairs beautifully with pork. This pork tastes delicious alongside Spiced Sweet Potato (page 313) and homemade Applesauce (page 122).

PREP TIME: 10 minutes
COOK TIME: 1 hour 20 minutes to 1 hour 40 minutes
SERVINGS: 8 to 10

INGREDIENTS:

- 3 tablespoons dried tarragon
- 2 teaspoons salt
- 1 (4- to 5-pound) pork roast (leg or loin)

SPECIAL EQUIPMENT

- Oven-safe meat thermometer
- Spice grinder or mortar and pestle

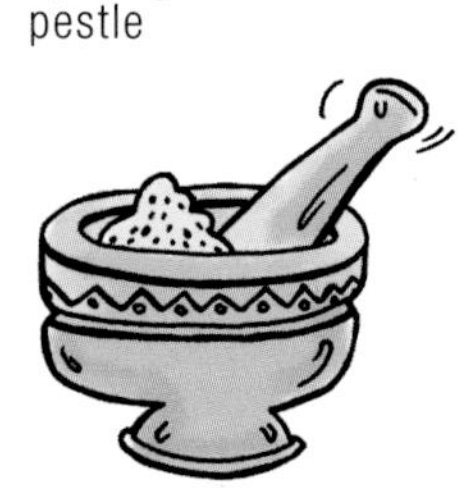

1. Preheat the oven to 350°F.
2. Combine the tarragon and salt in a spice grinder or mortar and pestle and grind until it's a fine powder.
3. Place the roast on the rack of a roasting pan. Pat dry with paper towels. Rub the tarragon and salt mixture over the entire surface of the roast. Insert an oven-safe meat thermometer.
4. Roast for 20 minutes per pound, until the internal temperature reaches a minimum of 145°F.
5. Let the roast rest for 10 minutes before carving.

VARIATIONS:

Using dried tarragon allows for a more even coating, but you can also use 3 tablespoons minced fresh tarragon.

Roasted Pork with Crackling. If you are lucky enough to get a roast with the skin on, here are directions for making crackling. Score the skin with a sharp knife (or ask your butcher to do this for you) in a grid pattern, approximately 1 by 1 inch. Before rubbing your pork with spices, "bloom" the crackling by pouring boiling water over the surface (you'll need a kettleful, and be careful!). Give the meat 5 minutes to cool before rubbing on the spices. Once the internal temperature of the meat reaches 130°F, turn the broiler on to high. Broil for 8 to 10 minutes to crisp up the crackling.

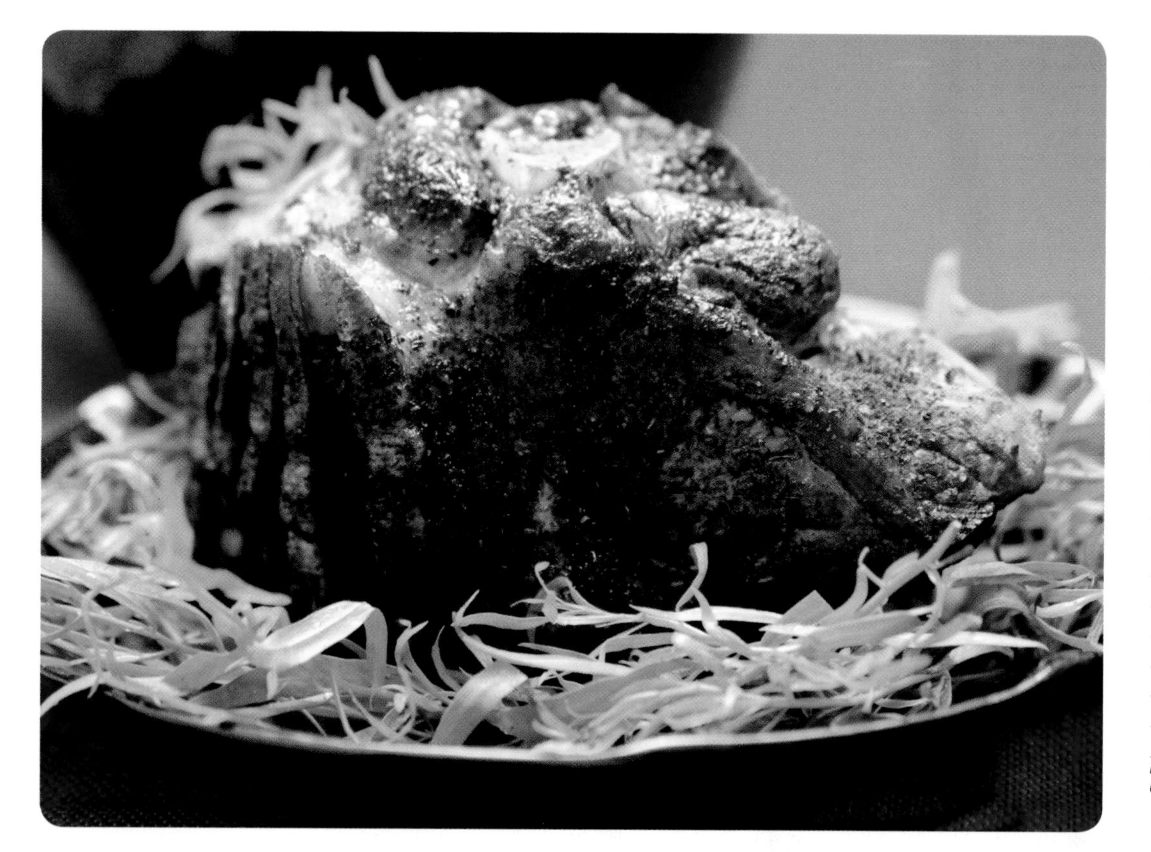

NUTRITION FACTS	
Serving Size	183 g
Recipe Yields	1831 g
Calories	**207**
Fats	**3.14 g**
MUFA	1.25 g
Omega-3	0.03 g
Omega-6	0.48 g
Saturated Fat	0.96 g
Carbohydrates	**0.27 g**
Fiber	0.04 g
Starch	0 g
Fructose	0 g
Glucose	0 g
Sucrose	0 g
Protein	**41.6 g**
Alanine	2.38 g
Arginine	2.68 g
Aspartic acid	3.88 g
Cystine	0.47 g
Glutamic acid	6.34 g
Glycine	1.88 g
Histidine	1.69 g
Isoleucine	1.97 g
Leucine	3.42 g
Lysine	3.69 g
Methionine	1.14 g
Phenylalanine	1.73 g
Proline	1.68 g
Serine	1.73 g
Threonine	1.83 g
Tryptophan	0.49 g
Tyrosine	1.65 g
Valine	2.1 g
Vitamins	
Vitamin B1	1.19 mg
Vitamin B12	0.96 mcg
Vitamin B2	0.65 mg
Vitamin B3	13.1 mg
Vitamin B5	1.63 mg
Vitamin B6	1.26 mg
Choline	145 mg
Folate	1.48 mcg
Vitamin A	1.13 mcg
Vitamin C	0.27 mg
Vitamin D	0 IU
Vitamin E	0.15 mg
Vitamin K	0 mcg
Minerals	
Calcium	17.6 mg
Copper	0.13 mg
Iron	2.83 mg
Magnesium	47.2 mg
Manganese	0.06 mg
Phosphorus	423 mg
Potassium	747 mg
Selenium	47.9 mcg
Sodium	296 mg
Zinc	3.74 mg

nutrition content estimated using the USDA database.

Roasted Chicken

Roasting two chickens at once is a great time-saving trick. Leftovers can be enjoyed as is, reinvented in stir-fries or soups, tossed into salads, or frozen for a quick midweek meal sometime in the future.

PREP TIME: 10 to 15 minutes
COOK TIME: 1 hour 20 minutes to 2 hours
SERVINGS: 10 to 18

INGREDIENTS:

2 (4- to 6-pound) whole chickens

3 to 4 tablespoons Poultry Seasoning (page 108)

1 tablespoon pink or gray salt or truffle salt

SPECIAL EQUIPMENT

- Oven-safe meat thermometer

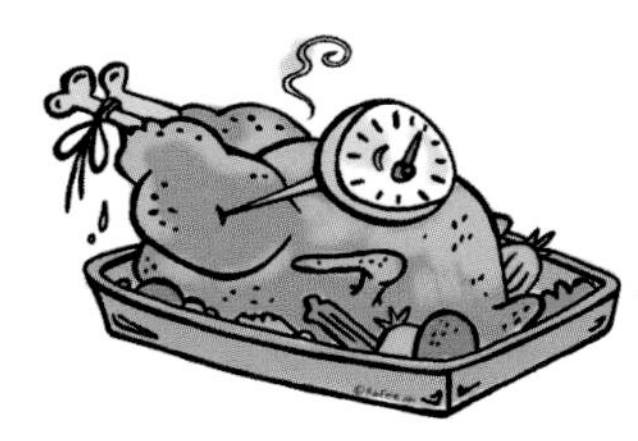

1. Preheat the oven to 350°F.
2. Place the chickens breast side up on a roasting pan. Remove the giblets and neck, if included (you can save them for making broth or save the giblets for Steak and Kidney Pot Pie, page 274). Sprinkle the entire surface of each chicken liberally with the seasoning mix and salt. Place an oven-safe meat thermometer into the breast or thigh of the larger chicken.
3. Bake for 20 minutes per pound (for your bigger chicken) or until the internal temperature reaches at least 165°F.
4. Let rest for 5 to 10 minutes before carving. Enjoy!

TIPS:

You can easily make the Poultry Seasoning ahead of time and store it for months in a spice shaker.

VARIATIONS:

Swap out the Poultry Seasoning for your favorite chopped fresh herbs and spices. Rosemary, thyme, savory, citrus zest, and garlic powder are all delicious seasonings for chicken.

Slow-Roasted Chicken. You can also slow-roast the chicken at 250°F for 5 hours for a meltingly juicy and tender meat (more like rotisserie chicken).

Roasted Chicken Pieces. Do you have just chicken thighs or a whole chicken cut into parts? Lay them skin side up on a roasting pan, sprinkle with seasoning, and roast using the guide on page 79. If you have a few different chicken parts (legs and thighs, for example), roast them for the longest time indicated. You can use the Poultry Seasoning or your favorite herbs. My kids particularly enjoy roasted chicken pieces simply seasoned with generous amounts of pink salt and garlic powder.

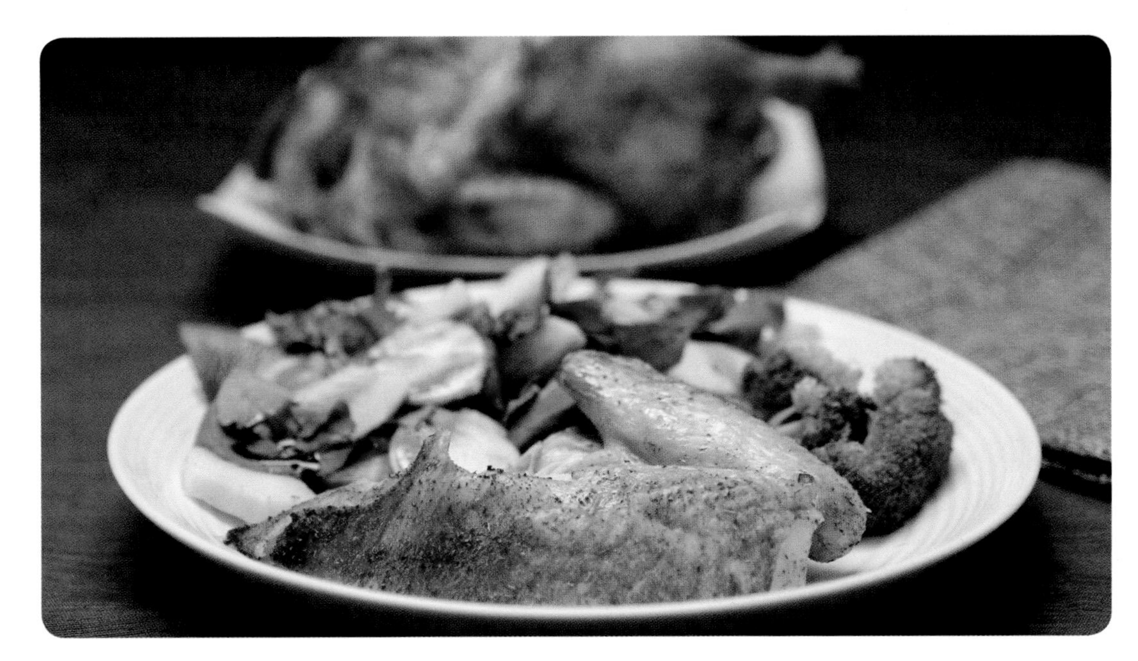

NUTRITION FACTS

Serving Size	203 g
Recipe Yields	3660 g
Calories	**483**
Fats	**27.4 g**
MUFA	10.8 g
Omega-3	0.37 g
Omega-6	5.4 g
Saturated Fat	7.65 g
Carbohydrates	**0.48 g**
Fiber	0.08 g
Starch	0.37 g
Fructose	0 g
Glucose	0 g
Sucrose	0 g
Protein	**55 g**
Alanine	3.2 g
Arginine	3.44 g
Aspartic acid	4.9 g
Cystine	0.73 g
Glutamic acid	8.03 g
Glycine	3.55 g
Histidine	1.61 g
Isoleucine	2.74 g
Leucine	4 g
Lysine	4.47 g
Methionine	1.46 g
Phenylalanine	2.14 g
Proline	2.66 g
Serine	1.94 g
Threonine	2.27 g
Tryptophan	0.61 g
Tyrosine	1.77 g
Valine	2.67 g
Vitamins	
Vitamin B1	0.13 mg
Vitamin B12	0.6 mcg
Vitamin B2	0.34 mg
Vitamin B3	17.1 mg
Vitamin B5	2.07 mg
Vitamin B6	0.81 mg
Choline	133 mg
Folate	11.1 mcg
Vitamin A	97.6 mcg
Vitamin C	0.09 mg
Vitamin D	4.03 IU
Vitamin E	0.55 mg
Vitamin K	10.7 mcg
Minerals	
Calcium	38.4 mg
Copper	0.14 mg
Iron	2.79 mg
Magnesium	48 mg
Manganese	0.09 mg
Phosphorus	368 mg
Potassium	454 mg
Selenium	48.2 mcg
Sodium	554 mg
Zinc	3.93 mg

nutrition content estimated using the USDA database.

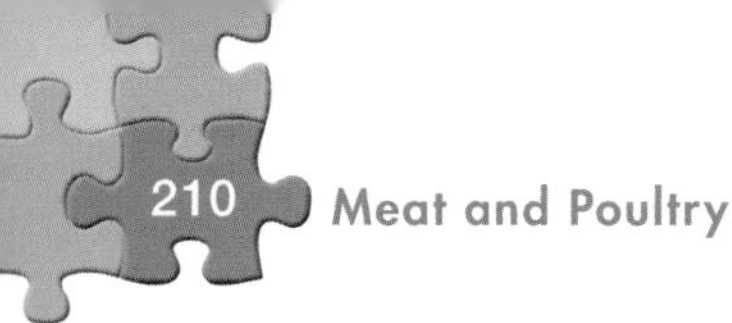

Whole Turkey with Mofongo Stuffing

I always loved turkey dinners, more for the stuffing than for the turkey itself. There is nothing like stuffing cooked inside a turkey. The wonderful thing about plantains is that they naturally absorb a substantial amount of liquid (comparable to other traditional stuffing ingredients, like bread or chestnuts), so the end result is moist and full of flavor. Green plantains have a very neutral starchy flavor as well, so all the flavor of the absorbed turkey juices shines through. For the complete turkey dinner experience, serve with Maple-Cranberry Sauce (page 222).

PREP TIME: 1 hour
COOK TIME: 4 to 5 hours
SERVINGS: 16 to 24

INGREDIENTS:

Mofongo Stuffing:

- 5 green plantains, peeled and cut into 1-inch-thick semicircles (see Tips)
- 4 cups Bone Broth (chicken or turkey, page 110) or water
- 10 ounces bacon, cut into small pieces
- 1 large onion, finely diced
- 7 to 10 stalks celery, chopped
- ¼ cup bacon fat, lard, duck fat, or goose fat
- 2 tablespoons dried savory or ⅓ cup fresh savory leaves

Turkey:

- 1 (12- to 15-pound) turkey
- 2 teaspoons salt
- 1 tablespoon dried savory

- 1 recipe Maple-Cranberry Sauce (page 222), for serving (optional)

FODMAP ALERT *Replace the onion with green onion or leek (green part only) or chives or omit.*

SPECIAL EQUIPMENT

- Oven-safe meat thermometer

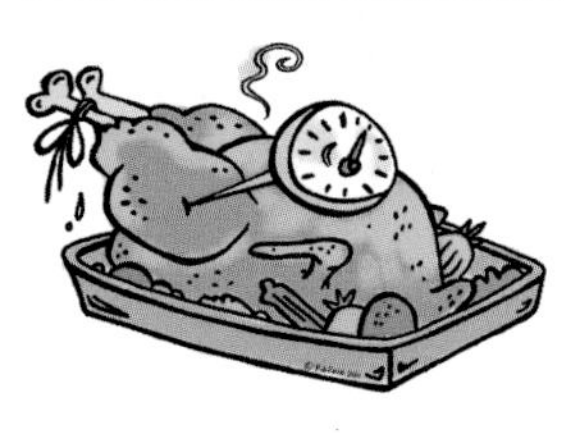

MOFONGO STUFFING:

1. Place the plantains in a pot with the broth or water (there should be enough to cover). Bring to a boil over high heat, then reduce the heat to maintain a simmer. Simmer, covered, until the plantains are tender when pierced with a knife, about 20 minutes.
2. Meanwhile, add the bacon to a cold skillet and turn on the heat to medium-high. Cook for 5 minutes, then add the onion and celery. Continue to cook, stirring occasionally, until the bacon is crisp and the onion is soft and caramelized, about 15 minutes.
3. Drain the plantains when they are done cooking, but reserve the cooking liquid.
4. Place the plantains in a bowl along with ½ cup of the cooking liquid. Mash with a wire potato masher to the desired consistency (I like it very lumpy). Add the bacon, onion, celery, and all the grease from the pan. Add the supplemental bacon fat and the savory and stir to incorporate.

TURKEY:

1. Preheat the oven to 325°F. Place the turkey in a large roasting pan. Position the rack in your oven appropriately low to accommodate the roasting pan.
2. Remove any giblets and the neck (sometimes they are both in the main cavity, sometimes the neck is in the neck cavity). Pat dry with paper towels. Fill the neck cavity and then the main cavity of the turkey with the stuffing (it's okay to really pack it in). If the skin around the main cavity does not cover the surface of the stuffing, place a little aluminum foil around the opening. Place an oven-safe meat thermometer in the deepest part of the breast or in the inner thigh near the breast.
3. Sprinkle the entire surface of the turkey with the salt and savory.
4. Roast for 3½ to 4 hours, until the meat temperature reaches a minimum of 165°F. (The stuffing should also reach 165°F, which may mean cooking the meat to a hotter temperature. Don't worry; your turkey should still be moist up to about 175°F to 180°F.) If you prefer crisp skin, don't baste. If you like moist skin, baste with the pan juices after the first hour and every 20 to 30 minutes thereafter throughout cooking.
5. Remove from the oven and let rest for 10 minutes before carving. Serve with maple-cranberry sauce, if desired.

NUTRITION FACTS	
Serving Size	308 g
Recipe Yields	7402 g
Calories	**462**
Fats	**20.2 g**
MUFA	7.37 g
Omega-3	0.23 g
Omega-6	3.22 g
Saturated Fat	5.9 g
Carbohydrates	**14 g**
Fiber	1.41 g
Starch	5.82 g
Fructose	0.35 g
Glucose	0.39 g
Sucrose	0.27 g
Protein	**54 g**
Alanine	2.98 g
Arginine	3.12 g
Aspartic acid	4.32 g
Cystine	0.51 g
Glutamic acid	7.24 g
Glycine	2.66 g
Histidine	1.48 g
Isoleucine	1.59 g
Leucine	3.69 g
Lysine	4.33 g
Methionine	1.36 g
Phenylalanine	1.75 g
Proline	3.02 g
Serine	2.1 g
Threonine	1.92 g
Tryptophan	0.55 g
Tyrosine	1.57 g
Valine	1.8 g
Vitamins	
Vitamin B1	0.18 mg
Vitamin B12	2.9 mcg
Vitamin B2	0.48 mg
Vitamin B3	18.9 mg
Vitamin B5	2.1 mg
Vitamin B6	1.54 mg
Choline	153 mg
Folate	31.1 mcg
Vitamin A	64.9 mcg
Vitamin C	8.45 mg
Vitamin D	29.3 IU
Vitamin E	0.35 mg
Vitamin K	4.44 mcg
Minerals	
Calcium	46.9 mg
Copper	0.24 mg
Iron	2.9 mg
Magnesium	78.6 mg
Manganese	0.09 mg
Phosphorus	495 mg
Potassium	815 mg
Selenium	55.9 mcg
Sodium	569 mg
Zinc	4.54 mg

nutrition content estimated using the USDA database.

TIPS:

Peeling green plantains can be an exercise in frustration. Cut them in half lengthwise and then in half crosswise. Get your thumbs under the peel and pry it off. If the peel breaks, use a paring knife to cut off whatever is stuck on.

If you purchase a frozen turkey for this recipe, make sure that it is completely thawed before roasting (see page 59).

You can save the giblets for making broth (which can be used to make pan gravy, below) and/or use the liver for pâté.

Pan Gravy. Simmer the whole giblets with enough water to cover for the entire turkey cooking time, or use chicken or turkey broth. After the turkey is done, remove the turkey and rack from the roasting pan, leaving the drippings in the pan. Place the pan on the stovetop over medium-high heat. If using giblet broth, strain the giblets from the broth and discard. Add 2 cups of the giblet broth or chicken or turkey broth and bring to a simmer before thickening. Arrowroot powder and kuzu starch make the best thickeners. Use them as you could cornstarch, mixing ¼ cup starch with ¼ cup cold water, then adding the slurry to the hot broth/drippings while stirring vigorously. Simmer until thick, about 3 to 4 minutes.

VARIATIONS:

Kufu Stuffing. Using very ripe plantains (the peels should be covered in black spots or almost entirely black) gives this stuffing a very different and delightful flavor. Simply swap ripe plantains for the green ones and note that they take less time to simmer, 5 to 10 minutes.

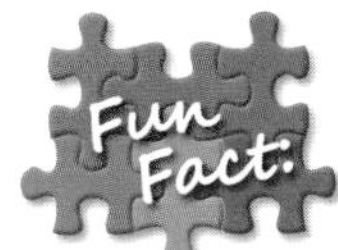

Contrary to popular belief, turkey is not that high in tryptophan, the essential amino acid scapegoated for making people sleepy. It does not even rank in the top 50 food sources. Organ meat and seafood, on the other hand, is a great source of tryptophan! And the sleepiness you feel after a turkey dinner is related to overeating rather than too much tryptophan.

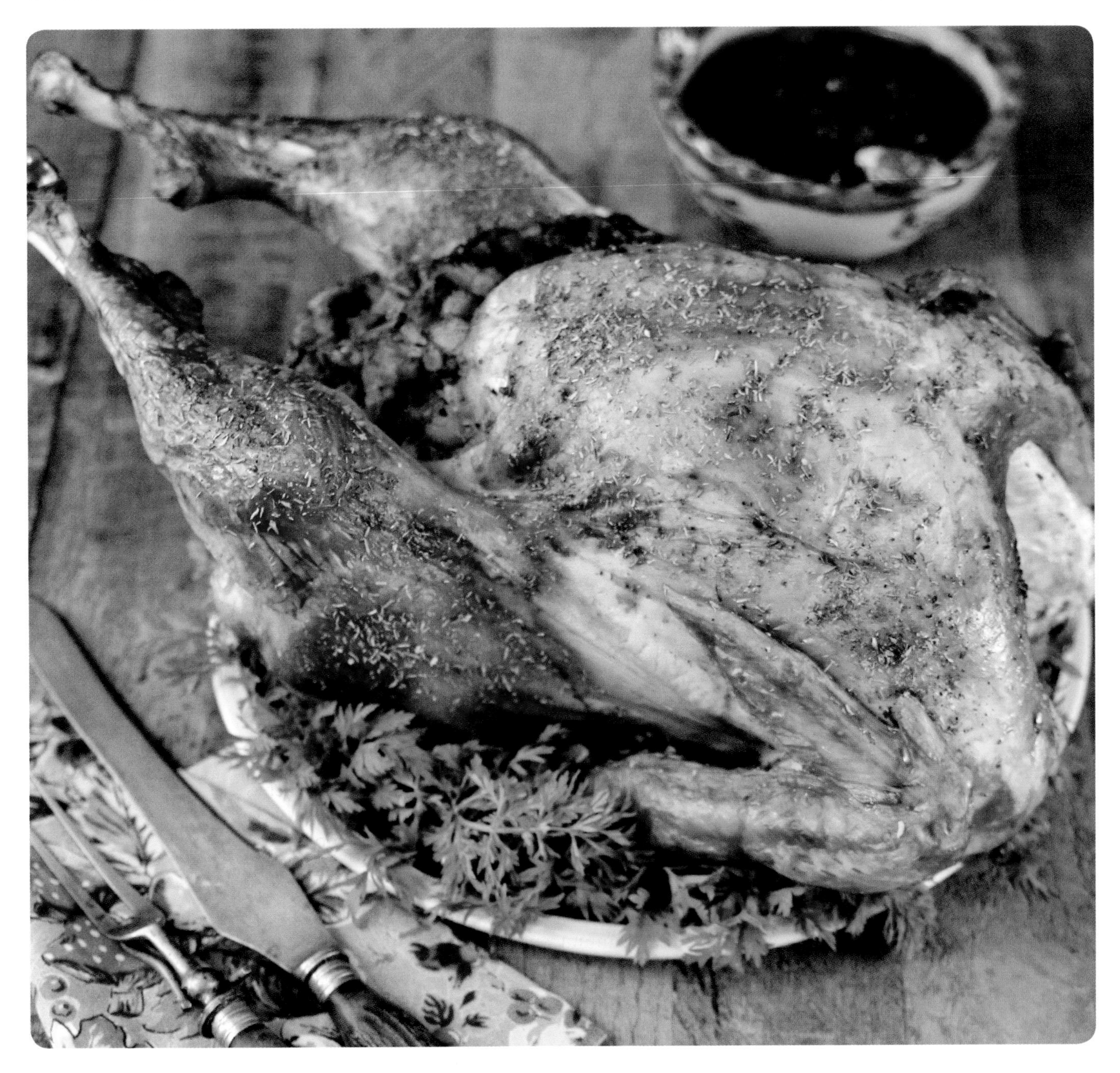

Rustic Bison Pot Roast

Pot roast is such a comforting meal, full of flavor with tender, fall-off-the-bone meat. Plus, it is very forgiving, meaning that you don't need to measure your ingredients particularly carefully, and you can cook it anywhere from 4 to 8 hours, depending on your schedule. While this recipe calls for bison, a rich and flavorful meat, you can easily substitute beef or tough cuts of meat from wild game.

PREP TIME: 15 to 20 minutes
COOK TIME: 4½ to 5½ hours
SERVINGS: 4 to 10

INGREDIENTS:

- 1½ teaspoons salt
- 1 teaspoon dried rosemary
- 1 teaspoon dried thyme leaves
- 1 teaspoon dried marjoram leaves
- 1 teaspoon dried savory
- 1 teaspoon dried oregano leaves
- 3 to 4 pounds bison chuck roast (bone-in or boneless)
- 2 to 3 tablespoons tallow or other cooking fat
- 2 onions, cut into thick wedges
- 1 pound carrots (about 3 medium), cut into large chunks
- 1 pound parsnips (about 3 medium), cut into large chunks
- 1 bay leaf
- ½ cup red wine or Bone Broth (beef, page 110)
- 6 to 8 cloves garlic, roughly chopped

FODMAP ALERT *Replace the garlic with green garlic or garlic scapes (green part only) or omit. Replace the onion with green onion or leek (green part only) or chives or omit.*

SPECIAL EQUIPMENT

- Spice grinder or mini food processor
- Dutch oven

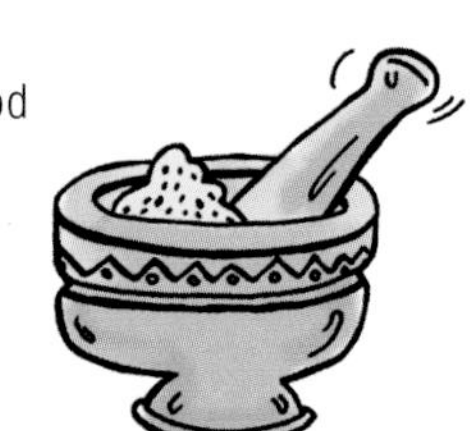

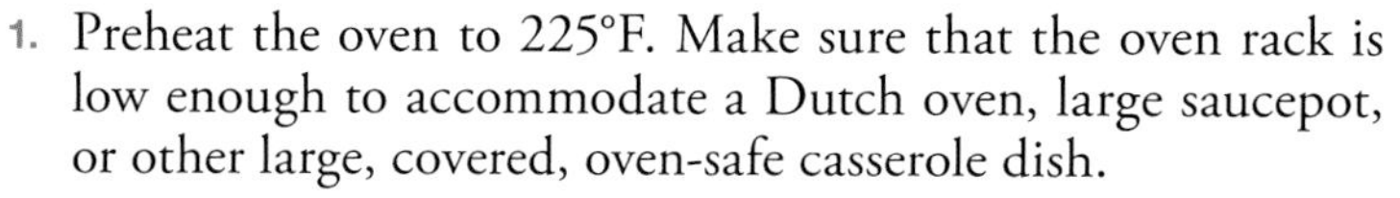

1. Preheat the oven to 225°F. Make sure that the oven rack is low enough to accommodate a Dutch oven, large saucepot, or other large, covered, oven-safe casserole dish.
2. Combine the salt, rosemary, thyme, marjoram, savory, and oregano in a spice grinder or mini food processor and grind to a powder.
3. Pat the roast dry with paper towels and season generously with the seasoning mix.
4. Heat 2 tablespoons of the tallow in a Dutch oven over medium-high heat. Brown the roast for 3 to 4 minutes on all sides. Once fully browned, remove from the pan and set aside.
5. Add the onions and cook for 5 minutes, until starting to brown. Add an additional tablespoon of tallow if they start to stick.
6. Add the carrots, parsnips, bay leaf, wine, and garlic and stir to incorporate. Place the roast on top of the vegetables and bring to a simmer. Cover and place in the oven for 4 to 5 hours.

TIPS:

Chuck roasts, also called "shoulder roasts," are the best roasts to choose for pot roast recipes. However, this recipe is also great for rump roast or any other tough cut of meat, such as cheek.

If you like your vegetables firmer, cut them into larger pieces. If you like them softer, cut them into smaller pieces.

VARIATIONS:

You can also cook this roast in a slow cooker for 4 to 8 hours, in a pressure cooker for 1 to 1½ hours, or simmer, covered, on the stovetop on low heat for 4 hours.

Beef Pot Roast. *You don't need to use bison for this recipe. If it's easier or more affordable for you to source beef, simply replace the bison chuck roast with beef.*

Pot Roast Gravy. *Instead or serving the vegetables on the side, you can purée them with the cooking liquid to make a flavorful gravy.*

NUTRITION FACTS	
Serving Size	253 g
Recipe Yields	2526 g
Calories	**318**
Fats	**12 g**
MUFA	5.92 g
Omega-3	0.06 g
Omega-6	0.43 g
Saturated Fat	4.01 g
Carbohydrates	**14.4 g**
Fiber	3.55 g
Starch	5.35 g
Fructose	0.44 g
Glucose	0.6 g
Sucrose	1.43 g
Protein	**36.7 g**
Alanine	2.19 g
Arginine	2.46 g
Aspartic acid	3.62 g
Cystine	0.42 g
Glutamic acid	5.86 g
Glycine	1.71 g
Histidine	1.16 g
Isoleucine	1.87 g
Leucine	3.18 g
Lysine	3.37 g
Methionine	1.01 g
Phenylalanine	1.57 g
Proline	1.53 g
Serine	1.45 g
Threonine	1.72 g
Tryptophan	0.39 g
Tyrosine	1.32 g
Valine	1.95 g
Vitamins	
Vitamin B1	0.2 mg
Vitamin B12	4.05 mcg
Vitamin B2	0.38 mg
Vitamin B3	5.34 mg
Vitamin B5	0.41 mg
Vitamin B6	0.53 mg
Choline	155 mg
Folate	49.1 mcg
Vitamin A	388 mcg
Vitamin C	9.36 mg
Vitamin D	8.9 IU
Vitamin E	1.26 mg
Vitamin K	10.2 mcg
Minerals	
Calcium	59.7 mg
Copper	0.23 mg
Iron	6.14 mg
Magnesium	52 mg
Manganese	0.3 mg
Phosphorus	359 mg
Potassium	851 mg
Selenium	42.4 mcg
Sodium	287 mg
Zinc	9.01 mg

nutrition content estimated using the USDA database.

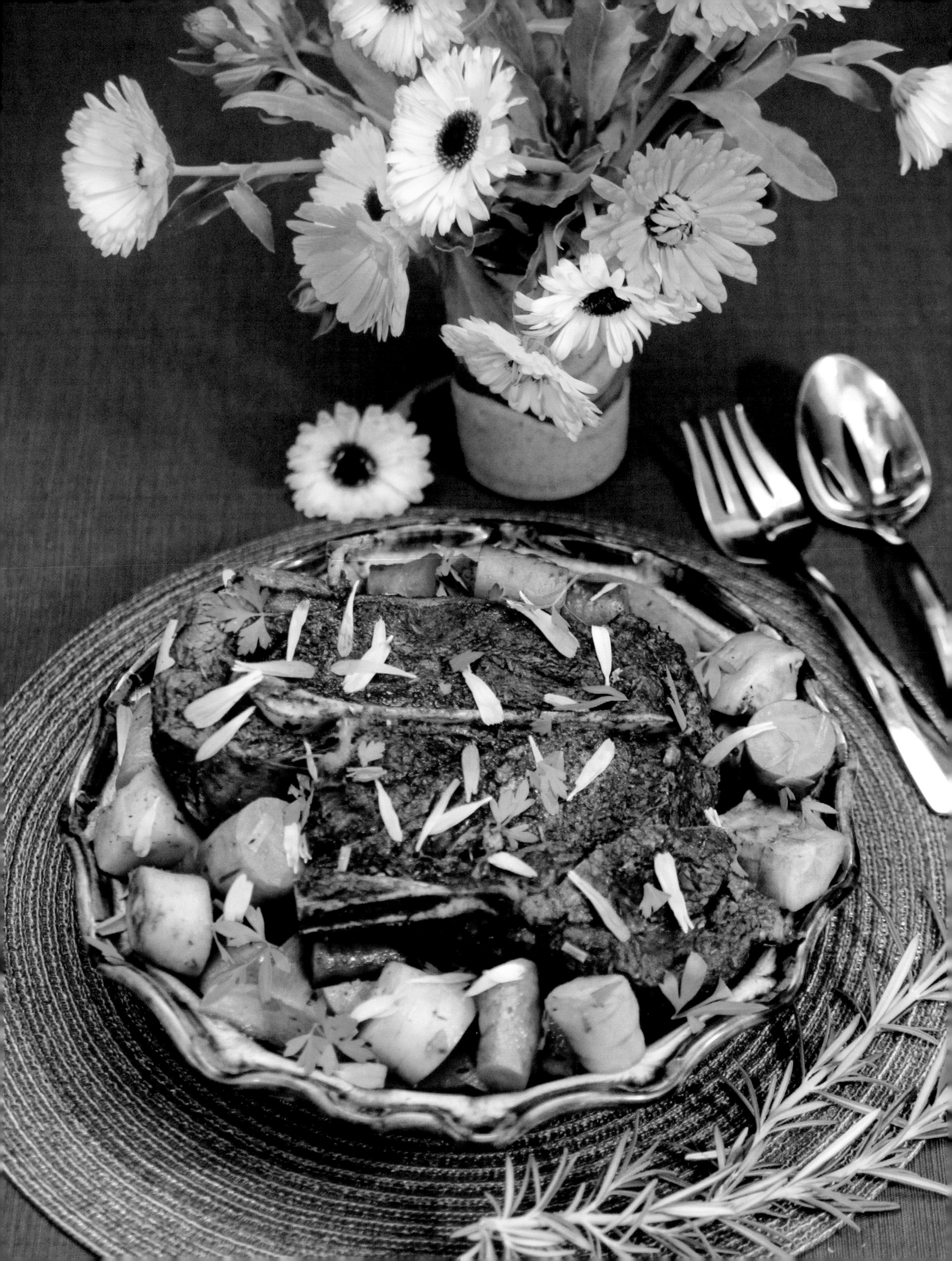

Garlic-Roasted Pork Shoulder

Pork shoulder is typically a very cheap cut of meat. When cooked "low and slow," it is also one of the most tender and delicious meals imaginable. This pork is delicious alongside squash, sweet potatoes, applesauce, baked apples, or fried plantains.

PREP TIME: 20 minutes, plus marinating overnight
COOK TIME: 6 hours
SERVINGS: 6 to 10

INGREDIENTS:

- 1 small head garlic, crushed
- 2 teaspoons salt
- 3 tablespoons minced fresh oregano
- 1½ tablespoons apple cider vinegar
- 1½ tablespoons fresh lemon juice
- 1 (3- to 4-pound) pork shoulder

FODMAP ALERT *This recipe cannot be made low-FODMAP. But a great alternative seasoning for pork shoulder is truffle salt and maple sugar.*

1. Combine the crushed garlic, salt, oregano, apple cider vinegar, and lemon juice in a small bowl.
2. Pat the pork shoulder dry with paper towels. Lay out several pieces of plastic wrap, overlapping (big enough to wrap the whole pork shoulder after the seasoning is rubbed on), and place the pork shoulder on top.
3. Rub the seasoning over the entire surface of the pork shoulder. Wrap tightly in the plastic wrap. Place in a dish or on a tray and refrigerate overnight.
4. Remove the pork shoulder from the refrigerator and let warm to room temperature for 1 hour before placing in the oven. Preheat the oven to 275°F.
5. Remove the plastic wrap and place the pork on a roasting pan. Roast for 6 hours, until the meat is fork-tender.

TIPS:

This recipe can be easily scaled up for larger shoulder roasts. For a 6- to 8-pound roast, double the rub ingredients and cook for 8 to 9 hours.

VARIATIONS:

Barbecue Pulled Pork. When the pork shoulder comes out of the oven, "pull" it using two forks, one to steady the meat and one to pull the meat apart into thin strips. Toss the shredded pork with Barbecue Sauce (page 124) and serve with Russ' Flatbread (page 326) and Cran-Apple Coleslaw (page 164), if desired.

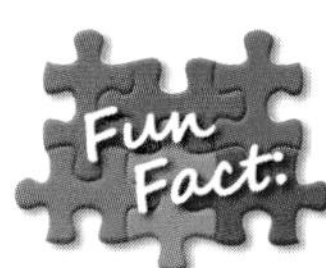

Pork shoulder is also called Boston butt. It can be boneless or contain a bone (which doesn't affect the recipe, but does affect the number of servings).

NUTRITION FACTS	
Serving Size	146 g
Recipe Yields	1462 g
Calories	**321**
Fats	**18.5 g**
MUFA	8.39 g
Omega-3	0.06 g
Omega-6	1.5 g
Saturated Fat	6.53 g
Carbohydrates	**1.99 g**
Fiber	0.46 g
Starch	1.37 g
Fructose	0.04 g
Glucose	0.04 g
Sucrose	0.02 g
Protein	**34.7 g**
Alanine	2.01 g
Arginine	2.17 g
Aspartic acid	3.22 g
Cystine	0.44 g
Glutamic acid	5.42 g
Glycine	1.65 g
Histidine	1.38 g
Isoleucine	1.62 g
Leucine	2.78 g
Lysine	3.11 g
Methionine	0.92 g
Phenylalanine	1.38 g
Proline	1.4 g
Serine	1.43 g
Threonine	1.58 g
Tryptophan	0.44 g
Tyrosine	1.21 g
Valine	1.88 g
Vitamins	
Vitamin B1	0.86 mg
Vitamin B12	1.17 mcg
Vitamin B2	0.51 mg
Vitamin B3	5.86 mg
Vitamin B5	0.92 mg
Vitamin B6	0.49 mg
Choline	119 mg
Folate	9.49 mcg
Vitamin A	3.48 mcg
Vitamin C	2.84 mg
Vitamin D	53 IU
Vitamin E	0.51 mg
Vitamin K	5.65 mcg
Minerals	
Calcium	47.9 mg
Copper	0.19 mg
Iron	3.64 mg
Magnesium	30.7 mg
Manganese	0.15 mg
Phosphorus	307 mg
Potassium	507 mg
Selenium	51.4 mcg
Sodium	308 mg
Zinc	5.72 mg

nutrition content estimated using the USDA database.

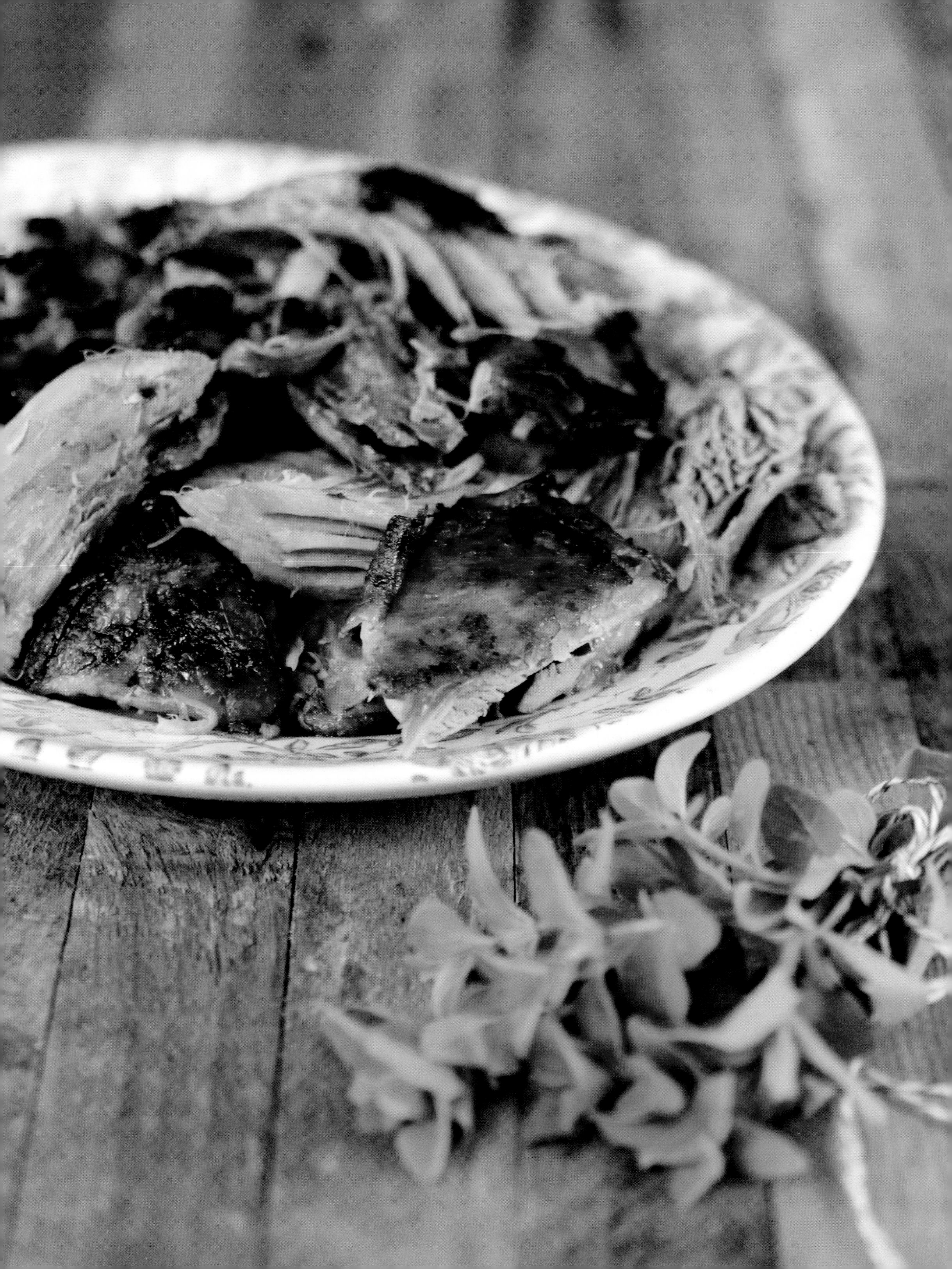

BBQ Pork Ribs

The secret to meltingly tender pork ribs is cooking them twice and marinating in between. Make sure to put plenty of napkins on the table for this meal!

PREP TIME: 20 minutes
COOK TIME: 40 to 42 minutes, plus up to 24 hours marinating time
SERVINGS: 8 to 14

INGREDIENTS:

7 to 8 pounds pork ribs
1½ cups Barbecue Sauce (page 124)

1. Preheat the oven to 350°F.
2. Arrange the racks of ribs on rimmed baking sheets or roasting pans. Bake for 30 minutes.
3. Remove the ribs from the oven and cover with barbecue sauce. Let cool.
4. Wrap the cooled ribs in plastic wrap or place in an airtight container. Refrigerate overnight and up to 24 hours.
5. Preheat a grill pan or a gas or charcoal grill. Once hot, place the racks of ribs on the grill (you may have to do this in batches). Grill for 5 to 6 minutes per side, depending on how hot your grill is.
6. Serve with additional barbecue sauce, if desired.

FODMAP ALERT *The Barbecue Sauce is not low-FODMAP. For a low-FODMAP option, try the Teriyaki Marinade (page 250), using green garlic or garlic scapes in place of crushed garlic.*

SPECIAL EQUIPMENT

- Gas or charcoal grill or grill pan

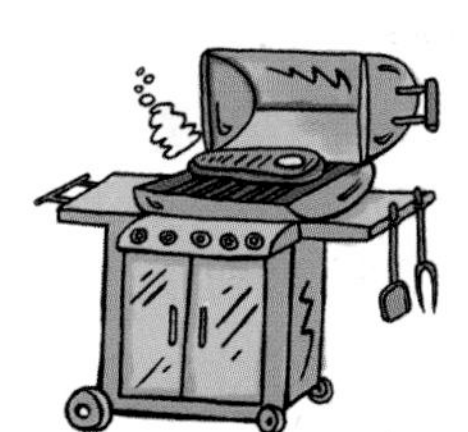

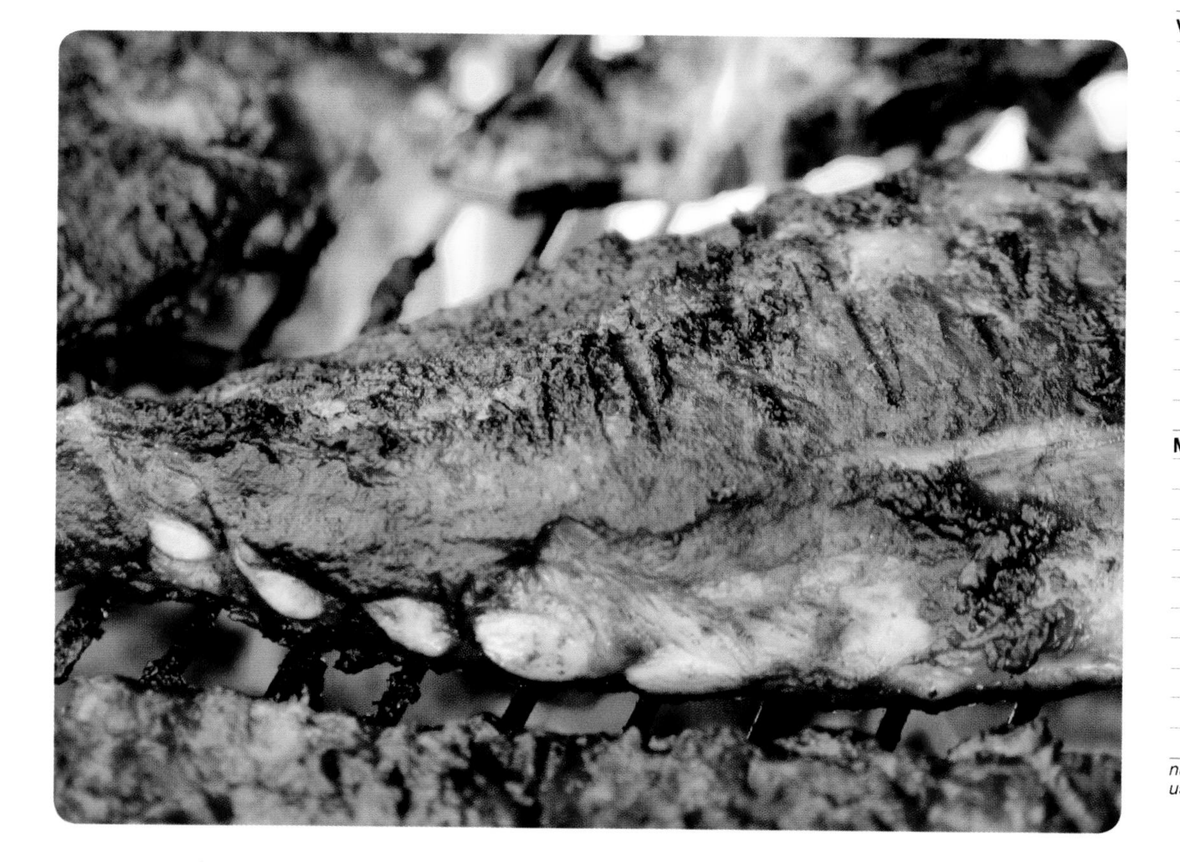

NUTRITION FACTS	
Serving Size	234 g
Recipe Yields	3269 g
Calories	**672**
Fats	**49.3 g**
MUFA	21.3 g
Omega-3	0.34 g
Omega-6	7.37 g
Saturated Fat	17.9 g
Carbohydrates	**1.32 g**
Fiber	0.06 g
Starch	0.06 g
Fructose	0.29 g
Glucose	0.23 g
Sucrose	0.37 g
Protein	**52.4 g**
Alanine	3 g
Arginine	3.37 g
Aspartic acid	4.9 g
Cystine	0.59 g
Glutamic acid	8 g
Glycine	2.37 g
Histidine	2.13 g
Isoleucine	2.48 g
Leucine	4.31 g
Lysine	4.65 g
Methionine	1.44 g
Phenylalanine	2.17 g
Proline	2.12 g
Serine	2.19 g
Threonine	2.3 g
Tryptophan	0.62 g
Tyrosine	2.07 g
Valine	2.65 g
Vitamins	
Vitamin B1	1.05 mg
Vitamin B12	1.68 mcg
Vitamin B2	0.75 mg
Vitamin B3	17.4 mg
Vitamin B5	2.88 mg
Vitamin B6	0.95 mg
Choline	179 mg
Folate	0.45 mcg
Vitamin A	13.7 mcg
Vitamin C	0.2 mg
Vitamin D	109 IU
Vitamin E	0.63 mg
Vitamin K	0.05 mcg
Minerals	
Calcium	108 mg
Copper	0.25 mg
Iron	2.17 mg
Magnesium	42.3 mg
Manganese	0.05 mg
Phosphorus	376 mg
Potassium	569 mg
Selenium	73.4 mcg
Sodium	242 mg
Zinc	6.99 mg

nutrition content estimated using the USDA database.

Greek-Inspired Lamb Chops

This Greek-inspired lamb recipe is the perfect accompaniment to Cauliflower Rice (page 298) and a simple salad of chopped cucumber, red onion, and olives tossed with Greek Salad Dressing (page 126).

PREP TIME: 5 to 10 minutes
COOK TIME: 8 to 16 minutes
SERVINGS: 4 to 6

INGREDIENTS:

- 3 cloves garlic, crushed
- 1 tablespoon finely grated lemon zest (about 1 lemon)
- 1 tablespoon minced fresh oregano
- ¼ teaspoon salt
- 2 pounds lamb chops (rib or loin)

FODMAP ALERT *Replace the garlic with green garlic or garlic scapes (green part only) or omit.*

1. Position an oven rack so that your lamb chops will be about 6 inches from the top element in your oven. Preheat the broiler on high for 10 minutes while you prepare the lamb.
2. Combine the crushed garlic, grated lemon zest, oregano, and salt.
3. Pat the lamb chops dry with paper towels and place on a roasting pan. Rub the seasoning mix all over the top and bottom of the chops.
4. Broil for 4 to 8 minutes per side (depending on the thickness of your lamb chops), until the internal temperature reaches 145°F for medium-rare or 160°F for medium.
5. Let the chops rest for 5 minutes. Enjoy!

VARIATIONS:

This Greek-style seasoning is very versatile. You can use it on chicken, pork, or lamb—from whole roasts to chunks for grilled kabobs, souvlaki style!

Chicken Souvlaki Skewers. Use this Greek-style seasoning on skewered chunks of chicken breast. Marinate for at least 2 hours, then grill over a hot barbecue until fully cooked. Serve with Tzatziki Sauce (page 258) and Russ' Flatbread (page 326).

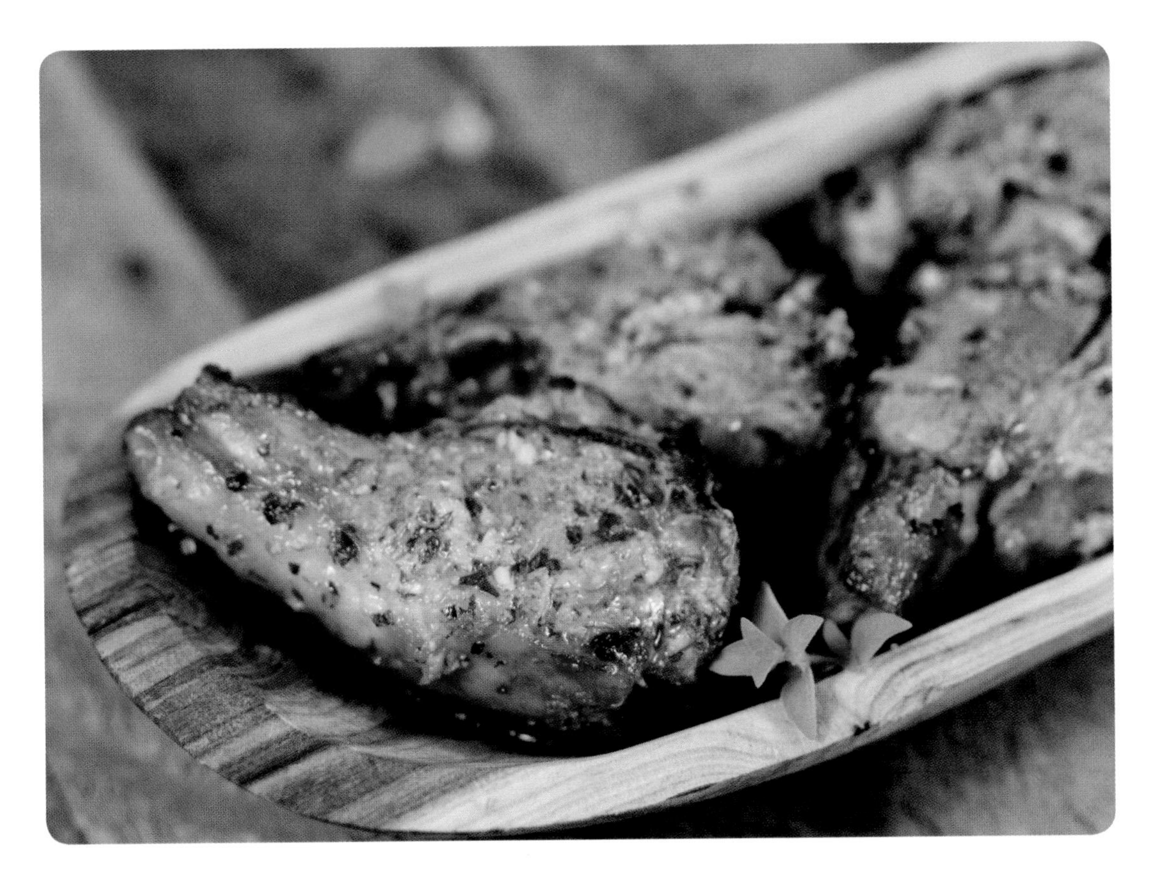

NUTRITION FACTS	
Serving Size	155 g
Recipe Yields	927 g
Calories	**204**
Fats	**7.46 g**
MUFA	3.08 g
Omega-3	0.11 g
Omega-6	0.24 g
Saturated Fat	2.96 g
Carbohydrates	**1 g**
Fiber	0.35 g
Starch	0.57 g
Fructose	<0.01 g
Glucose	<0.01 g
Sucrose	<0.01 g
Protein	**31.1 g**
Alanine	1.86 g
Arginine	1.85 g
Aspartic acid	2.73 g
Cystine	0.37 g
Glutamic acid	4.5 g
Glycine	1.51 g
Histidine	0.98 g
Isoleucine	1.5 g
Leucine	2.41 g
Lysine	2.74 g
Methionine	0.79 g
Phenylalanine	1.26 g
Proline	1.3 g
Serine	1.15 g
Threonine	1.32 g
Tryptophan	0.36 g
Tyrosine	1.04 g
Valine	1.67 g
Vitamins	
Vitamin B1	0.24 mg
Vitamin B12	4.55 mcg
Vitamin B2	0.49 mg
Vitamin B3	8.45 mg
Vitamin B5	0.82 mg
Vitamin B6	0.64 mg
Choline	0.59 mg
Folate	1.36 mcg
Vitamin A	0.46 mcg
Vitamin C	1.77 mg
Vitamin D	0 IU
Vitamin E	0.1 mg
Vitamin K	3.14 mcg
Minerals	
Calcium	26.2 mg
Copper	0.24 mg
Iron	3.4 mg
Magnesium	39.7 mg
Manganese	0.07 mg
Phosphorus	327 mg
Potassium	533 mg
Selenium	12.3 mcg
Sodium	140 mg
Zinc	5.45 mg

nutrition content estimated using the USDA database.

Simple Grilled Steak with Rhubarb Chutney

This chutney relies on fresh apple and orange juice to cut the sour rhubarb flavor. Pick a sweet variety of apple such as Fuji, Gala, or Honeycrisp. This recipe makes enough Rhubarb Chutney for about eight servings. If you wish, you can cook less steak and simply store the leftover chutney in the freezer or reinvent it as a dessert accompaniment for Parsnip Vanilla Custard (page 351).

PREP TIME: 15 minutes
COOK TIME: 30 to 40 minutes, plus 1 hour chilling time if desired
SERVINGS: 4

INGREDIENTS:

Rhubarb Chutney:

- 8 ounces rhubarb, cut into ½-inch-thick slices
- ¼ medium yellow onion, finely diced
- ½ apple, peeled, cored, and grated
- 1½ teaspoons finely grated orange zest
- 2 tablespoons fresh orange juice
- 2 tablespoons coconut water vinegar
- ¼ teaspoon peeled and grated fresh ginger
- ½ teaspoon ground cinnamon
- Pinch of ground cloves
- ¼ teaspoon salt

Steak:

- 4 (4- to 8-ounce) steaks
- 1 to 2 tablespoons Steak Spice (page 108)

FODMAP ALERT *Rhubarb chutney cannot be made low-FODMAP, so just stick with steak and season simply with truffle salt.*

SPECIAL EQUIPMENT

- Gas or charcoal grill or grill pan

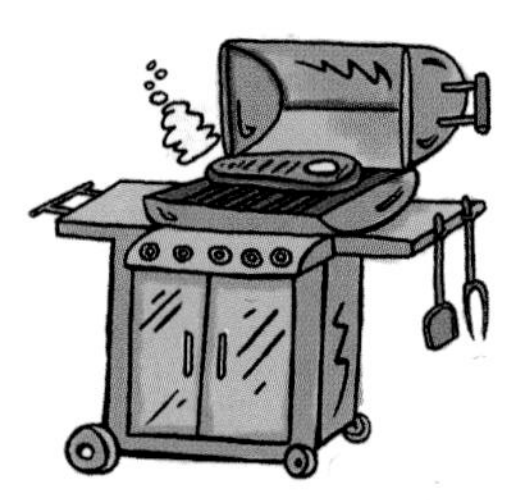

RHUBARB CHUTNEY:

1. Combine all the chutney ingredients in a saucepan.
2. Bring to a simmer over medium-high heat. Reduce the heat to medium-low and simmer uncovered until thick, approximately 30 minutes.
3. Serve warm or chill for 1 hour to serve cold.

STEAK:

1. Pat the steaks dry with paper towels and season with the steak spice.
2. Preheat a grill pan or a gas or charcoal grill. Once hot, place the steaks on the grill. Grill for 3 to 5 minutes per side, depending on how you like your steak cooked (see Tips) and how thick the steaks are.
3. Let the steaks rest for at least 5 minutes before serving.

TIPS:

You can use a barbecue-safe meat thermometer to check the temperature of your steak to guarantee that it's cooked to your liking.

Rare: 120°F to 125°F

Medium-rare: 130°F to 135°F

Medium: 140°F to 145°F

Medium-well: 150°F to 155°F

Well-done: 160°F and above

VARIATIONS:

Want to keep it simple? Instead of Steak Spice, use plain salt or truffle salt.

Instead of Rhubarb Chutney, try serving with Mango Salsa (page 242), Arugula Pesto (page 310), or Barbecue Sauce (page 124).

NUTRITION FACTS	
Serving Size	210 g
Recipe Yields	840 g
Calories	**259**
Fats	**10.5 g**
MUFA	4.24 g
Omega-3	0.07 g
Omega-6	0.35 g
Saturated Fat	4.04 g
Carbohydrates	**7.62 g**
Fiber	1.81 g
Starch	1.93 g
Fructose	1.33 g
Glucose	0.8 g
Sucrose	0.25 g
Protein	**32 g**
Alanine	1.9 g
Arginine	2.04 g
Aspartic acid	2.87 g
Cystine	0.4 g
Glutamic acid	4.71 g
Glycine	1.9 g
Histidine	1 g
Isoleucine	1.42 g
Leucine	2.49 g
Lysine	2.64 g
Methionine	0.81 g
Phenylalanine	1.24 g
Proline	1.5 g
Serine	1.23 g
Threonine	1.25 g
Tryptophan	0.21 g
Tyrosine	1 g
Valine	1.55 g
Vitamins	
Vitamin B1	0.11 mg
Vitamin B12	1.84 mcg
Vitamin B2	0.18 mg
Vitamin B3	8.56 mg
Vitamin B5	0.71 mg
Vitamin B6	0.69 mg
Choline	124 mg
Folate	17.8 mcg
Vitamin A	4.26 mcg
Vitamin C	10.9 mg
Vitamin D	7.44 IU
Vitamin E	0.65 mg
Vitamin K	18.9 mcg
Minerals	
Calcium	86 mg
Copper	0.13 mg
Iron	2.78 mg
Magnesium	37.9 mg
Manganese	0.29 mg
Phosphorus	260 mg
Potassium	622 mg
Selenium	34.7 mcg
Sodium	1148 mg
Zinc	5.78 mg

nutrition content estimated using the USDA database.

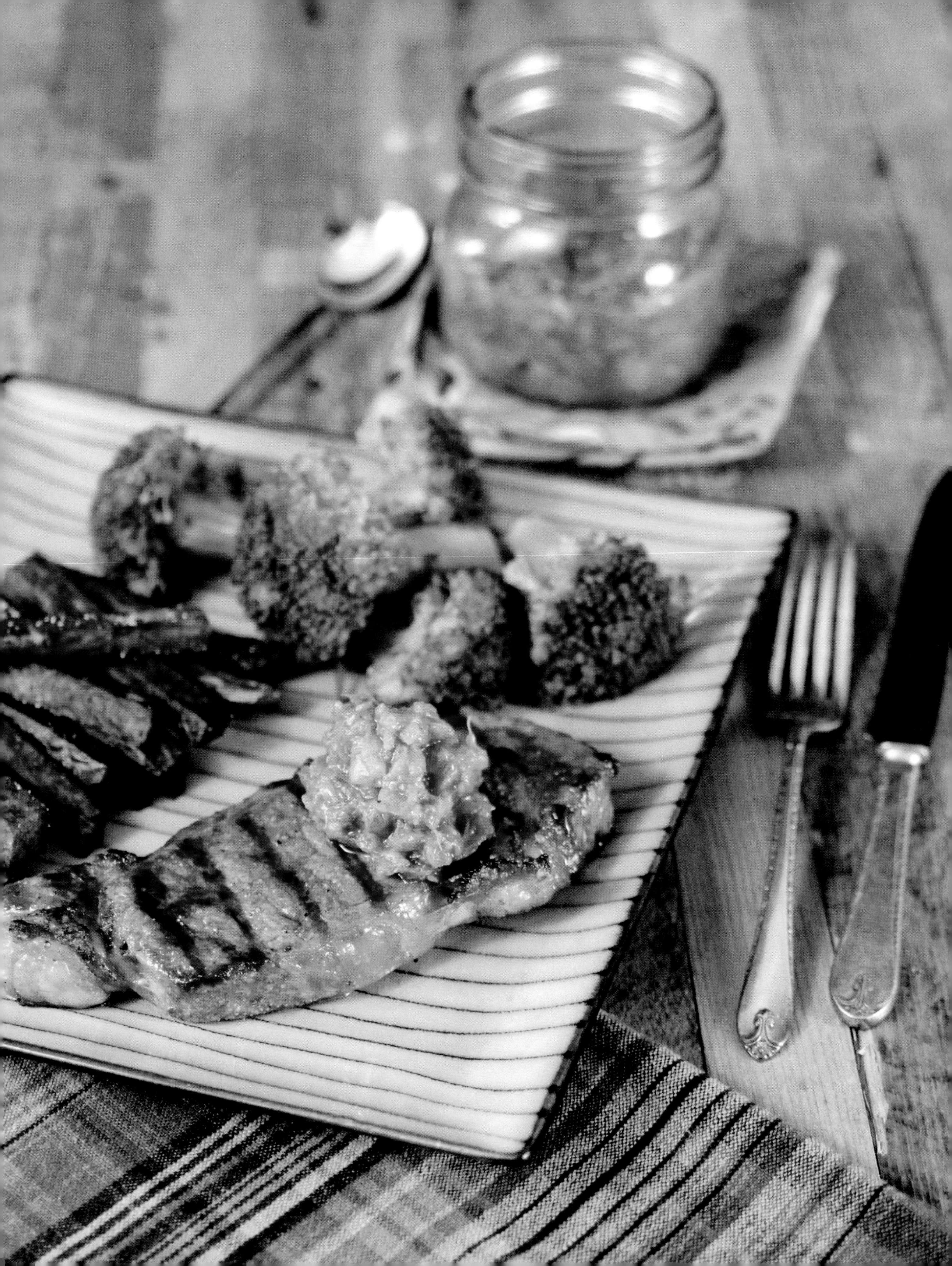

Braised Pork Chops with Apple and Fennel

Pork, apple, and fennel are about the most perfect flavor combination ever devised. This dish has all the comforts of pot roast and is equally good made with chops or uncured ham steaks. This recipe can also be made with pork shank, hocks, or even neck bones. These tougher cuts of meat require a slightly longer cooking time to become tender—try 1½ to 2 hours instead (you may want to set the vegetables aside and then add them to the pot for the last hour of cooking so they don't get mushy).

PREP TIME: 15 minutes
COOK TIME: 1 hour 15 minutes
SERVINGS: 4 to 6

INGREDIENTS:

- 2 pounds pork chops or uncured ham steaks (about 4 chops)
- 1 teaspoon ground mace
- 1 teaspoon ground cinnamon
- ½ teaspoon salt
- 2 to 4 tablespoons lard or other cooking fat
- 4 or 5 slices peeled fresh ginger
- 1 onion, cut into thick wedges
- 2 large fennel bulbs (approximately 1¼ to 1½ pounds), sliced into ½-inch- to ¾-inch-thick wedges (see Tips)
- 2 apples, peeled, cored, and cut into 1- to 2-inch chunks
- 1 bay leaf
- 1 cup dry white wine or Bone Broth (chicken, page 110)

FODMAP ALERT

This recipe cannot be made low-FODMAP.

SPECIAL EQUIPMENT

- Dutch oven

1. Preheat the oven to 300°F.
2. Pat the pork chops dry and season with the mace, cinnamon, and salt.
3. Heat 2 to 3 tablespoons of the lard in a large Dutch oven or saucepot over medium-high heat. Add the ginger slices and sauté for 3 to 4 minutes, until fragrant and starting to brown. Remove the ginger, if desired.
4. Brown the pork chops in batches, 2 to 3 minutes per side. Once browned, remove from the pot and set aside.
5. Add the onion and fennel to the pot (you may want to add an extra 1 to 2 tablespoons of cooking fat if the onion or fennel starts sticking to the pot). Cook, stirring frequently, until the onion and fennel are slightly browned and starting to soften, 8 to 10 minutes.
6. Add the apples, bay leaf, and wine and stir. Nestle the pork chops in among the vegetables, adding any juices the pork chops produced while they were set aside.
7. Place the pot in the oven and bake uncovered for 1 hour.

TIPS:

To slice fennel bulb, cut it into quarters. Slice out and discard the core. Slice the quarters into ½- to ¾-inch wedges. If the slices stick, gently pull them apart with your fingers. Fennel greens can be saved for salad or added to the pot for the last 20 minutes of cooking.

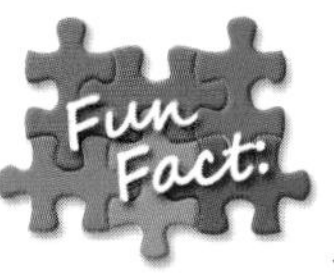

The best cooking apple varieties are Granny Smith, Fuji, and Rome Beauty because they hold their shape during cooking.

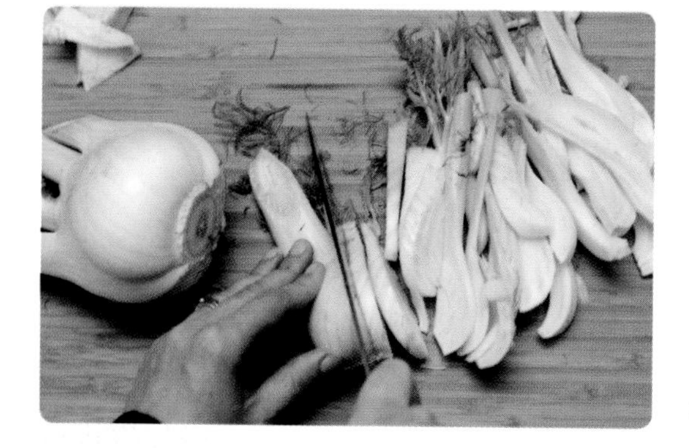

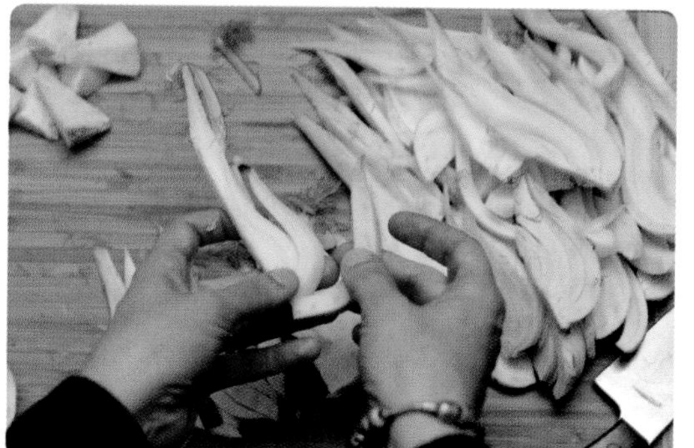

NUTRITION FACTS

Serving Size	313 g
Recipe Yields	1875 g
Calories	**409**
Fats	**21.5 g**
MUFA	7.95 g
Omega-3	0.11 g
Omega-6	1.81 g
Saturated Fat	6.77 g
Carbohydrates	**16.5 g**
Fiber	3.78 g
Starch	1.93 g
Fructose	3.48 g
Glucose	2.11 g
Sucrose	0.62 g
Protein	**38.9 g**
Alanine	2.16 g
Arginine	2.44 g
Aspartic acid	3.56 g
Cystine	0.42 g
Glutamic acid	5.79 g
Glycine	1.7 g
Histidine	1.53 g
Isoleucine	1.78 g
Leucine	3.1 g
Lysine	3.35 g
Methionine	1.03 g
Phenylalanine	1.57 g
Proline	1.52 g
Serine	1.58 g
Threonine	1.66 g
Tryptophan	0.45 g
Tyrosine	1.49 g
Valine	1.91 g
Vitamins	
Vitamin B1	0.99 mg
Vitamin B12	1.03 mcg
Vitamin B2	0.43 mg
Vitamin B3	12.3 mg
Vitamin B5	1.98 mg
Vitamin B6	0.87 mg
Choline	124 mg
Folate	25.3 mcg
Vitamin A	45.1 mcg
Vitamin C	13.1 mg
Vitamin D	48.3 IU
Vitamin E	0.84 mg
Vitamin K	49.6 mcg
Minerals	
Calcium	64.8 mg
Copper	0.19 mg
Iron	2.64 mg
Magnesium	55.6 mg
Manganese	0.3 mg
Phosphorus	463 mg
Potassium	1032 mg
Selenium	68.2 mcg
Sodium	216 mg
Zinc	3.76 mg

nutrition content estimated using the USDA database.

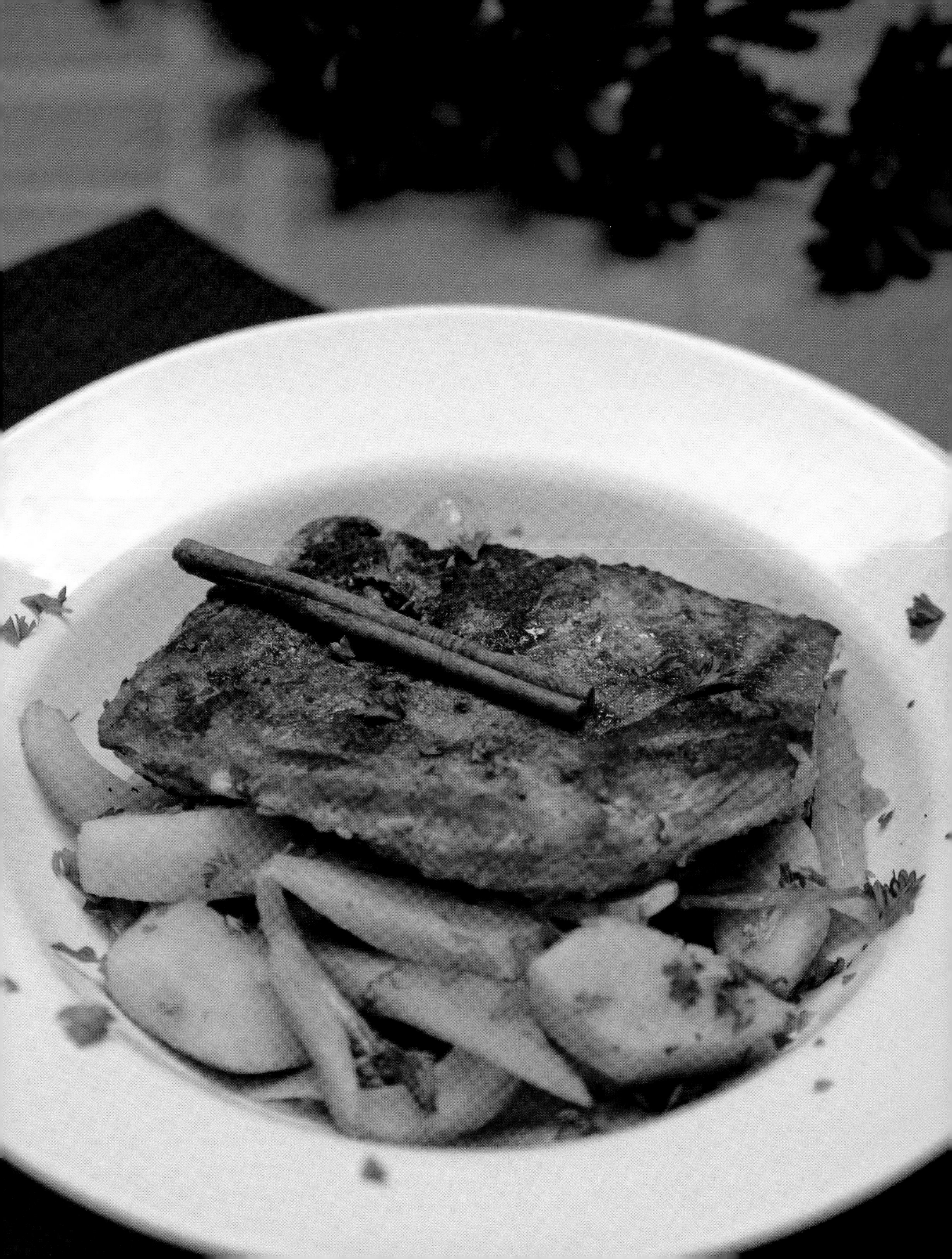

Bacon-Apple Chicken Burgers with Maple-Cranberry Sauce

The words "life-changing" have been used to describe these burgers. The combination of flavors is absolutely exquisite. And the best part? The leftovers make an amazing breakfast!

PREP TIME: 15 minutes
COOK TIME: 1 hour 15 minutes
SERVINGS: 4 to 6

INGREDIENTS:

Maple-Cranberry Sauce:

2 cups fresh or frozen cranberries

½ cup grade B maple syrup

¼ cup water

Bacon-Apple Chicken Burgers:

8 to 10 ounces bacon (if using 2½ pounds ground chicken, use 10 ounces bacon)

1 medium onion, minced

1 large cooking apple, peeled, cored, and minced

2 teaspoons minced fresh rosemary

2 to 2½ pounds ground chicken

½ teaspoon salt or truffle salt

1 tablespoon bacon fat or other cooking fat, if needed

FODMAP ALERT

Bacon-Apple Chicken Burgers cannot be made low-FODMAP.

MAPLE-CRANBERRY SAUCE:

1. Combine the cranberries, maple syrup, and water in a small saucepan.
2. Bring to a boil over high heat, then reduce the heat to maintain a simmer.
3. Simmer uncovered for 8 to 10 minutes, stirring occasionally, until most of the berries have popped and the sauce has thickened.
4. Transfer to a serving bowl and refrigerate for at least 1 hour before serving.

BACON-APPLE CHICKEN BURGERS:

1. Place the bacon in a cold skillet, then turn on the heat to medium-high. Cook, flipping once or twice, until the bacon is crispy.
2. When the bacon is crispy, remove it from the pan. Add the onion to the bacon fat in the pan and sauté for 5 minutes over medium-high heat, stirring occasionally, until the onion is starting to soften. Add the apple and rosemary and continue sautéing until the onion is browned and both the onion and apple are soft, 5 to 8 more minutes. Remove from the pan with a slotted spoon and allow to cool slightly. Do not clean the pan; you will be using it to cook the burgers.
3. Once the bacon has cooled enough to handle, chop into small pieces (think bacon bit size).
4. Combine the ground chicken, bacon, apple and onion mix, and salt in a bowl. Mix well with your hands and form into 6- to 8-ounce patties.
5. Preheat the pan over medium heat. If there is no more bacon fat left in the pan, add a tablespoon of bacon fat or other cooking fat. Fry the patties in the pan, in batches if needed so as not to overcrowd, until fully cooked, 15 to 25 minutes total, flipping once. To be sure that the meat is fully cooked, check the internal temperature with a meat thermometer; it should read 160°F.
6. Serve with chilled maple-cranberry sauce!

TIPS:

Good cooking apple varieties are Granny Smith, Fuji, and Rome Beauty. They hold their shape when cooked rather than turning to mush, which yields a nicer texture in the finished burgers.

VARIATIONS:

You can also make these burgers with ground turkey or ground pork.

NUTRITION FACTS

Serving Size	308 g
Recipe Yields	1848 g
Calories	**600**
Fats	**33 g**
MUFA	14.6 g
Omega-3	0.3 g
Omega-6	4.41 g
Saturated Fat	10.1 g
Carbohydrates	**28.1 g**
Fiber	2.61 g
Starch	1.83 g
Fructose	2.37 g
Glucose	2.61 g
Sucrose	16.2 g
Protein	**49.1 g**
Alanine	2.89 g
Arginine	3.19 g
Aspartic acid	4.63 g
Cystine	0.53 g
Glutamic acid	7.36 g
Glycine	2.66 g
Histidine	1.59 g
Isoleucine	2.25 g
Leucine	3.82 g
Lysine	4.19 g
Methionine	1.2 g
Phenylalanine	1.93 g
Proline	2.08 g
Serine	2.01 g
Threonine	2.01 g
Tryptophan	0.41 g
Tyrosine	1.66 g
Valine	2.41 g
Vitamins	
Vitamin B1	0.35 mg
Vitamin B12	1.21 mcg
Vitamin B2	0.9 mg
Vitamin B3	14.9 mg
Vitamin B5	2.55 mg
Vitamin B6	0.99 mg
Choline	139 mg
Folate	8.76 mcg
Vitamin A	6.41 mcg
Vitamin C	7.24 mg
Vitamin D	0 IU
Vitamin E	1.17 mg
Vitamin K	5.65 mcg
Minerals	
Calcium	53.1 mg
Copper	0.2 mg
Iron	2.67 mg
Magnesium	64.8 mg
Manganese	0.95 mg
Phosphorus	559 mg
Potassium	1375 mg
Selenium	44.2 mcg
Sodium	1033 mg
Zinc	4.64 mg

nutrition content estimated using the USDA database.

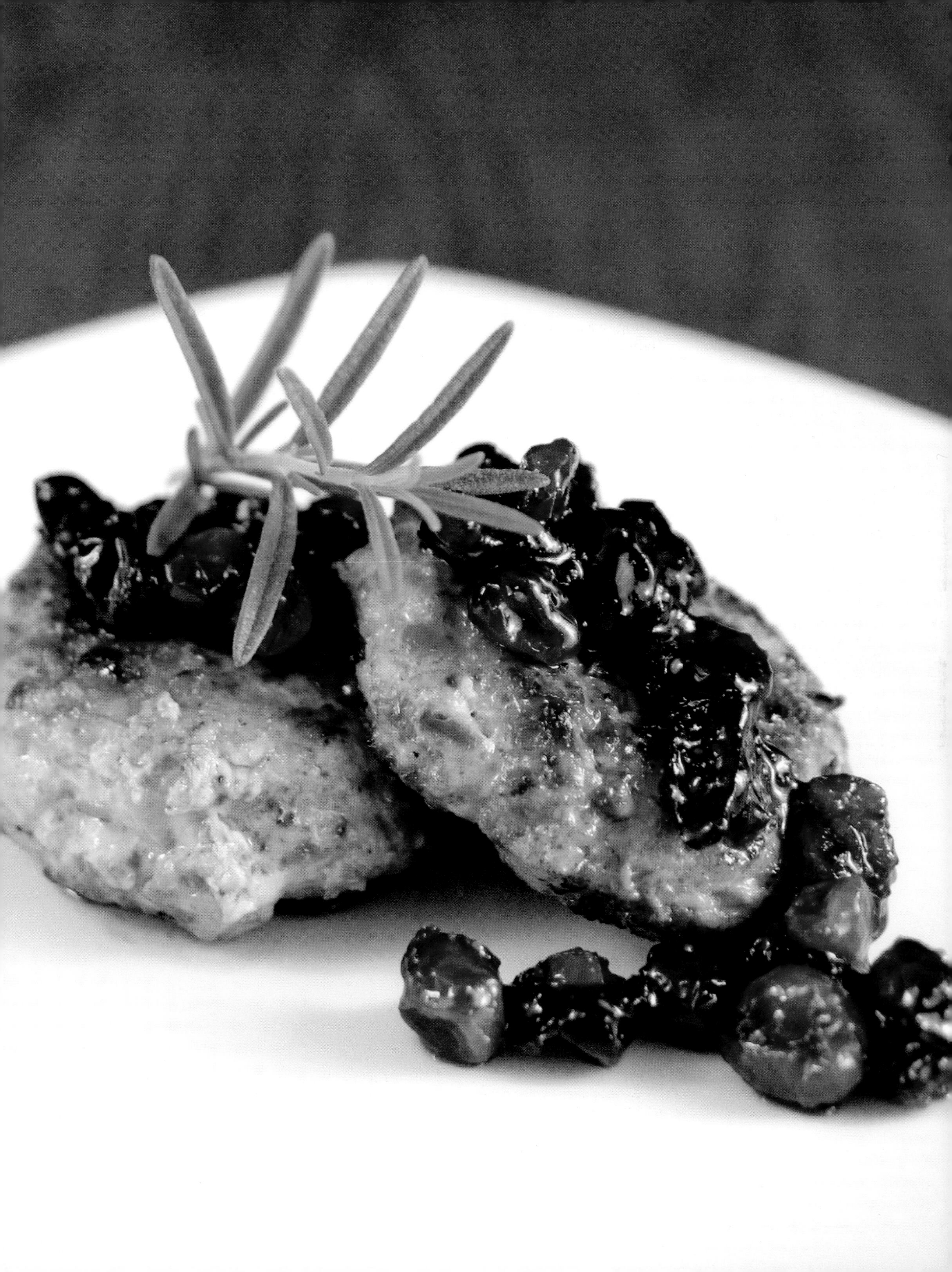

"Spaghetti"

Don't think that spaghetti without tomatoes is pointless! Red wine and/or fish sauce give this dish that great umami flavor that tomatoes typically provide, and the combination of oregano, basil, garlic, and olives lend a wonderful familiarity to the sauce.

Spaghetti squash is a very mild-tasting squash with naturally long strings that mimic spaghetti noodles very well. If you prefer, you could use your favorite spiral-cut or julienned vegetables instead. Or just chop some of your favorite vegetables and add them to the pot at the same time as the mushrooms (zucchini, carrots, butternut squash, sweet potatoes, and even kale and spinach are all great additions) to turn this into more of a one-pot meal.

PREP TIME: 15 minutes
COOK TIME: 30 minutes to 1½ hours
SERVINGS: 4 to 5

INGREDIENTS:

- 3 to 4 pounds spaghetti squash (2 small or 1 large)
- 1 pound ground beef
- 1 pound ground lamb
- 1 medium onion
- 10 to 12 cloves garlic, sliced
- ½ pound mushrooms, sliced
- ½ cup red wine or Bone Broth (beef, page 110)
- 1 teaspoon fish sauce
- 1 cup sliced black olives (1 [4-ounce] can)
- ¼ cup chopped fresh basil
- ¼ cup chopped fresh oregano
- 2 tablespoons kuzu starch or arrowroot powder
- 2 tablespoons cold water
- Salt, to taste

FODMAP ALERT *Replace the garlic with green garlic or garlic scapes (green part only) or omit. Replace the onion with green onion or leek (green part only) or chives or omit. Omit the mushrooms.*

SPECIAL EQUIPMENT

- Large skillet

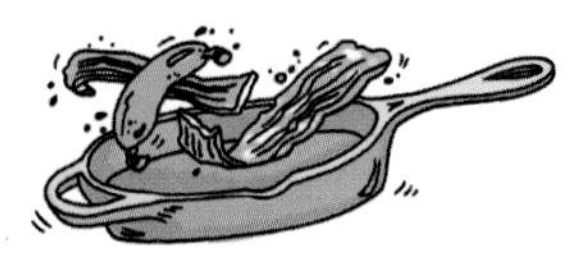

1. Pierce the spaghetti squash all over with a fork. Cook the squash whole in the microwave for 10 to 15 minutes or in a preheated 375°F oven for 45 minutes to 1 hour.
2. Let the spaghetti squash cool. Cut in half lengthwise. Spoon out the seeds and discard. Scrape out the noodlelike strings with a fork (a fun way to serve this is right in the rind!).
3. Meanwhile, brown the meat, onion, and garlic in a large skillet over medium-high heat, about 10 minutes.
4. Once the meat is cooked, add the mushrooms, wine, and fish sauce.
5. Reduce the heat to medium. Cook for 7 to 10 minutes, until the mushrooms are cooked, stirring occasionally.
6. Add the olives, basil, and oregano. Simmer for 1 to 2 minutes.
7. Mix the kuzu starch with the cold water. Add to the meat, stirring quickly. Simmer for 1 to 2 more minutes, until the liquid has completely thickened. Taste and season with salt if desired. Serve on the spaghetti squash noodles.

TIPS:

Simmering the wine removes the majority of the alcohol. However, if you know that you are very sensitive to alcohol, use broth instead.

VARIATIONS:

This dish is an excellent opportunity to hide some organ meat. Replace one-quarter to one-half of the ground meat with ground liver or ground heart.

Serve with Zucchini Noodles (page 310) instead of spaghetti squash.

Spaghetti Squash Noodles. *Want to use spaghetti squash as a noddle substitute in another dish? Simply follow steps 1 and 2! They make a delicious side dish tossed with Bacon Bits (page 120) and with fresh chopped sage leaves that have been sautéed in a little bacon fat until crispy.*

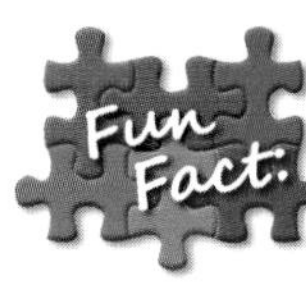

Olives, apricots, spinach, and dandelion greens are excellent plant sources of vitamin E.

NUTRITION FACTS	
Serving Size	693 g
Recipe Yields	3467 g
Calories	**605**
Fats	**31 g**
MUFA	14 g
Omega-3	0.55 g
Omega-6	1.48 g
Saturated Fat	11.5 g
Carbohydrates	**37.2 g**
Fiber	7.76 g
Starch	13.1 g
Fructose	0.37 g
Glucose	1.12 g
Sucrose	0.22 g
Protein	**42.8 g**
Alanine	2.6 g
Arginine	2.67 g
Aspartic acid	3.79 g
Cystine	0.44 g
Glutamic acid	6.26 g
Glycine	2.63 g
Histidine	1.28 g
Isoleucine	1.9 g
Leucine	3.18 g
Lysine	3.37 g
Methionine	1 g
Phenylalanine	1.68 g
Proline	2.05 g
Serine	1.66 g
Threonine	1.65 g
Tryptophan	0.33 g
Tyrosine	1.31 g
Valine	2.18 g
Vitamins	
Vitamin B1	0.32 mg
Vitamin B12	3.9 mcg
Vitamin B2	0.61 mg
Vitamin B3	13.3 mg
Vitamin B5	3.11 mg
Vitamin B6	0.96 mg
Choline	176 mg
Folate	66 mcg
Vitamin A	32.7 mcg
Vitamin C	19.2 mg
Vitamin D	11.7 IU
Vitamin E	1.49 mg
Vitamin K	17.8 mcg
Minerals	
Calcium	176 mg
Copper	0.53 mg
Iron	6.36 mg
Magnesium	92.2 mg
Manganese	0.7 mg
Phosphorus	401 mg
Potassium	1169 mg
Selenium	42 mcg
Sodium	479 mg
Zinc	9.67 mg

nutrition content estimated using the USDA database.

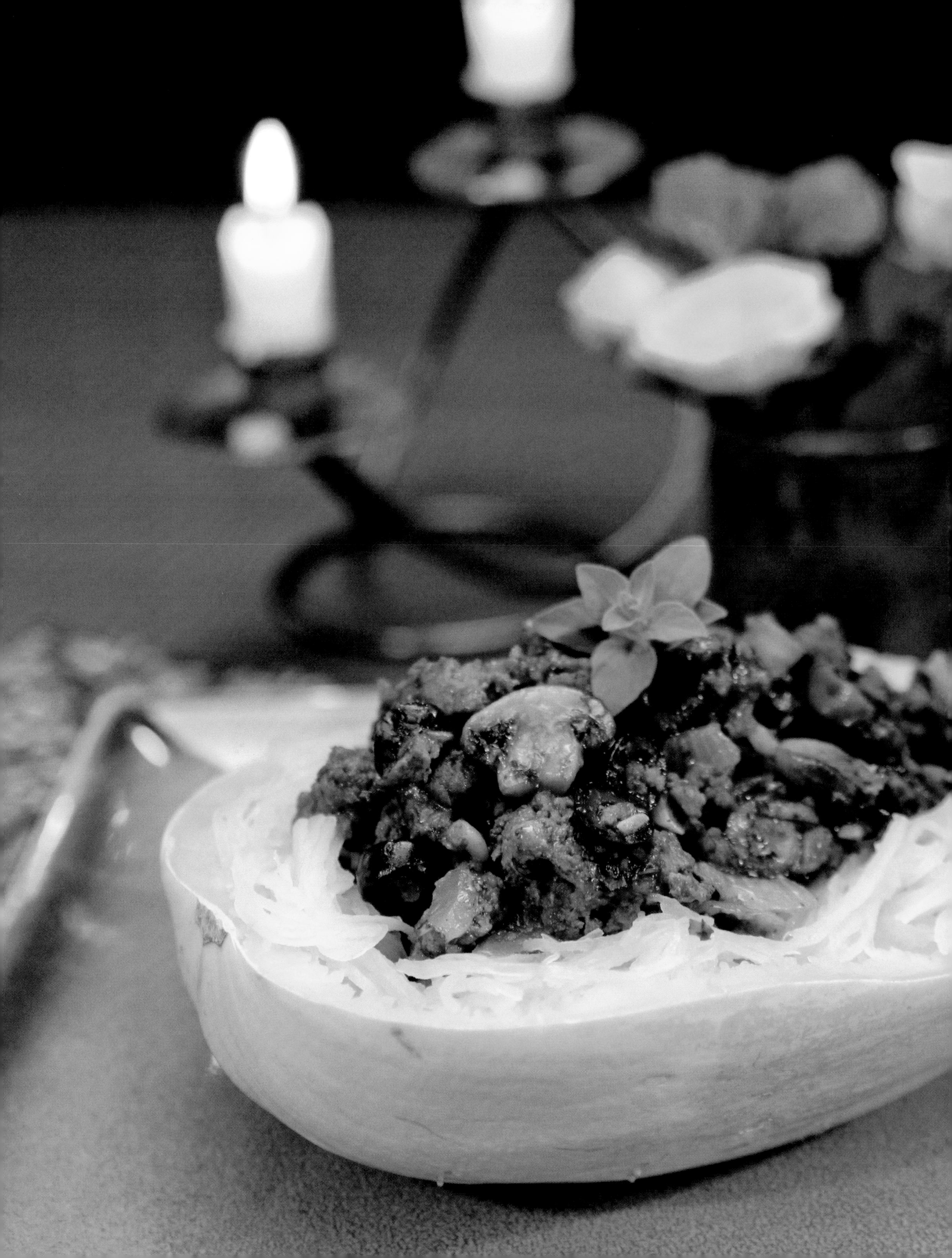

Sweet Potato Linguine with Bolognese Sauce

This modification of a traditional Bolognese sauce relies on umeboshi paste and tamarind paste to replace tomatoes, while employing traditional cooking techniques to fully embrace the flavors. Sweet potato noodles make a great pasta substitute.

PREP TIME: 20 to 30 minutes
COOK TIME: 4½ hours
SERVINGS: 6 to 8

INGREDIENTS:

Bolognese Sauce:

- 2 tablespoons tallow or other cooking fat
- 1 large onion, finely diced
- 4 carrots, finely diced
- 4 stalks celery, finely diced
- 4 cloves garlic, minced
- 1½ teaspoons salt, plus more to taste
- 4 ounces pancetta, ham, or Canadian bacon, finely diced
- 2 pounds lean ground beef (or a combination of veal, pork, and beef)
- 1 cup dry white wine
- 2 cups Bone Broth (beef, page 110)
- 1⅔ cups homemade Coconut Milk (page 116) or 1 (13½-ounce) can full-fat coconut milk
- ⅓ cup umeboshi paste
- ⅓ cup tamarind paste

Sweet Potato Linguine:

- 6 to 8 sweet potatoes (look for long ones)
- ½ cup coconut oil (or use oil from Bolognese Sauce)
- ½ cup nutritional yeast, for serving (optional)

FODMAP ALERT

This recipe cannot be made low-FODMAP.

BOLOGNESE SAUCE:

1. Heat the tallow in a large saucepan over medium heat. Once hot, add the onion, carrots, celery, garlic, and ½ teaspoon of the salt. Sauté for 5 minutes, stirring often.
2. Add the diced pancetta and cook for 10 more minutes, until the vegetables are softened and the pancetta is golden.
3. Increase the heat to high and add the meat a third at a time, stirring and breaking up lumps with a spoon after each addition.
4. Once the meat is fully browned, continue to cook for 15 minutes, stirring frequently, to caramelize.
5. Reduce the heat to medium and add the white wine. With a wooden spoon, scrape all the brown bits stuck to the bottom of the pan.
6. Add the broth, coconut milk, umeboshi paste, tamarind paste, and 1 teaspoon of the salt. Bring to a boil, then lower the heat to the lowest setting and simmer very slowly, half-covered, for 4 hours. Stir once in a while. If the sauce starts sticking before the end of the cooking time, add a bit of broth or water.
7. Taste and add a little more salt if desired. Set aside while you make the linguine.

SWEET POTATO LINGUINE:

1. Peel the sweet potatoes and slice lengthwise as thinly as possible (a mandoline slicer works well, but you can do this with a sharp chef's knife, too). Then cut each slice into long, thin strips about ¼ to ½ inch wide. The longer your sweet potato, the longer your "linguine" noodles will be.
2. Heat the coconut oil in a large skillet over medium heat. Add the sweet potato strips to the oil. Stir gently until the sweet potatoes are tender, 3 to 5 minutes.
3. Serve the sauce tossed with the sweet potato noodles. Add 1 to 2 tablespoons of the nutritional yeast per serving, if desired.

TIPS:

The Sweet Potato Linguine has the best texture when freshly made. If you do not plan on serving the entire batch in one meal, make only enough sweet potatoes for each meal (about 1 sweet potato per person).

VARIATIONS:

This recipe is also excellent with ground heart—beef, lamb, or pork—instead of ground beef.

NUTRITION FACTS	
Serving Size	453 g
Recipe Yields	3627 g
Calories	**701**
Fats	**48.1 g**
MUFA	12 g
Omega-3	0.14 g
Omega-6	1.29 g
Saturated Fat	30.2 g
Carbohydrates	**30.9 g**
Fiber	5.03 g
Starch	7.55 g
Fructose	0.94 g
Glucose	1.28 g
Sucrose	5.23 g
Protein	**33.6 g**
Alanine	2.04 g
Arginine	2.19 g
Aspartic acid	3.26 g
Cystine	0.37 g
Glutamic acid	4.93 g
Glycine	2.21 g
Histidine	1.03 g
Isoleucine	1.43 g
Leucine	2.5 g
Lysine	2.6 g
Methionine	0.81 g
Phenylalanine	1.33 g
Proline	1.66 g
Serine	1.36 g
Threonine	1.34 g
Tryptophan	0.2 g
Tyrosine	0.98 g
Valine	1.62 g
Vitamins	
Vitamin B1	0.31 mg
Vitamin B12	3.19 mcg
Vitamin B2	0.38 mg
Vitamin B3	9.44 mg
Vitamin B5	1.76 mg
Vitamin B6	0.82 mg
Choline	124 mg
Folate	40.9 mcg
Vitamin A	1080 mcg
Vitamin C	21.7 mg
Vitamin D	13.64 IU
Vitamin E	1.51 mg
Vitamin K	14 mcg
Minerals	
Calcium	101 mg
Copper	0.38 mg
Iron	4.54 mg
Magnesium	81.2 mg
Manganese	0.98 mg
Phosphorus	371 mg
Potassium	1214 mg
Selenium	28.3 mcg
Sodium	1089 mg
Zinc	7.91 mg

nutrition content estimated using the USDA database.

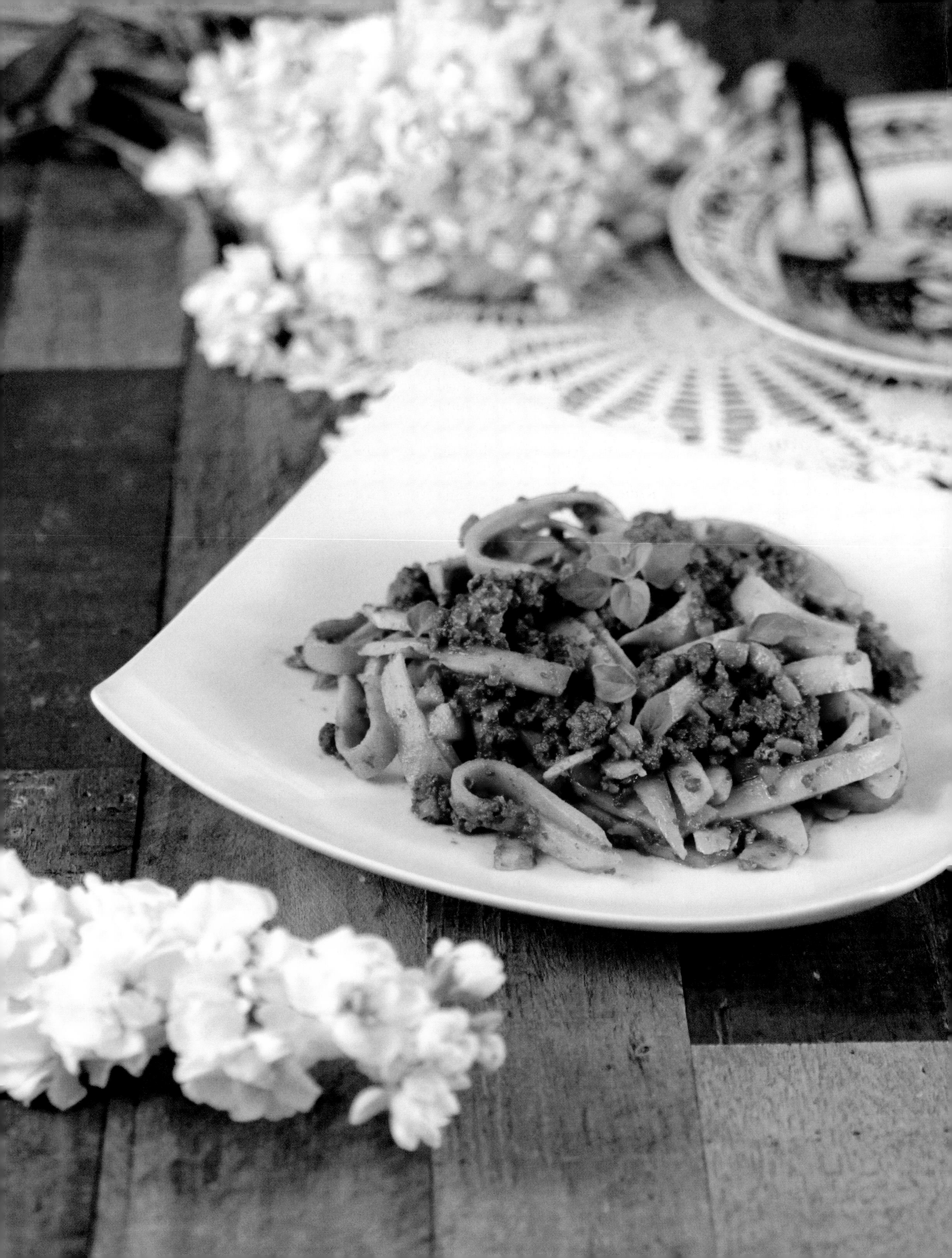

Burgers with Caramelized Onions and Portobello "Buns"

Bunless burgers are a super easy and quick meal to prepare. Adding caramelized onions and portobello mushroom cap "buns" turns this staple into something very special. And if you are mourning the loss of ketchup and mustard as condiments, these burgers are fantastic when served with Guacamole (page 171), Marrow Spread (page 267), or Barbecue Sauce (page 124).

PREP TIME: 20 minutes
COOK TIME: 12 to 25 minutes
SERVINGS: 2 to 3

INGREDIENTS:

Caramelized Onions:

- 2 to 3 tablespoons tallow, lard, or duck fat
- 2 large onions, cut into ¼-inch half-moons

Portobello "Buns":

- 3 tablespoons avocado oil
- 3 tablespoons balsamic vinegar
- 4 to 6 portobello mushroom caps, stems removed (see Tips)

Hamburgers:

- 1 pound ground beef
- Truffle salt (optional)

FODMAP ALERT

This recipe cannot be made low FODMAP.

SPECIAL EQUIPMENT

- Gas or charcoal grill or grill pan

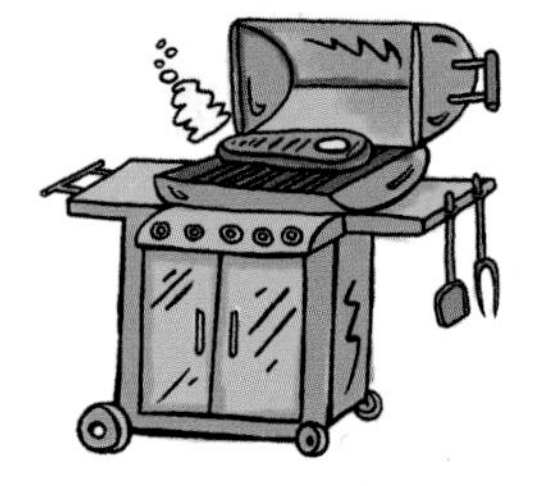

CARAMELIZED ONIONS AND PORTOBELLO "BUNS":

1. Preheat a grill pan or a gas or charcoal grill to medium-high heat.
2. Make the caramelized onions: Heat 2 tablespoons of the tallow in a large skillet over medium-high heat.
3. Add the onions and cook, stirring occasionally, until soft and browned, 10 to 12 minutes. If they start to stick, add an extra tablespoon of tallow.
4. Meanwhile, grill the portobellos: Mix the avocado oil and balsamic vinegar in a small bowl. Use a marinating or pastry brush to brush both sides of each mushroom cap, being most generous on the lamella (gill) side.
5. Grill for 3 to 5 minutes per side, until grill marks form and the mushrooms are fully cooked.

HAMBURGERS:

1. Maintain the grill at medium-high heat. Form 5- to 8-ounce hamburger patties with your hands. Sprinkle with the truffle salt, if desired.
2. Grill for 6 to 8 minutes per side, until cooked to your liking.
3. Serve the burgers inside the portobello "buns" with the caramelized onions and your favorite extras.

TIPS:

Save the portobello mushroom stems for stew, or chop them and add them to the skillet at the same time as the onions.

If you find the portobello mushroom caps to be a little slippery as "buns," try putting the whole burger into a couple of leaves of lettuce. Or just eat it with a knife and fork.

VARIATIONS:

Ground heart meat can easily replace some or all of the ground beef when you are making burgers.

You can also fry the burgers and portobello mushroom caps in a skillet on the stovetop if you don't have a grill pan or an outdoor grill.

Brush both sides of the burgers with Barbecue Sauce (page 124) before grilling.

NUTRITION FACTS	
Serving Size	402 g
Recipe Yields	1206 g
Calories	**723**
Fats	**60.8 g**
MUFA	30.1 g
Omega-3	0.3 g
Omega-6	2.94 g
Saturated Fat	20.4 g
Carbohydrates	**16.4 g**
Fiber	3.16 g
Starch	3.48 g
Fructose	3.02 g
Glucose	5.43 g
Sucrose	0.99 g
Protein	**27.4 g**
Alanine	1.76 g
Arginine	1.8 g
Aspartic acid	2.48 g
Cystine	0.25 g
Glutamic acid	4.15 g
Glycine	1.96 g
Histidine	0.83 g
Isoleucine	1.17 g
Leucine	2.03 g
Lysine	2.14 g
Methionine	0.63 g
Phenylalanine	1.06 g
Proline	1.44 g
Serine	1.1 g
Threonine	1.04 g
Tryptophan	0.15 g
Tyrosine	0.74 g
Valine	1.28 g
Vitamins	
Vitamin B1	0.18 mg
Vitamin B12	3.25 mcg
Vitamin B2	0.39 mg
Vitamin B3	10.9 mg
Vitamin B5	2.09 mg
Vitamin B6	0.74 mg
Choline	115 mg
Folate	62.5 mcg
Vitamin A	0 mcg
Vitamin C	7.4 mg
Vitamin D	21.2 IU
Vitamin E	0.95 mg
Vitamin K	4.03 mcg
Minerals	
Calcium	62.9 mg
Copper	0.45 mg
Iron	3.63 mg
Magnesium	34.6 mg
Manganese	0.24 mg
Phosphorus	372 mg
Potassium	942 mg
Selenium	43 mcg
Sodium	162 mg
Zinc	6.63 mg

nutrition content estimated using the USDA database.

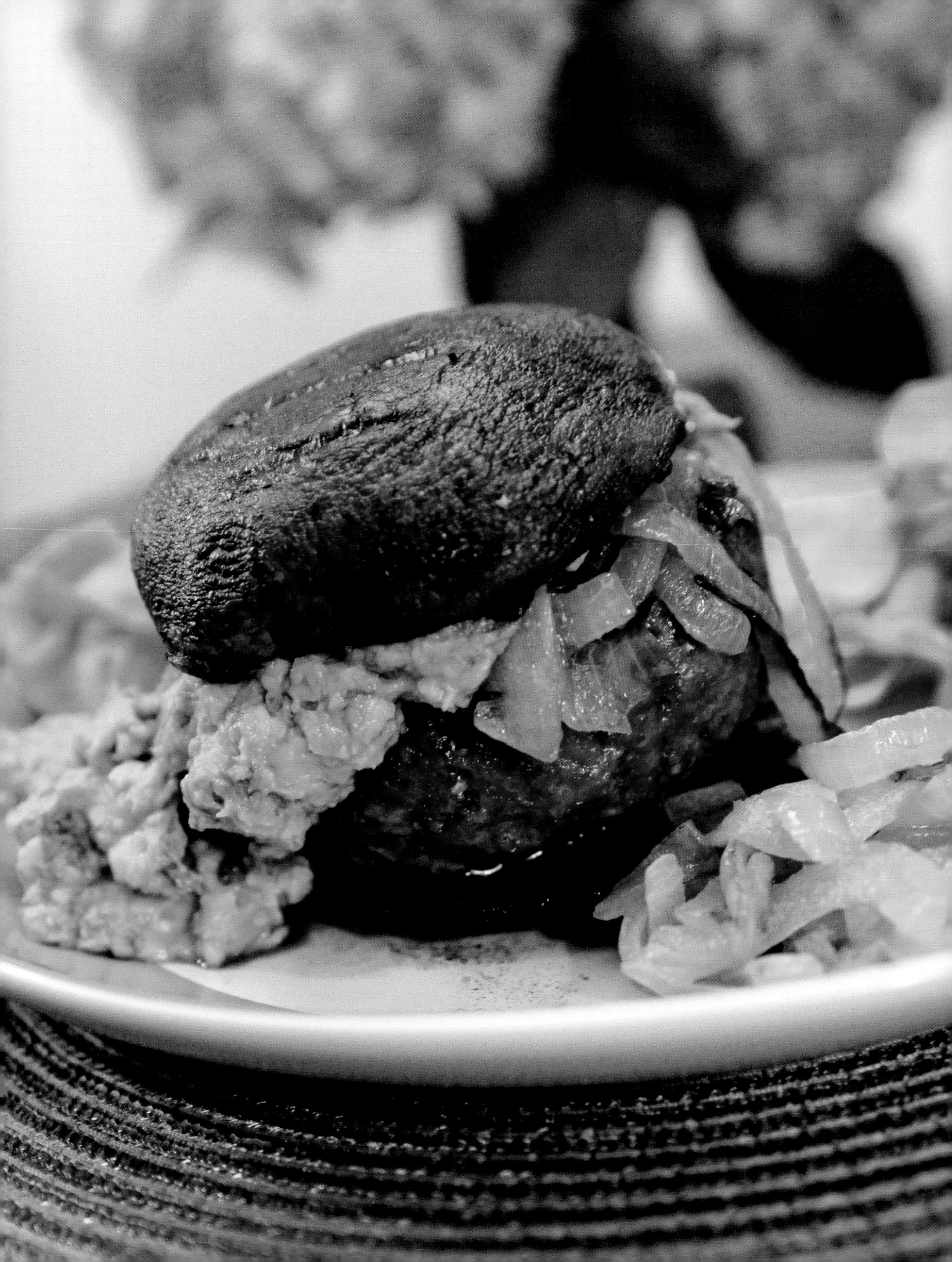

Lemon and Thyme Broiled Pork Chops

The best part about these pork chops (besides the fact that they taste delicious!) is that they are very quick to prepare and cook. They are absolutely delicious with homemade Applesauce (page 122).

PREP TIME: 5 to 10 minutes
COOK TIME: 10 to 16 minutes
SERVINGS: 4 to 6

INGREDIENTS:

- 1 tablespoon chopped fresh thyme
- 1 tablespoon finely grated lemon zest (about 1 lemon)
- ½ teaspoon salt
- 2 pounds pork chops (bone-in or boneless)

1. Position an oven rack so that the pork chops will be about 6 inches from the top element. Preheat the broiler on high for 10 minutes while you prepare the chops.
2. Combine the thyme, lemon zest, and salt.
3. Pat the pork chops dry with paper towels and place on a roasting pan. Rub the seasoning all over the chops.
4. Broil for 5 to 8 minutes per side (depending on the thickness of the pork chops), until the internal temperature reaches at least 145°F.
5. Let rest for 5 minutes. Enjoy!

VARIATIONS:

This seasoning also works very well with poultry and fish.

You can easily substitute other seasonings on these pork chops, too. Tarragon Salt (page 108) is particularly good.

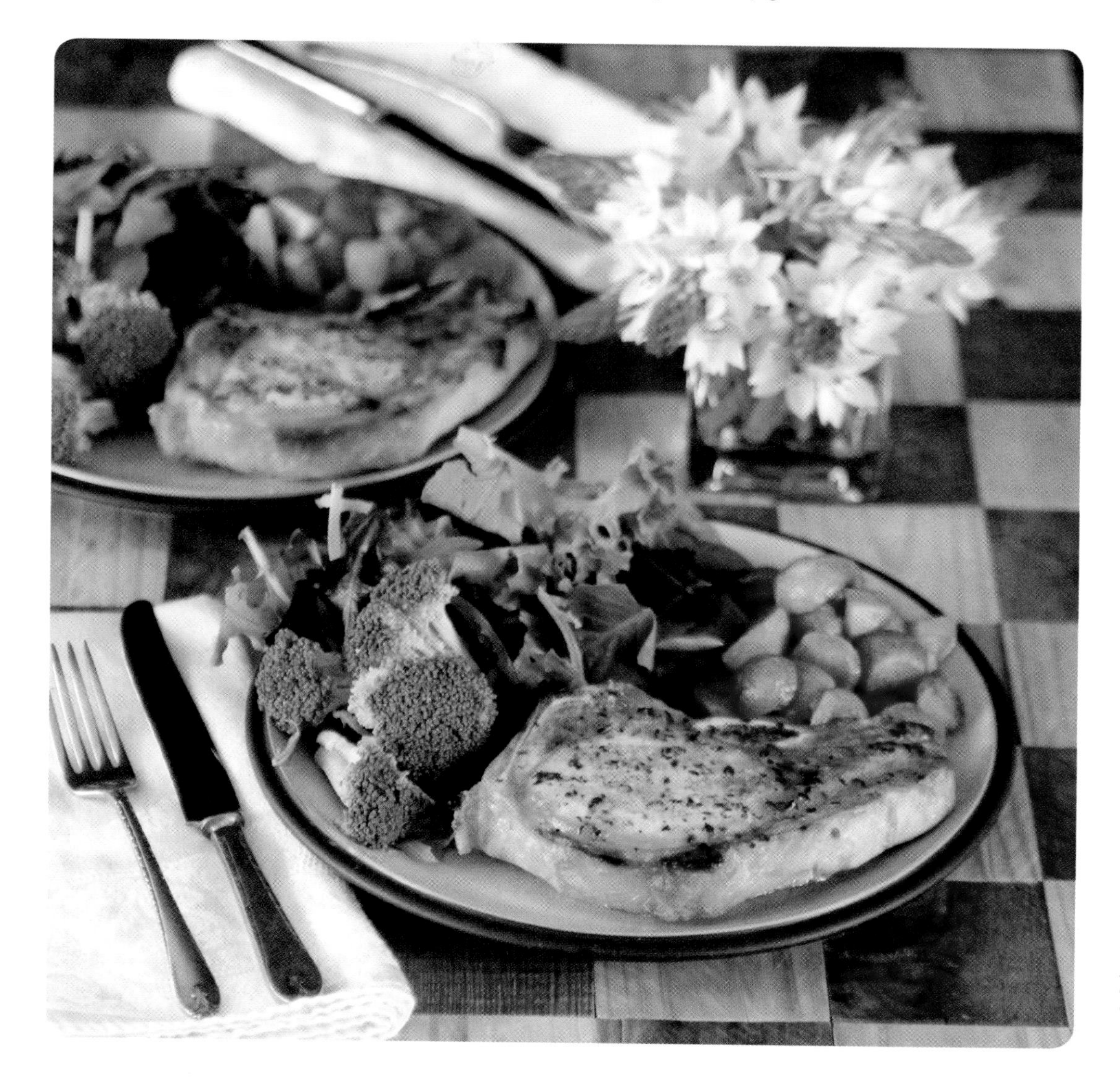

NUTRITION FACTS	
Serving Size	153 g
Recipe Yields	918 g
Calories	**306**
Fats	**16.8 g**
MUFA	5.91 g
Omega-3	0.06 g
Omega-6	1.2 g
Saturated Fat	4.96 g
Carbohydrates	**1.51 g**
Fiber	0.16 g
Starch	0.01 g
Fructose	0 g
Glucose	0 g
Sucrose	0 g
Protein	**37.4 g**
Alanine	2.14 g
Arginine	2.41 g
Aspartic acid	3.5 g
Cystine	0.42 g
Glutamic acid	5.71 g
Glycine	1.69 g
Histidine	1.52 g
Isoleucine	1.77 g
Leucine	3.08 g
Lysine	3.32 g
Methionine	1.02 g
Phenylalanine	1.55 g
Proline	1.51 g
Serine	1.56 g
Threonine	1.64 g
Tryptophan	0.44 g
Tyrosine	1.48 g
Valine	1.89 g
Vitamins	
Vitamin B1	0.96 mg
Vitamin B12	1.03 mcg
Vitamin B2	0.38 mg
Vitamin B3	11.6 mg
Vitamin B5	1.74 mg
Vitamin B6	0.78 mg
Choline	108 mg
Folate	0.31 mcg
Vitamin A	7.03 mcg
Vitamin C	1.93 mg
Vitamin D	43.8 IU
Vitamin E	0.32 mg
Vitamin K	0 mcg
Minerals	
Calcium	16 mg
Copper	0.11 mg
Iron	1.92 mg
Magnesium	37.1 mg
Manganese	0.02 mg
Phosphorus	410 mg
Potassium	622 mg
Selenium	67.4 mcg
Sodium	173 mg
Zinc	3.52 mg

nutrition content estimated using the USDA database.

Pork Pie–Stuffed Acorn Squash

This dish combines the flavors of my mom's tourtière (a French-Canadian meat pie) with the sweetness of acorn squash for a fun meal to eat and an outstanding comfort food.

PREP TIME: 20 minutes
COOK TIME: 1 hour 10 minutes
SERVINGS: 4 to 5

INGREDIENTS:

- Lard or coconut oil, for greasing the baking sheet
- 2 small acorn squash (about 1 pound each)
- 2 pounds ground pork
- 1 medium onion, finely diced
- 3 or 4 stalks celery, finely diced
- 1 teaspoon salt
- 2 sprigs fresh rosemary
- 2 or 3 bay leaves
- 2 tablespoons arrowroot powder or kuzu starch

FODMAP ALERT *Replace the onion with green onion or leek (green part only) or chives or omit.*

1. Preheat the oven to 350°F. Grease a rimmed baking sheet with lard or coconut oil or line it with parchment paper or a silicone liner.
2. Cut the acorn squash in half and scoop out the seeds. Place cut side down on the baking sheet and bake for 50 minutes.
3. Meanwhile, place the ground pork, onion, celery, salt, rosemary, and bay leaves in a large skillet over medium-high heat. Cook, stirring occasionally to break up the ground pork, until the meat is cooked throughout and the onion and celery are soft, 20 to 25 minutes. Sprinkle the arrowroot powder over the meat and cook for 5 more minutes, stirring frequently.
4. Remove the squash from the oven and turn cut side up. Spoon the meat mixture into the squash halves, discarding the bay leaves and rosemary stems. Return to the oven for 20 more minutes.

VARIATIONS:

You can also make this dish with ground chicken or turkey or with other winter squashes.

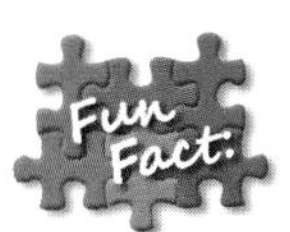

Pungent-tasting onions have 8 times more phytonutrients than sweet ones.

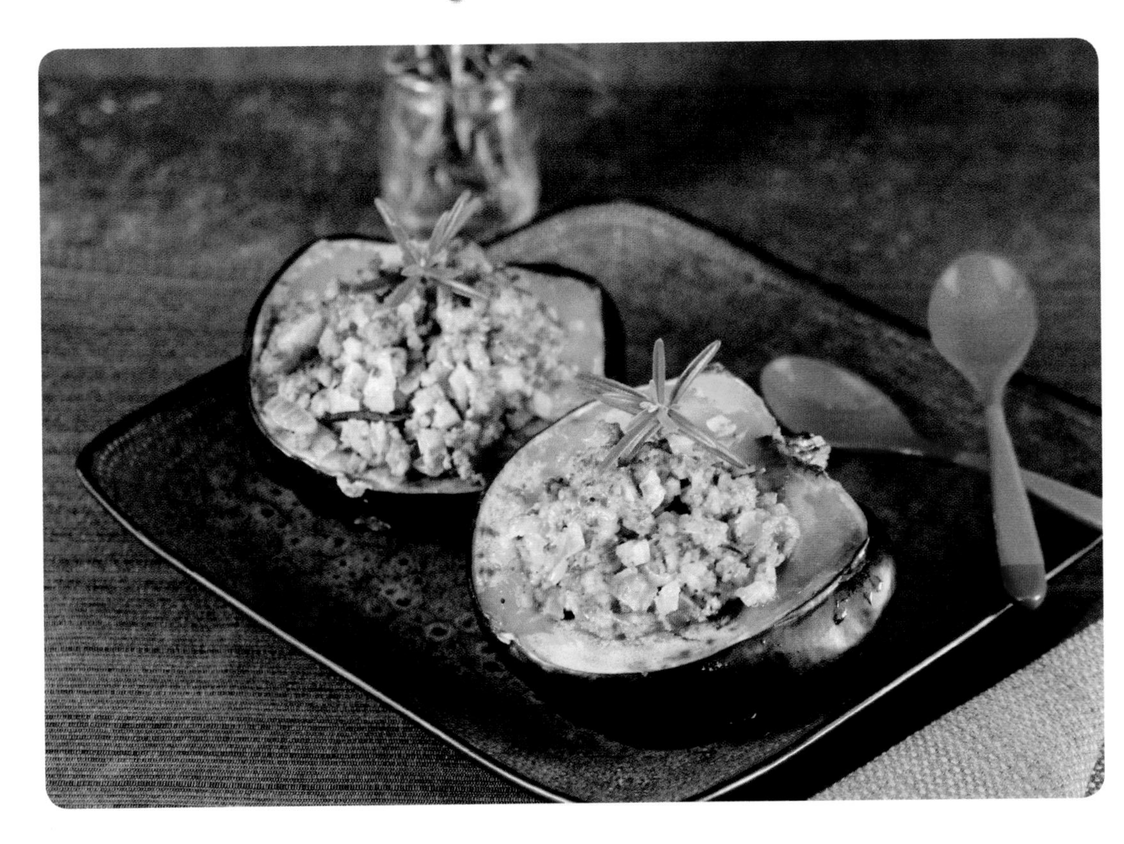

NUTRITION FACTS

Serving Size	412 g
Recipe Yields	2061 g
Calories	**665**
Fats	**38 g**
MUFA	16.8 g
Omega-3	0.2 g
Omega-6	3.04 g
Saturated Fat	14.1 g
Carbohydrates	**32.4 g**
Fiber	8.91 g
Starch	0.75 g
Fructose	0.43 g
Glucose	0.59 g
Sucrose	0.25 g
Protein	**49.1 g**
Alanine	2.81 g
Arginine	3.04 g
Aspartic acid	4.59 g
Cystine	0.62 g
Glutamic acid	7.73 g
Glycine	2.3 g
Histidine	1.9 g
Isoleucine	2.27 g
Leucine	3.87 g
Lysine	4.28 g
Methionine	1.26 g
Phenylalanine	1.95 g
Proline	1.95 g
Serine	2.01 g
Threonine	2.2 g
Tryptophan	0.63 g
Tyrosine	1.7 g
Valine	2.63 g
Vitamins	
Vitamin B1	1.6 mg
Vitamin B12	0.98 mcg
Vitamin B2	0.45 mg
Vitamin B3	9.34 mg
Vitamin B5	1.96 mg
Vitamin B6	1.11 mg
Choline	163 mg
Folate	57.7 mcg
Vitamin A	48.7 mcg
Vitamin C	24 mg
Vitamin D	38.1 IU
Vitamin E	0.46 mg
Vitamin K	8.59 mcg
Minerals	
Calcium	139 mg
Copper	0.25 mg
Iron	5.49 mg
Magnesium	127 mg
Manganese	0.53 mg
Phosphorus	504 mg
Potassium	1555 mg
Selenium	65.8 mcg
Sodium	366 mg
Zinc	6.21 mg

nutrition content estimated using the USDA database.

Lamb "Biryani"

Indian flavors without seeds and nightshades? Is that possible? Yes! And you will love this dish!

PREP TIME: 30 minutes
COOK TIME: 1 hour
SERVINGS: 4 to 8

INGREDIENTS:

Lamb:

- 2 pounds lamb stew meat
- 1 onion, sliced into half-moons
- 1 cup homemade Coconut Cream (page 116)
- 1 tablespoon fresh lemon juice
- ¼ cup raisins
- 6 to 7 cloves garlic, crushed
- 1 tablespoon peeled and grated fresh ginger
- 1 tablespoon chopped fresh curry leaves or crushed dried curry leaves
- 1 bay leaf
- 1 teaspoon ground turmeric
- 1 teaspoon salt
- 1 cinnamon stick
- 1 teaspoon Horseradish Sauce (page 205) or peeled and grated fresh horseradish

"Rice":

- 1 head cauliflower (about 2 pounds)
- 3 to 4 tablespoons red palm oil
- 1 carrot, very finely diced
- 1 medium onion, very finely diced
- 3 cloves garlic, crushed
- 1 teaspoon Horseradish Sauce (page 205) or peeled and grated fresh horseradish
- ½ teaspoon ground turmeric
- Pinch of ground cloves
- Pinch of ground cinnamon

Garnishes:

- 2 tablespoons chopped fresh mint
- 2 to 3 tablespoons chopped fresh cilantro

FODMAP ALERT

This recipe cannot be made low-FODMAP.

SPECIAL EQUIPMENT

- Pressure cooker

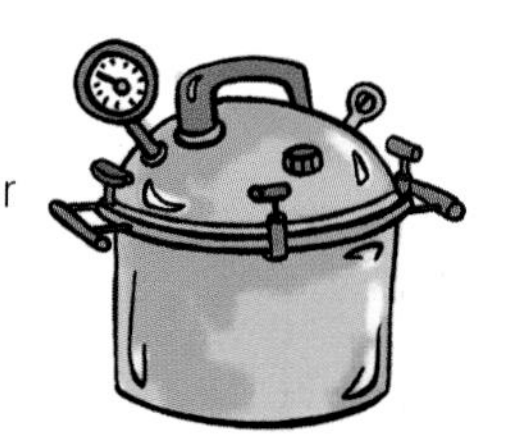

LAMB:

1. Combine all the ingredients for the lamb in a pressure cooker. Stir to mix and coat the meat. (See Tips for alternative cooking methods.)
2. Cook on high pressure for 30 minutes. While the lamb is cooking, prepare the "rice."
3. When the lamb is done, carefully release the pressure, allowing all the steam to escape before unlocking the lid.

"RICE":

1. Core the cauliflower and cut into florets. Place the florets in a food processor (you may have to do this in batches) and pulse until chopped to rice-grain size. Set aside. Alternatively, you can grate the cauliflower with a box grater.
2. Heat 3 tablespoons of the palm oil in a large skillet or wok over medium-high heat.
3. Add the carrot and onion to pan and cook until starting to soften, 6 to 7 minutes.
4. Add the cauliflower, garlic, horseradish sauce, and spices and cook, stirring frequently, until the cauliflower is cooked al dente, 6 to 8 minutes. If the rice starts sticking to the pan or the pan looks very dry during cooking, add an additional tablespoon of palm oil.

"BIRYANI":

1. Pour the lamb over the rice and garnish with the mint and cilantro. Serve!

TIPS:

If you don't own a pressure cooker, you can stew the lamb on the stovetop for 2 to 3 hours (or in a slow cooker for 4 to 6 hours). If the liquid level needs topping up during cooking, use Bone Broth (lamb, beef, or chicken; page 110).

VARIATIONS:

Substitute goat, mutton, or beef for the lamb.

NUTRITION FACTS

Serving Size	242 g
Recipe Yields	1933 g
Calories	**455**
Fats	**26.9 g**
MUFA	8.7 g
Omega-3	0.23 g
Omega-6	1.4 g
Saturated Fat	14.7 g
Carbohydrates	**32.6 g**
Fiber	2.95 g
Starch	3.94 g
Fructose	2.47 g
Glucose	2.54 g
Sucrose	19.6 g
Protein	**22.1 g**
Alanine	1.3 g
Arginine	1.36 g
Aspartic acid	1.95 g
Cystine	0.26 g
Glutamic acid	3.24 g
Glycine	1.04 g
Histidine	0.68 g
Isoleucine	1.03 g
Leucine	1.65 g
Lysine	1.93 g
Methionine	0.53 g
Phenylalanine	0.88 g
Proline	0.91 g
Serine	0.83 g
Threonine	0.93 g
Tryptophan	0.26 g
Tyrosine	0.72 g
Valine	1.19 g
Vitamins	
Vitamin B1	0.15 mg
Vitamin B12	2.05 mcg
Vitamin B2	0.28 mg
Vitamin B3	5.81 mg
Vitamin B5	1.15 mg
Vitamin B6	0.36 mg
Choline	113 mg
Folate	71 mcg
Vitamin A	51.9 mcg
Vitamin C	40.4 mg
Vitamin D	1.57 IU
Vitamin E	1.15 mg
Vitamin K	18.2 mcg
Minerals	
Calcium	62.6 mg
Copper	0.27 mg
Iron	3.26 mg
Magnesium	44.8 mg
Manganese	0.78 mg
Phosphorus	221 mg
Potassium	656 mg
Selenium	25 mcg
Sodium	239 mg
Zinc	4.25 mg

nutrition content estimated using the USDA database.

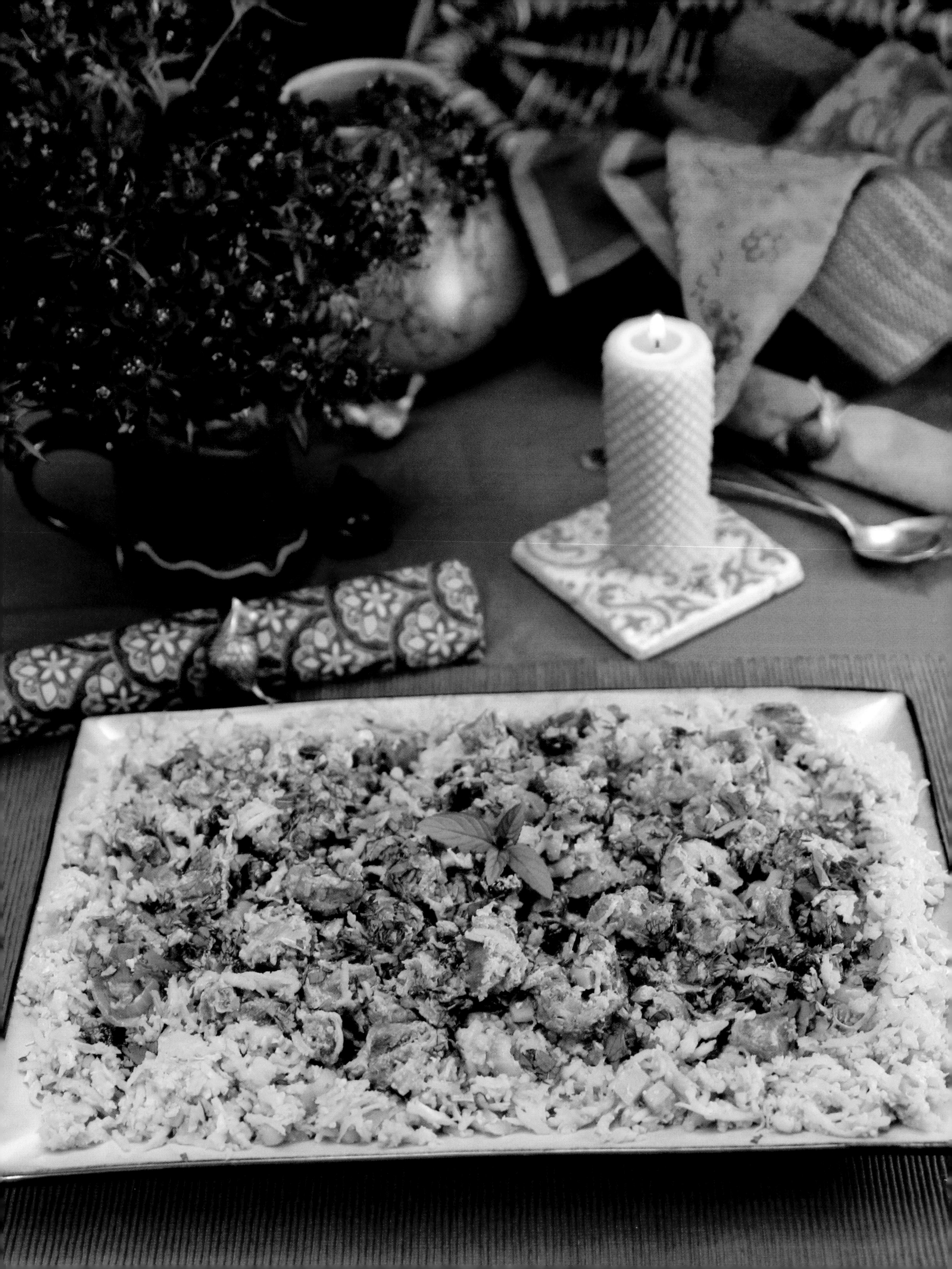

Pork Pad Thai

The flavor of this pad Thai is very traditional, with just one major substitution: spiral-cut and/or julienned vegetables take the place of rice noodles.

PREP TIME: 20 to 30 minutes
COOK TIME: 20 to 28 minutes
SERVINGS: 2 to 4

INGREDIENTS:

- 2 pounds kohlrabi, peeled
- ½ pound carrots
- 1 pound ground pork or boneless pork chops, trimmed and thinly sliced
- 5 cloves garlic, finely chopped
- 3 tablespoons fish sauce
- 1 tablespoon coconut aminos
- ¼ cup fresh lime juice
- 1½ teaspoons coconut water vinegar
- 4 to 5 green onions, finely chopped
- ⅓ cup chopped fresh cilantro

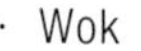

FODMAP ALERT *Replace the garlic with green garlic or garlic scapes (green part only) or omit. Use only the green parts of the green onions.*

SPECIAL EQUIPMENT

- Spiral vegetable slicer or mandoline slicer
- Wok

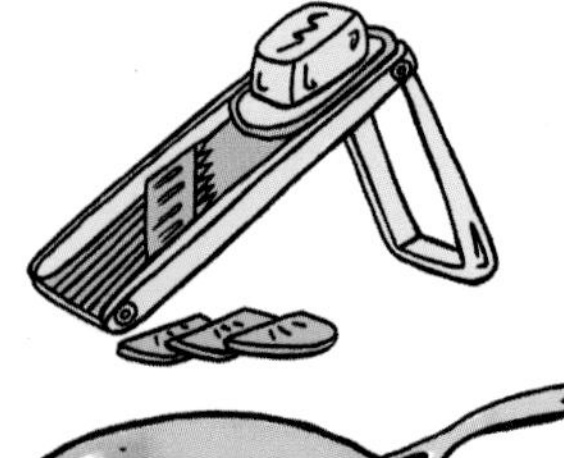

1. Use a spiral vegetable slicer to spiral-cut the kohlrabi into long noodles. Alternatively, you can julienne the kohlrabi using a mandoline slicer, julienne peeler, or sharp knife. Use a mandoline slicer, julienne peeler, or sharp knife to julienne the carrots into long strips.
2. Heat a wok or large skillet over medium-high heat. Add the pork and garlic and cook until the meat is completely browned, 5 to 8 minutes.
3. Add the fish sauce, coconut aminos, lime juice, and vinegar. Cook at a rapid simmer until the liquid is reduced by at least three-quarters, 7 to 10 minutes.
4. Add the spiral-cut kohlrabi and julienned carrot. Cook over medium-high heat, stirring frequently, until the vegetables are cooked al dente, 7 to 8 minutes.
5. Toss or garnish with the green onions and cilantro. Enjoy!

TIPS:

If you can't source coconut aminos, you can replace it with extra fish sauce and lime juice (half and half).

VARIATIONS:

Many different vegetables can be julienned or spiral-cut to act as noodles in this dish, including celery root, sweet potato, and parsnip. Another great option is to use two 12-ounce bags of broccoli slaw (typically found in the refrigerated coolers in the produce section of your grocery store, which also makes this a very fast meal to prepare). You could also use kelp noodles or sweet potato noodles.

Chicken Pad Thai. Replace the ground pork with very thinly sliced boneless chicken breast or thigh. It's easiest to slice chicken while it's still partially frozen. Allow to thaw in the fridge for 6 to 8 hours before slicing.

Shrimp Pad Thai. Replace the ground pork with shrimp and add the sauce ingredients at the same time as the shrimp (instead of cooking the shrimp first). Add the spiral-cut vegetables once the shrimp are opaque throughout.

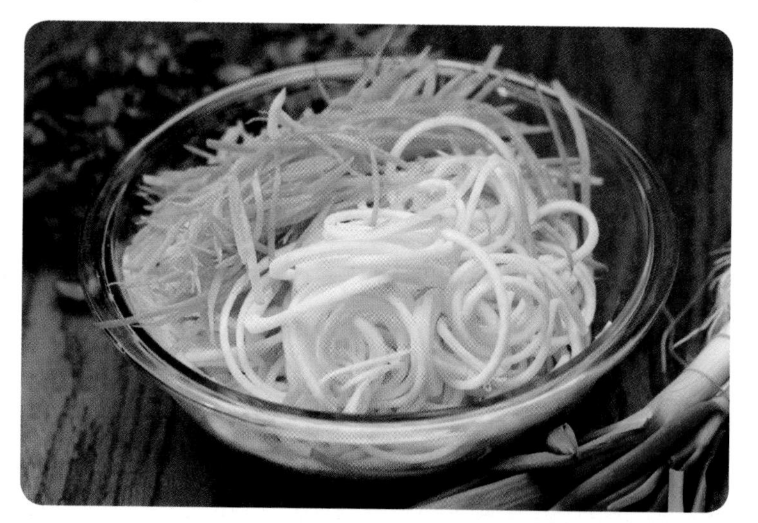

NUTRITION FACTS	
Serving Size	449 g
Recipe Yields	1794 g
Calories	**448**
Fats	**24.1 g**
MUFA	10.5 g
Omega-3	0.15 g
Omega-6	1.99 g
Saturated Fat	8.83 g
Carbohydrates	**25.2 g**
Fiber	4.48 g
Starch	9.25 g
Fructose	0.73 g
Glucose	0.68 g
Sucrose	2.14 g
Protein	**34.9 g**
Alanine	1.77 g
Arginine	2.14 g
Aspartic acid	2.85 g
Cystine	0.44 g
Glutamic acid	4.82 g
Glycine	1.42 g
Histidine	1.24 g
Isoleucine	1.61 g
Leucine	2.57 g
Lysine	2.83 g
Methionine	0.82 g
Phenylalanine	1.3 g
Proline	1.21 g
Serine	1.25 g
Threonine	1.56 g
Tryptophan	0.4 g
Tyrosine	1.04 g
Valine	1.76 g
Vitamins	
Vitamin B1	0.95 mg
Vitamin B12	0.68 mcg
Vitamin B2	0.35 mg
Vitamin B3	6.63 mg
Vitamin B5	1.19 mg
Vitamin B6	0.99 mg
Choline	139 mg
Folate	57.8 mcg
Vitamin A	510 mcg
Vitamin C	135 mg
Vitamin D	23.9 IU
Vitamin E	1.89 mg
Vitamin K	30.5 mcg
Minerals	
Calcium	122 mg
Copper	0.4 mg
Iron	2.81 mg
Magnesium	105 mg
Manganese	0.54 mg
Phosphorus	391 mg
Potassium	1464 mg
Selenium	43.9 mcg
Sodium	1319 mg
Zinc	4.6 mg

nutrition content estimated using the USDA database.

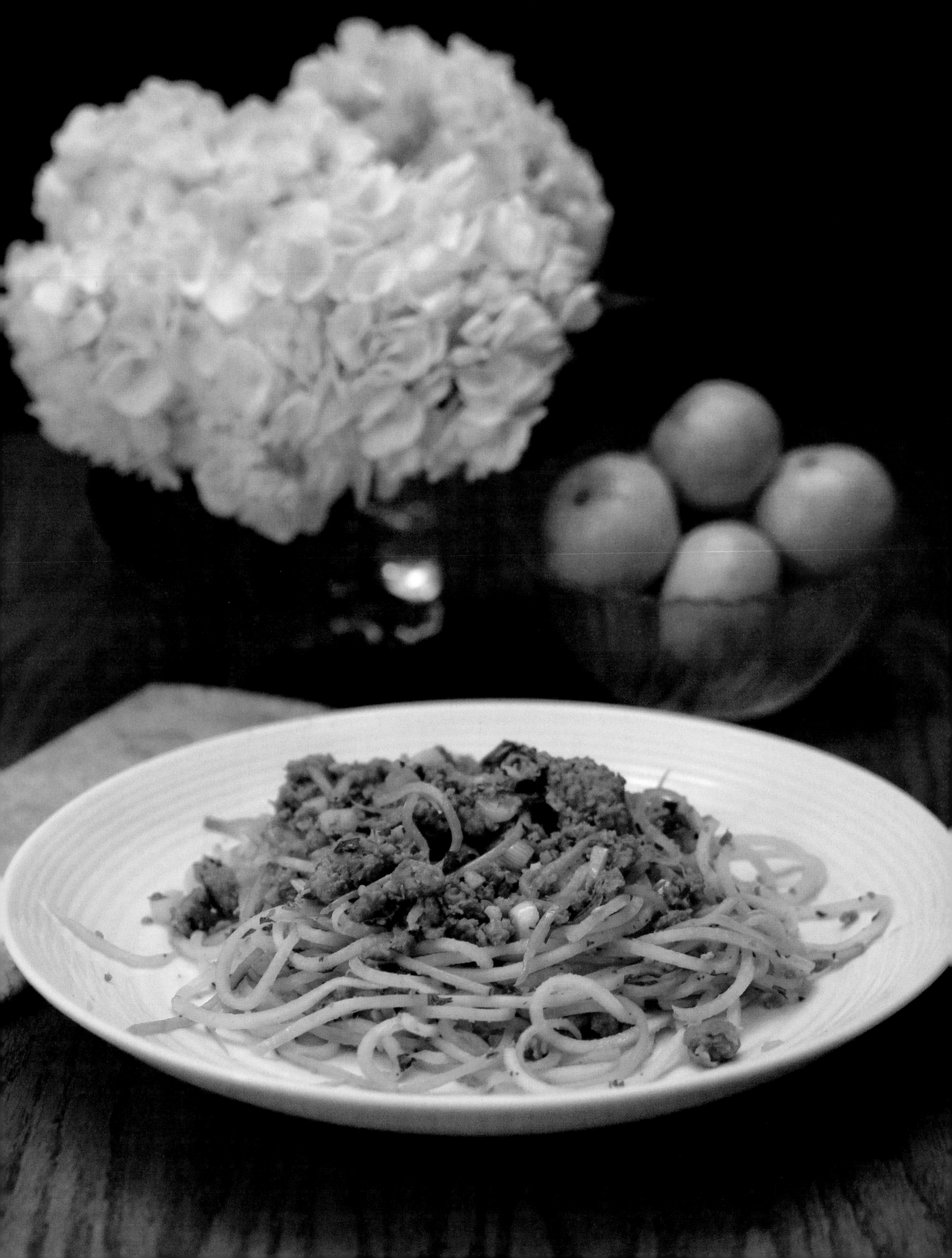

Chapter 9

Fish and Shellfish

When it comes to fish recipes, don't feel restricted to the type of fish called for in the recipe. It is simple to switch out types of fish or even types of shellfish. As a general rule, whitefish can be subbed for other whitefish, and oily fish can be subbed for other oily fish. Prawns and shrimp can be used interchangeably. Muscles, oysters, and clams can often be used interchangeably.

If you're a seafood lover, you'll be happy to know that seafood can be found in some other recipes in this book, including Ahi Tuna Ceviche (page 150), Shrimp and Avocado Skewers (page 154), Har Gow–Inspired Shrimp Balls (page 156), Smoked Salmon and Roe Endive Boats (page 174), Smoked Salmon and Mango Salsa Nori Wraps (page 175), Vietnamese-Style Fresh "Spring Rolls" (page 176), "Wonton" Soup (page 184), Seafood and Leek Soup (page 190), and Deep-Fried Fish Heads (page 285).

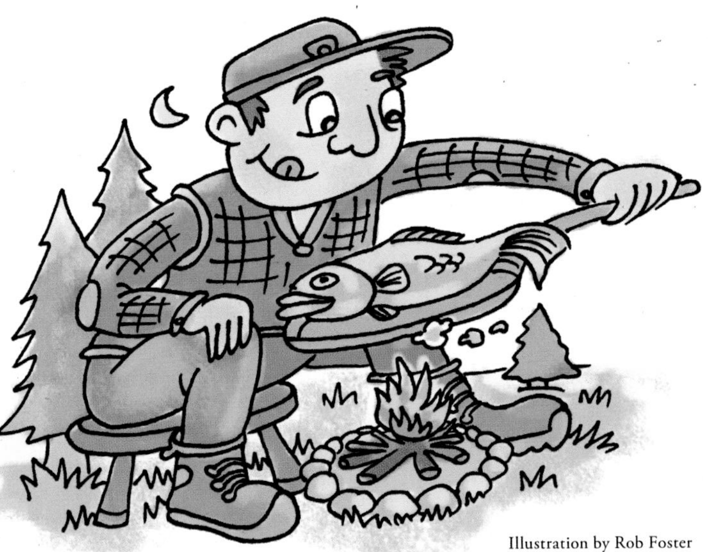

Illustration by Rob Foster

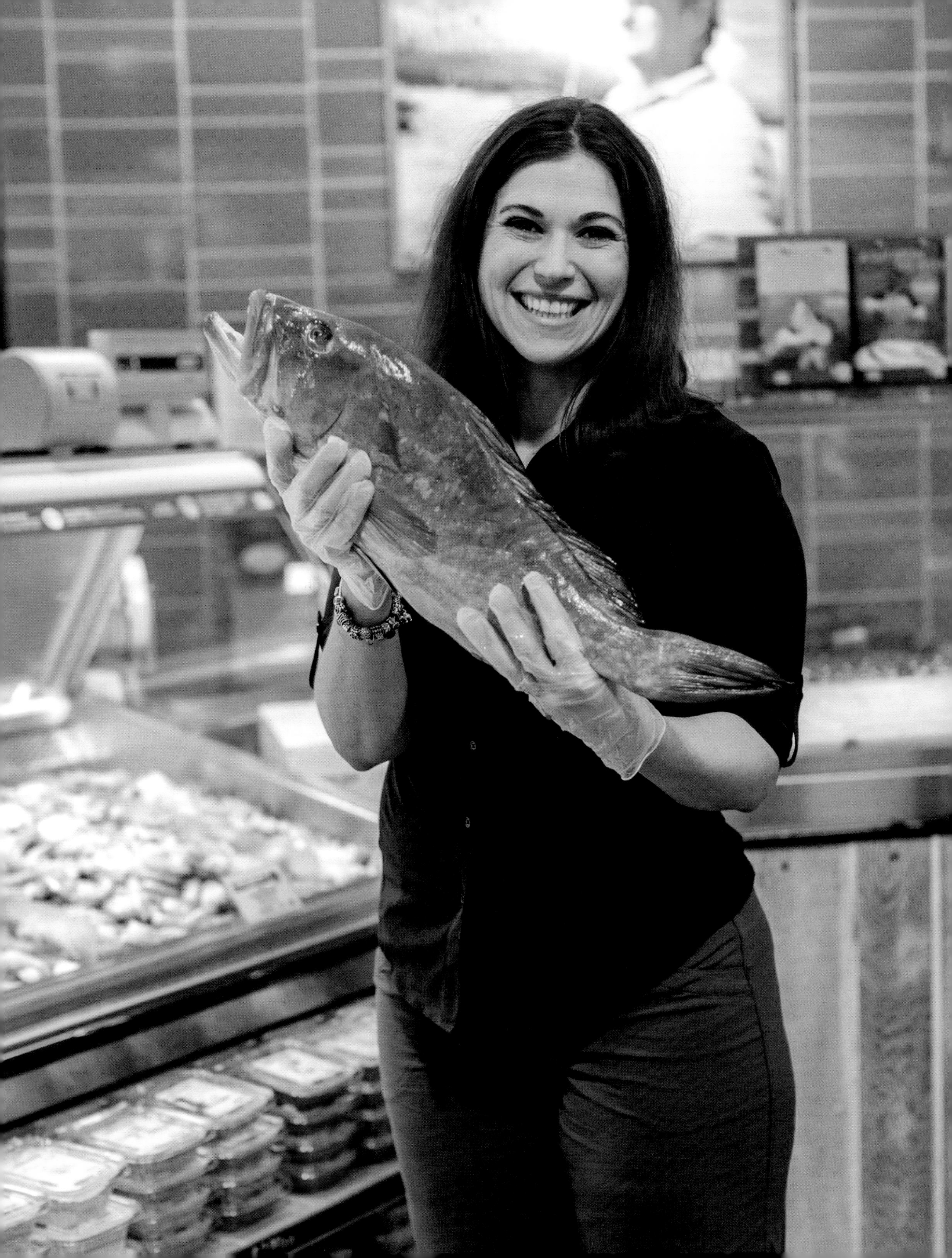

Pomegranate Molasses–Glazed Salmon

Pomegranate molasses is simply pomegranate juice that has been simmered until it has developed a syrupy consistency. It has a lovely sweet-and-sour tang, and its flavor works beautifully with fish, chicken, and lamb.

PREP TIME: 20 minutes
COOK TIME: 15 minutes
SERVINGS: 3 to 5

INGREDIENTS:

- 1 tablespoon avocado oil, for greasing the baking sheet (if needed)
- 1 tablespoon peeled and finely grated fresh ginger
- 3 or 4 cloves garlic, crushed
- ¼ cup fresh orange juice
- 2 tablespoons pomegranate molasses, plus 1 to 2 tablespoons for the glaze
- 3 or 4 (6- to 8-ounce) salmon fillets

FODMAP ALERT *Replace the garlic with green garlic or garlic scapes (green part only) or omit.*

1. Preheat the oven to 425°F. Line a rimmed baking sheet with parchment paper, aluminum foil, or a silicone liner. Lightly grease with avocado oil (you can skip the greasing if you are using a silicone liner).
2. Combine the ginger, garlic, orange juice, and 2 tablespoons of the pomegranate molasses in a small bowl. Pour over the salmon in a resealable bag or a nonreactive container and marinate at room temperature for 15 minutes.
3. Remove the salmon from the marinade and place on the prepared baking sheet, skin side down if your salmon has skin. Discard any remaining marinade.
4. Drizzle about 1 teaspoon of the additional pomegranate molasses over the top of each piece of salmon and spread with the back of a spoon or a pastry brush. Wipe up any pomegranate molasses that drips over the side of the salmon, since it would likely burn during cooking.
5. Bake for 12 to 15 minutes, until the salmon is fully cooked. It should be opaque throughout, and the segments should come apart easily.

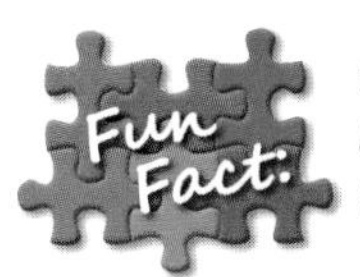

Pomegranate molasses is a staple in Middle Eastern cuisine.

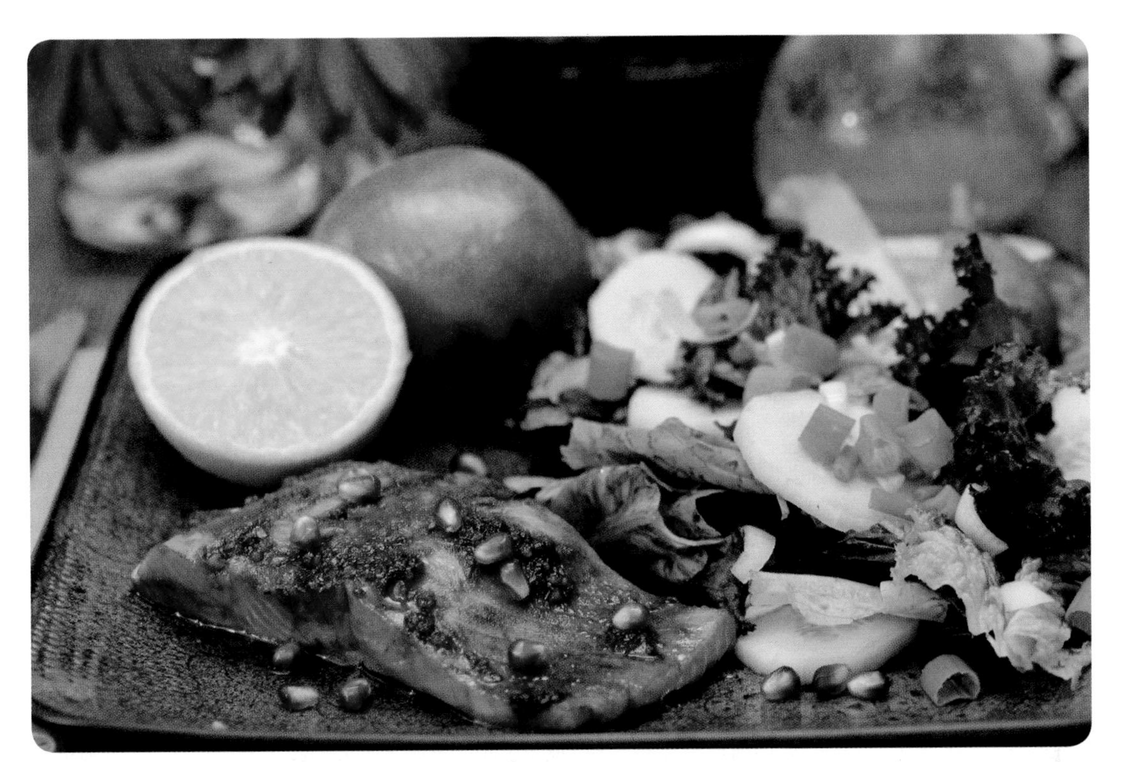

NUTRITION FACTS	
Serving Size	128 g
Recipe Yields	641 g
Calories	**242**
Fats	**11.1 g**
MUFA	4.73 g
Omega-3	2.66 g
Omega-6	0.59 g
Saturated Fat	1.61 g
Carbohydrates	**8.06 g**
Fiber	0.09 g
Starch	0.93 g
Fructose	1.02 g
Glucose	0.95 g
Sucrose	2.35 g
Protein	**26.1 g**
Alanine	1.57 g
Arginine	1.57 g
Aspartic acid	2.67 g
Cystine	0.28 g
Glutamic acid	3.89 g
Glycine	1.25 g
Histidine	0.77 g
Isoleucine	1.2 g
Leucine	2.11 g
Lysine	2.39 g
Methionine	0.77 g
Phenylalanine	1.02 g
Proline	0.92 g
Serine	1.06 g
Threonine	1.14 g
Tryptophan	0.29 g
Tyrosine	0.88 g
Valine	1.34 g
Vitamins	
Vitamin B1	0.3 mg
Vitamin B12	3.11 mcg
Vitamin B2	0.5 mg
Vitamin B3	10.4 mg
Vitamin B5	2.06 mg
Vitamin B6	1.04 mg
Choline	2.59 mg
Folate	33.4 mcg
Vitamin A	14.5 mcg
Vitamin C	6.81 mg
Vitamin D	0 IU
Vitamin E	<0.01 mg
Vitamin K	0.04 mcg
Minerals	
Calcium	36.5 mg
Copper	0.38 mg
Iron	1.49 mg
Magnesium	59.3 mg
Manganese	0.18 mg
Phosphorus	268 mg
Potassium	793 mg
Selenium	49.4 mcg
Sodium	60.6 mg
Zinc	0.89 mg

nutrition content estimated using the USDA database.

Baked Whole Fish

Baked whole fish is a beautiful and impressive dish to serve, even though it's actually very simple to make. Any variety of fish—provided it's in the 1- to 5-pound range—can be used for this dish, including trout, red snapper, Coho salmon, bass, pike, perch, cod, and grouper. You can enjoy it warm out of the oven or chilled with salad for a special lunch.

Remember to keep the head, fins, and bones for making fish Bone Broth (page 110)!

PREP TIME: 15 to 30 minutes
COOK TIME: 20 minutes per inch thick
SERVINGS: 3 to 6

INGREDIENTS:

1 (1- to 5-pound) whole fish, gutted and scaled (see Tips)

6 to 12 sprigs fresh parsley

1 to 2 lemons, sliced into thin circles

1. Preheat the oven to 375°F.
2. Lay the fish flat on a cutting board. Use a sharp knife to cut through the skin and flesh down to the spine. Make 3 or 4 slices, parallel to the gills and spaced about 1½ inches apart, down the body from head to tail. (The slits can be either straight up and down or slightly angled—it's up to you.) Flip the fish over and repeat on the other side.
3. Stuff sprigs of parsley into the cuts you made on both sides of the fish.
4. Place a sheet of aluminum foil about 2½ times longer than the fish on a rimmed baking sheet (if you have a large fish, you may want to use 2 sheets of foil side by side, slightly overlapping). Alternately, you can use a Dutch oven or clay baker. Line up half of the lemon slices on the foil and place the fish on top of them. Line up the rest of the lemon slices on top of the fish. Fold the foil over the fish and fold the end and sides over a couple of times to create a sealed cocoon for the fish to bake in.
5. Bake for 20 minutes per inch thick at the thickest part, until the fish is opaque throughout and the segments flake apart easily. To serve, use a metal spatula or cake knife to gently pry the meat away from the spine. Once you have served the top half of the fish, you can either peel the spine off the bottom half or flip the fish over to access the other half.
6. Enjoy—and watch for bones!

TIPS:

When purchasing a whole fish, ask your fishmonger to scale it for you and make the slices along the sides. If the fish is already scaled, this meal is very quick to prepare.

If the fish was not scaled for you when you purchased it, scale it in the sink (preferably one with a disposal; otherwise, you'll want to line the sink with newsprint or something similar to make cleaning up the scales easier) or outside by scraping a sharp knife against the grain of the scales—that is, from tail to head. An occasional scrape in the opposite direction can help loosen stubborn scales. Remember to do both sides. You can tell that the fish is completely scaled when it has a very smooth texture when you rub it with your hand.

If you caught the fish yourself, you will need to gut it, too.

VARIATIONS:

Use any citrus fruit in place of the lemons—Meyer lemons, tangerines, and oranges are particularly nice. Substitute fresh sage, thyme, marjoram, dill, or tarragon in place of the parsley, or a mix of your favorite herbs.

NUTRITION FACTS	
Serving Size	106 g
Recipe Yields	532 g
Calories	**143**
Fats	**4.84 g**
MUFA	1.48 g
Omega-3	0.66 g
Omega-6	0.12 g
Saturated Fat	0.89 g
Carbohydrates	**1.33 g**
Fiber	0.46 g
Starch	0.55 g
Fructose	0 g
Glucose	0 g
Sucrose	0 g
Protein	**22.5 g**
Alanine	1.43 g
Arginine	1.4 g
Aspartic acid	2.8 g
Cystine	0.17 g
Glutamic acid	3.16 g
Glycine	1.38 g
Histidine	0.59 g
Isoleucine	1.04 g
Leucine	1.7 g
Lysine	1.92 g
Methionine	0.63 g
Phenylalanine	0.92 g
Proline	0.95 g
Serine	0.99 g
Threonine	1.16 g
Tryptophan	0.24 g
Tyrosine	0.81 g
Valine	1.2 g
Vitamins	
Vitamin B1	0.09 mg
Vitamin B12	4.28 mcg
Vitamin B2	0.12 mg
Vitamin B3	8.74 mg
Vitamin B5	1.15 mg
Vitamin B6	0.64 mg
Choline	104 mg
Folate	11.9 mcg
Vitamin A	54.9 mcg
Vitamin C	11.4 mg
Vitamin D	472 IU
Vitamin E	0.48 mg
Vitamin K	65.8 mcg
Minerals	
Calcium	15.7 mg
Copper	0.08 mg
Iron	0.72 mg
Magnesium	31.9 mg
Manganese	0.02 mg
Phosphorus	287 mg
Potassium	435 mg
Selenium	34.1 mcg
Sodium	83.9 mg
Zinc	0.47 mg

nutrition content estimated using the USDA database.

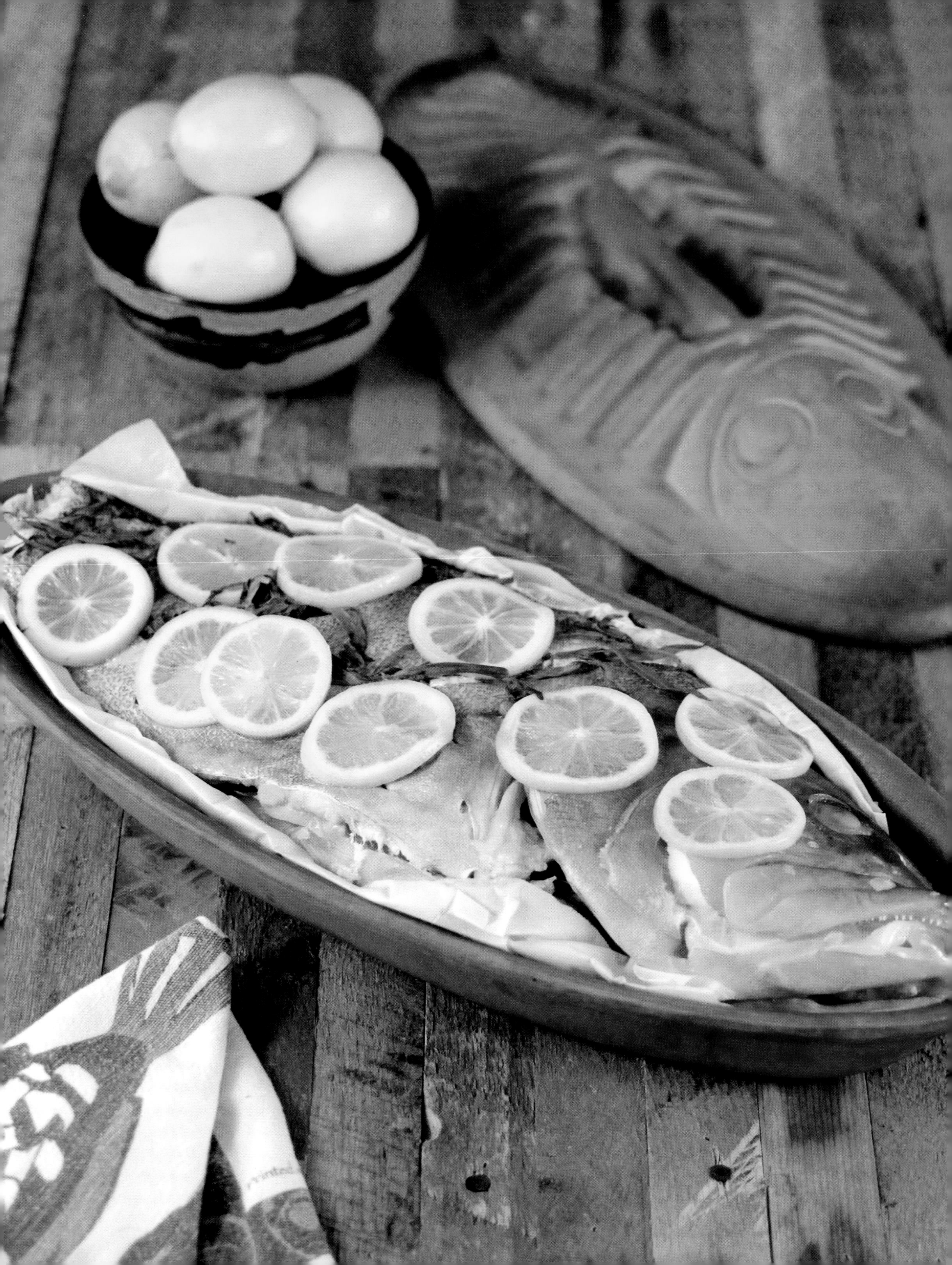

Lemon and Thyme Broiled Salmon with Blood Orange Salsa

Fruit salsa is a wonderful companion to fish or chicken. This salmon is very simple to prepare and cook, but the resulting dish has a sophisticated flavor and beautiful colors on your plate.

PREP TIME: 30 minutes
COOK TIME: 10 to 12 minutes
SERVINGS: 4 to 8

INGREDIENTS:

Salsa:

- 2 pounds blood oranges, segmented (see Tips)
- Finely grated zest of 1 lime
- Juice of 1 lime
- ½ medium red onion, diced
- 3 stalks celery, diced
- ¼ cup chopped fresh cilantro

Salmon:

- 4 to 6 (6- to 8-ounce) salmon fillets
- 1 tablespoon finely grated lemon zest (about 1 lemon)
- ¼ cup fresh lemon juice
- 1 tablespoon chopped fresh thyme
- ½ cup white wine, fresh orange juice, or apple juice

FODMAP ALERT *Replace the red onion with green onion (green part only) or chives or omit.*

SALSA:

1. Combine the salsa ingredients in a bowl and refrigerate until it's time to eat.

SALMON:

1. Combine the lemon zest and juice, thyme, and wine in a small bowl. Pour over the salmon fillets in a resealable bag or nonreactive container. Marinate 15 minutes.
2. Meanwhile, adjust an oven rack so that salmon will be 6 to 8 inches from the top element in the oven. Preheat the broiler on high for 10 minutes. Line a rimmed baking sheet with foil.
3. Remove the salmon from the marinade and place on the prepared baking sheet (if the fillets have skin, lay them skin side down). Discard the remaining marinade.
4. Broil 10 to 12 minutes, until the salmon is opaque throughout and the segments flake apart easily.
5. Serve with the salsa.

TIPS:

To segment an orange, use a sharp paring knife to cut off the top and bottom. Lay the orange on a cutting board and cut off the peel all the way around. Then, holding the orange in your hand, use the knife to carefully cut out each segment by cutting down one side of the segment close to the membrane and then twisting the knife to pry the segment off the membrane on the other side.

VARIATIONS:

You can easily substitute just about any other type of fish in this recipe—trout, halibut, and amberjack work particularly well.

Mango Salsa. In place of the blood oranges, use 2 pounds mango, peeled, seeded, and diced. Mango Salsa is a great accompaniment to chicken, pork, and beef.

Actually, this salsa tastes delicious with many different types of fruits. Other fruits that work particularly well are papaya, pear, peach, apricot, orange, grapefruit, and strawberries.

Lemon and Thyme Baked Chicken. Instead of using fish fillets, use chicken breasts, thighs, or tenders. Bake at 375°F for 20 to 40 minutes, until fully cooked.

Truffle Salt Broiled Salmon. Want to skip the wine? Broiled salmon seasoned simply with a sprinkle of truffle salt is absolutely divine!

NUTRITION FACTS	
Serving Size	229 g
Recipe Yields	1835 g
Calories	**184**
Fats	**5.6 g**
MUFA	1.83 g
Omega-3	1.72 g
Omega-6	0.41 g
Saturated Fat	0.86 g
Carbohydrates	**16 g**
Fiber	2.97 g
Starch	2.71 g
Fructose	2.75 g
Glucose	2.49 g
Sucrose	4.96 g
Protein	**18.1 g**
Alanine	1.06 g
Arginine	1.15 g
Aspartic acid	1.91 g
Cystine	0.19 g
Glutamic acid	2.83 g
Glycine	0.84 g
Histidine	0.51 g
Isoleucine	0.8 g
Leucine	1.41 g
Lysine	1.6 g
Methionine	0.51 g
Phenylalanine	0.69 g
Proline	0.81 g
Serine	0.74 g
Threonine	0.76 g
Tryptophan	0.2 g
Tyrosine	0.59 g
Valine	0.9 g
Vitamins	
Vitamin B1	0.28 mg
Vitamin B12	2.7 mcg
Vitamin B2	0.39 mg
Vitamin B3	7.23 mg
Vitamin B5	1.77 mg
Vitamin B6	0.81 mg
Choline	11.4 mg
Folate	67.6 mcg
Vitamin A	28.9 mcg
Vitamin C	71 mg
Vitamin D	217 IU
Vitamin E	0.24 mg
Vitamin K	6 mcg
Minerals	
Calcium	68.8 mg
Copper	0.27 mg
Iron	0.9 mg
Magnesium	40.3 mg
Manganese	0.08 mg
Phosphorus	203 mg
Potassium	665 mg
Selenium	31.1 mcg
Sodium	51.2 mg
Zinc	0.68 mg

nutrition content estimated using the USDA database.

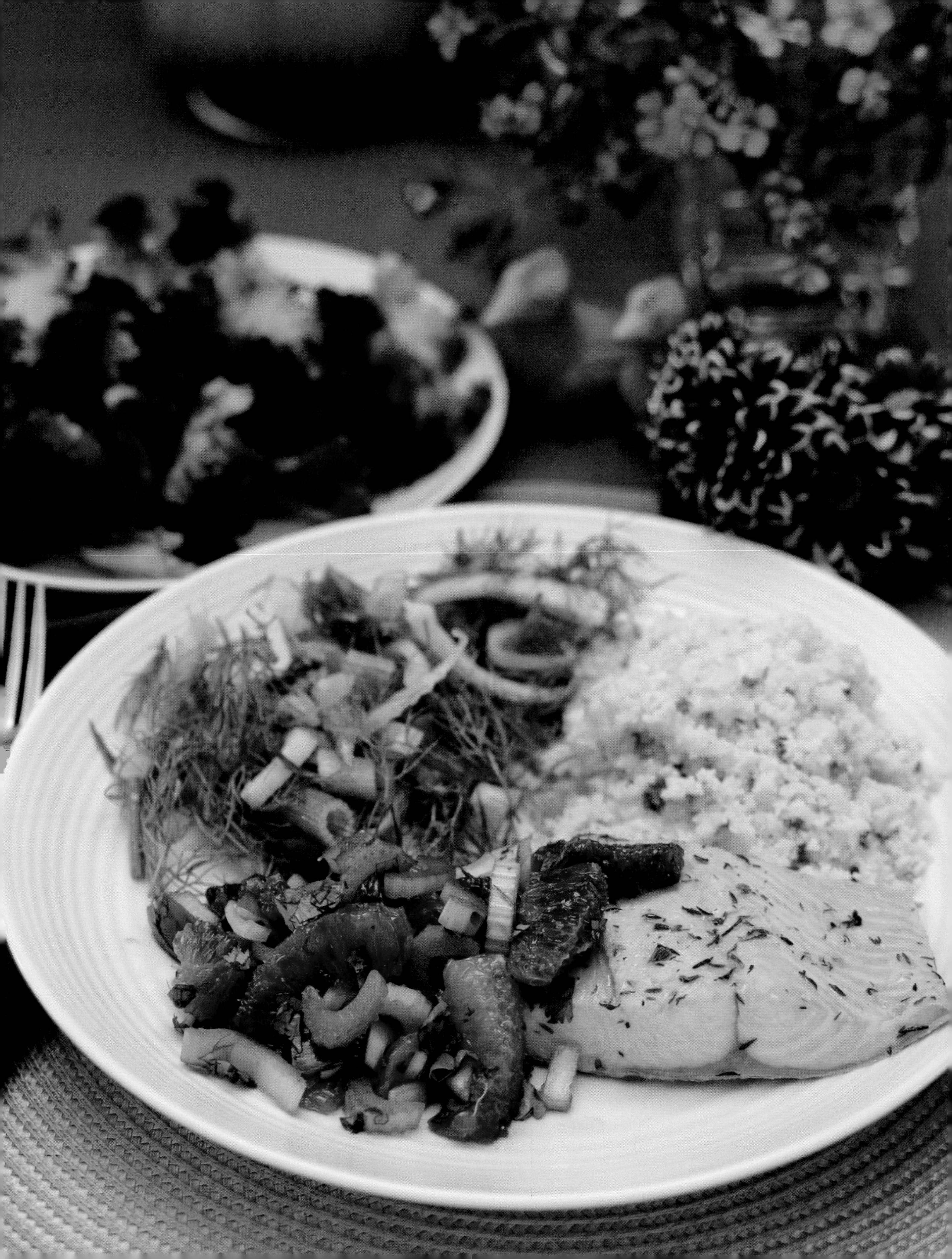

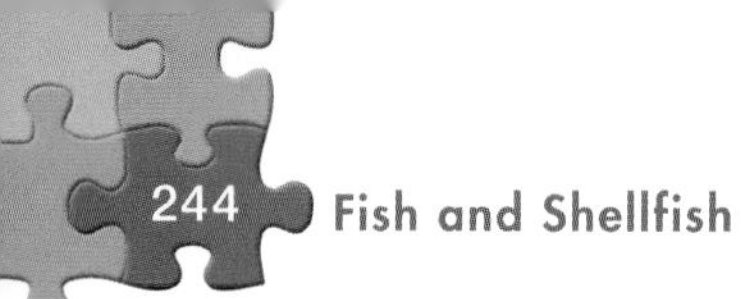

Simple Baked Whitefish

This recipe works beautifully with hake, cod, halibut, sea bass, mahi mahi, or any other whitefish. You can also play around with the seasonings to make this dish a little different every time you prepare it!

PREP TIME: 10 minutes, plus 30 minutes to 1 hour marinating time
COOK TIME: 20 minutes
SERVINGS: 3 to 5

INGREDIENTS:

- 1 tablespoon chopped fresh oregano leaves
- 1 tablespoon chopped fresh parsley
- 1 clove garlic, crushed
- Finely grated zest of 1 lemon
- Juice of 1 lemon
- ¼ teaspoon salt
- 3 tablespoons avocado oil
- 3 or 4 (6- to 8-ounce) whitefish fillets

FODMAP ALERT *Replace the garlic with green garlic or garlic scapes (green part only) or omit.*

1. Combine the oregano, parsley, garlic, lemon zest and juice, salt, and avocado oil.
2. Pour over the whitefish fillets in a resealable bag or a non-reactive container and marinate in the refrigerator for 30 minutes to 1 hour.
3. Preheat the oven to 350°F. Line a rimmed baking sheet with parchment paper, aluminum foil, or a silicone liner.
4. Place the fish fillets on the prepared baking sheet. Discard any extra marinade, but make sure that each piece of fish has a good amount of herbs stuck to it.
5. Bake for 20 minutes, until the fish is opaque throughout and the segments flake apart easily.

TIPS:

Marinating in a resealable plastic bag is very convenient. Simply flipping the bag over halfway through the marinating time helps redistribute the marinade so the fish marinates evenly.

VARIATIONS:

You can replace the oregano in this recipe with your favorite fresh herbs. Herbes de Provence (page 108), thyme, tarragon, and dill are all lovely options.

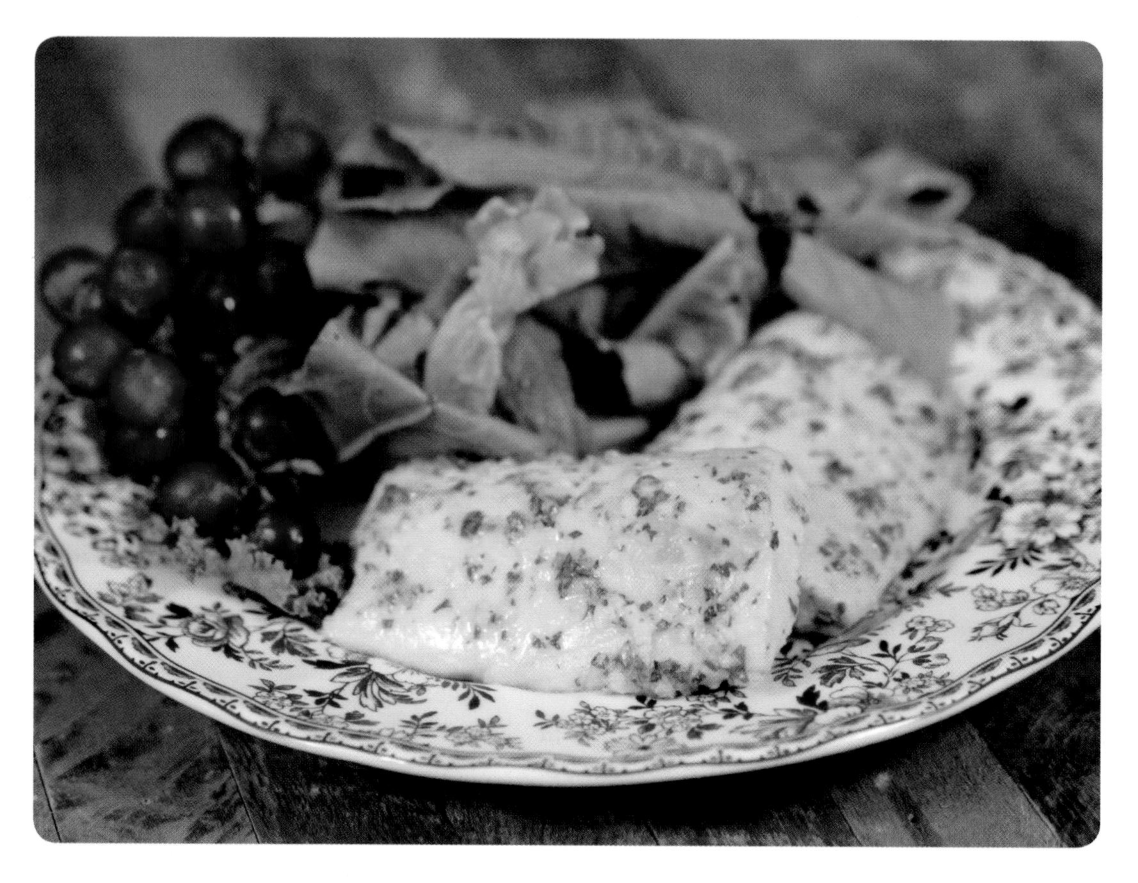

NUTRITION FACTS	
Serving Size	104 g
Recipe Yields	521 g
Calories	**144**
Fats	**6.81 g**
MUFA	2.63 g
Omega-3	1.64 g
Omega-6	0.38 g
Saturated Fat	1.02 g
Carbohydrates	**0.12 g**
Fiber	0.03 g
Starch	0.06 g
Fructose	0.01 g
Glucose	<0.01 g
Sucrose	<0.01 g
Protein	**19.5 g**
Alanine	1.18 g
Arginine	1.16 g
Aspartic acid	1.99 g
Cystine	0.21 g
Glutamic acid	2.9 g
Glycine	0.93 g
Histidine	0.57 g
Isoleucine	0.9 g
Leucine	1.58 g
Lysine	1.79 g
Methionine	0.58 g
Phenylalanine	0.76 g
Proline	0.69 g
Serine	0.79 g
Threonine	0.85 g
Tryptophan	0.22 g
Tyrosine	0.66 g
Valine	1 g
Vitamins	
Vitamin B1	0.14 mg
Vitamin B12	1.02 mcg
Vitamin B2	0.12 mg
Vitamin B3	3.06 mg
Vitamin B5	0.77 mg
Vitamin B6	0.31 mg
Choline	66.3 mg
Folate	15.7 mcg
Vitamin A	37 mcg
Vitamin C	0.65 mg
Vitamin D	487 IU
Vitamin E	0.21 mg
Vitamin K	1.47 mcg
Minerals	
Calcium	27 mg
Copper	0.07 mg
Iron	0.42 mg
Magnesium	33.8 mg
Manganese	0.07 mg
Phosphorus	275 mg
Potassium	325 mg
Selenium	12.9 mcg
Sodium	57.2 mg
Zinc	1.01 mg

nutrition content estimated using the USDA database.

Salmon with Maître D' "Butter"

If you make a big batch of Maitre D' "Butter" and keep it in the freezer, this becomes a quick and easy midweek meal. This recipe makes enough Maitre D' "Butter" for sixteen to eighteen servings of fish. When freezing the Maitre D' "Butter," spoon tablespoonfuls onto a plate or lined baking sheet. Freeze until hard (about 1 hour), then move to a resealable plastic bag or container for long-term freezer storage. No need to thaw before popping in the oven. This "butter" will also keep for up to a week in the fridge.

PREP TIME: 20 minutes
COOK TIME: 20 minutes
SERVINGS: 16 to 18

INGREDIENTS:

- 1 tablespoon finely grated lemon zest (about 1 lemon)
- 4 large cloves garlic, crushed
- ⅔ cup chopped fresh dill
- ½ cup minced fresh parsley
- ½ teaspoon salt
- 1 cup lard, at room temperature
- 6- to 8-ounce salmon fillets (as many as desired)
- Water

FODMAP ALERT *Replace the garlic with green garlic or garlic scapes (green part only) or omit.*

SPECIAL EQUIPMENT

- Parchment paper or aluminum foil to make "envelopes"
- Microplane or fine zester

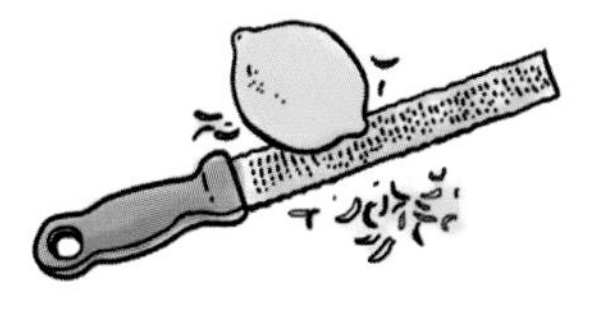

TIPS:

You can really use any cooking fat for the "butter." Lard is delicious, but bacon fat (omit the salt), coconut oil, tallow, palm shortening, or a mix of all of the above can be used instead.

VARIATIONS:

This Maitre D' "Butter" is very versatile. It's delicious melted on grilled steak or chicken, and it can be used to sauté vegetables.

1. Combine the lemon zest, garlic, herbs, and salt with the lard in a small bowl. Mix until well combined.
2. Preheat the oven to 350°F.
3. Prepare a parchment or foil "envelope" for each piece of fish. Place a large sheet of parchment paper or aluminum foil on a rimmed baking sheet. The parchment or foil should measure a little over twice the length of the fish fillet. (You can also place all of your fillets in one large parchment envelope. To create an envelope for more than one fillet, place them side by side and ensure that there is 3 to 4 inches of extra parchment width at the top and bottom.)
4. Place the salmon fillet on the bottom half of the parchment or foil, leaving 3 to 4 inches of space (in addition to one long side) around it for folding over. Spoon a tablespoonful of herb butter onto each fillet (you can spread it out or leave it as a ball). Also add approximately 1 tablespoon of water around the fillets (add 2 tablespoons if placing more than one fillet in each envelope). Fold over the long top portion of the parchment or foil to cover the fish. Then triple-fold the edges on all three unsealed sides to form a fully sealed envelope or pocket.
5. Place in the oven (still on the baking sheet) and bake for 20 minutes, until the fish is opaque throughout and the segments flake apart easily. Be careful when opening the envelopes to avoid steam burns.

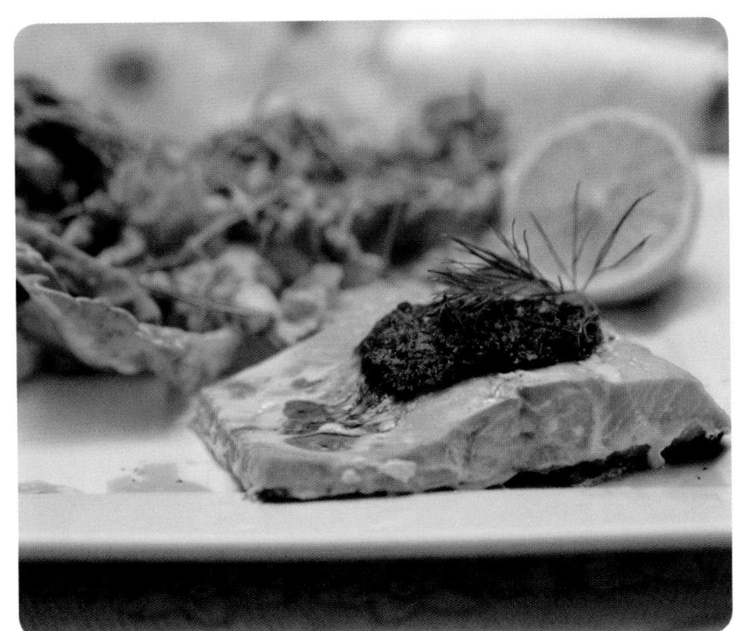

NUTRITION FACTS	
Serving Size	166 g
Recipe Yields	2983 g
Calories	**320**
Fats	**21 g**
MUFA	8.34 g
Omega-3	3.16 g
Omega-6	1.82 g
Saturated Fat	5.96 g
Carbohydrates	**0.4 g**
Fiber	0.11 g
Starch	0.24 g
Fructose	0 g
Glucose	0 g
Sucrose	0 g
Protein	**30.2 g**
Alanine	1.82 g
Arginine	1.8 g
Aspartic acid	3.09 g
Cystine	0.32 g
Glutamic acid	4.5 g
Glycine	1.45 g
Histidine	0.89 g
Isoleucine	1.39 g
Leucine	2.45 g
Lysine	2.76 g
Methionine	0.89 g
Phenylalanine	1.18 g
Proline	1.07 g
Serine	1.23 g
Threonine	1.32 g
Tryptophan	0.34 g
Tyrosine	1.02 g
Valine	1.55 g
Vitamins	
Vitamin B1	0.35 mg
Vitamin B12	4.82 mcg
Vitamin B2	0.58 mg
Vitamin B3	11.9 mg
Vitamin B5	2.53 mg
Vitamin B6	1.25 mg
Choline	6.07 mg
Folate	41 mcg
Vitamin A	26.5 mcg
Vitamin C	3.14 mg
Vitamin D	398 IU
Vitamin E	0.08 mg
Vitamin K	27.4 mcg
Minerals	
Calcium	23.2 mg
Copper	0.38 mg
Iron	1.52 mg
Magnesium	45.2 mg
Manganese	0.04 mg
Phosphorus	305 mg
Potassium	758 mg
Selenium	55.4 mcg
Sodium	96.5 mg
Zinc	1.01 mg

nutrition content estimated using the USDA database.

Mediterranean Mahi Mahi

Mediterranean flavors don't have to mean tomatoes, and this combination of herbs and vegetables is proof! An added benefit is that this dish is one of those where you throw everything into a baking dish and, an hour later, an amazing meal is served!

PREP TIME: 20 minutes
COOK TIME: 1 hour
SERVINGS: 4 to 6

INGREDIENTS:

- 1½ tablespoons Herbes de Provence (page 108)
- 1 medium zucchini (6 to 8 ounces), cut into ½- to ¾-inch chunks
- 2 medium carrots, cut into ½-inch rounds
- 1 bunch radishes (about 8 ounces), cut in half or quartered if large
- ½ head cauliflower, cored and cut into small florets
- ¾ cup whole olives (green or black)
- 2 cloves garlic, chopped
- Finely grated zest of 1 lemon
- Juice of 1 lemon
- 1 tablespoon coconut oil or avocado oil
- 4 to 6 (6-ounce) mahi mahi fillets

FODMAP ALERT *Replace the cauliflower with cubed peeled turnip or green plantain. Replace the garlic with green garlic or garlic scapes (green part only) or omit.*

1. Preheat the oven to 375°F.
2. Combine all the ingredients except the mahi mahi in a bowl and toss to combine.
3. Place the mahi mahi in a large casserole dish or lasagna pan. Pour the vegetable mixture over the top of the fish and cover. If your casserole dish doesn't come with a lid, cover with aluminum foil instead.
4. Bake for 1 hour, until the mahi mahi is opaque throughout, the segments flake apart easily, and the vegetables are cooked but still slightly firm.

VARIATIONS:

Peeled and cubed green plantain makes a lovely starchy addition to this dish, or you can use it as a replacement for the cauliflower.

NUTRITION FACTS	
Serving Size	249 g
Recipe Yields	1495 g
Calories	**170**
Fats	**4.9 g**
MUFA	1.42 g
Omega-3	0.03 g
Omega-6	0.2 g
Saturated Fat	2.45 g
Carbohydrates	**7.74 g**
Fiber	2.84 g
Starch	1.45 g
Fructose	0.94 g
Glucose	1.06 g
Sucrose	0.8 g
Protein	**24.1 g**
Alanine	0.1 g
Arginine	0.09 g
Aspartic acid	0.18 g
Cystine	0.03 g
Glutamic acid	0.29 g
Glycine	0.07 g
Histidine	0.05 g
Isoleucine	0.07 g
Leucine	0.1 g
Lysine	0.15 g
Methionine	0.02 g
Phenylalanine	0.07 g
Proline	0.06 g
Serine	0.07 g
Threonine	0.09 g
Tryptophan	0.02 g
Tyrosine	0.04 g
Valine	0.1 g
Vitamins	
Vitamin B1	0.05 mg
Vitamin B12	0 mcg
Vitamin B2	0.06 mg
Vitamin B3	0.58 mg
Vitamin B5	0.48 mg
Vitamin B6	0.17 mg
Choline	28.1 mg
Folate	43.8 mcg
Vitamin A	174 mcg
Vitamin C	35.9 mg
Vitamin D	0 IU
Vitamin E	0.42 mg
Vitamin K	11 mcg
Minerals	
Calcium	44.7 mg
Copper	0.09 mg
Iron	2.05 mg
Magnesium	16 mg
Manganese	0.16 mg
Phosphorus	40.9 mg
Potassium	829 mg
Selenium	0.83 mcg
Sodium	255 mg
Zinc	0.36 mg

nutrition content estimated using the USDA database.

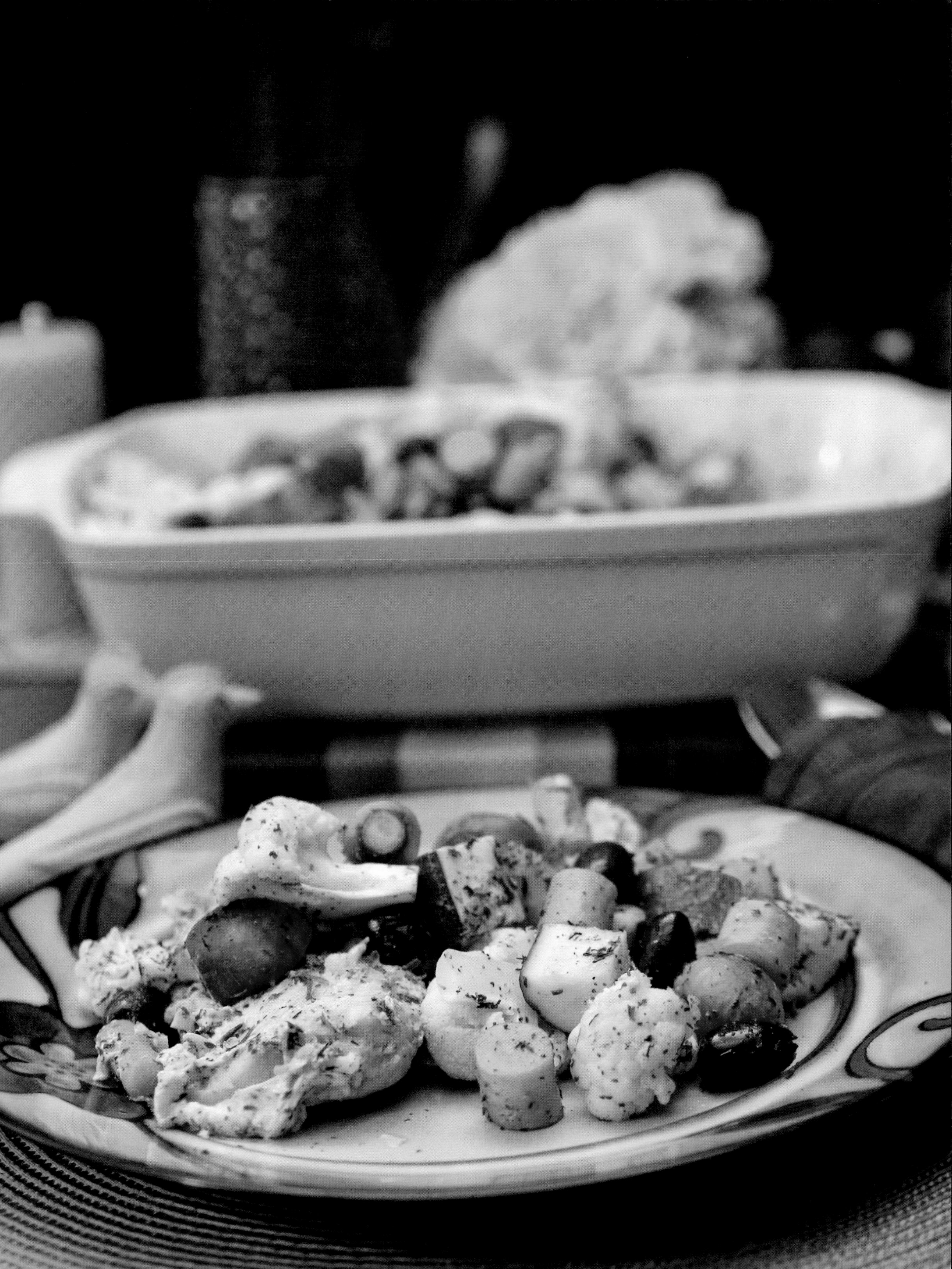

Scalloped Hake and Oysters

This may just be one of the most decadent meals you've ever made. Even if you think you don't like oysters, this is an amazing dish to try! Look for preshucked oysters to save time. If you're intimidated by the number of servings (or the price of oysters), simply halve the recipe. The hake can be baked and flaked one day ahead, and the sauce, Plantain Crackers, and Bacon Bits can all be premade, speeding up the process on the day of assembly.

PREP TIME: 30 minutes
COOK TIME: 1 hour 10 minutes
SERVINGS: 8 to 12

INGREDIENTS:

- 2½ pounds hake fillets
- 2 tablespoons lard
- 1 shallot, finely diced
- 2 cups Bone Broth (chicken, page 110)
- ½ head cauliflower, cored and cut into florets
- Pinch of saffron
- 1 clove garlic, minced
- ¼ cup white wine
- ½ teaspoon finely grated lemon zest
- 1 cup (about ¾ batch) Plantain Crackers (page 149)
- ¼ cup Bacon Bits (page 120)
- 2 pounds shucked oysters

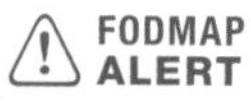

FODMAP ALERT

This recipe cannot be made low-FODMAP.

SPECIAL EQUIPMENT

- Immersion blender or blender
- Lasagna pan or deep casserole dish

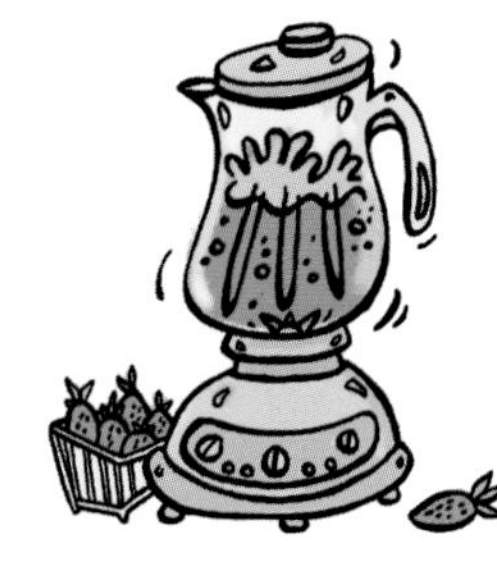

1. Preheat the oven to 350°F. Line a rimmed baking sheet with parchment paper or a silicone liner.
2. Place the hake fillets on the prepared baking sheet and bake for 15 to 20 minutes, until the fish is opaque throughout and the segments flake apart easily. Set aside to cool until easy to handle. Leave the oven on.
3. Meanwhile, make the sauce: Heat the lard in a saucepot over medium-high heat. Add the shallot and sauté until caramelized, 7 to 8 minutes.
4. Add the broth, cauliflower, saffron, garlic, wine, and lemon zest. Bring to a boil, then cover and reduce the heat to maintain a simmer. Simmer until the cauliflower is soft, 10 to 15 minutes. Remove from the heat and let cool. Purée with an immersion blender or in a countertop blender until smooth.
5. To make the crumb topping, process the plantain crackers in a food processor to a fine crumb. Add the bacon bits and pulse to combine.
6. Flake the hake: Using your fingers or a butter knife, break apart the fish into flakes.
7. To assemble, lay half of the flaked cooked hake in a large casserole dish. Layer half of the oysters in a flat layer over the hake. Layer the remaining hake over the oysters. Finish with the remaining oysters. Pour the cauliflower sauce over the entire dish. Sprinkle the crumb topping evenly over the top of the casserole.
8. Bake for 20 minutes, until the sauce is bubbling and the oysters are cooked through.

VARIATIONS:

Replace the hake with any whitefish. This is a great way to reinvent leftover fish.

You can replace the wine with more broth if you prefer.

NUTRITION FACTS	
Serving Size	264 g
Recipe Yields	3165 g
Calories	**283**
Fats	**14.5 g**
MUFA	3.81 g
Omega-3	2.11 g
Omega-6	0.68 g
Saturated Fat	5.8 g
Carbohydrates	**9.55 g**
Fiber	0.83 g
Starch	2.22 g
Fructose	0.24 g
Glucose	0.23 g
Sucrose	0 g
Protein	**27 g**
Alanine	1.61 g
Arginine	1.69 g
Aspartic acid	2.68 g
Cystine	0.3 g
Glutamic acid	3.88 g
Glycine	1.4 g
Histidine	0.72 g
Isoleucine	1.21 g
Leucine	2.07 g
Lysine	2.33 g
Methionine	0.72 g
Phenylalanine	1.02 g
Proline	1 g
Serine	1.12 g
Threonine	1.16 g
Tryptophan	0.3 g
Tyrosine	0.88 g
Valine	1.33 g
Vitamins	
Vitamin B1	0.22 mg
Vitamin B12	13.1 mcg
Vitamin B2	0.34 mg
Vitamin B3	4.93 mg
Vitamin B5	1.31 mg
Vitamin B6	0.42 mg
Choline	78.7 mg
Folate	39.5 mcg
Vitamin A	103 mcg
Vitamin C	20.6 mg
Vitamin D	454 IU
Vitamin E	0.27 mg
Vitamin K	6.62 mcg
Minerals	
Calcium	40.4 mg
Copper	1.29 mg
Iron	4.61 mg
Magnesium	58.2 mg
Manganese	0.61 mg
Phosphorus	408 mg
Potassium	593 mg
Selenium	72.1 mcg
Sodium	361 mg
Zinc	13.7 mg

nutrition content estimated using the USDA database.

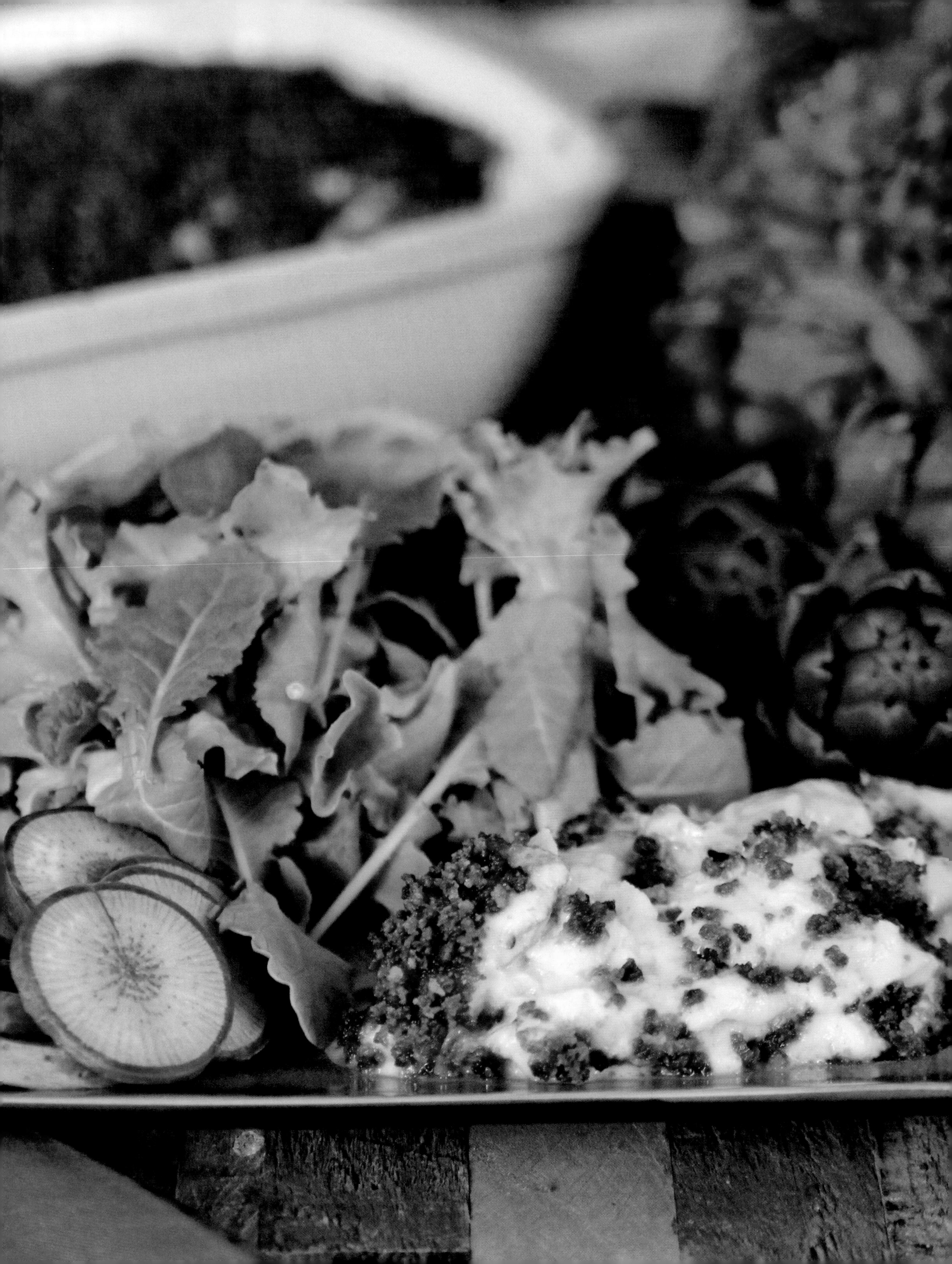

Teriyaki-Poached Trout

Poaching is one of the quickest and easiest ways to prepare fish. You can even poach frozen fish in a pinch (increasing the cooking time slightly), although it's better if your fish has thawed first. The flavor of this teriyaki-inspired poaching liquid is lovely with trout, salmon, mackerel, or any fatty fish. Asian-Inspired Cauliflower Rice (page 298) is the perfect accompaniment.

PREP TIME: 10 minutes, plus 15 minutes marinating time
COOK TIME: 10 to 12 minutes
SERVINGS: 3 to 5

INGREDIENTS:

- ½ cup fresh orange juice
- 1 teaspoon finely grated orange zest (optional)
- ¼ cup coconut aminos
- 2 teaspoons peeled and finely grated fresh ginger
- 3 or 4 cloves garlic, crushed
- 3 or 4 (6- to 8-ounce) trout fillets

FODMAP ALERT *Replace the garlic with green garlic or garlic scapes (green part only) or omit.*

1. Combine the orange juice, orange zest (if using), coconut aminos, ginger, and garlic in a small bowl.
2. Place the trout fillets in a large skillet or saucepan (it's okay if they overlap). Pour the poaching liquid over the top and let sit for 15 minutes before turning on the heat.
3. Bring to a boil over high heat, then cover and reduce the temperature to maintain a simmer. Simmer for 8 to 10 minutes, until the trout is fully cooked and opaque throughout. Enjoy!

VARIATIONS:

Teriyaki Marinade. *You can use the poaching liquid as a marinade for many uses. Simply combine the orange juice and zest, coconut aminos, ginger, and garlic and use it to marinate beef, pork, or chicken or as a stir-fry sauce!*

Teriyaki Salmon Jerky. *Slice salmon as thinly as possible, and marinate it in the Teriyaki Marinade in the refrigerator for 1 to 2 days. Then dry in a dehydrator for 3 to 6 hours.*

Lemon and Herb Poached Salmon. *Want to keep it super simple? Another lovely poaching liquid for fish is water or broth with 1 tablespoon lemon juice per ½ cup water, plus 1 to 2 teaspoons lemon zest and 3 or 4 sprigs fresh thyme. And fresh dill is a lovely herb to add instead of thyme.*

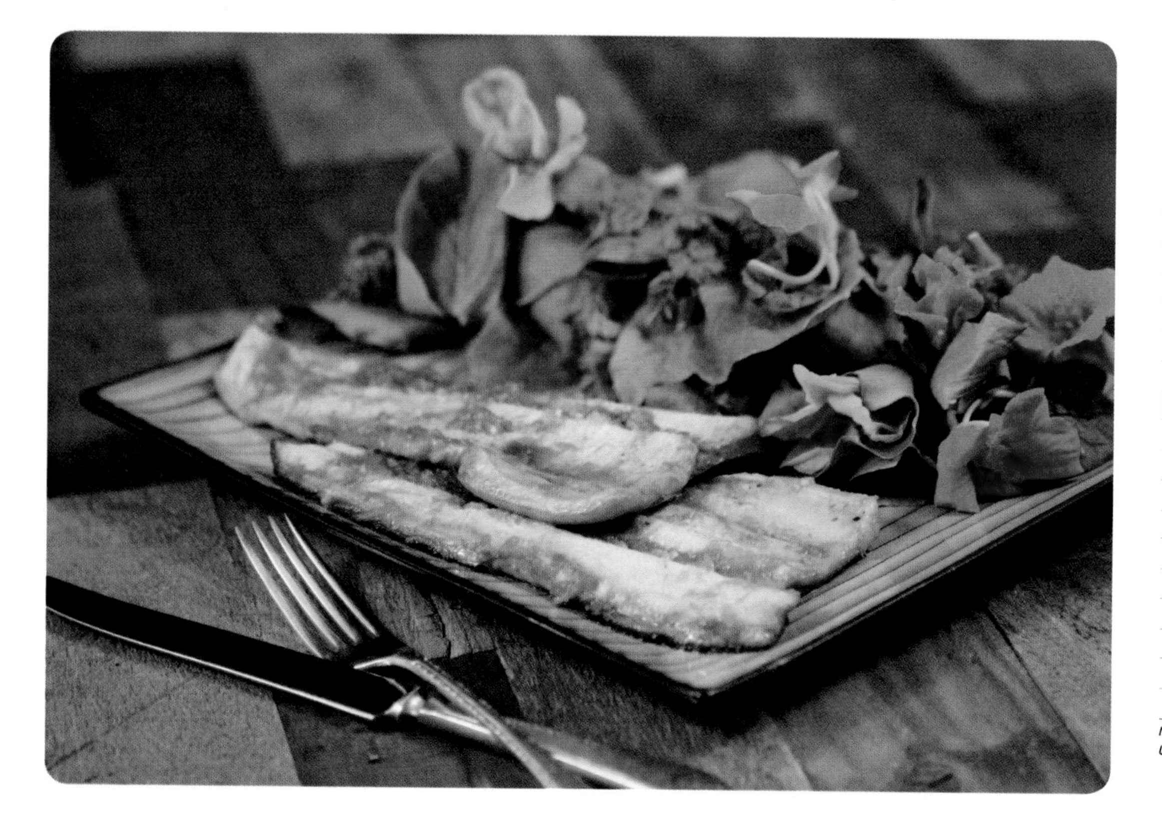

NUTRITION FACTS	
Serving Size	142 g
Recipe Yields	709 g
Calories	**213**
Fats	**8.37 g**
MUFA	2.77 g
Omega-3	2.64 g
Omega-6	0.24 g
Saturated Fat	1.29 g
Carbohydrates	**5.82 g**
Fiber	0.15 g
Starch	1.1 g
Fructose	0 g
Glucose	.0 g
Sucrose	0 g
Protein	**26.3 g**
Alanine	1.58 g
Arginine	1.58 g
Aspartic acid	2.69 g
Cystine	0.28 g
Glutamic acid	3.9 g
Glycine	1.25 g
Histidine	0.77 g
Isoleucine	1.2 g
Leucine	2.12 g
Lysine	2.39 g
Methionine	0.77 g
Phenylalanine	1.02 g
Proline	0.93 g
Serine	1.07 g
Threonine	1.14 g
Tryptophan	0.29 g
Tyrosine	0.88 g
Valine	1.35 g
Vitamins	
Vitamin B1	0.31 mg
Vitamin B12	3.12 mcg
Vitamin B2	0.51 mg
Vitamin B3	10.4 mg
Vitamin B5	2.02 mg
Vitamin B6	1 mg
Choline	2.19 mg
Folate	37.3 mcg
Vitamin A	15.9 mcg
Vitamin C	13.6 mg
Vitamin D	0 IU
Vitamin E	0.01 mg
Vitamin K	0.06 mcg
Minerals	
Calcium	22.1 mg
Copper	0.35 mg
Iron	1.14 mg
Magnesium	41.4 mg
Manganese	0.06 mg
Phosphorus	269 mg
Potassium	703 mg
Selenium	48.1 mcg
Sodium	330 mg
Zinc	0.87 mg

nutrition content estimated using the USDA database.

Smoked Salmon

Homemade smoked salmon is incredible—you'll never want to buy it from the store again! Plus, once you own a smoker, an entire world of delicious foods is suddenly at your fingertips.

PREP TIME: 5 to 10 minutes
COOK TIME: 1 hour 15 minutes
SERVINGS: 8 to 16

INGREDIENTS:

- 1 teaspoon avocado oil or melted coconut oil
- 4 pounds salmon fillets, skin on
- 1 tablespoon maple sugar
- 1 teaspoon salt

1. Line a smoker rack with aluminum foil. Spread the avocado oil over the foil. Place the salmon skin side down on the oiled aluminum foil.
2. Sprinkle the maple sugar and salt over the top of the salmon.
3. Preheat the smoker to 225°F following the manufacturer's directions. Cherry wood chips are especially lovely to use with salmon, but any type of wood works well.
4. Place the salmon in the smoker. Smoke for 1 hour 15 minutes.

TIPS:

While using a smoker is the easiest way to smoke salmon, you can also use a gas or charcoal grill. Place soaked wood chips in a foil pie plate and cover it with aluminum foil. Poke a few holes in the foil. If using a gas grill, place the pie plate on the burners on one side of your grill before lighting, and smoke the salmon on the opposite side of the grill. If using a charcoal grill, move the lit coals to one side of the grill and place the pie plate in the middle. Keep the vents closed to keep the smoke inside the grill as much as possible. Alternatively, see the directions for making your own smoker on page 54 of Beyond Bacon *by Stacy Toth and Matthew McCarry.*

VARIATIONS:

You can also use this recipe to smoke trout. Simply reduce the smoking time to 45 minutes to 1 hour.

Photo credit: Mickey Trescott of Autoimmune-Paleo.com

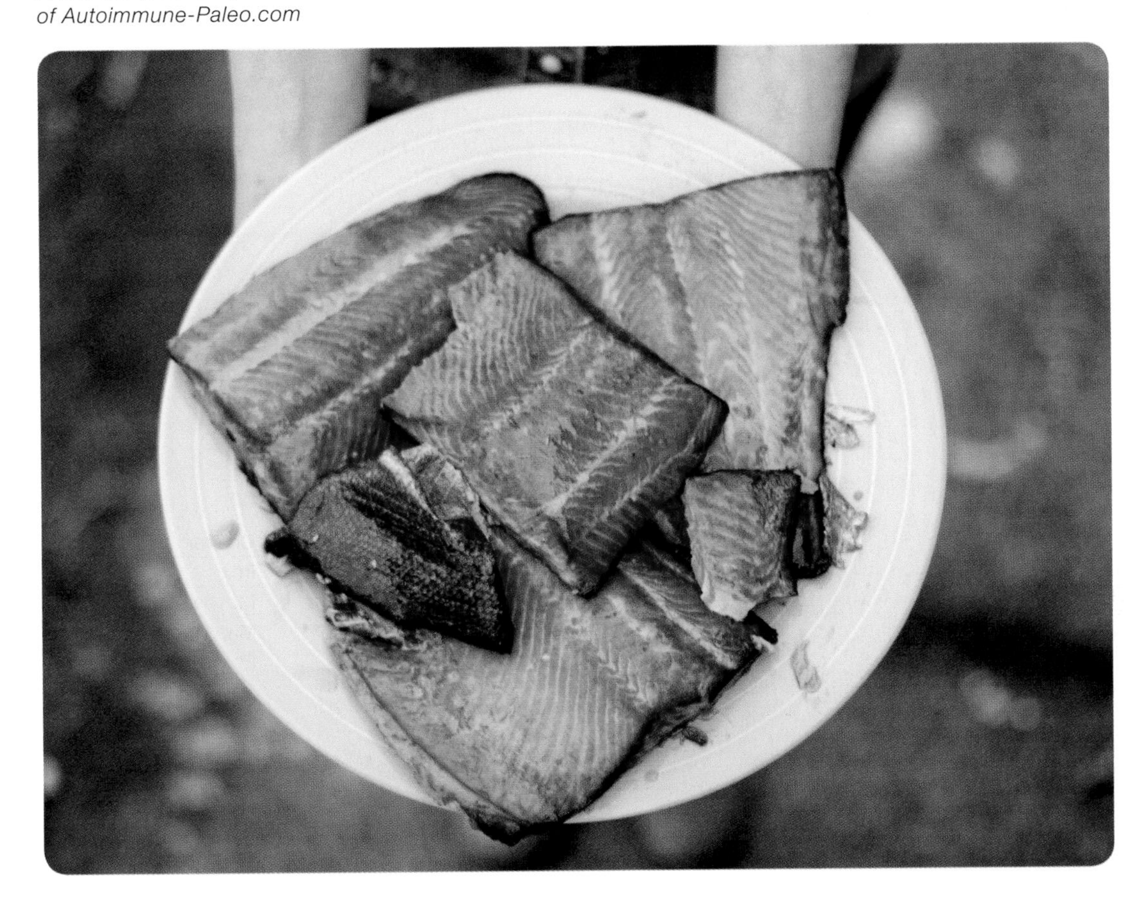

NUTRITION FACTS	
Serving Size	115 g
Recipe Yields	1834 g
Calories	**138**
Fats	**5.2 g**
MUFA	2.5 g
Omega-3	0.6 g
Omega-6	0.57 g
Saturated Fat	1.09 g
Carbohydrates	**0.51 g**
Fiber	0 g
Starch	0 g
Fructose	0 g
Glucose	0 g
Sucrose	0 g
Protein	**20.8 g**
Alanine	1.26 g
Arginine	1.24 g
Aspartic acid	2.13 g
Cystine	0.22 g
Glutamic acid	3.1 g
Glycine	1 g
Histidine	0.61 g
Isoleucine	0.96 g
Leucine	1.69 g
Lysine	1.91 g
Methionine	0.62 g
Phenylalanine	0.81 g
Proline	0.73 g
Serine	0.85 g
Threonine	0.91 g
Tryptophan	0.23 g
Tyrosine	0.7 g
Valine	1.07 g
Vitamins	
Vitamin B1	0.03 mg
Vitamin B12	3.71 mcg
Vitamin B2	0.11 mg
Vitamin B3	5.37 mg
Vitamin B5	0.99 mg
Vitamin B6	0.32 mg
Choline	101 mg
Folate	2.28 mcg
Vitamin A	29.6 mcg
Vitamin C	0 mg
Vitamin D	51.9 IU
Vitamin E	1.57 mg
Vitamin K	0.37 mcg
Minerals	
Calcium	13.4 mg
Copper	0.26 mg
Iron	0.98 mg
Magnesium	20.6 mg
Manganese	0.04 mg
Phosphorus	187 mg
Potassium	201 mg
Selenium	36.9 mcg
Sodium	1039 mg
Zinc	0.39 mg

nutrition content estimated using the USDA database.

Pan-Fried Sardines

If you don't enjoy sardines straight out of the can, trying them fried is definitely worthwhile! The tapioca coating leaves an incredibly light batter, just enough for a crisp outside. It's a very different flavor and texture and, in many ways, a more familiar flavor for most people.

PREP TIME: 10 to 15 minutes
COOK TIME: 10 to 20 minutes
SERVINGS: 2

INGREDIENTS:

- 2 (4-ounce) cans sardines (preferably packed in olive oil)
- ¼ cup tapioca starch or Water Chestnut Flour (page 121)
- ½ teaspoon salt
- 1 cup coconut oil
- Lemon wedges, for serving
- Chopped fresh parsley, for serving

1. Rinse, drain, and pat dry the sardines. If using larger sardines, split open (don't cut through) and open flat like a book.
2. Mix together the tapioca starch and salt in a shallow bowl. Toss the sardines in the tapioca mixture, shaking off the excess.
3. Heat the oil in a sauté pan or skillet over medium heat.
4. Fry the sardines until golden brown and crisp, about 2 minutes per side. Do this in batches so as not to overcrowd the pan.
5. Transfer the sardines to a paper towel–lined plate. Serve with lemon wedges and chopped parsley.

VARIATIONS:

You can easily make this recipe with fresh sardines or mackerel. Fresh fish will need to be gutted and scaled first and will take an extra minute or two per side to cook, depending on the size of the fish.

Pan-Fried Oysters. This is a great way to cook large oysters! Fresh shucked oysters will need to be cooked for 2 to 4 minutes per side, depending on their size.

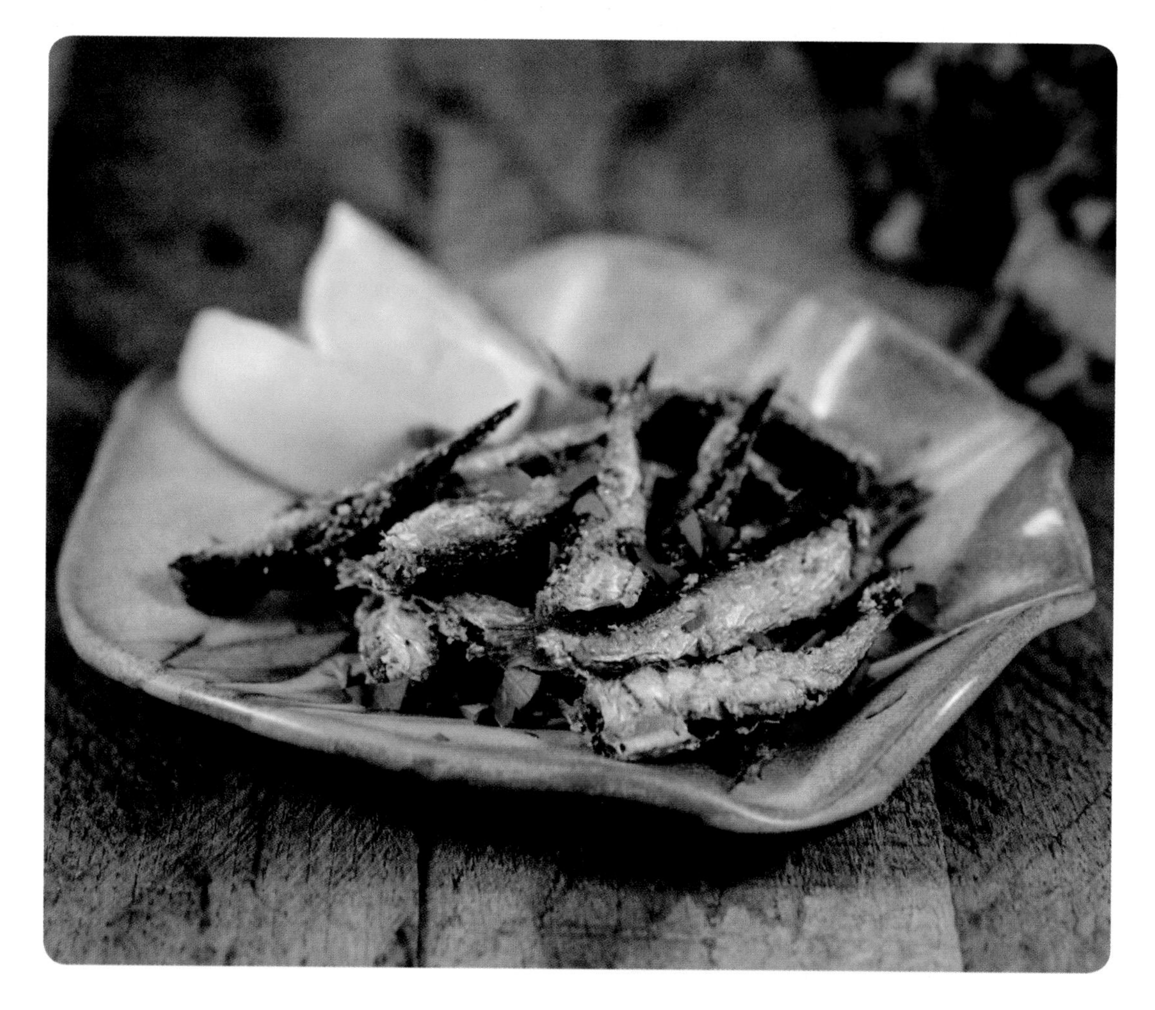

NUTRITION FACTS	
Serving Size	138 g
Recipe Yields	275 g
Calories	**336**
Fats	**21.8 g**
MUFA	4.91 g
Omega-3	1.83 g
Omega-6	4.19 g
Saturated Fat	9.31 g
Carbohydrates	**6.18 g**
Fiber	0.31 g
Starch	5.42 g
Fructose	0.08 g
Glucose	0.1 g
Sucrose	0.19 g
Protein	**28.1 g**
Alanine	1.7 g
Arginine	1.68 g
Aspartic acid	2.88 g
Cystine	0.3 g
Glutamic acid	4.19 g
Glycine	1.35 g
Histidine	0.83 g
Isoleucine	1.29 g
Leucine	2.28 g
Lysine	2.58 g
Methionine	0.83 g
Phenylalanine	1.1 g
Proline	1 g
Serine	1.15 g
Threonine	1.23 g
Tryptophan	0.32 g
Tyrosine	0.95 g
Valine	1.45 g
Vitamins	
Vitamin B1	0.1 mg
Vitamin B12	10.2 mcg
Vitamin B2	0.26 mg
Vitamin B3	6 mg
Vitamin B5	0.76 mg
Vitamin B6	0.2 mg
Choline	86 mg
Folate	15.3 mcg
Vitamin A	44.5 mcg
Vitamin C	6.25 mg
Vitamin D	219 IU
Vitamin E	2.35 mg
Vitamin K	34.2 mcg
Minerals	
Calcium	440 mg
Copper	0.22 mg
Iron	3.58 mg
Magnesium	46 mg
Manganese	0.13 mg
Phosphorus	560 mg
Potassium	472 mg
Selenium	60 mcg
Sodium	786 mg
Zinc	1.53 mg

nutrition content estimated using the USDA database.

Steamed Clams

Steamed clams are a wonderful nutrient-dense treat on their own or when served with salad, steamed vegetables, or Zucchini Noodles (page 310).

PREP TIME: 10 minutes
COOK TIME: 8 to 12 minutes
SERVINGS: 2 to 6

INGREDIENTS:

- 4 to 5 pounds littleneck clams
- 3 tablespoons lard, bacon fat, or coconut oil
- 5 cloves garlic, minced
- 1 tablespoon finely grated lemon zest (about 1 lemon)
- ½ cup white wine or a combination of 6 tablespoons Bone Broth (chicken, page 110) and 2 tablespoons fresh lemon juice
- 3 tablespoons chopped fresh parsley
- 1 lemon, halved

FODMAP ALERT *Replace the garlic with green garlic or garlic scapes (green part only) or omit.*

SPECIAL EQUIPMENT

- Large pot or skillet with a tight-fitting lid

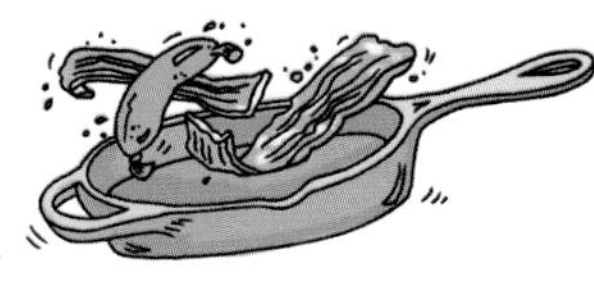

1. Rinse the clams under cool water. Discard any that do not close when gently tapped.
2. Heat the lard, garlic, and lemon zest in a large pot (one that has a tight-fitting lid, ideally glass) over medium-high heat. Cook for 3 to 4 minutes, until fragrant.
3. Place the clams in the pot. Add the wine, cover, and cook until the clams open, 5 to 8 minutes. Stir and check frequently to remove individual clams as they open, adding a little water if necessary.
4. Remove the clams from the pot. Remove and discard any clams that did not open. Sprinkle with parsley and drizzle with fresh lemon juice. Enjoy!

TIPS:

Serve with Russ' Flatbread (page 326) or Root Vegetable Biscuits (page 328) to mop up all those yummy juices! Alternatively, save the juices to substitute for broth in New England Clam Chowder (page 196).

VARIATIONS:

You can use any type of clam for this recipe. Depending on how big they are, you may need to adjust the cooking time.

Steamed Mussels. This recipe is ideal for cooking fresh mussels. To clean mussels, soak them in fresh water for about 20 minutes. Remove the beard by holding the mussel in one hand, covering the beard with a dry towel, and giving it a sharp yank toward the hinge end of the mussel. Use a firm brush to brush off any additional sand or barnacles. Also, replace the chopped parsley with chopped fresh tarragon.

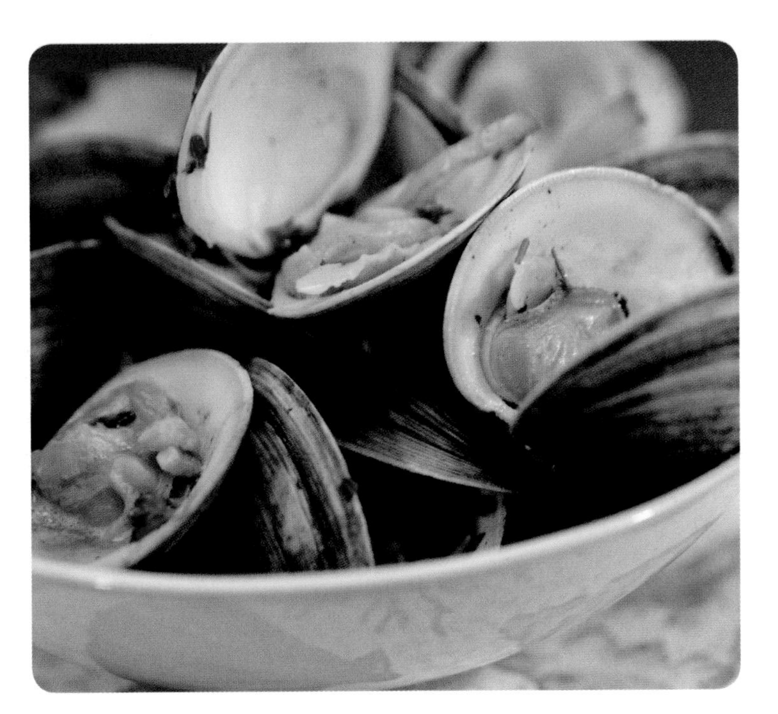

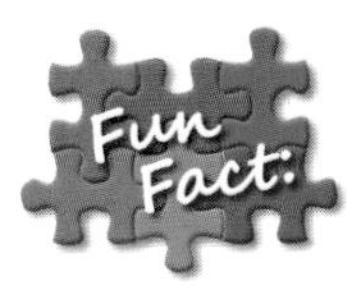

Clams, liver, and kidneys are excellent sources of vitamin B_{12}.

NUTRITION FACTS	
Serving Size	60 g
Recipe Yields	359 g
Calories	**50.4**
Fats	**1.12 g**
MUFA	0.35 g
Omega-3	0.07 g
Omega-6	0.09 g
Saturated Fat	0.34 g
Carbohydrates	**2.8 g**
Fiber	0.35 g
Starch	1.14 g
Fructose	0 g
Glucose	0 g
Sucrose	0 g
Protein	**6.85 g**
Alanine	0.41 g
Arginine	0.55 g
Aspartic acid	0.74 g
Cystine	0.08 g
Glutamic acid	1.03 g
Glycine	0.29 g
Histidine	0.14 g
Isoleucine	0.32 g
Leucine	0.55 g
Lysine	0.51 g
Methionine	0.19 g
Phenylalanine	0.26 g
Proline	0.23 g
Serine	0.32 g
Threonine	0.32 g
Tryptophan	0.09 g
Tyrosine	0.27 g
Valine	0.34 g
Vitamins	
Vitamin B1	0.01 mg
Vitamin B12	5.13 mcg
Vitamin B2	0.02 mg
Vitamin B3	0.2 mg
Vitamin B5	0.1 mg
Vitamin B6	0.02 mg
Choline	30.8 mg
Folate	6.27 mcg
Vitamin A	49 mcg
Vitamin C	7.88 mg
Vitamin D	1.11 IU
Vitamin E	0.34 mg
Vitamin K	31.3 mcg
Minerals	
Calcium	23.6 mg
Copper	0.03 mg
Iron	0.92 mg
Magnesium	10.6 mg
Manganese	0.05 mg
Phosphorus	93.4 mg
Potassium	47.4 mg
Selenium	14 mcg
Sodium	275 mg
Zinc	0.26 mg

nutrition content estimated using the USDA database.

Bacon-Braised Whitefish and Brussels

Sometimes it's nice to be able to throw a bunch of ingredients in a single pot or pan and have dinner at the end of it. While this is a common way to cook ground beef or reinvent leftover chicken, it's also a wonderful way to cook whitefish.

PREP TIME: 15 minutes
COOK TIME: 50 minutes
SERVINGS: 3 to 6

INGREDIENTS:

8 ounces bacon, cut into small pieces

1 pound Brussels sprouts, halved if large

1 small bunch kale, chopped (about 5 cups)

1½ to 2 pounds whitefish fillets, such as cod, hake, tilapia, or halibut, cut into 2-inch-wide pieces

3 cloves garlic, crushed

1 teaspoon finely grated lemon zest

Juice of 1 lemon

1 cup Bone Broth (fish or chicken, page 110)

FODMAP ALERT

This recipe cannot be made low-FODMAP.

SPECIAL EQUIPMENT

- Large skillet

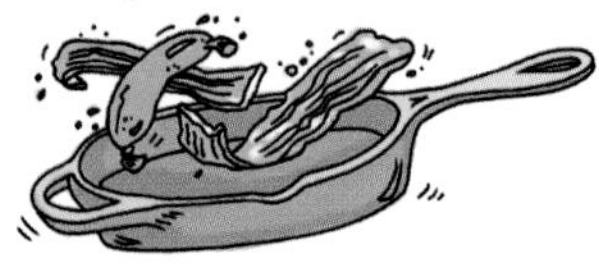

1. Place the bacon in a big saucepot or extra-large skillet, then turn on the heat to medium-high. Cook the bacon until it is crisp, stirring occasionally, about 10 minutes. If the bacon is very fatty, drain off a little fat, leaving 2 to 3 tablespoons of fat in the pan.
2. Add the Brussels sprouts and 2 to 3 tablespoons of the broth to the pan. Cook, stirring frequently, until the Brussels sprouts are fully cooked, about 20 minutes. When the broth evaporates, add another 2 to 3 tablespoons to the pan (this will likely happen 3 to 5 times). Try to maintain 1⁄16 to 1⁄8 inch of liquid in the pan. If you run out of broth before the Brussels sprouts are fully cooked, just use water.
3. Once the Brussels sprouts are done, add the kale (and a little more broth or water if needed). Once the kale starts to wilt (3 to 4 minutes), move the vegetables to the side of the pan and add the fish to the middle (again, add 1 to 2 tablespoons of broth or water, if needed).
4. Stir the fish gently and minimally. Once cooked (4 to 10 minutes, depending on how thick the pieces are), add the crushed garlic, lemon zest, and lemon juice and cook for 1 to 2 more minutes. Enjoy!

VARIATIONS:

You can use any vegetables you want in this dish; however, braising is a particularly nice way to cook cruciferous vegetables. You can try it with cabbage, broccoli, turnips, collards, or even add a little taro root for a starchy vegetable contribution. (If using taro, prepare it by following steps 1 and 3 for making Taro Hash on page 138, but cut the steamed and peeled taro into large pieces rather than ¼-inch dice.)

Bacon-Braised Scallops and Brussels. *Replace the whitefish with scallops. Depending on the size of the scallops, they may need only 3 to 4 minutes to cook before adding the garlic and lemon.*

Bacon-Braised Squid and Brussels. *Replace the whitefish with chopped squid rounds and tentacles. Squid pieces typically take 4 to 5 minutes to cook before adding the garlic and lemon.*

NUTRITION FACTS	
Serving Size	297 g
Recipe Yields	1779 g
Calories	**462**
Fats	**25.8 g**
MUFA	10.2 g
Omega-3	2.65 g
Omega-6	2.16 g
Saturated Fat	6.82 g
Carbohydrates	**11.9 g**
Fiber	4.07 g
Starch	4.49 g
Fructose	0.09 g
Glucose	0.08 g
Sucrose	0.03 g
Protein	**45.8 g**
Alanine	2.64 g
Arginine	2.76 g
Aspartic acid	4.29 g
Cystine	0.48 g
Glutamic acid	6.36 g
Glycine	2.38 g
Histidine	1.41 g
Isoleucine	2.11 g
Leucine	3.53 g
Lysine	3.88 g
Methionine	1.16 g
Phenylalanine	1.77 g
Proline	1.84 g
Serine	1.73 g
Threonine	1.9 g
Tryptophan	0.47 g
Tyrosine	1.43 g
Valine	2.34 g
Vitamins	
Vitamin B1	0.47 mg
Vitamin B12	1.53 mcg
Vitamin B2	0.41 mg
Vitamin B3	9.43 mg
Vitamin B5	1.64 mg
Vitamin B6	0.82 mg
Choline	77.2 mg
Folate	146 mcg
Vitamin A	358 mcg
Vitamin C	118 mg
Vitamin D	0 IU
Vitamin E	1.32 mg
Vitamin K	500 mcg
Minerals	
Calcium	156 mg
Copper	1.08 mg
Iron	2.87 mg
Magnesium	101 mg
Manganese	0.67 mg
Phosphorus	681 mg
Potassium	1195 mg
Selenium	42.6 mcg
Sodium	957 mg
Zinc	3.3 mg

nutrition content estimated using the USDA database.

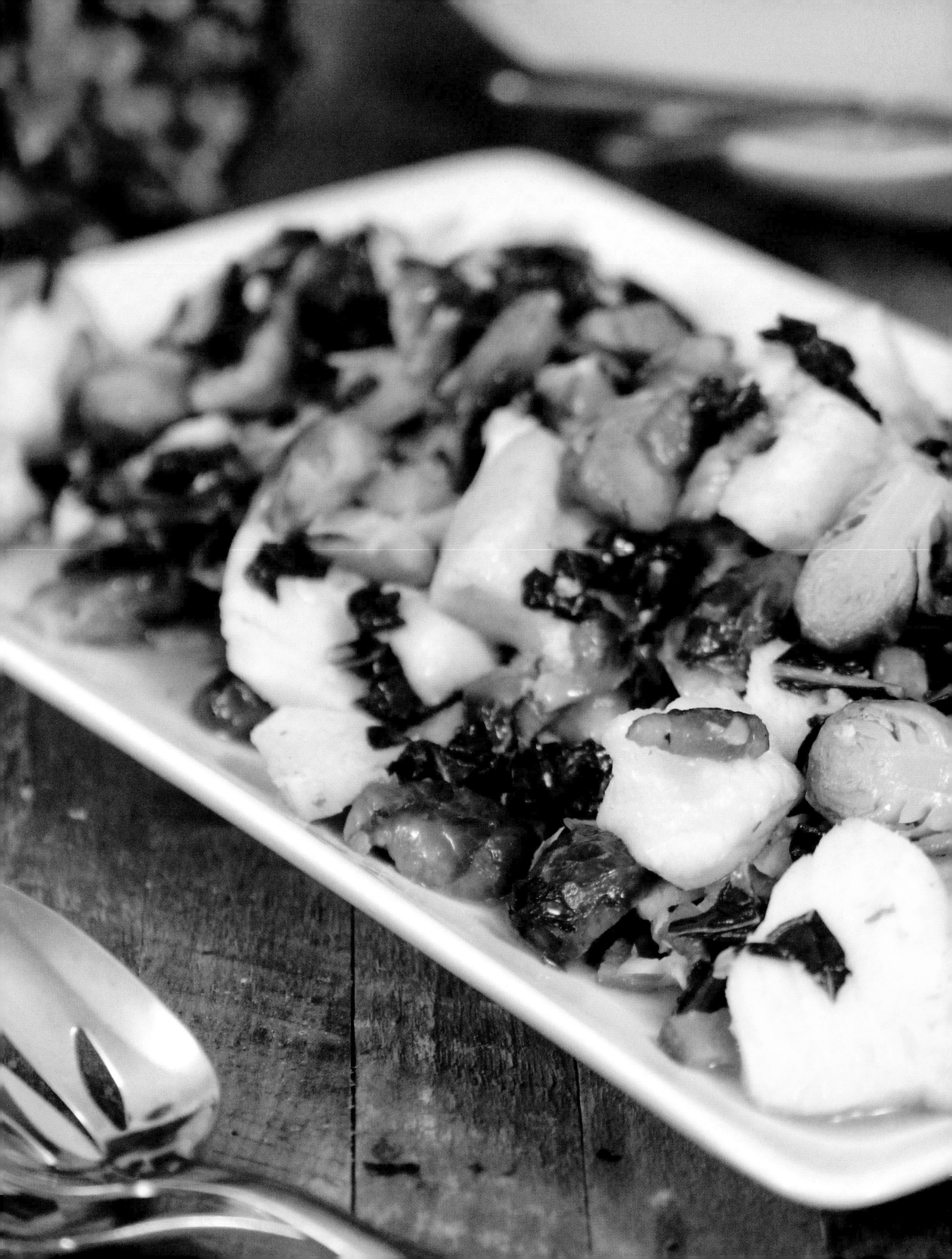

Deep-Fried Whole Shrimp with Cocktail Sauce

Finding out that deep-frying shrimp in the shell turns the shell into a crisp, edible outer coating was one of the most amazing discoveries! It's as though shrimp have their own natural breading! The shell is full of minerals that promote bone health, and the heads are the most nutrient-dense part of the whole shrimp.

PREP TIME: 15 minutes
COOK TIME: 30 minutes
SERVINGS: 2 to 4

INGREDIENTS:

Cocktail Sauce:

- 3 tablespoons peeled and finely grated fresh horseradish
- 1 tablespoon apple cider vinegar
- 2 tablespoons umeboshi paste
- 1 tablespoon tamarind paste

Shrimp:

- Lard or other fat, for deep-frying
- 1 pound whole shrimp, with heads and shells on

SPECIAL EQUIPMENT

- Countertop deep-fryer or large heavy-bottomed pot with an oil thermometer

COCKTAIL SAUCE:

1. Combine all the ingredients in a small bowl and chill in the refrigerator for at least 1 hour.

SHRIMP:

1. Heat the lard to 360°F to 365°F in a countertop deep-fryer or a large heavy-bottomed pot over medium heat with a deep-fry thermometer attached to the side. Use enough fat to fill the deep-fryer to the fill line or to have 2 inches in the bottom of the pot.
2. Carefully drop the shrimp into the hot lard, cooking in batches and being careful not to overcrowd.
3. Deep-fry until the shrimp has turned pink, 4 to 5 minutes, depending on the size of the shrimp.
4. Remove and drain on paper towels. Serve warm with the cocktail sauce.

TIPS:

For spicier cocktail sauce, let the horseradish sit for 30 minutes after grating before combining it with the remaining ingredients.

If you can't get whole fresh shrimp, or if you just aren't ready to eat shrimp heads, you can use cleaned shrimp (with the heads removed) that still have their shells on. The cocktail sauce is also delicious with steamed or sautéed shrimp.

There will be a lot of gritty bits in your deep-fryer when you're done. Filter them out by pouring your fat through a paper towel–lined sieve. Deep-frying seafood can leave a slightly fishy flavor in your fat. Use separate fat to deep-fry seafood versus vegetables.

NUTRITION FACTS

Nutrient	Amount
Serving Size	142 g
Recipe Yields	566 g
Calories	**155**
Fats	**2.05 g**
MUFA	0.44 g
Omega-3	0.35 g
Omega-6	0.33 g
Saturated Fat	0.62 g
Carbohydrates	**7.06 g**
Fiber	0.66 g
Starch	1.73 g
Fructose	0.02 g
Glucose	0.05 g
Sucrose	0.48 g
Protein	**26.2 g**
Alanine	1.61 g
Arginine	2.56 g
Aspartic acid	2.9 g
Cystine	0.31 g
Glutamic acid	4.58 g
Glycine	1.53 g
Histidine	0.57 g
Isoleucine	1.2 g
Leucine	2.22 g
Lysine	2.48 g
Methionine	0.76 g
Phenylalanine	1.13 g
Proline	1.19 g
Serine	1.06 g
Threonine	1.03 g
Tryptophan	0.3 g
Tyrosine	0.98 g
Valine	1.22 g
Vitamins	
Vitamin B1	0.06 mg
Vitamin B12	1.89 mcg
Vitamin B2	0.04 mg
Vitamin B3	3.2 mg
Vitamin B5	0.61 mg
Vitamin B6	0.29 mg
Choline	155 mg
Folate	34.5 mcg
Vitamin A	102 mcg
Vitamin C	3.01 mg
Vitamin D	4.55 IU
Vitamin E	2.51 mg
Vitamin K	0.76 mcg
Minerals	
Calcium	114 mg
Copper	0.31 mg
Iron	0.58 mg
Magnesium	50.5 mg
Manganese	0.08 mg
Phosphorus	358 mg
Potassium	264 mg
Selenium	56.7 mcg
Sodium	1321 mg
Zinc	1.95 mg

nutrition content estimated using the USDA database.

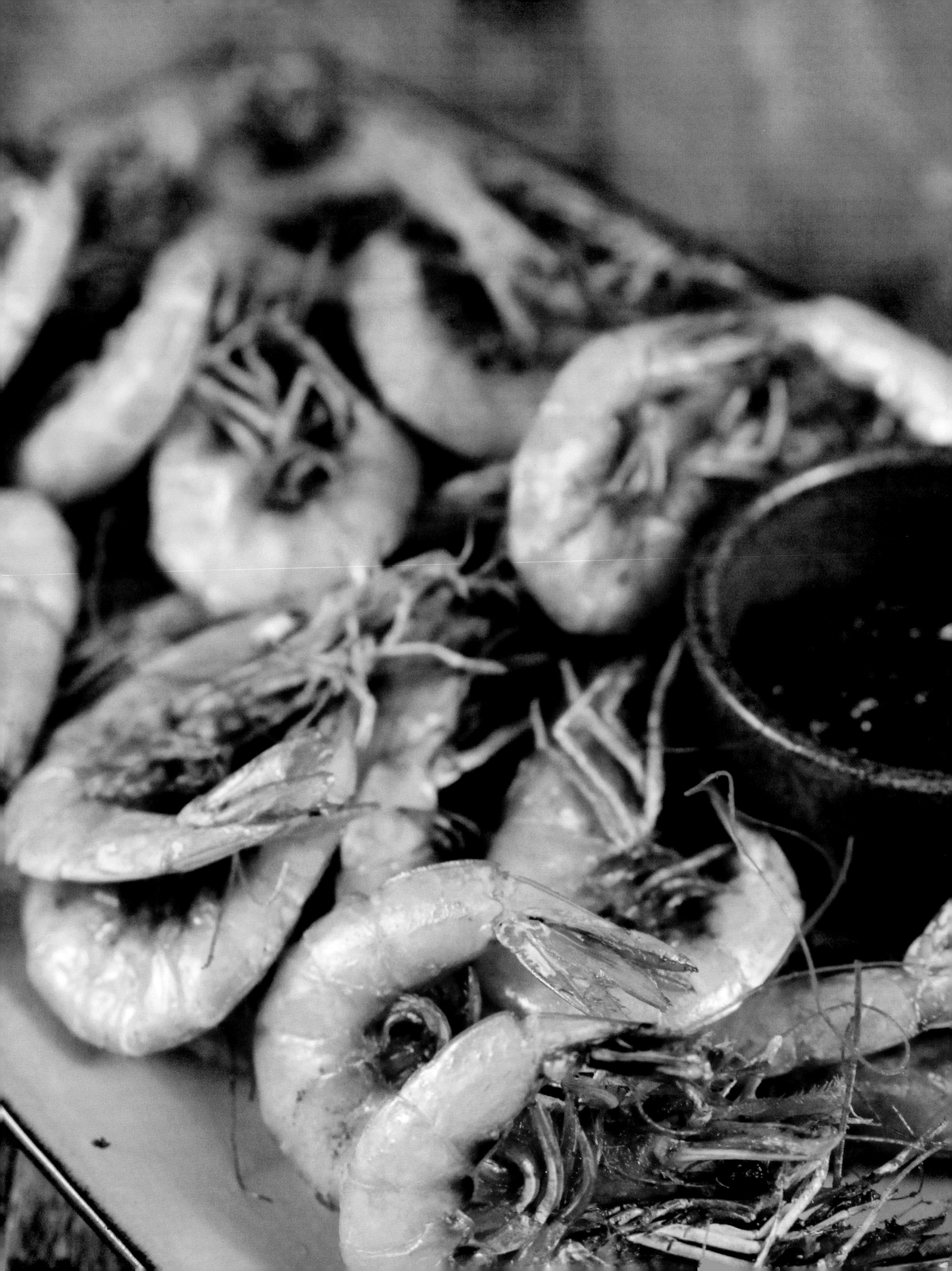

Calamari with Tzatziki Sauce

Calamari was always the highlight of any restaurant visit for me. But now I don't have to negotiate the gluten-filled batters in restaurants, because this calamari is absolutely delicious!

PREP TIME: 20 to 30 minutes
COOK TIME: 20 to 30 minutes
SERVINGS: 2 to 4

INGREDIENTS:

Tzatziki:

½ cup Coconut Milk Yogurt (page 118)

3 tablespoons chopped fresh dill

½ cup minced cucumber

1 clove garlic, crushed

1 tablespoon fresh lemon juice

Calamari:

Lard, for deep-frying

1 pound squid, tubes and tentacles

½ cup tapioca starch

¼ teaspoon salt

Lemon wedges, for serving

FODMAP ALERT *Replace the garlic with green garlic or garlic scapes (green part only) or omit. If you do not tolerate Coconut Milk Yogurt, skip the Tzatziki Sauce.*

SPECIAL EQUIPMENT

- Countertop deep-fryer or heavy-bottomed pot with an oil thermometer

TZATZIKI:

1. Place all the ingredients in a bowl and mix to thoroughly combine. Chill in the fridge for 1 hour.

CALAMARI:

1. Heat the lard to 360°F in a countertop deep-fryer or a heavy-bottomed pot over medium heat with a deep-fry thermometer attached to the side. Use enough lard to fill your deep-fryer to the fill line or to have 2 inches in the bottom of your pot.
2. Pat the squid dry with a clean kitchen towel or paper towels. If the tubes are whole, cut into ½-inch-wide rounds.
3. Mix together the tapioca and salt in shallow bowl. Dust the squid pieces with the tapioca and salt mixture, shaking off the excess, and carefully drop them into the hot lard, cooking in batches and being careful not to overcrowd.
4. Cook for 4 to 5 minutes, until golden brown and crisp on the outside. Drain on paper towels or newsprint.
5. Serve with lemon wedges and tzatziki sauce.

TIPS:

If you don't want to make homemade yogurt for the tzatziki sauce, you can use store-bought plain coconut milk yogurt or kefir.

The tapioca starch doesn't stick to the squid as well as traditional batters. While you can't tell from eating the finished product, there will be a lot of tapioca crumbs in your deep-fryer when you're done. Filter them out by pouring your fat through a paper towel–lined sieve.

Deep-frying seafood can leave a slightly fishy flavor to your fat. Use separate fat to deep-fry seafood versus vegetables.

NUTRITION FACTS	
Serving Size	206 g
Recipe Yields	825 g
Calories	**252**
Fats	**11.9 g**
MUFA	0.57 g
Omega-3	0.65 g
Omega-6	0.14 g
Saturated Fat	9.35 g
Carbohydrates	**15.1 g**
Fiber	1.21 g
Starch	10.4 g
Fructose	0.96 g
Glucose	0.86 g
Sucrose	0.19 g
Protein	**21.8 g**
Alanine	1.31 g
Arginine	1.68 g
Aspartic acid	2.08 g
Cystine	0.29 g
Glutamic acid	3.08 g
Glycine	1.39 g
Histidine	0.42 g
Isoleucine	0.93 g
Leucine	1.52 g
Lysine	1.58 g
Methionine	0.48 g
Phenylalanine	0.79 g
Proline	0.92 g
Serine	0.97 g
Threonine	0.92 g
Tryptophan	0.24 g
Tyrosine	0.68 g
Valine	0.96 g
Vitamins	
Vitamin B1	0.04 mg
Vitamin B12	1.27 mcg
Vitamin B2	0.44 mg
Vitamin B3	2.63 mg
Vitamin B5	0.81 mg
Vitamin B6	0.1 mg
Choline	90.8 mg
Folate	15.7 mcg
Vitamin A	14.8 mcg
Vitamin C	8.6 mg
Vitamin D	0 IU
Vitamin E	1.64 mg
Vitamin K	6.22 mcg
Minerals	
Calcium	58.7 mg
Copper	2.47 mg
Iron	1.79 mg
Magnesium	59.7 mg
Manganese	0.49 mg
Phosphorus	283 mg
Potassium	433 mg
Selenium	61.2 mcg
Sodium	98.9 mg
Zinc	2.37 mg

nutrition content estimated using the USDA database.

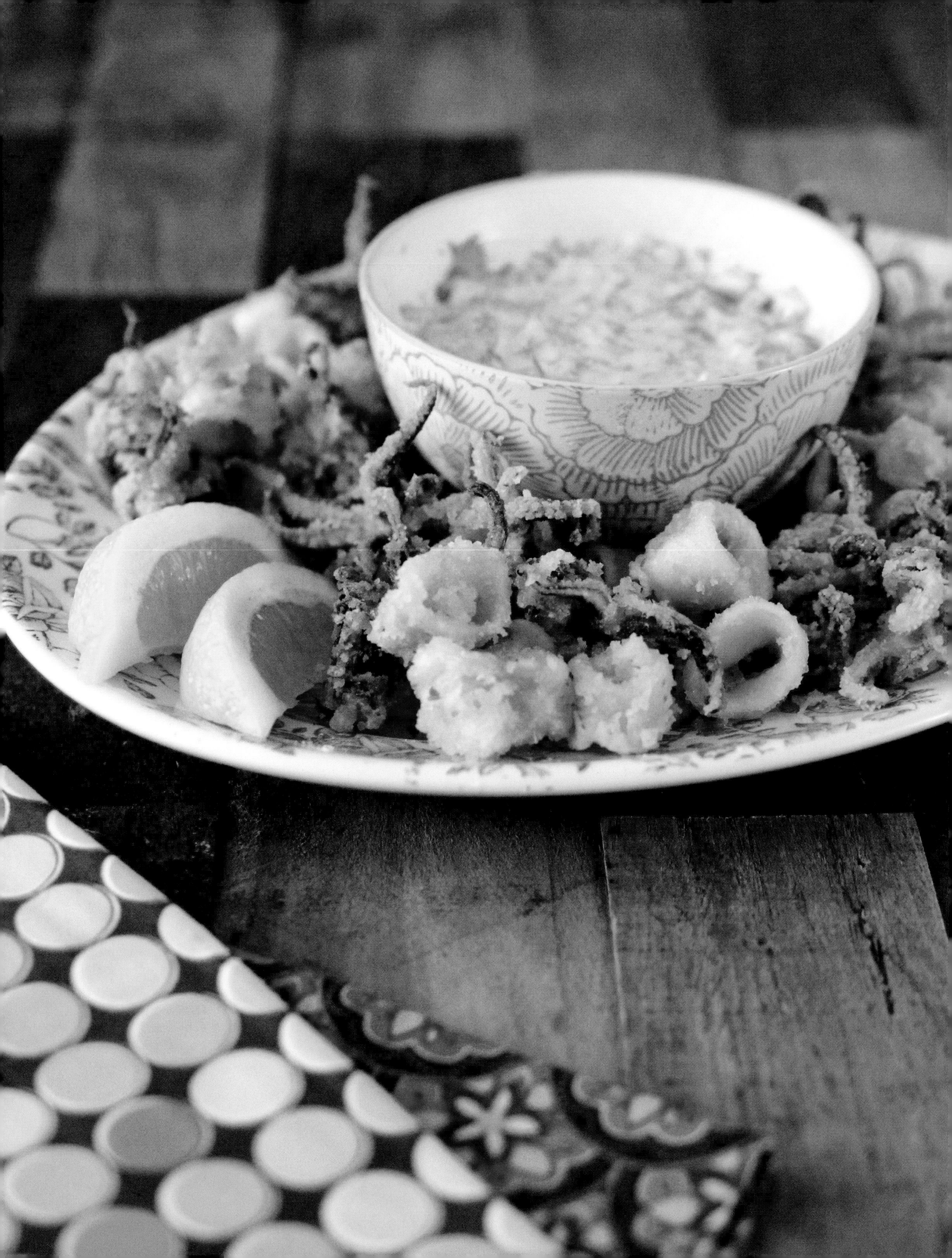

Tuna Salad Wraps

Avocado and lemon juice replace mayonnaise in these easy and delicious tuna salad wraps!

PREP TIME: 10 minutes
COOK TIME: none
SERVINGS: 1 to 2

INGREDIENTS:

1 (5-ounce) can albacore tuna (preferably no salt added), drained

½ avocado, peeled, pitted, and diced

2 teaspoons capers, minced

3 tablespoons chopped Green Tea and Garlic Pickles (page 114)

2 tablespoons finely diced red onion

1 stalk celery, finely diced

1 tablespoon fresh lemon juice

Pinch of ground turmeric

Pinch of salt, plus more to taste

Large lettuce leaves, for serving

1. Combine the tuna, avocado, capers, pickles, red onion, celery, lemon juice, turmeric, and salt. Mix to combine (minimally to keep it chunkier, or more thoroughly to make a smoother tuna salad, depending on your preference). Taste and season with additional salt, if desired.
2. Carefully slide a knife through the rib of each lettuce leaf to remove it (this makes it easier to fold the lettuce leaves into wraps). Add a spoonful of tuna salad and wrap the lettuce around it.

VARIATIONS:

Instead of wrapping in lettuce leaves, you can use large collard or chard leaves, coconut wraps, or nori. Or serve the tuna salad in celery sticks; in cucumber cups (see page 150); on slices of jicama, kohlrabi, cucumber, turnip, or radish; on Plantain Crackers (page 149); or on Russ' Flatbread (page 326).

You can use store-bought pickles for this tuna salad, too, or omit the pickles if you prefer.

FODMAP ALERT

This recipe cannot be made low-FODMAP.

NUTRITION FACTS	
Serving Size	189 g
Recipe Yields	378 g
Calories	**150**
Fats	**6.11 g**
MUFA	3.45 g
Omega-3	0.25 g
Omega-6	0.63 g
Saturated Fat	0.93 g
Carbohydrates	**6.64 g**
Fiber	3.67 g
Starch	0.41 g
Fructose	0.66 g
Glucose	0.68 g
Sucrose	0.2 g
Protein	**18 g**
Alanine	1.07 g
Arginine	1.06 g
Aspartic acid	1.86 g
Cystine	0.19 g
Glutamic acid	2.71 g
Glycine	0.86 g
Histidine	0.52 g
Isoleucine	0.81 g
Leucine	1.43 g
Lysine	1.6 g
Methionine	0.51 g
Phenylalanine	0.71 g
Proline	0.64 g
Serine	0.74 g
Threonine	0.77 g
Tryptophan	0.2 g
Tyrosine	0.59 g
Valine	0.92 g
Vitamins	
Vitamin B1	0.37 mg
Vitamin B12	0.37 mcg
Vitamin B2	0.12 mg
Vitamin B3	7.8 mg
Vitamin B5	1.15 mg
Vitamin B6	0.79 mg
Choline	56.7 mg
Folate	81.5 mcg
Vitamin A	143 mcg
Vitamin C	9.53 mg
Vitamin D	77.9 IU
Vitamin E	1.17 mg
Vitamin K	47.7 mcg
Minerals	
Calcium	43.3 mg
Copper	0.15 mg
Iron	1.19 mg
Magnesium	55.1 mg
Manganese	0.16 mg
Phosphorus	173 mg
Potassium	649 mg
Selenium	26.3 mcg
Sodium	322 mg
Zinc	0.74 mg

nutrition content estimated using the USDA database.

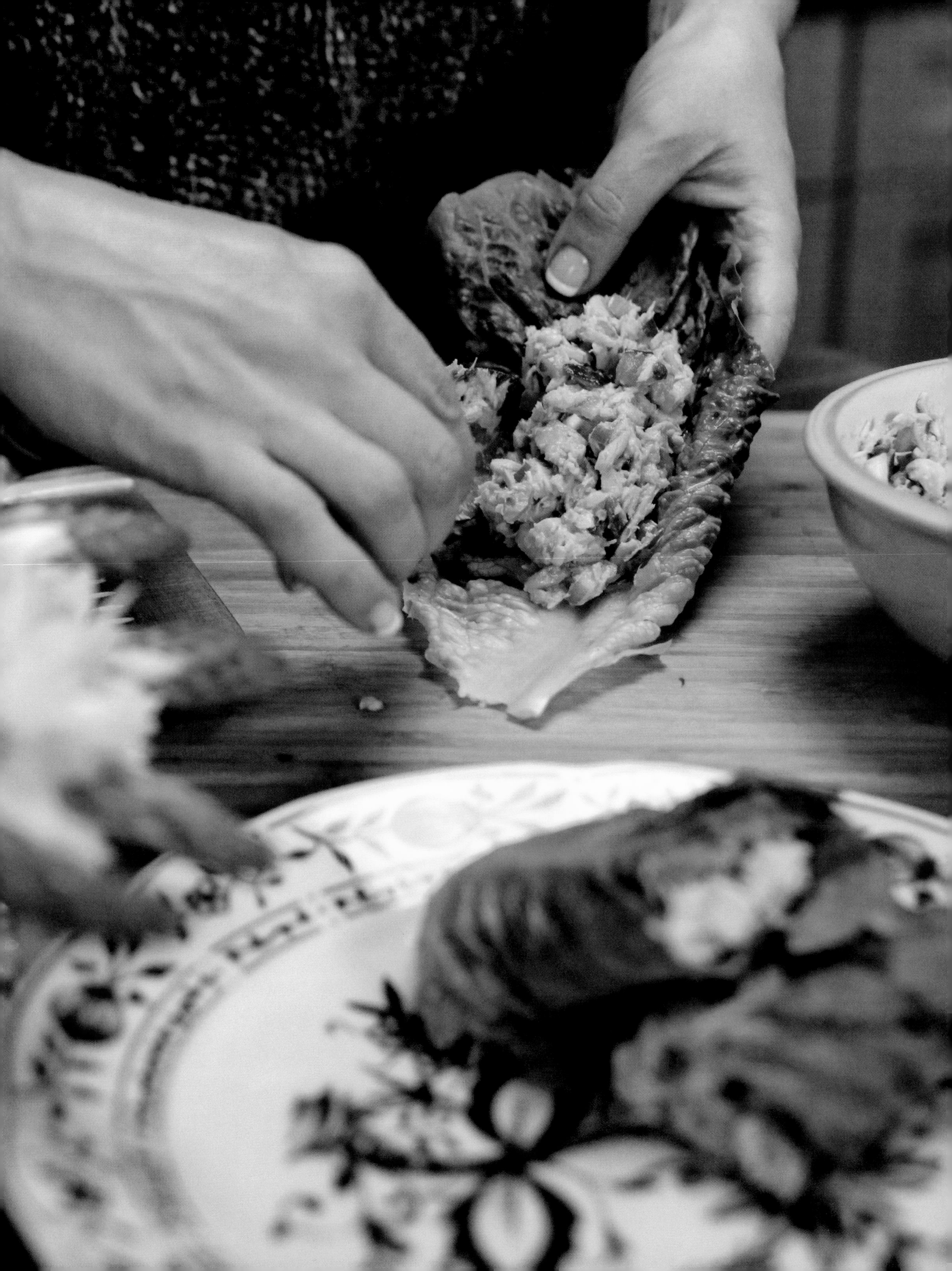

Asian-Inspired Salmon en Papillote

Doesn't the term en Papillote *sound elegant? All it really means is that the ingredients are baked in a pouch made from parchment paper (you can also use aluminum foil). Cooking this way retains moisture and allows the flavors to combine beautifully. It's a fancy term for a very straightforward cooking technique!*

Cucumber is actually wonderful when cooked, and it works well with both seafood and Asian-inspired flavors.

PREP TIME: 10 to 15 minutes
COOK TIME: 12 to 15 minutes
SERVINGS: 2 to 3

INGREDIENTS:

- 1 cucumber, peeled, seeded, and cut into bite-sized pieces
- 3 green onions, chopped
- 2 tablespoons coconut water vinegar
- ½ teaspoon peeled and finely grated fresh ginger
- 1 clove garlic, crushed
- 2 or 3 (6- to 8-ounce) salmon fillets

FODMAP ALERT *Replace the garlic with green garlic or garlic scapes (green part only) or omit. Use only the green parts of the green onions.*

SPECIAL EQUIPMENT

- Parchment paper or aluminum foil to make "envelopes"

1. Preheat the oven to 450°F.
2. Combine the cucumber, green onions, coconut water vinegar, ginger, and garlic in a bowl. Set aside.
3. Prepare a parchment or foil "envelope" for each piece of fish. Place a large sheet of parchment paper or aluminum foil on a rimmed baking sheet. The parchment or foil should measure a little over twice the length of the fish fillet. (You can also place all of your fillets in one parchment envelope. To create an envelope for more than one fillet, place them side by side, ensuring that there is 3 to 4 inches of extra parchment width at the top and bottom.)
4. Place the salmon on the bottom half of the parchment or foil, leaving 3 to 4 inches of space (in addition to one long side) around it for folding over. Spoon the cucumber mixture and liquid in the bowl over the salmon, dividing it equally among the envelopes. Fold over the long top portion of the parchment paper to cover the fish. Then triple-fold the edges on all 3 unsealed sides to form a fully sealed envelope or pocket.
5. Place in the oven (still on the baking sheet) and bake for 12 to 15 minutes, until the fish is opaque throughout and the segments flake apart easily. Be careful when opening the envelopes to avoid steam burns.

VARIATIONS:

Asian-Inspired Shellfish en Papillote. *Try this recipe with large prawns or a mix of shellfish instead of salmon.*

Har Gow–Inspired Shrimp Balls en Papillote. *Replace the salmon with uncooked Har Gow–Inspired Shrimp Balls (page 156) and spoon the cucumber mixture on top. As an alternative, you can form the shrimp ball mixture into patties rather than balls.*

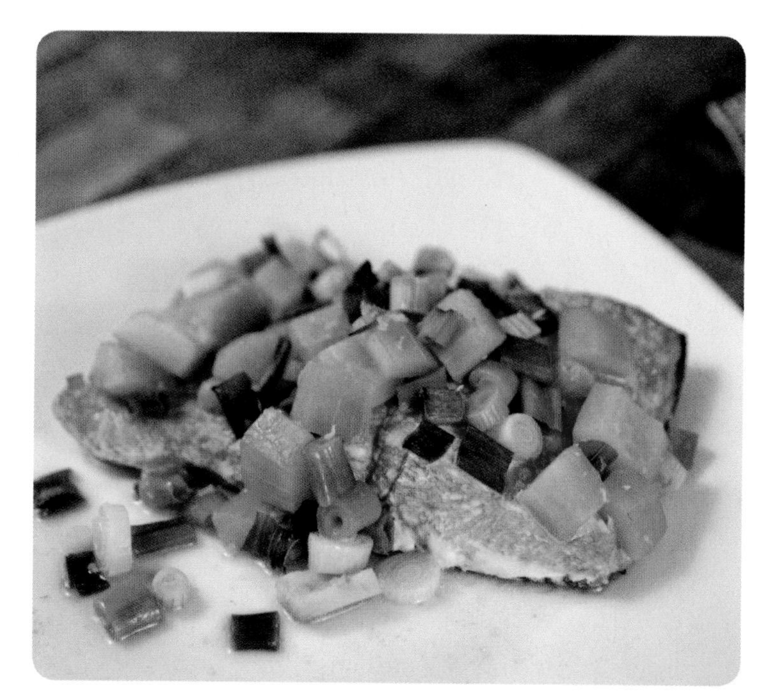

NUTRITION FACTS	
Serving Size	204 g
Recipe Yields	611 g
Calories	**189**
Fats	**6.17 g**
MUFA	1.84 g
Omega-3	0.83 g
Omega-6	0.14 g
Saturated Fat	1.12 g
Carbohydrates	**2.62 g**
Fiber	0.71 g
Starch	0.4 g
Fructose	0.86 g
Glucose	0.68 g
Sucrose	0.02 g
Protein	**28.5 g**
Alanine	1.8 g
Arginine	1.78 g
Aspartic acid	3.54 g
Cystine	0.22 g
Glutamic acid	4.1 g
Glycine	1.74 g
Histidine	0.74 g
Isoleucine	1.31 g
Leucine	2.15 g
Lysine	2.42 g
Methionine	0.79 g
Phenylalanine	1.17 g
Proline	1.19 g
Serine	1.25 g
Threonine	1.46 g
Tryptophan	0.31 g
Tyrosine	1.01 g
Valine	1.51 g
Vitamins	
Vitamin B1	0.13 mg
Vitamin B12	5.37 mcg
Vitamin B2	0.16 mg
Vitamin B3	11 mg
Vitamin B5	1.59 mg
Vitamin B6	0.85 mg
Choline	133 mg
Folate	18.8 mcg
Vitamin A	74.4 mcg
Vitamin C	4.09 mg
Vitamin D	593 IU
Vitamin E	0.59 mg
Vitamin K	24.2 mcg
Minerals	
Calcium	27.3 mg
Copper	0.14 mg
Iron	0.76 mg
Magnesium	47.2 mg
Manganese	0.12 mg
Phosphorus	375 mg
Potassium	622 mg
Selenium	43 mcg
Sodium	106 mg
Zinc	0.68 mg

nutrition content estimated using the USDA database.

Oysters on the Half Shell

Oysters are one of the most nutrient-dense foods available. Some types of oysters are better for cooking, while others are absolutely delectable raw. When in doubt, ask your fishmonger for suggestions.

PREP TIME: 20 to 30 minutes, plus at least 1 hour marinating time
COOK TIME: none
SERVINGS: 2 to 4

INGREDIENTS:

- ¼ cup coconut water vinegar or white wine vinegar
- 2 tablespoons fresh lemon juice
- 1 small shallot, minced
- 1½ teaspoons peeled and grated fresh ginger
- ⅓ English cucumber, minced (about 1 cup; peel if desired)
- 2 tablespoons chopped fresh cilantro leaves
- 12 oysters, cleaned and shucked (see Tips)

SPECIAL EQUIPMENT

- Shucking knife

1. In a bowl, combine the vinegar, lemon juice, shallot, ginger, cucumber, and cilantro. Chill in the fridge for at least 1 hour and up to overnight.
2. Place an even layer of crushed ice on the bottom of a serving platter. Place the shucked oysters on the bed of ice.
3. Spoon a dollop of the cucumber sauce over the top of each oyster, and serve immediately.

TIPS:

When you buy oysters, ask your fishmonger to shuck them for you; otherwise, you will need to shuck them yourself. To shuck an oyster, scrub the outside under cold water, then stick a shucking knife or the tip of a sturdy knife into the hinge and pry it open.

FODMAP ALERT *Replace the shallot with chopped green onion (green part only) or chives.*

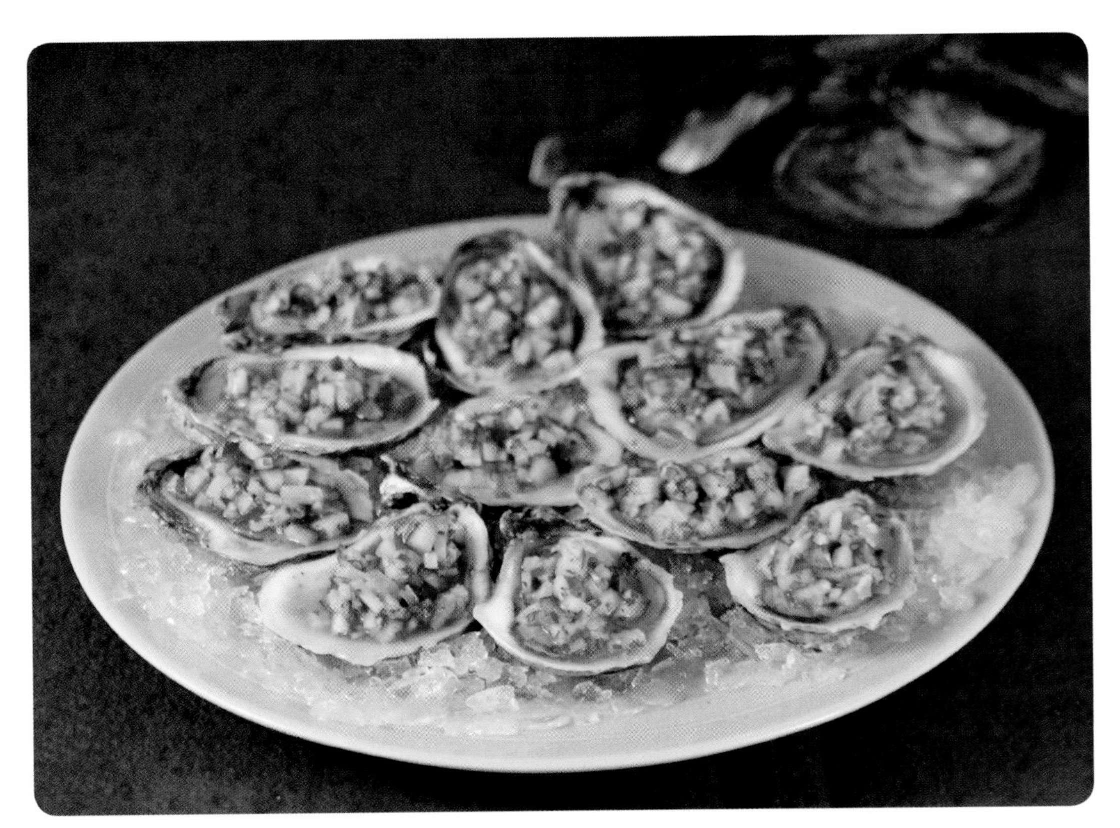

NUTRITION FACTS

Serving Size	148 g
Recipe Yields	593 g
Calories	**89.6**
Fats	**2.29 g**
MUFA	0.35 g
Omega-3	0.8 g
Omega-6	0.08 g
Saturated Fat	0.51 g
Carbohydrates	**6.93 g**
Fiber	0.26 g
Starch	5.56 g
Fructose	0.34 g
Glucose	0.28 g
Sucrose	0.04 g
Protein	**9.44 g**
Alanine	0.56 g
Arginine	0.68 g
Aspartic acid	0.9 g
Cystine	0.12 g
Glutamic acid	1.31 g
Glycine	0.58 g
Histidine	0.18 g
Isoleucine	0.41 g
Leucine	0.66 g
Lysine	0.7 g
Methionine	0.21 g
Phenylalanine	0.34 g
Proline	0.38 g
Serine	0.42 g
Threonine	0.4 g
Tryptophan	0.1 g
Tyrosine	0.3 g
Valine	0.41 g
Vitamins	
Vitamin B1	0.08 mg
Vitamin B12	15.5 mcg
Vitamin B2	0.24 mg
Vitamin B3	2 mg
Vitamin B5	0.57 mg
Vitamin B6	0.07 mg
Choline	57.9 mg
Folate	14.2 mcg
Vitamin A	81.5 mcg
Vitamin C	11.8 mg
Vitamin D	0.97 IU
Vitamin E	0.86 mg
Vitamin K	6.6 mcg
Minerals	
Calcium	14.6 mg
Copper	1.55 mg
Iron	5.1 mg
Magnesium	26.7 mg
Manganese	0.69 mg
Phosphorus	167 mg
Potassium	232 mg
Selenium	74.8 mcg
Sodium	105 mg
Zinc	16.2 mg

nutrition content estimated using the USDA database.

Chapter 10

Offal

Eating snout-to-tail is important for nutrient-density reasons, ecological reasons, and economic reasons. While there are organs and other unusual cuts that are not represented here, this chapter attempts to provide a good cross-section of those that are more easily obtained.

Some of these recipes are designed to hide organ meat. Others are designed to embrace it. And many of these recipes can be made with more familiar muscle meats if you want to try a non-offal variation.

Offal is actually found in some other recipes throughout this book, and many recipes can be made with offal as a variation. For example, organ meat can easily be hidden in sausage (see page 131), spaghetti (see page 224 and page 310), and generally any recipe that calls for ground meat or stew meat. Offal recipes found in other chapters include Bone Broth (page 110), Bacon and Bison Liver Pâté (page 152), Pork Rinds (page 167), Sweet-and-Sour Beef Heart Jerky (page 178), Oxtail and Pearl Onion Soup (page 191), Beef Heart Borscht (page 192), Beef Cheek and Daikon Radish Stew (page 198), Rabbit and Wild Mushroom Stew (page 200), and Deep-Fried Whole Shrimp with Cocktail Sauce (page 256).

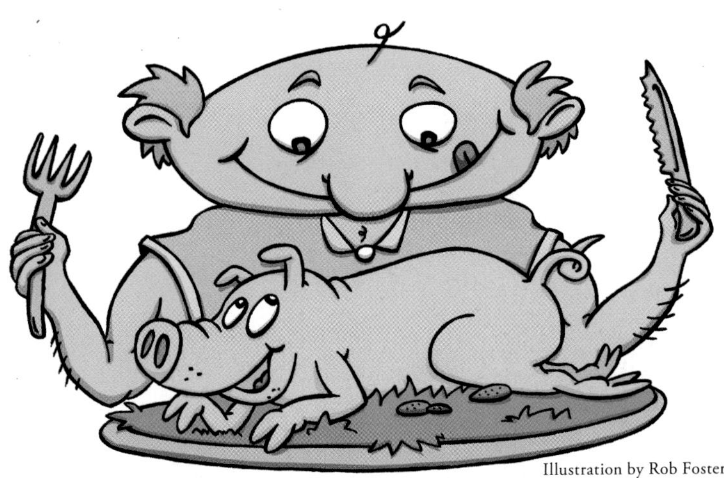

Illustration by Rob Foster

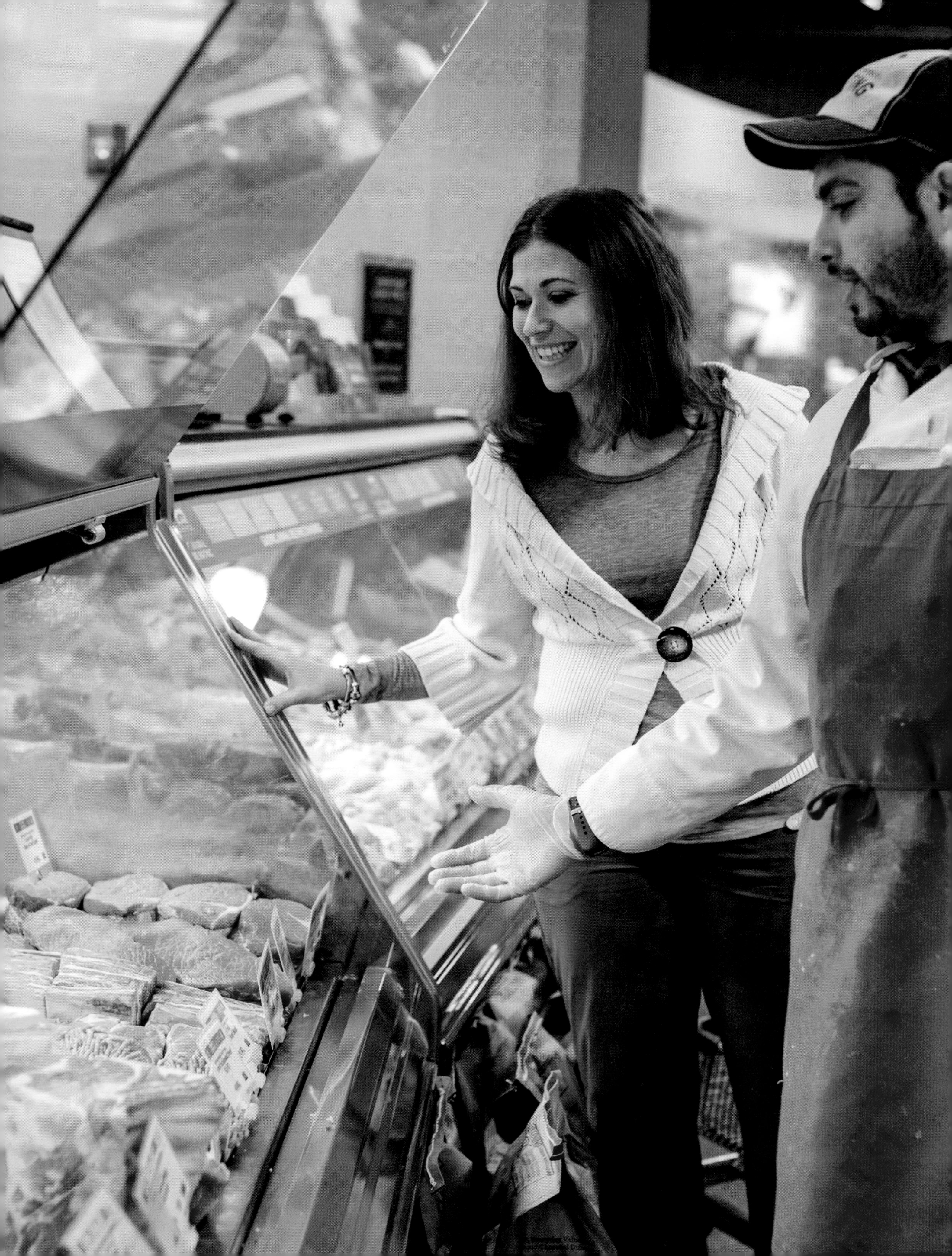

Marrow Spread with Parsley Salad

Bone marrow is one of the most luxurious and delicious foods available. In addition to Plantain Crackers (page 149), roasted marrow is also delicious served on Russ' Flatbread (page 326), sliced cucumber, or Belgian endive leaves, and it is an amazing topping for Hamburgers (page 222 and page 289). It's also really good with a spoon!

PREP TIME: 10 minutes
COOK TIME: 20 minutes
SERVINGS: 2 to 5

INGREDIENTS:

Parsley Salad:

- ½ cup chopped fresh parsley
- 1 shallot, thinly sliced
- 1 teaspoon capers
- 1 tablespoon extra-virgin olive oil
- 1 teaspoon fresh lemon juice
- Dash of salt

Marrow:

- 2 pounds marrow bones (either center-cut or narrow cross-cut)
- Plantain Crackers, for serving (page 149)

PARSLEY SALAD:

1. Combine all the ingredients in a small bowl.

MARROW:

1. Preheat the oven to 450°F.
2. If the marrow bones are center-cut, stand them up on end in a baking dish. If they are cross-cut, arrange them marrow side up in a baking dish.
3. Roast for 20 minutes.
4. Spread the marrow on a cracker or other base, and add a spoonful of the parsley salad on top.

FODMAP ALERT *Replace the shallot with chopped green onion (green part only) or chives.*

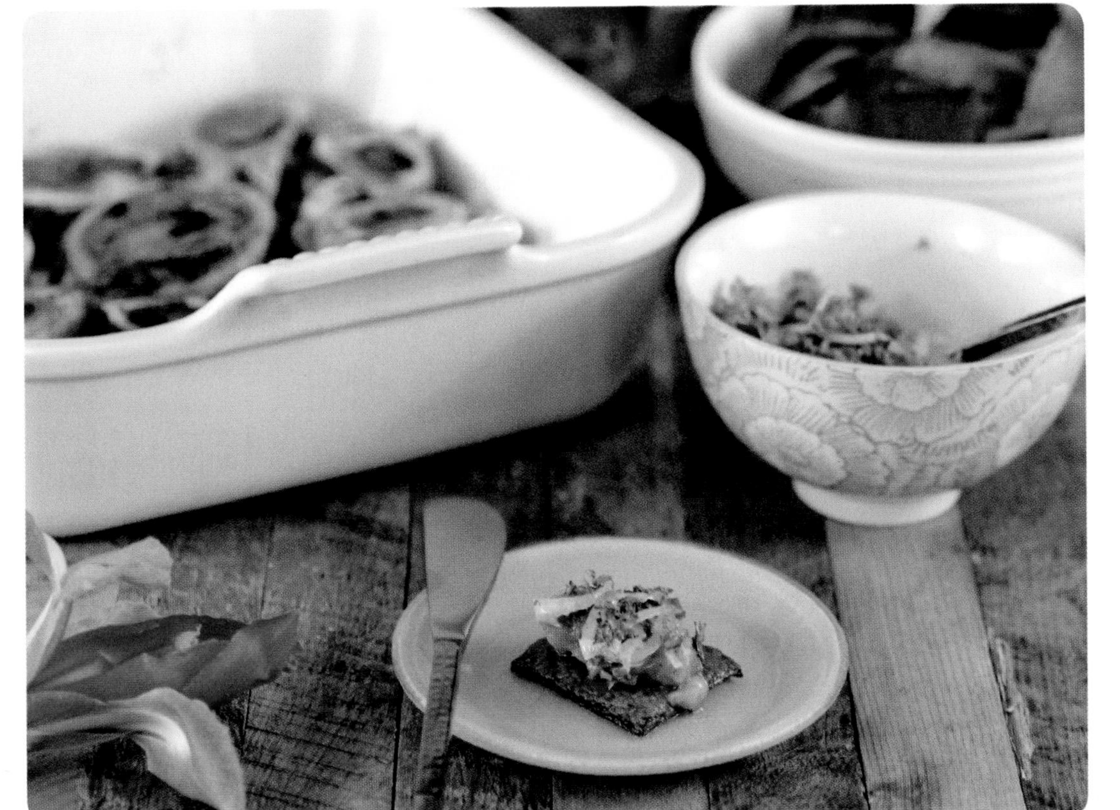

NUTRITION FACTS	
Serving Size	154 g
Recipe Yields	768 g
Calories	**679**
Fats	**66.2 g**
MUFA	3.28 g
Omega-3	0.04 g
Omega-6	0.7 g
Saturated Fat	19.4 g
Carbohydrates	**23.8 g**
Fiber	1.94 g
Starch	10.8 g
Fructose	0.03 g
Glucose	0.03 g
Sucrose	0.01 g
Protein	**1.59 g**
Alanine	0.05 g
Arginine	0.09 g
Aspartic acid	0.1 g
Cystine	0.02 g
Glutamic acid	0.11 g
Glycine	0.04 g
Histidine	0.05 g
Isoleucine	0.04 g
Leucine	0.06 g
Lysine	0.06 g
Methionine	0.02 g
Phenylalanine	0.04 g
Proline	0.05 g
Serine	0.04 g
Threonine	0.03 g
Tryptophan	0.01 g
Tyrosine	0.03 g
Valine	0.05 g
Vitamins	
Vitamin B1	0.04 mg
Vitamin B12	0 mcg
Vitamin B2	0.05 mg
Vitamin B3	0.76 mg
Vitamin B5	0.22 mg
Vitamin B6	0.23 mg
Choline	11 mg
Folate	26.3 mcg
Vitamin A	65.5 mcg
Vitamin C	22.6 mg
Vitamin D	0 IU
Vitamin E	0.56 mg
Vitamin K	101 mcg
Minerals	
Calcium	32.9 mg
Copper	0.09 mg
Iron	2.37 mg
Magnesium	41.7 mg
Manganese	0.02 mg
Phosphorus	29.4 mg
Potassium	405 mg
Selenium	5.66 mcg
Sodium	163 mg
Zinc	0.63 mg

nutrition content estimated using the USDA database.

Fried Kidney with Kumquat and Cranberry Chutney

This is one of my favorite breakfasts, especially with some homemade sauerkraut on the side.

PREP TIME: 10 minutes
COOK TIME: 20 minutes
SERVINGS: 2 to 6

INGREDIENTS:

Kumquat and Cranberry Chutney:

- 1 tablespoon coconut oil
- 1 red onion, finely chopped
- 1 clove garlic, crushed
- 10 ounces kumquats, sliced into rounds
- 5 ounces cranberries (fresh or frozen)
- 1 tablespoon port or Madeira (optional)
- ⅓ cup red wine vinegar
- 3 tablespoons grade B maple syrup

Kidney:

- 3 to 4 tablespoons bacon fat
- 1 to 1½ pounds beef kidney, cut crosswise into 1-inch-thick slices

FODMAP ALERT *Replace the garlic with green garlic or garlic scapes (green part only) or omit. Replace the red onion with green onion or leek (green part only) or chives or omit.*

CHUTNEY:

1. Heat the oil in a skillet over medium-high heat. Sauté the onion and garlic for 4 to 5 minutes, until softened.
2. Stir in the kumquats, cranberries, port, red wine vinegar, and maple syrup. Bring the mixture to the boil, then reduce to a simmer. Simmer for 15 to 20 minutes, until the mixture reaches a jamlike consistency. Enjoy warm or chilled.

KIDNEY:

1. Heat the bacon fat in a large skillet over medium-high heat.
2. Add the slices of kidney to the hot fat, taking care not to overcrowd the pan. Fry for 3 to 4 minutes per side, until browned and cooked through.
3. Serve with the chutney.

TIPS:

This chutney is delicious with steak, pork chops, burgers, chicken, and turkey, too!

VARIATIONS:

You can serve this dish as an appetizer by cutting the kidney into smaller pieces and serving it on Plantain Crackers (page 149) or Russ' Flatbread (page 326).

NUTRITION FACTS

Serving Size	189 g
Recipe Yields	1132 g
Calories	**241**
Fats	**8.4 g**
MUFA	1.72 g
Omega-3	0.06 g
Omega-6	0.93 g
Saturated Fat	3.67 g
Carbohydrates	**18.8 g**
Fiber	4.35 g
Starch	1.01 g
Fructose	0.45 g
Glucose	1.23 g
Sucrose	5.99 g
Protein	**21.8 g**
Alanine	1.26 g
Arginine	1.33 g
Aspartic acid	1.94 g
Cystine	0.23 g
Glutamic acid	3.17 g
Glycine	1.14 g
Histidine	0.71 g
Isoleucine	0.94 g
Leucine	1.65 g
Lysine	1.74 g
Methionine	0.53 g
Phenylalanine	0.82 g
Proline	0.92 g
Serine	0.81 g
Threonine	0.91 g
Tryptophan	0.23 g
Tyrosine	0.7 g
Valine	1.02 g
Vitamins	
Vitamin B1	0.15 mg
Vitamin B12	18.9 mcg
Vitamin B2	2.43 mg
Vitamin B3	3.23 mg
Vitamin B5	1.37 mg
Vitamin B6	0.35 mg
Choline	396 mg
Folate	73.4 mcg
Vitamin A	7.82 mcg
Vitamin C	25 mg
Vitamin D	36.3 IU
Vitamin E	0.43 mg
Vitamin K	1.27 mcg
Minerals	
Calcium	60.4 mg
Copper	0.5 mg
Iron	4.97 mg
Magnesium	24.1 mg
Manganese	0.61 mg
Phosphorus	248 mg
Potassium	258 mg
Selenium	127 mcg
Sodium	82.7 mg
Zinc	2.44 mg

nutrition content estimated using the USDA database.

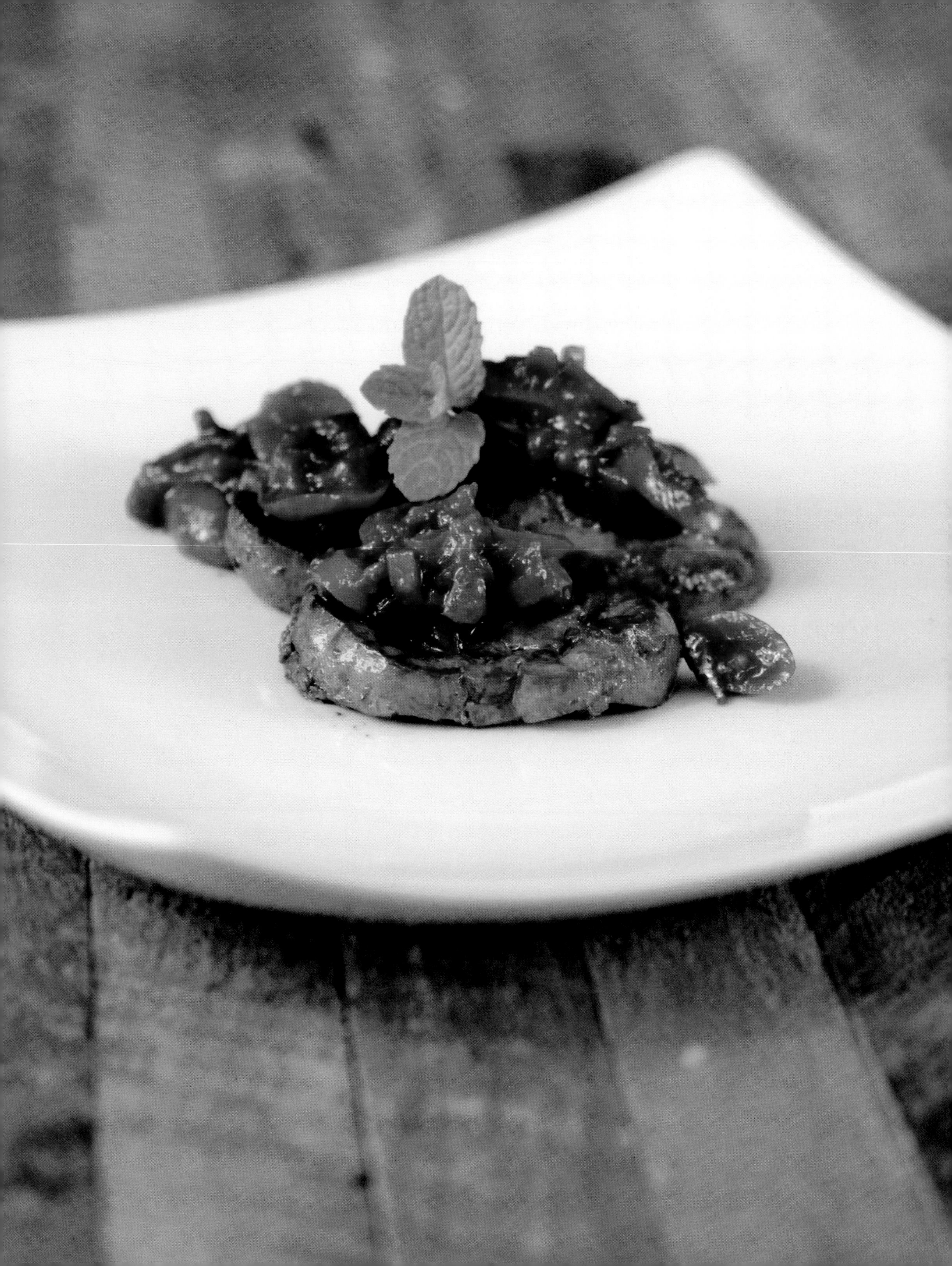

Beef Tongue with Celery Root and Fennel Slaw

Tongue is probably the most universally enjoyed offal. While it can look a little intimidating, when properly prepared, it is tender with a delightful and familiar flavor. (It is a muscle, after all!) This slaw takes advantage of how well the flavor of tongue works with pickling spices. And it tastes even better as leftovers.

PREP TIME: 30 minutes
COOK TIME: 3 hours
SERVINGS: 5 to 8

INGREDIENTS:

- 2½ to 3 pounds beef tongue
- 4 bay leaves
- 1 cup chopped fresh dill
- 2 teaspoons ground mace or 3 to 4 whole mace avrils, plus 1 pinch of ground mace
- 1 teaspoon plus 1 pinch of salt
- 6 to 8 cloves garlic, sliced
- 5 to 6 slices fresh ginger (about 1 inch in diameter)
- 1 stick cinnamon
- ¼ teaspoon whole cloves
- 2 tablespoons fresh lemon juice
- 3 tablespoons apple cider vinegar
- ⅓ cup extra-virgin olive oil
- Pinch of bay leaf powder (see Tips)
- Pinch of ground cinnamon
- 2 small fennel bulbs (about 1½ pounds), julienned
- 1 large celery root (about 1 pound), peeled and julienned

1. Place the tongue in a large stockpot with enough water to cover. Add the bay leaves, ¾ cup of the dill, 2 teaspoons of the mace, 1 teaspoon of the salt, garlic, ginger, cinnamon stick, and cloves. Bring to a boil, then reduce the heat to a rapid simmer. Cook, covered, for 3 hours, topping off the water level to keep the tongue covered, if needed.
2. Meanwhile, in a large bowl, combine the lemon juice, vinegar, olive oil, remaining ¼ cup of dill, pinch of ground mace, bay leaf powder, ground cinnamon, and pinch of salt. Add the julienned fennel and celery root and toss to coat evenly. Cover and refrigerate until the tongue is ready.
3. Remove the tongue from the pot. Let cool until just barely cool enough to handle, about 5 minutes.
4. Peel off the white outer layer, or "skin," of the tongue and discard. It should peel off very easily (you may need a paring knife to get it started or to cut it off in a few stubborn places). You can slice the tongue meat while warm or let it cool completely before slicing. Thinly slice it crosswise, then cut each of those slices into thin strips, mimicking the size of the julienned vegetable pieces.
5. Toss the tongue strips with the vegetables and serve.

TIPS:

The most efficient and precise way to julienne the fennel bulbs and celery root is with a mandoline slicer. If you don't have a mandoline slicer, you can use a knife. A large grater or grater attachment on a food processor is another option.

If you don't have ground bay leaf, you can easily grind dried bay leaves into a powder using a spice grinder or mortar and pestle.

FODMAP ALERT

This recipe cannot be made low-FODMAP.

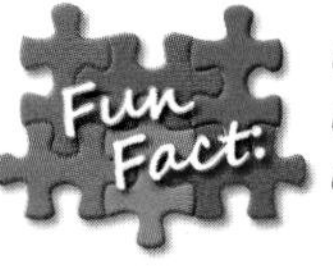

Celery root is also called celeriac. It is actually the corm of the celery plant.

NUTRITION FACTS	
Serving Size	276 g
Recipe Yields	2209 g
Calories	**527**
Fats	**40.9 g**
MUFA	21 g
Omega-3	0.17 g
Omega-6	1.81 g
Saturated Fat	12.9 g
Carbohydrates	**9.99 g**
Fiber	2.89 g
Starch	3.7 g
Fructose	0.06 g
Glucose	0.04 g
Sucrose	0.02 g
Protein	**29 g**
Alanine	<0.01 g
Arginine	<0.01 g
Aspartic acid	<0.01 g
Cystine	<0.01 g
Glutamic acid	<0.01 g
Glycine	<0.01 g
Histidine	<0.01 g
Isoleucine	<0.01 g
Leucine	<0.01 g
Lysine	<0.01 g
Methionine	<0.01 g
Phenylalanine	<0.01 g
Proline	<0.01 g
Serine	<0.01 g
Threonine	<0.01 g
Tryptophan	<0.01 g
Tyrosine	<0.01 g
Valine	<0.01 g
Vitamins	
Vitamin B1	0.07 mg
Vitamin B12	4.43 mcg
Vitamin B2	0.47 mg
Vitamin B3	5.73 mg
Vitamin B5	1.4 mg
Vitamin B6	0.35 mg
Choline	233 mg
Folate	31.5 mcg
Vitamin A	29.3 mcg
Vitamin C	15.2 mg
Vitamin D	21.3 IU
Vitamin E	2.27 mg
Vitamin K	67.1 mcg
Minerals	
Calcium	62.7 mg
Copper	0.29 mg
Iron	4.71 mg
Magnesium	43.4 mg
Manganese	0.26 mg
Phosphorus	301 mg
Potassium	685 mg
Selenium	19.6 mcg
Sodium	193 mg
Zinc	6.11 mg

nutrition content estimated using the USDA database.

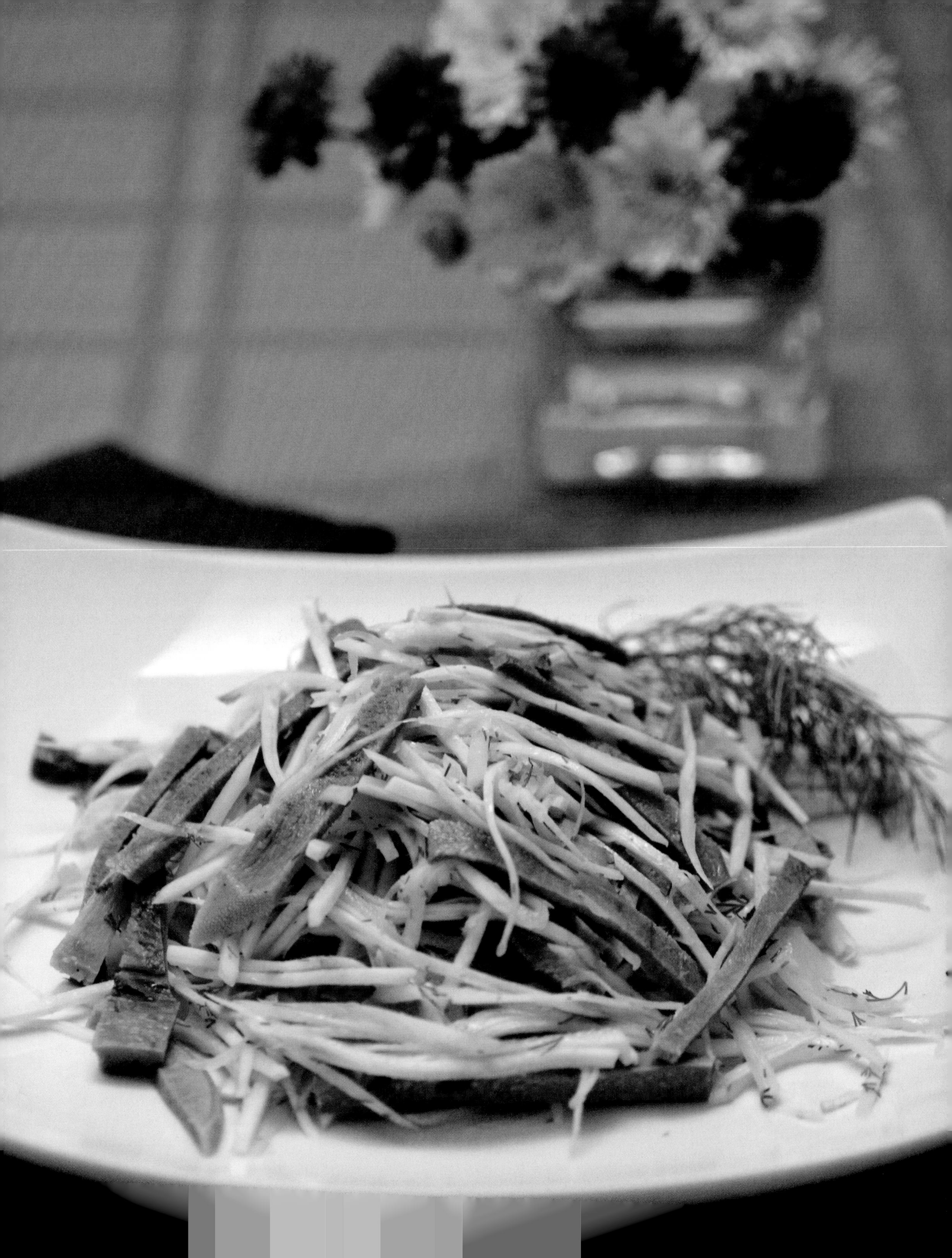

Hidden Liver Meatloaf

This meatloaf is so good that A) you won't miss the tomatoes or ketchup at all, and B) you won't even notice that you are eating liver.

The easiest livers to "hide" are bison, lamb, and chicken. If you use a stronger-tasting liver like beef or pork, you will be able to taste it (not necessarily a bad thing, but it depends on your preferences). Ask your butcher to grind the liver for you. Otherwise, you can grind it using a home meat grinder or food processor.

PREP TIME: 20 to 30 minutes, plus 4 to 6 hours chilling time
COOK TIME: 1 hour 40 minutes
SERVINGS: 6 to 8

INGREDIENTS:

- 2 to 3 tablespoons tallow or other cooking fat
- 1 medium onion, very finely chopped
- 2 stalks celery, very finely chopped
- 1 medium carrot, very finely chopped
- 1 pound ground pork
- 1 pound ground beef
- 1 pound liver, ground
- 4 cloves garlic, crushed
- ⅓ cup fresh parsley, finely chopped
- 3 tablespoons fresh basil, finely chopped
- 3 tablespoons fresh oregano, finely chopped
- 1 tablespoon fresh thyme, finely chopped
- 1 tablespoon fresh chives, finely chopped
- 1½ tablespoons fresh tarragon, finely chopped
- 1 tablespoon blackstrap molasses
- 2 tablespoons coconut aminos
- 3 tablespoons apple cider vinegar
- 1 tablespoon fish sauce

FODMAP ALERT *Replace the garlic with green garlic or garlic scapes (green part only) or omit. Replace the onion with green onion or leek (green part only) or chives or omit.*

1. Heat the tallow in a skillet over medium-high heat. Add the onion, celery, and carrot and sauté until soft and starting to brown, 8 to 10 minutes. Let cool for at least 5 minutes.
2. In a large bowl, combine the sautéed vegetables with the remaining ingredients. Stir until fully incorporated, or mix with your hands.
3. Cover and refrigerate for 4 to 6 hours and up to overnight to let the flavors combine.
4. Preheat the oven to 350°F.
5. Press the meat mixture into a large (9-by-5-inch) loaf pan. Place the loaf pan on a rimmed baking sheet or in a larger baking pan before placing in the oven.
6. Bake for 1 hour 40 minutes, until the internal temperature reaches 160°F.
7. Let the meatloaf rest for 5 to 10 minutes before serving. Enjoy!

TIPS:

The more finely you chop the onion, carrots, and celery, the better this meatloaf will hold together. You can even julienne the vegetables with a mandoline slicer and then chop them.

VARIATIONS:

Try serving this meatloaf with Barbecue Sauce (page 124). You can also spread some Barbecue Sauce over the top in lieu of ketchup before baking.

SPECIAL EQUIPMENT

- Food processor or meat grinder

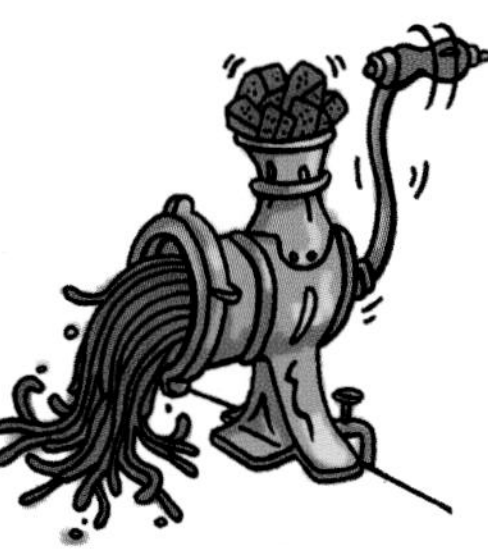

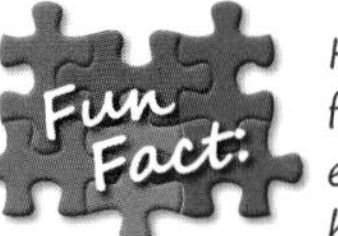

Herbs, especially fresh herbs, are an excellent way to boost a meal's fiber, vitamin, and mineral content.

NUTRITION FACTS	
Serving Size	223 g
Recipe Yields	1785 g
Calories	**469**
Fats	**26.8 g**
MUFA	11.5 g
Omega-3	0.09 g
Omega-6	1.65 g
Saturated Fat	11.2 g
Carbohydrates	**8.78 g**
Fiber	0.85 g
Starch	1.03 g
Fructose	0.59 g
Glucose	0.66 g
Sucrose	1.04 g
Protein	**45.3 g**
Alanine	2.69 g
Arginine	2.85 g
Aspartic acid	4.14 g
Cystine	0.62 g
Glutamic acid	6.43 g
Glycine	2.75 g
Histidine	1.51 g
Isoleucine	2.07 g
Leucine	3.76 g
Lysine	3.71 g
Methionine	1.15 g
Phenylalanine	2 g
Proline	2.17 g
Serine	1.9 g
Threonine	1.88 g
Tryptophan	0.45 g
Tyrosine	1.55 g
Valine	2.48 g
Vitamins	
Vitamin B1	0.56 mg
Vitamin B12	41.7 mcg
Vitamin B2	2.19 mg
Vitamin B3	14.9 mg
Vitamin B5	4.72 mg
Vitamin B6	1.07 mg
Choline	343 mg
Folate	165 mcg
Vitamin A	5420 mcg
Vitamin C	7.86 mg
Vitamin D	40.6 IU
Vitamin E	0.9 mg
Vitamin K	54.4 mcg
Minerals	
Calcium	66.3 mg
Copper	8.21 mg
Iron	6.39 mg
Magnesium	53 mg
Manganese	0.39 mg
Phosphorus	520 mg
Potassium	686 mg
Selenium	52.4 mcg
Sodium	404 mg
Zinc	8.27 mg

nutrition content estimated using the USDA database.

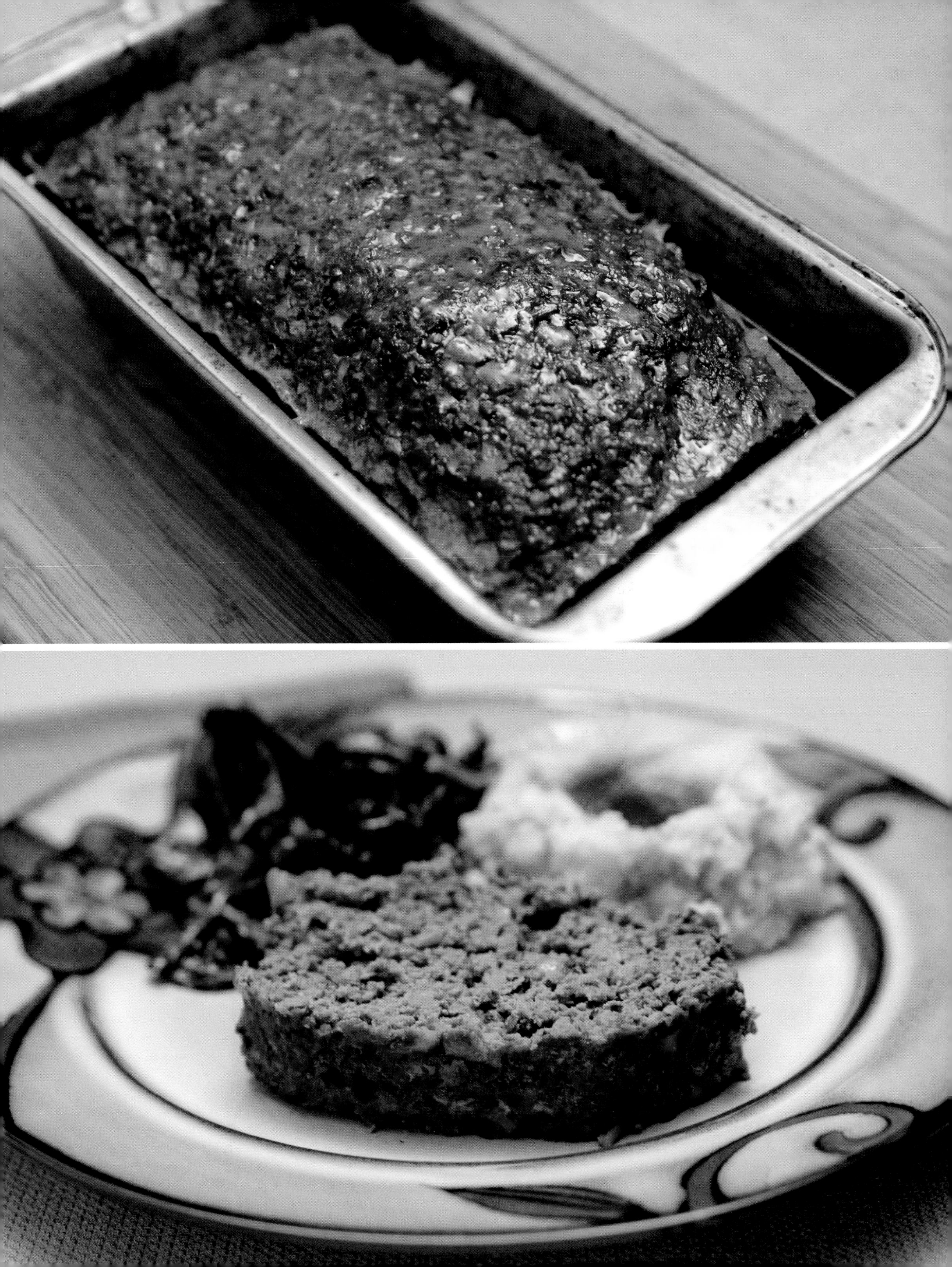

Steak and Kidney Pot Pie

Part pot pie, part shepherd's pie, part stew, and all flavor—you will probably be surprised by just how delicious offal can be when you try this recipe.

PREP TIME: 20 minutes
COOK TIME: 1 hour 45 minutes
SERVINGS: 4 to 6

INGREDIENTS:

- 2 to 5 tablespoons tallow or lard
- 1 pound steak (any cheaper cut) or beef stew meat, cut crosswise into ¼-inch-thick slices
- 1 pound kidney, cut into ¼-inch-thick slices
- 1 medium onion, cut into ¼-inch-thick half-moons
- 3 medium carrots, cut into ½-inch rounds
- 6 ounces portobello mushrooms, chopped
- 2 tablespoons arrowroot powder or kuzu starch
- 1 cup cold Bone Broth (beef, page 110) or red wine
- 1½ teaspoons fish sauce
- 1 bay leaf
- Truffle salt, to taste
- 1 batch Cauliflower Mash (page 295) or Kufu (page 318)

FODMAP ALERT

This recipe cannot be made low-FODMAP.

1. Heat 2 to 3 tablespoons of the tallow in a large saucepot or Dutch oven over medium-high heat. Brown the steak and kidney separately in batches. Set aside.
2. Add the remaining 1 to 2 tablespoons of tallow to the pot if needed. Brown the onion slices for 7 to 8 minutes. Add the carrots and mushrooms and cook for 3 to 4 more minutes.
3. Return the meat to the pot. Whisk the arrowroot powder into the cold beef stock and add to the pot while stirring quickly to incorporate. Add the fish sauce and bay leaf. Simmer uncovered for 1½ hours.
4. Meanwhile, make the cauliflower mash or kufu.
5. Preheat the oven to 425°F.
6. Taste the steak and kidney filling and season with truffle salt as needed. Pour the filling into a 9-by-9-inch casserole dish or lasagna pan. (Alternatively, you can make this in individual 10- to 14-ounce ramekins.)
7. Gently spread a thick layer of cauliflower mash or kufu over the top.
8. Place the casserole dish on a rimmed baking sheet. Bake for 15 minutes, until it is bubbling around the edges and the topping has browned.

VARIATIONS:

You can make this pot pie with chicken or turkey giblets instead of kidney. If you don't want to bother with the topping, you can also serve it as a stew.

In place of Cauliflower Mash or Kufu, try Mashed Acorn Squash with Forty Cloves of Garlic (page 307), other mashed winter squash, Sweet Potato Mash (page 121), or ripe plantain sliced and sautéed in coconut oil.

Add some veggies in the last 10 minutes of stovetop cooking. Broccoli, kale, collards, and spinach are all wonderful additions.

NUTRITION FACTS	
Serving Size	440 g
Recipe Yields	2642 g
Calories	**441**
Fats	**22.9 g**
MUFA	8.7 g
Omega-3	0.3 g
Omega-6	1.49 g
Saturated Fat	9.24 g
Carbohydrates	**12 g**
Fiber	3.61 g
Starch	1.27 g
Fructose	0.31 g
Glucose	1.07 g
Sucrose	0.79 g
Protein	**46.1 g**
Alanine	1.45 g
Arginine	1.53 g
Aspartic acid	2.24 g
Cystine	0.32 g
Glutamic acid	3.63 g
Glycine	1.39 g
Histidine	0.74 g
Isoleucine	1.07 g
Leucine	1.85 g
Lysine	1.94 g
Methionine	0.59 g
Phenylalanine	0.94 g
Proline	1.13 g
Serine	0.97 g
Threonine	0.98 g
Tryptophan	0.18 g
Tyrosine	0.74 g
Valine	1.27 g
Vitamins	
Vitamin B1	0.33 mg
Vitamin B12	21.5 mcg
Vitamin B2	2.62 mg
Vitamin B3	9.51 mg
Vitamin B5	2.33 mg
Vitamin B6	0.83 mg
Choline	521 mg
Folate	120 mcg
Vitamin A	202 mcg
Vitamin C	40.4 mg
Vitamin D	49.5 IU
Vitamin E	0.65 mg
Vitamin K	36.6 mcg
Minerals	
Calcium	56.1 mg
Copper	0.7 mg
Iron	8.8 mg
Magnesium	47.3 mg
Manganese	0.39 mg
Phosphorus	527 mg
Potassium	761 mg
Selenium	158 mcg
Sodium	764 mg
Zinc	7.26 mg

nutrition content estimated using the USDA database.

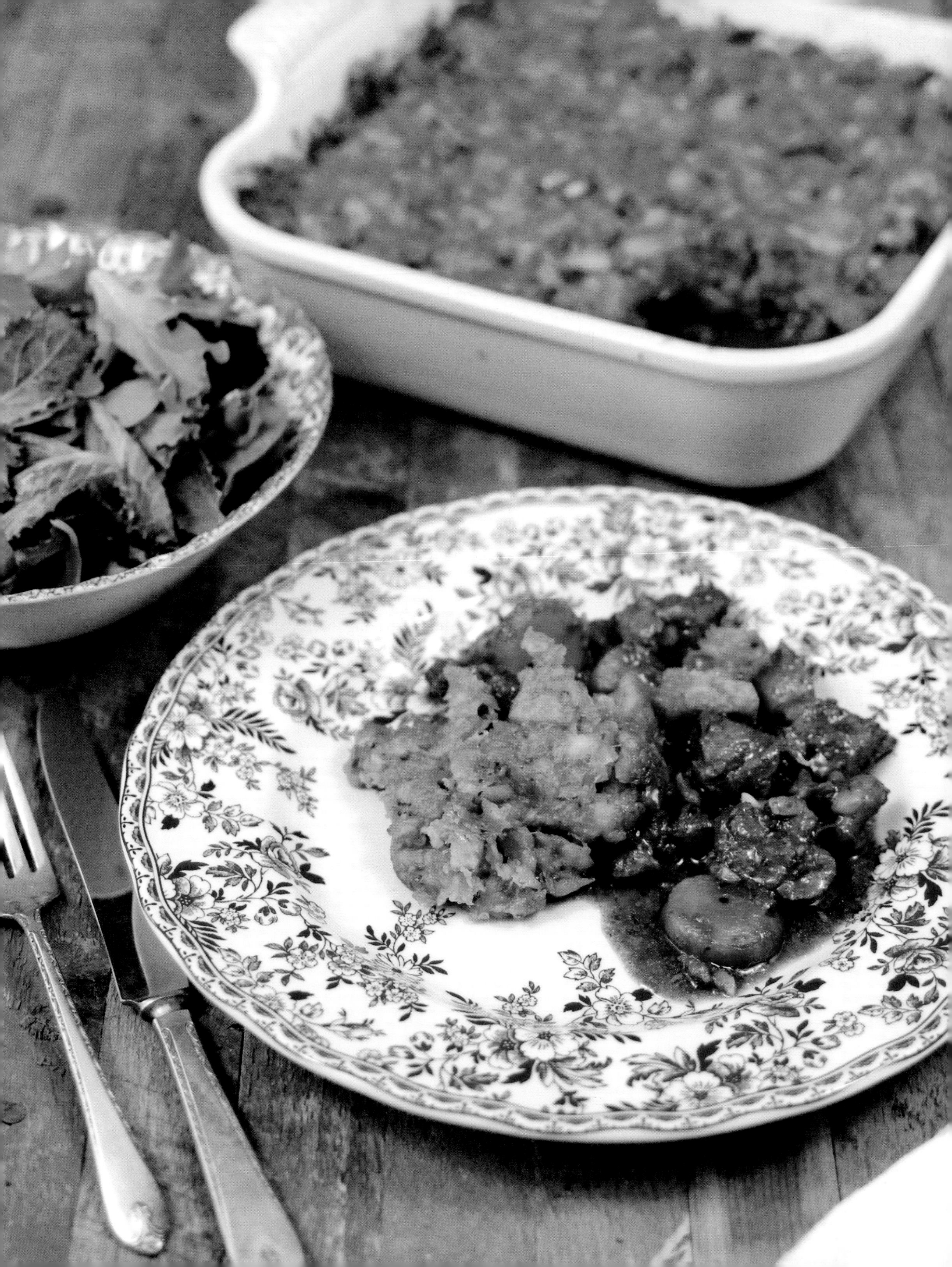

Stuffed Heart Roast

Heart may be daunting to both cook and eat, but it shouldn't be. Because heart is a muscle, it has a familiar flavor, like a very rich steak. When cooked at a relatively low temperature and cooked rare to medium-rare, it can be extremely tender.

PREP TIME: 30 minutes
COOK TIME: 1 to 1½ hours
SERVINGS: 6 to 10

INGREDIENTS:

- 4 tablespoons bacon fat or other cooking fat
- 1 medium onion, finely diced
- 1 pound wild mushrooms, finely chopped
- ½ cup Bacon Bits (page 120)
- 5 ounces fresh spinach (about 8 cups)
- 5 or 6 cloves garlic, crushed
- 1 (3- to 4-pound) whole beef heart, trimmed of any large blood vessels and thick silver skin (see Tips)
- ½ teaspoon salt or truffle salt

FODMAP ALERT *Replace the garlic with green garlic or garlic scapes (green part only) or omit. Replace the onion with green onion or leek (green part only) or chives or omit. Omit the mushrooms.*

1. Heat 2 tablespoons of the bacon fat in an oven-safe skillet over medium-high heat. Add the onion and mushrooms and cook until soft and browned, about 15 minutes. Add the bacon bits, spinach, and garlic and cook for 2 more minutes. Remove from the heat.
2. Hearts are typically cut open when you buy them (this is part of the USDA inspection). If not completely open, finish the cut so the meat can lie flat. If the heart is completely intact, you can simply cut a small slit in one side and stuff it that way.
3. Prepare some lengths of butcher's twine. You'll want 1 piece of twine to go around the length of the heart and 3 or 4 lengths of twine to go around the width of the heart, spaced about 1 inch apart. Slide 1 lengthwise and 3 or 4 widthwise under the heart.
4. Spoon the stuffing onto the heart and spread to cover evenly. Roll the heart back up and use the butcher's twine to tie it closed. It may be easiest to tie the lengthwise truss first, then start tying the widthwise trusses every inch or so down the length of the heart, tucking in any bits as you go. This does take some practice, so don't worry if it's not perfect the first time you attempt it. (You can always cut a truss and redo it if you need to.) Once the heart is trussed, sprinkle the outside with the salt.
5. Preheat the oven to 275°F.
6. Heat the remaining 2 tablespoons of bacon fat in the same skillet in which you cooked the stuffing.
7. Place the heart in the pan and sear for 3 to 4 minutes on each side. Once completely browned, place in the oven and bake for 15 minutes per pound for rare (125°F) or 20 minutes per pound for medium-rare (135°F).
8. Remove from the oven and let rest for 10 minutes. Remove the trusses as you slice and enjoy!

TIPS:

If buying a heart from a butcher, ask the butcher to leave it whole but trim it (this means cutting off any big blood vessels and thick silver skin). Otherwise, you can do this yourself with a sharp paring knife or boning knife. Vessels look like white tubes and are usually at the top of the heart where it is widest, embedded in the fat. You can easily cut them off. Silver skin is gray or white and covers the meat of the heart. Most of the silver skin on a heart is thin enough that it isn't a problem (thick silver skin can be tough), so you only need to trim it off if it's thick enough to be opaque.

VARIATIONS:

This stuffing can also be used to stuff a beef roast, spread onto butterflied flank steak and rolled up pinwheel-style, or even stuffed into a large turkey breast.

NUTRITION FACTS	
Serving Size	219 g
Recipe Yields	2192 g
Calories	**321**
Fats	**14.2 g**
MUFA	4.77 g
Omega-3	0.1 g
Omega-6	1.87 g
Saturated Fat	4.76 g
Carbohydrates	**3.79 g**
Fiber	0.98 g
Starch	1.09 g
Fructose	0.24 g
Glucose	0.9 g
Sucrose	0.12 g
Protein	**42.8 g**
Alanine	0.24 g
Arginine	0.21 g
Aspartic acid	0.33 g
Cystine	0.03 g
Glutamic acid	0.54 g
Glycine	0.21 g
Histidine	0.11 g
Isoleucine	0.04 g
Leucine	0.25 g
Lysine	0.25 g
Methionine	0.07 g
Phenylalanine	0.14 g
Proline	0.16 g
Serine	0.14 g
Threonine	0.15 g
Tryptophan	0.04 g
Tyrosine	0.1 g
Valine	0.24 g
Vitamins	
Vitamin B1	0.21 mg
Vitamin B12	14.8 mcg
Vitamin B2	1.87 mg
Vitamin B3	11.4 mg
Vitamin B5	2.94 mg
Vitamin B6	0.46 mg
Choline	332 mg
Folate	44.2 mcg
Vitamin A	67 mcg
Vitamin C	6.21 mg
Vitamin D	12.5 IU
Vitamin E	0.74 mg
Vitamin K	69.1 mcg
Minerals	
Calcium	28.6 mg
Copper	0.94 mg
Iron	9.72 mg
Magnesium	47 mg
Manganese	0.23 mg
Phosphorus	425 mg
Potassium	575 mg
Selenium	60.8 mcg
Sodium	278 mg
Zinc	4.44 mg

nutrition content estimated using the USDA database.

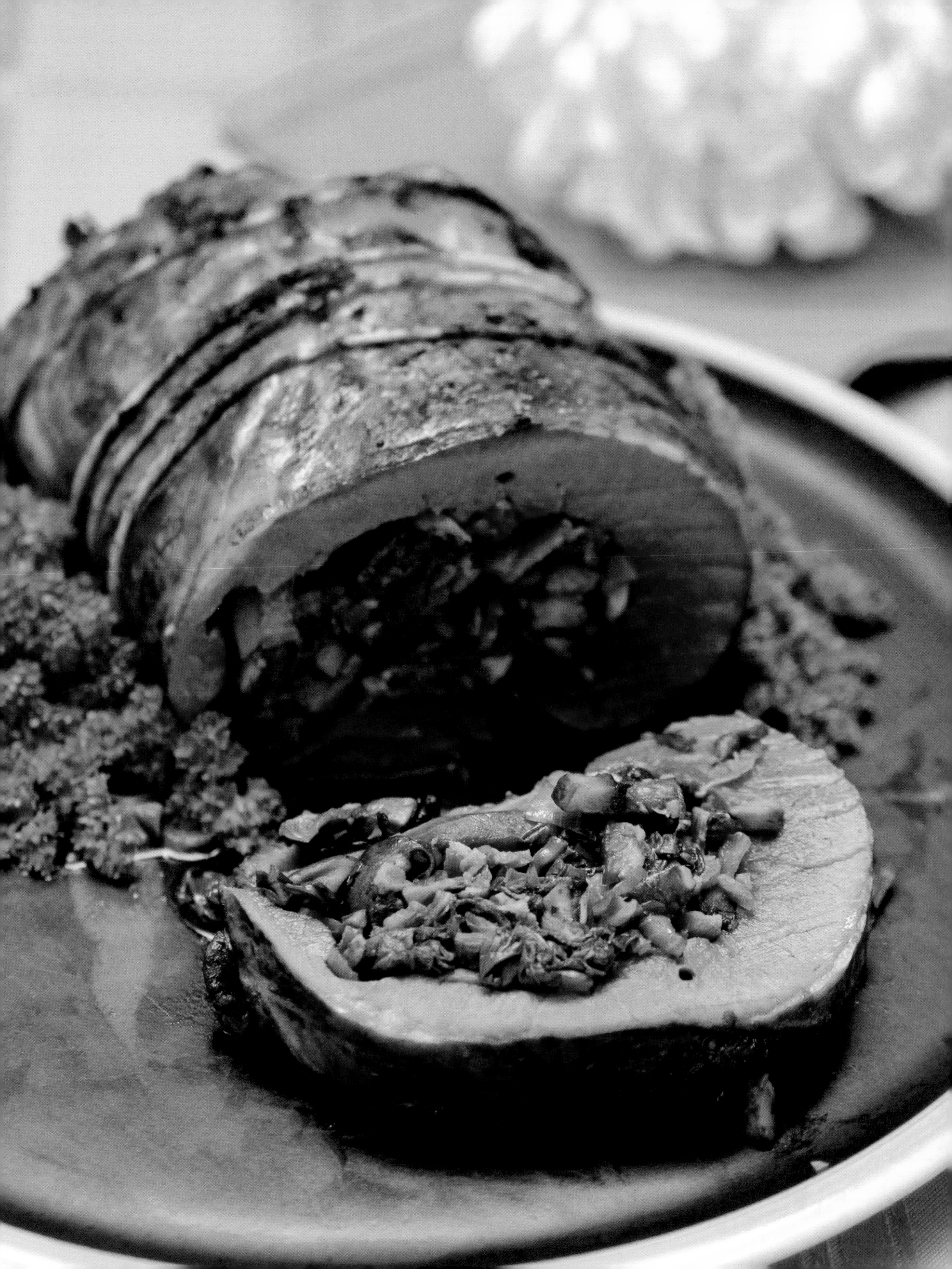

Beef Heart "Chow Mein"

It can be very difficult (if not impossible) to source Asian food that is compliant with the Paleo Approach. Fortunately, delicious Asian-inspired food is quite simple to make! Plus, it's a great opportunity to eat some offal. In this dish, beef heart cooks up tender, with a rich beefy flavor.

PREP TIME: 20 minutes
COOK TIME: 20 to 25 minutes
SERVINGS: 2 to 3

INGREDIENTS:

- 3 tablespoons coconut oil
- 3 or 4 slices fresh ginger (about 1 inch in diameter)
- 1 pound beef heart, trimmed of any large blood vessels and thick silver skin (see Tips, page 276), and cut into thin strips
- 1 medium yellow onion, cut into ½-inch wedges
- 2 medium carrots, sliced
- ½ cup Bone Broth (beef, pork, or chicken, page 110)
- 2 tablespoons coconut water vinegar
- 1 bunch bok choy, leaves separated and sliced if very large
- 1 (5-ounce) can sliced water chestnuts, drained and rinsed
- 1 (5-ounce) can sliced bamboo shoots, drained and rinsed
- 1 pound kelp noodles
- 2 to 3 green onions, chopped

FODMAP ALERT *Replace the yellow onion with leek (green part only) and use only the green parts of the green onions.*

SPECIAL EQUIPMENT

- Wok

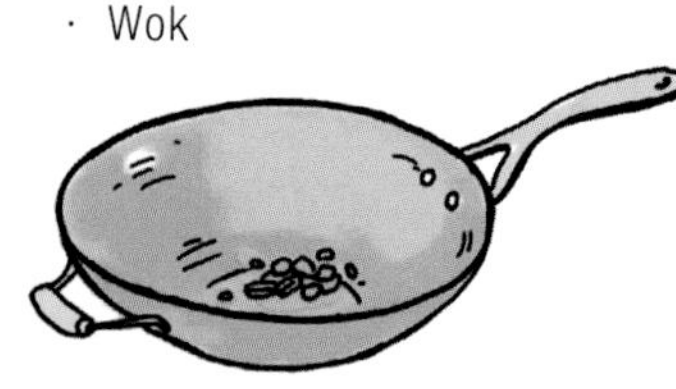

1. Heat a wok over medium-high heat. When the wok is hot, add the coconut oil and ginger slices. Cook for 2 to 3 minutes, until the ginger is browned and fragrant. Remove the ginger slices, if desired.
2. Add the beef heart strips. Cook, stirring frequently, until completely browned, about 5 minutes.
3. Add the onion, carrots, bone broth, and coconut water vinegar. Cook, stirring frequently, for 5 minutes.
4. Add the bok choy, water chestnuts, and bamboo. Cook for another 4 to 7 minutes, until the beef heart is cooked through and the vegetables are cooked al dente. The broth should be boiling. If not, turn up the heat to high.
5. Meanwhile, remove the kelp noodles from the package and rinse with cold water (or follow the package directions). Kelp noodles are naturally very long, which makes them fun to eat. If you prefer shorter noodles, use scissors to cut the mass of noodles in half.
6. Push the beef heart and veggies to the side of the wok to create a little hole in the middle. Place the kelp noodles in the hole. Let them simmer in the remaining broth for 2 to 3 minutes, then start stirring to break up the kelp noodles and distribute them throughout the chow mein, another 1 to 2 minutes.
7. Garnish with the chopped green onions and enjoy!

TIPS:

Kelp noodles and coconut water vinegar can be found in many specialty and ethnic grocery stores or ordered online.

VARIATIONS:

This stir-fry recipe is very versatile. You can make it with thinly sliced beef, pork, or chicken or even with shrimp. Sui choy cabbage, shiitake mushrooms, and kai-lan (Chinese broccoli) are all delightful additions or substitutions.

Instead of kelp noodles, try using sweet potato noodles, julienned or spiral-cut vegetables, or broccoli slaw.

NUTRITION FACTS	
Serving Size	819 g
Recipe Yields	2456 g
Calories	**504**
Fats	**22 g**
MUFA	2.42 g
Omega-3	0.28 g
Omega-6	1.63 g
Saturated Fat	14.1 g
Carbohydrates	**26.2 g**
Fiber	7.95 g
Starch	9.24 g
Fructose	0.83 g
Glucose	1.02 g
Sucrose	1.21 g
Protein	**50.4 g**
Alanine	0.32 g
Arginine	0.33 g
Aspartic acid	0.52 g
Cystine	0.08 g
Glutamic acid	1.28 g
Glycine	0.17 g
Histidine	0.1 g
Isoleucine	0.29 g
Leucine	0.33 g
Lysine	0.33 g
Methionine	0.04 g
Phenylalanine	0.18 g
Proline	0.17 g
Serine	0.2 g
Threonine	0.22 g
Tryptophan	0.06 g
Tyrosine	0.1 g
Valine	0.25 g
Vitamins	
Vitamin B1	0.38 mg
Vitamin B12	16.4 mcg
Vitamin B2	2.17 mg
Vitamin B3	12.9 mg
Vitamin B5	3.07 mg
Vitamin B6	1.24 mg
Choline	391 mg
Folate	217 mcg
Vitamin A	903 mcg
Vitamin C	134 mg
Vitamin D	4.54 IU
Vitamin E	1.98 mg
Vitamin K	145 mcg
Minerals	
Calcium	546 mg
Copper	1.16 mg
Iron	13.4 mg
Magnesium	107 mg
Manganese	0.86 mg
Phosphorus	565 mg
Potassium	1541 mg
Selenium	61.6 mcg
Sodium	479 mg
Zinc	5.61 mg

nutrition content estimated using the USDA database.

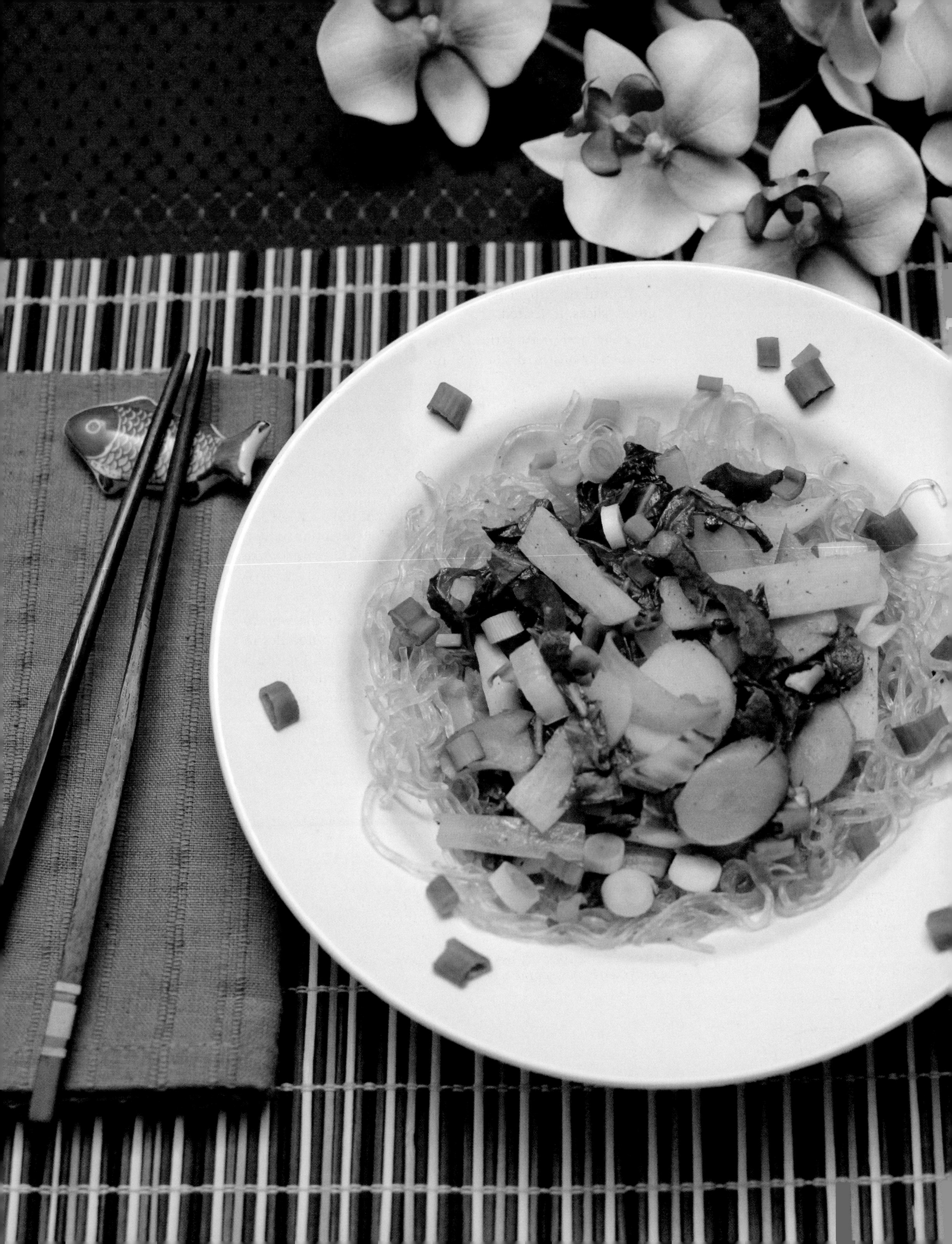

Thai-Inspired Pork Jowl

Jowl is arguably the most delicious cut of pork. Considered a delicacy in many parts of the world, it can typically be purchased very inexpensively in Western countries.

The flavors of this dish work beautifully when served with celery leaves, cucumber, and spring or green onions. Another delicious side dish is plain Cauliflower Rice (page 298) drizzled with Thai Salad Dressing (page 126).

PREP TIME: 15 to 20 minutes, plus at least 6 hours marinating time
COOK TIME: 27 to 28 minutes
SERVINGS: 4 to 8

INGREDIENTS:

- 1 stalk lemongrass (fresh or dried)
- 3 to 4 spring onions or green onions, chopped
- 1 cup Bone Broth (chicken, page 110)
- 1 tablespoon peeled and grated fresh ginger
- 2 tablespoons fish sauce
- 1 tablespoon coconut water vinegar
- 2 cloves garlic, crushed
- Finely grated zest of 1 lime
- Juice of 1 lime
- 2 to 3 pounds pork jowl, cut into ¼- to ⅜-inch slices (see Tips)

1. If using fresh lemongrass, peel off the tough outer layers of the stalk, chop off the top two-thirds of the stalk, and discard. Chop the tender white part. If using dried lemongrass, chop the entire stalk. Combine with the onions, broth, ginger, fish sauce, coconut water vinegar, and garlic in a saucepan.
2. Bring to a simmer over high heat. Reduce the temperature to maintain a simmer and simmer uncovered for 20 minutes.
3. Remove from the heat and let cool. Stir in the lime zest and juice. Place the mixture in a blender or food processor and blend until smooth.
4. Place the sliced jowl in a resealable plastic bag or nonreactive container and pour the marinade over it. Marinate in the fridge for at least 6 hours and up to 24 hours.
5. Arrange an oven rack so that the jowl will be 6 to 8 inches from the top element. Preheat the broiler on high for 10 minutes. Arrange the jowl slices on a rimmed baking sheet lined with aluminum foil or in a roasting pan. If the jowl does not all fit in your pan, you may need to cook it in 2 batches.
6. Broil for 7 to 8 minutes, until the jowl is starting to brown and crisp around the edges. Enjoy!

FODMAP ALERT *Replace the garlic with green garlic or garlic scapes (green part only) or omit. Use only the green parts of the green onions.*

TIPS:

Jowl often comes presliced, but if you are buying it whole, ask your butcher to remove the skin (and slice it for Pork Rinds, page 167) and slice the meat ¼ to ⅜ inch thick. You can also do this job yourself with a sharp knife.

SPECIAL EQUIPMENT

- Blender or food processor

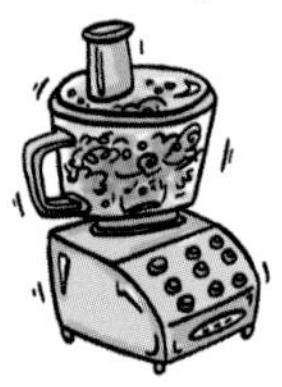

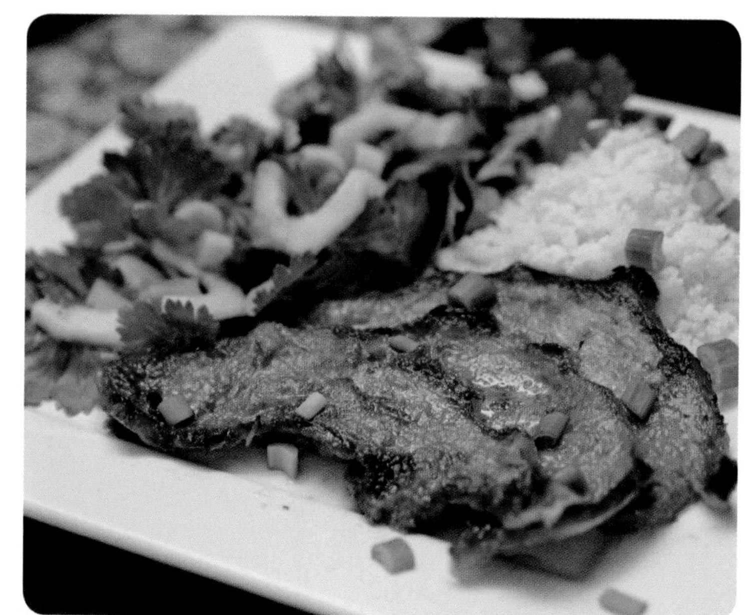

VARIATIONS:

If you can't get pork jowl, this marinade is equally delicious with pork chops, uncured ham steaks, chicken, or even whitefish!

Instead of broiling, you can grill the slices of jowl.

NUTRITION FACTS	
Serving Size	125 g
Recipe Yields	998 g
Calories	**748**
Fats	**79.1 g**
MUFA	37.4 g
Omega-3	0.66 g
Omega-6	8.47 g
Saturated Fat	28.7 g
Carbohydrates	**0.86 g**
Fiber	0.11 g
Starch	0.39 g
Fructose	0.05 g
Glucose	0.04 g
Sucrose	0.03 g
Protein	**7.35 g**
Alanine	0.43 g
Arginine	0.75 g
Aspartic acid	0.68 g
Cystine	0.06 g
Glutamic acid	1.13 g
Glycine	0.33 g
Histidine	0.08 g
Isoleucine	0.19 g
Leucine	0.51 g
Lysine	0.6 g
Methionine	0.11 g
Phenylalanine	0.27 g
Proline	0.28 g
Serine	0.3 g
Threonine	0.24 g
Tryptophan	0.02 g
Tyrosine	0.12 g
Valine	0.35 g
Vitamins	
Vitamin B1	0.44 mg
Vitamin B12	0.93 mcg
Vitamin B2	0.27 mg
Vitamin B3	5.19 mg
Vitamin B5	0.3 mg
Vitamin B6	0.11 mg
Choline	0.49 mg
Folate	2.69 mcg
Vitamin A	4.46 mcg
Vitamin C	2.73 mg
Vitamin D	0 IU
Vitamin E	0.35 mg
Vitamin K	0.74 mcg
Minerals	
Calcium	7.5 mg
Copper	0.05 mg
Iron	0.56 mg
Magnesium	5.34 mg
Manganese	0.05 mg
Phosphorus	99.8 mg
Potassium	184 mg
Selenium	1.79 mcg
Sodium	75.7 mg
Zinc	0.98 mg

nutrition content estimated using the USDA database.

Liver and Onions

Liver and onions is a classic dish and one that I remember vehemently disliking as a child, but greatly enjoy now. There are two secrets to making it delicious. First, it is important not to overcook the liver; it should still be pink on the inside. Second, choosing a mild-tasting liver like lamb or bison makes a big difference. (Chicken liver and calf's liver have a stronger flavor than lamb or bison but are still much milder than beef liver or pork liver.)

PREP TIME: 10 minutes
COOK TIME: 17 to 22 minutes
SERVINGS: 2 to 4

INGREDIENTS:

3 to 4 tablespoons bacon fat, lard, tallow, or duck fat

2 pounds yellow onions (4 to 5 medium), halved and sliced into ¼-inch-thick half-moons

1 pound liver, sliced

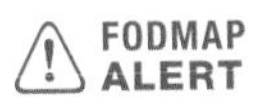

This recipe cannot be made low-FODMAP.

1. Heat 2 to 3 tablespoons of the bacon fat in a skillet over medium-high heat. Add the onions and sauté, stirring frequently, until soft and caramelized, about 15 minutes.
2. Meanwhile, pat the liver dry with paper towels.
3. Remove the onions from the pan and set aside. Add 1 to 2 tablespoons more bacon fat to the skillet and heat until quite hot, but not so hot that the bacon fat smokes.
4. Lay the liver slices in the skillet without overcrowding (you may have to cook it in batches). For ¼-inch-thick slices, cook for 30 seconds to 1 minute per side. For ½- to ¾-inch-thick slices, cook for 2 to 3 minutes per side.
5. Serve the liver and onions together. Enjoy!

TIPS:

Liver typically comes already prepared. However, if you find yourself faced with a whole liver, remove the membrane, trim away any large vessels (if the gallbladder is attached, discard it, being careful not to spill any bile on the meat), then slice with a sharp knife. You can also ask your butcher to trim and slice the liver for you.

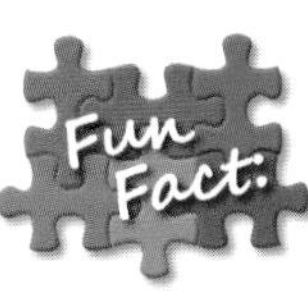

Liver of all kinds is an excellent source of vitamin A—better than any vegetable.

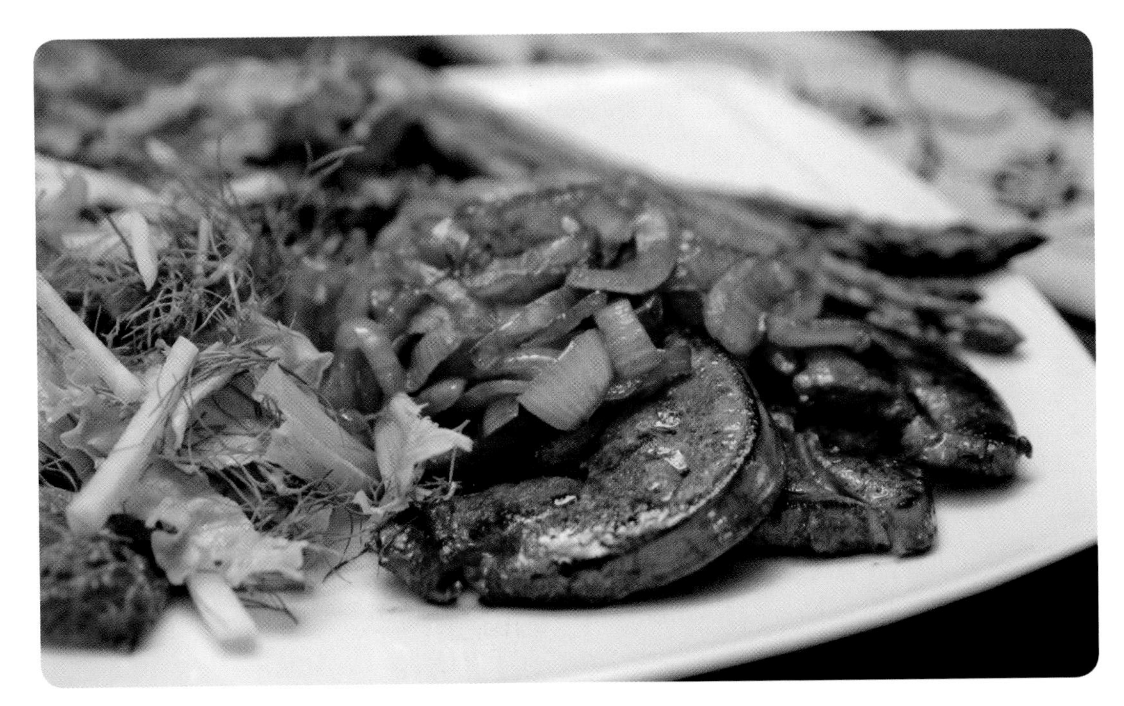

NUTRITION FACTS

Serving Size	350 g
Recipe Yields	1399 g
Calories	**385**
Fats	**15.4 g**
MUFA	5.66 g
Omega-3	0.12 g
Omega-6	1.89 g
Saturated Fat	6.72 g
Carbohydrates	**28.9 g**
Fiber	3.18 g
Starch	9.12 g
Fructose	3.27 g
Glucose	4.97 g
Sucrose	2.5 g
Protein	**33.2 g**
Alanine	1.77 g
Arginine	2.21 g
Aspartic acid	2.95 g
Cystine	0.6 g
Glutamic acid	4.28 g
Glycine	1.81 g
Histidine	0.96 g
Isoleucine	1.51 g
Leucine	2.87 g
Lysine	2.47 g
Methionine	0.81 g
Phenylalanine	1.65 g
Proline	1.48 g
Serine	1.4 g
Threonine	1.33 g
Tryptophan	0.43 g
Tyrosine	1.24 g
Valine	1.89 g
Vitamins	
Vitamin B1	0.3 mg
Vitamin B12	94.3 mcg
Vitamin B2	3.94 mg
Vitamin B3	20.2 mg
Vitamin B5	8.13 mg
Vitamin B6	1.46 mg
Choline	494 mg
Folate	329 mcg
Vitamin A	8785 mcg
Vitamin C	12.6 mg
Vitamin D	65.4 IU
Vitamin E	0.63 mg
Vitamin K	5.56 mcg
Minerals	
Calcium	56.7 mg
Copper	16.7 mg
Iron	7.54 mg
Magnesium	49.9 mg
Manganese	0.75 mg
Phosphorus	630 mg
Potassium	775 mg
Selenium	38.6 mcg
Sodium	109 mg
Zinc	6.42 mg

nutrition content estimated using the USDA database.

Hidden Offal Swedish Meatballs

The easiest livers to "hide" are bison, lamb, and chicken. If you use a stronger-tasting liver like beef or pork, you will be able to taste it (not necessarily a bad thing, but it depends on your preferences). Ask your butcher to grind the heart and liver for you (he or she may or may not be able to depending on the available equipment). Otherwise, you can easily grind it yourself using a home meat grinder or food processor. The great thing about grinding heart meat is that you don't need to bother trimming it first.

These meatballs are delicious served with Braised Savoy Cabbage (page 300), as pictured, but are also delicious with Spaghetti Squash Noodles (page 224), Cauliflower Mash (page 295), or Zucchini Noodles (page 310).

PREP TIME: 20 minutes, plus time for the onions to cool
COOK TIME: 35 minutes
SERVINGS: 5 to 8

INGREDIENTS:

- 1 to 2 tablespoons tallow or other cooking fat
- 2 medium yellow onions, very finely diced
- 1 pound ground beef
- 1 pound beef heart, ground
- ½ pound liver, ground
- 2½ teaspoons ground mace
- Pinch of ground cloves
- ½ teaspoon salt, plus more to taste
- 2 tablespoons arrowroot powder
- 2 cups Bone Broth (beef, page 110), cold or at room temperature
- 1 tablespoon chopped fresh parsley

1. Heat the tallow in a skillet over medium-high heat. Add the onions and sauté until completely cooked and starting to brown, 10 to 12 minutes. Let cool.
2. Preheat the oven to 400°F. Line a rimmed baking sheet with parchment paper, aluminum foil, or a silicone liner.
3. Mix the ground beef, ground heart, ground liver, sautéed onions, mace, cloves, and salt in a bowl. Using your hands, form the mixture into 1½-inch meatballs and place them on the prepared baking sheet (you should get approximately 40 meatballs).
4. Bake for 20 minutes, or until cooked through.
5. While the meatballs are cooking, whisk the arrowroot powder into the cold broth in a small saucepan, then bring to a simmer over medium-high heat. Stir frequently until thick, approximately 3 to 4 minutes.
6. Season the gravy with salt, if desired. Stir in the parsley and remove from the heat.
7. Gently toss the cooked meatballs with the gravy, or pour the gravy over the meatballs as you serve them.

FODMAP ALERT *Replace the yellow onion with green onion or leek (green part only), chives, or other finely chopped vegetables, such as celery and carrots.*

SPECIAL EQUIPMENT

- Meat grinder or food processor

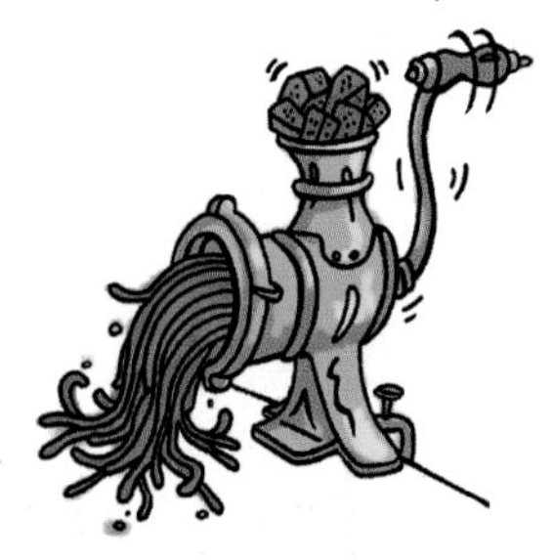

TIPS:

When you first add arrowroot powder to the broth, it will seem cloudy, but it will turn translucent as it cooks. The resulting gravy is clearer than what you're used to, but is still thick and tastes great. Kuzu starch can be used in place of the arrowroot powder for an extremely similar result.

VARIATIONS:

You can also make these meatballs with regular ground beef or bison in place of the heart meat and/or liver.

As an alternative to the gravy used in this recipe, serve the meatballs with Cauliflower Gravy (page 123).

NUTRITION FACTS	
Serving Size	237 g
Recipe Yields	1896 g
Calories	**336**
Fats	**15.1 g**
MUFA	5.92 g
Omega-3	0.17 g
Omega-6	0.9 g
Saturated Fat	6.08 g
Carbohydrates	**7.98 g**
Fiber	0.73 g
Starch	0.95 g
Fructose	0.36 g
Glucose	0.54 g
Sucrose	0.27 g
Protein	**39.5 g**
Alanine	1.37 g
Arginine	1.45 g
Aspartic acid	2.01 g
Cystine	0.28 g
Glutamic acid	3.1 g
Glycine	1.59 g
Histidine	0.67 g
Isoleucine	1 g
Leucine	1.82 g
Lysine	1.76 g
Methionine	0.55 g
Phenylalanine	0.98 g
Proline	1.19 g
Serine	0.93 g
Threonine	0.85 g
Tryptophan	0.16 g
Tyrosine	0.72 g
Valine	1.17 g
Vitamins	
Vitamin B1	0.16 mg
Vitamin B12	27.6 mcg
Vitamin B2	1.78 mg
Vitamin B3	11.9 mg
Vitamin B5	3.26 mg
Vitamin B6	0.64 mg
Choline	305 mg
Folate	87.6 mcg
Vitamin A	2680 mcg
Vitamin C	3.32 mg
Vitamin D	16 IU
Vitamin E	0.71 mg
Vitamin K	10.9 mcg
Minerals	
Calcium	52.3 mg
Copper	4.47 mg
Iron	7.44 mg
Magnesium	32.2 mg
Manganese	0.21 mg
Phosphorus	406 mg
Potassium	461 mg
Selenium	43.7 mcg
Sodium	357 mg
Zinc	6.57 mg

nutrition content estimated using the USDA database.

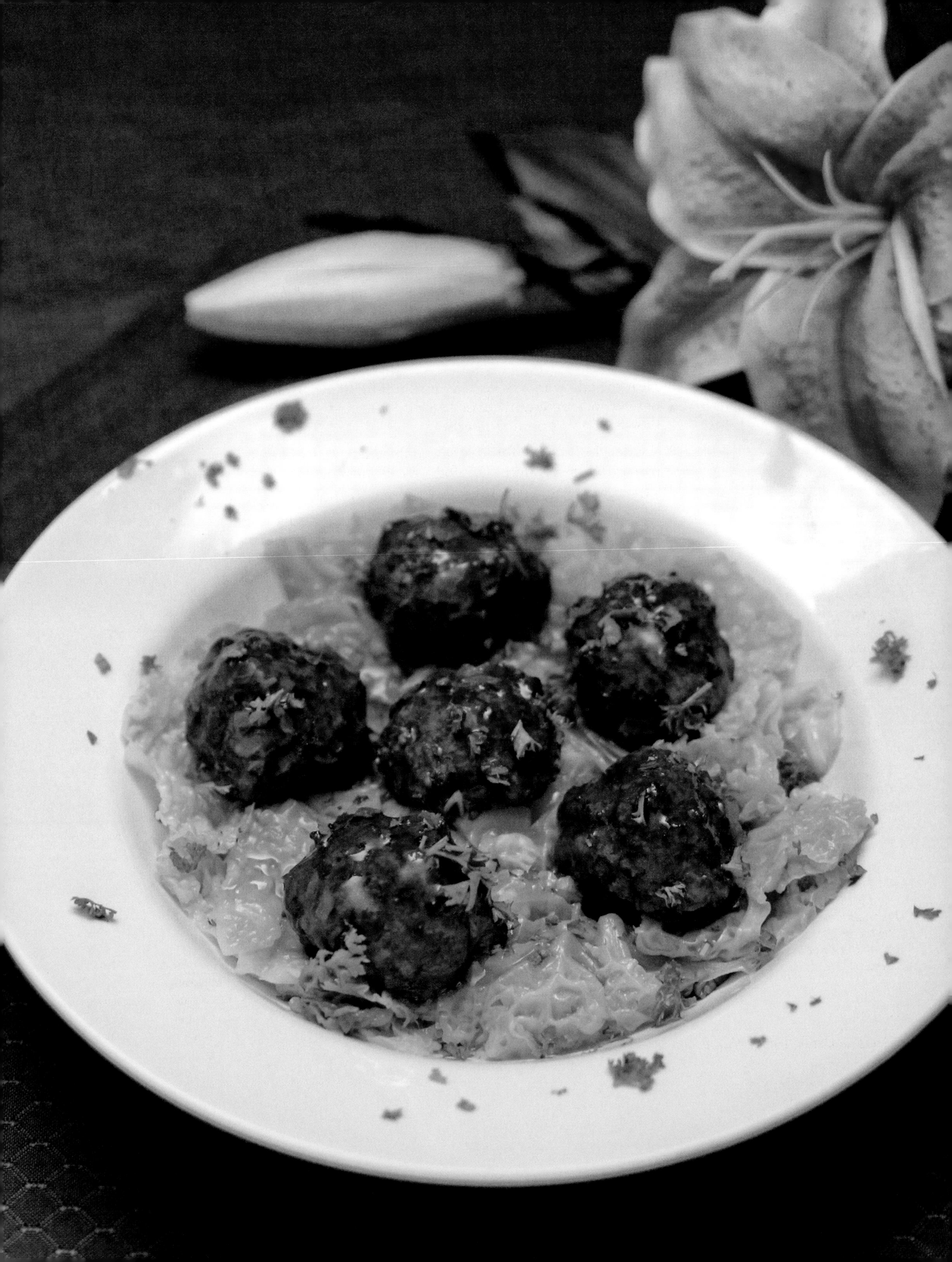

Oxtail-Braised Greens

This treatment of braising greens, inspired by one of my favorite recipes in The Ancestral Table *by Russ Crandall, is a wonderful way to make use of oxtail, and it is a nice change of pace from the ubiquitous oxtail stew. Make sure to keep the oxtail bones to make broth, as there will still be lots of collagen on them!*

PREP TIME: 20 minutes
COOK TIME: 1 hour 30 minutes
SERVINGS: 5 to 8

INGREDIENTS:

- 2 pounds oxtail
- 1 cup red wine, Bone Broth (beef, page 110), or water
- 1 medium yellow onion, diced
- 4 or 5 whole cloves
- 1 teaspoon salt, plus more to taste
- 12 cups mixed greens (collards, broccoli greens, cauliflower greens, kale, mustard greens, or turnip greens), chopped

FODMAP ALERT *Replace the yellow onion with green onion or leek (green part only) or chives or omit.*

SPECIAL EQUIPMENT

- Pressure cooker (optional)

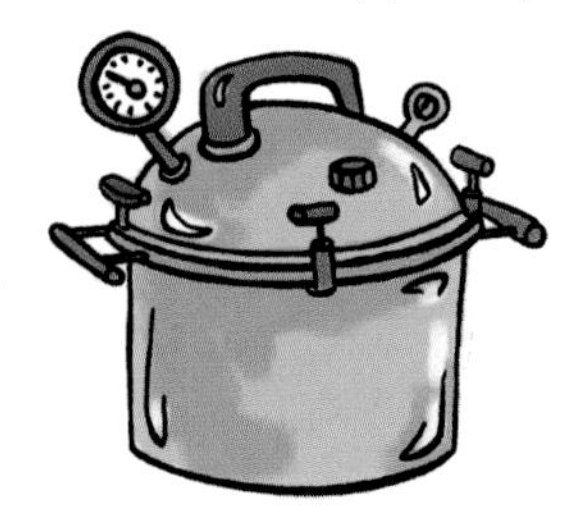

1. Combine the oxtail, wine, onion, cloves, and salt in a pressure cooker. Cook on high pressure for 45 minutes. (See Tips, below, for alternative cooking methods.)
2. Carefully release the pressure, allowing all the steam to escape before unlocking the lid. Remove the oxtail and let cool. Fish out the whole cloves and discard them.
3. Remove the meat from the oxtail bones. Chop and add back to the juices and onion in the pressure cooker. Add the chopped greens to the pressure cooker and stir to combine.
4. Cook on high pressure for 15 minutes. Carefully release the pressure, allowing all the steam to escape before unlocking the lid. Taste and season with additional salt, if desired, and serve!

TIPS:

If you don't own a pressure cooker, you can stew the oxtail on the stovetop with wine and 2 to 3 cups water for 2 to 3 hours (or 4 to 6 hours in a slow cooker). Top off with water as needed to keep the oxtail covered. When you remove the oxtail, simmer the liquid to reduce it before adding the greens. Cook the greens for 40 minutes on the stovetop or 1 to 1½ hours in a slow cooker.

VARIATIONS:

You can also make these greens with beef shanks, beef short ribs, pork shanks, or ham hocks (if using smoked ham hocks, omit the salt).

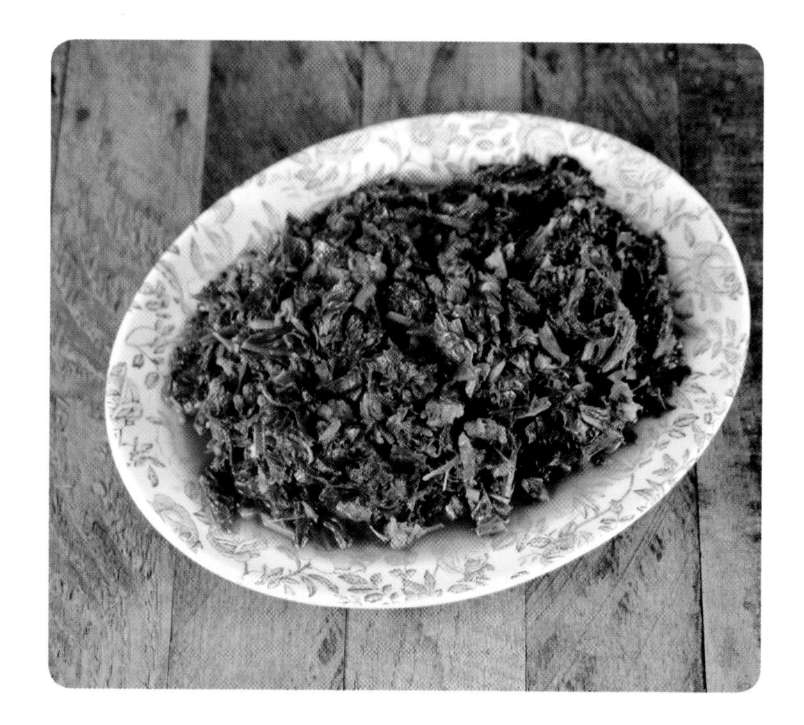

NUTRITION FACTS	
Serving Size	183 g
Recipe Yields	1463 g
Calories	**308**
Fats	**17.5 g**
MUFA	7.36 g
Omega-3	0.21 g
Omega-6	0.54 g
Saturated Fat	6.8 g
Carbohydrates	**4.41 g**
Fiber	2.49 g
Starch	1.07 g
Fructose	0.18 g
Glucose	0.27 g
Sucrose	0.14 g
Protein	**32.1 g**
Alanine	1.88 g
Arginine	2.02 g
Aspartic acid	2.84 g
Cystine	0.4 g
Glutamic acid	4.64 g
Glycine	1.88 g
Histidine	0.98 g
Isoleucine	1.42 g
Leucine	2.47 g
Lysine	2.6 g
Methionine	0.8 g
Phenylalanine	1.23 g
Proline	1.49 g
Serine	1.23 g
Threonine	1.25 g
Tryptophan	0.22 g
Tyrosine	0.99 g
Valine	1.55 g
Vitamins	
Vitamin B1	0.12 mg
Vitamin B12	1.57 mcg
Vitamin B2	0.23 mg
Vitamin B3	8.34 mg
Vitamin B5	0.76 mg
Vitamin B6	0.77 mg
Choline	129 mg
Folate	81.5 mcg
Vitamin A	136 mcg
Vitamin C	20.1 mg
Vitamin D	31.8 IU
Vitamin E	1.76 mg
Vitamin K	238 mcg
Minerals	
Calcium	156 mg
Copper	0.11 mg
Iron	2.17 mg
Magnesium	42.9 mg
Manganese	0.55 mg
Phosphorus	260 mg
Potassium	525 mg
Selenium	33.5 mcg
Sodium	368 mg
Zinc	5.65 mg

nutrition content estimated using the USDA database.

Deep-Fried Fish Heads

I owe a debt of gratitude to Stacy Toth of PaleoParents.com for accidentally introducing me to deep-fried fish heads. (It was, in fact, the Japanese restaurant she took me to that introduced me to this delicacy.) It may seem a bit strange (okay, a lot strange), but deep-frying small fish heads turns the bones crisp and edible, so not only are you eating some of the most tender meat on the whole fish, but you're eating the whole kit 'n' caboodle and all those amazing nutrients to boot. This truly is a magical transformation of a part of the animal that, in the West, is typically tossed aside. It may end up becoming your favorite!

PREP TIME: 20 minutes
COOK TIME: 1 hour 30 minutes
SERVINGS: 2 to 3

INGREDIENTS:

Lard, for deep-frying

4 to 6 whole fish heads from small fish (such as mackerel, herring, sardine, or branzini), gills removed, rinsed and patted dry with a paper towel

Salt, to taste

SPECIAL EQUIPMENT

- Countertop deep-fryer or heavy-bottomed pot with an oil thermometer

1. Heat the lard to 360°F in a countertop deep-fryer or heavy-bottomed pot over medium heat with a deep-fry thermometer attached to the side. Use enough lard to fill the deep-fryer to the fill line or to have 2 to 3 inches in the bottom of the pot.
2. Deep-fry the fish heads for 6 to 8 minutes.
3. Drain on paper towels or newsprint. Sprinkle with a little salt and serve.

TIPS:

The smaller the fish heads, the better. When deep-frying larger fish heads, some of the bigger bones won't crisp up. They are still tasty but are more work to eat.

When you're done deep-frying, let the fat cool, then filter by pouring it through a paper towel–lined sieve. Deep-frying seafood can leave a slightly fishy flavor in your fat, so use separate fat to deep-fry seafood versus vegetables.

VARIATIONS:

You can also deep-fry the skeletons of small fish. Smaller fish like sardines can be deep-fried whole!

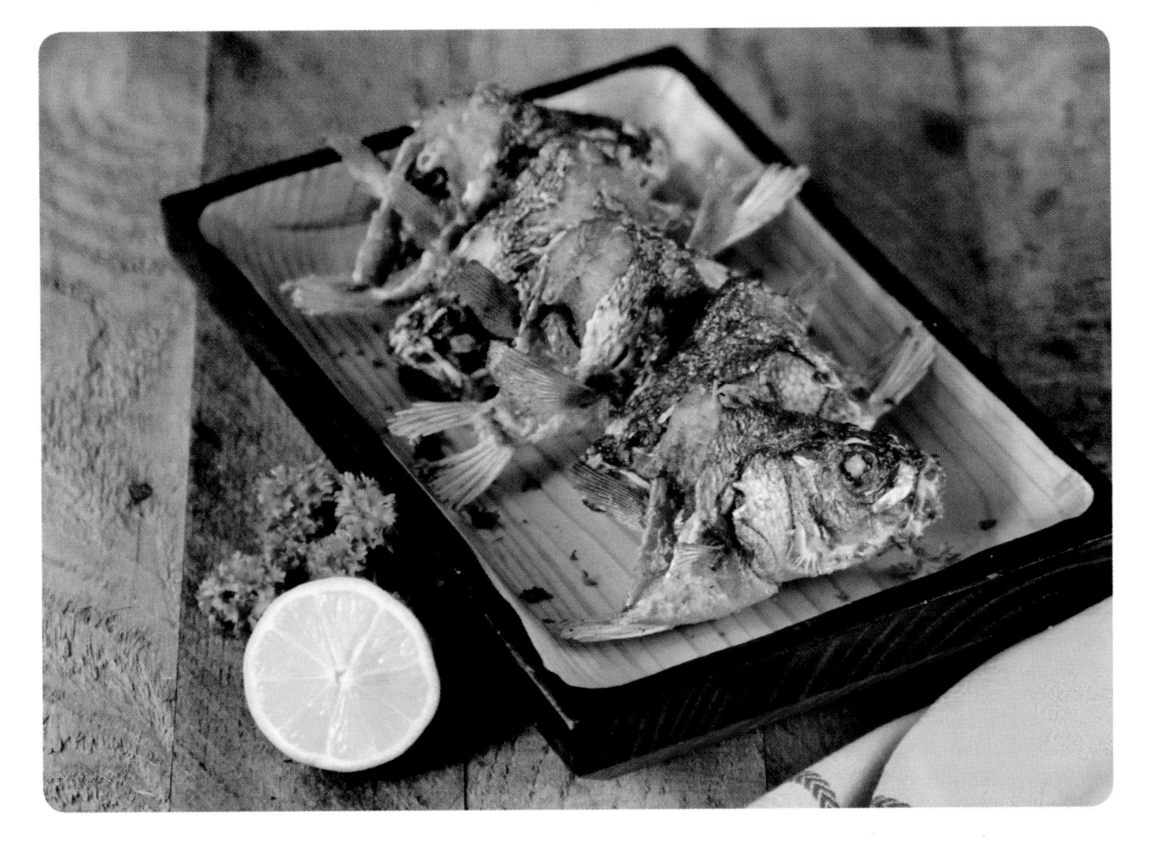

NUTRITION FACTS	
Serving Size	109 g
Recipe Yields	326 g
Calories	**225**
Fats	**16 g**
MUFA	3.86 g
Omega-3	1.13 g
Omega-6	1.23 g
Saturated Fat	3.36 g
Carbohydrates	**0 g**
Fiber	0 g
Starch	0 g
Fructose	0 g
Glucose	0 g
Sucrose	0 g
Protein	**19.1 g**
Alanine	0 g
Arginine	0 g
Aspartic acid	0 g
Cystine	0 g
Glutamic acid	0 g
Glycine	0 g
Histidine	0 g
Isoleucine	0 g
Leucine	0 g
Lysine	0 g
Methionine	0 g
Phenylalanine	0 g
Proline	0 g
Serine	0 g
Threonine	0 g
Tryptophan	0 g
Tyrosine	0 g
Valine	0 g
Vitamins	
Vitamin B1	0 mg
Vitamin B12	0 mcg
Vitamin B2	0 mg
Vitamin B3	0 mg
Vitamin B5	0 mg
Vitamin B6	0 mg
Choline	4.25 mg
Folate	0 mcg
Vitamin A	0 mcg
Vitamin C	0 mg
Vitamin D	8.73 IU
Vitamin E	0.05 mg
Vitamin K	0 mcg
Minerals	
Calcium	546 mg
Copper	0.07 mg
Iron	4.82 mg
Magnesium	24.1 mg
Manganese	0.18 mg
Phosphorus	366 mg
Potassium	218 mg
Selenium	0.02 mcg
Sodium	164 mg
Zinc	5.03 mg

nutrition content estimated using the USDA database.

French-Inspired Stewed Tripe with Saffron

This tripe stew is inspired by the traditional French braising method. Cooked very slowly, the tripe becomes tender and absorbs the flavors of the aromatic vegetables and herbs it's cooked with. You can make this recipe either in the oven or in a slow cooker.

PREP TIME: 40 minutes
COOK TIME: 13 hours
SERVINGS: 4 to 8

INGREDIENTS:

- 2 pounds beef or lamb tripe
- 3 cups cold water
- 3 tablespoons white wine vinegar
- 1 bouquet garni:
  - 4 or 5 sprigs fresh parsley
  - 7 or 8 sprigs fresh thyme
  - 1 or 2 bay leaves
- 2 medium carrots, sliced
- 1 medium onion, sliced
- 1 leek, cleaned and sliced
- 1 stalk celery, sliced
- 2 cups dry white wine or Bone Broth (chicken, page 110)
- 1 teaspoon anchovy paste or 2 anchovy fillets, minced
- ¼ teaspoon saffron threads
- 1 teaspoon salt, plus more to taste

FODMAP ALERT *Replace the onion with additional leek and use only the green parts.*

SPECIAL EQUIPMENT

- Slow cooker or 7- to 9-quart Dutch oven with a tight-fitting lid

1. Soak the tripe in the cold water and vinegar for 1 hour. Make the bouquet garni by tying butcher's twine around the bouquet of herbs to hold them together.
2. Drain and rinse the tripe. Place it in a stockpot, cover with cold water, and bring to a boil. Simmer for 15 minutes, then drain and discard the water. As soon as the tripe is cool enough to handle, cut it into 1½-inch pieces.
3. If using a 7- to 9-quart Dutch oven with a tight-fitting lid, preheat the oven to 210°F. Place the vegetables in the Dutch oven. Add the tripe, bouquet garni, wine, anchovy paste, and saffron. Cover, place the pot on the center oven rack, and cook for 12 hours.

   If using a slow cooker, place the vegetables in the slow cooker, followed by tripe, bouquet garni, wine, anchovy paste, and saffron. Cook for 12 hours.
4. Remove the bouquet garni. Taste and season with additional salt, if needed. Serve.

TIPS:

Honeycomb tripe, which comes from only the first chamber of the cow's stomach, has the mildest flavor.

If you buy tripe presliced, you can skip the first two steps.

This stew is delicious with Russ' Flatbread (page 326) or Root Vegetable Biscuits (page 328) to soak up the juices.

VARIATIONS:

The more traditional French version of this dish also includes two pig's feet. Simmer the pig's feet with the tripe after the tripe has been soaked and drained. Add the pig's feet to the Dutch oven whole. To serve, remove the feet and separate the meat from the bones. Give the meat a quick chop and add it back to the pot. Discard the bones or save them for making stock.

As an alternative method for serving the tripe, you can remove it (and the trotters, if using) from the stew, discard the bouquet garni and the bay leaf, and then purée the vegetables to make a gravy to serve with the tripe.

NUTRITION FACTS	
Serving Size	258 g
Recipe Yields	2061 g
Calories	**205**
Fats	**4.82 g**
MUFA	1.9 g
Omega-3	0.03 g
Omega-6	0.21 g
Saturated Fat	1.58 g
Carbohydrates	**9.43 g**
Fiber	1.06 g
Starch	0.83 g
Fructose	0.47 g
Glucose	0.55 g
Sucrose	0.78 g
Protein	**14 g**
Alanine	0.04 g
Arginine	0.04 g
Aspartic acid	0.07 g
Cystine	0.02 g
Glutamic acid	0.14 g
Glycine	0.02 g
Histidine	0.01 g
Isoleucine	0.03 g
Leucine	0.04 g
Lysine	0.04 g
Methionine	<0.01 g
Phenylalanine	0.02 g
Proline	0.02 g
Serine	0.03 g
Threonine	0.05 g
Tryptophan	<0.01 g
Tyrosine	0.02 g
Valine	0.03 g
Vitamins	
Vitamin B1	0.03 mg
Vitamin B12	0.82 mcg
Vitamin B2	0.06 mg
Vitamin B3	0.92 mg
Vitamin B5	0.25 mg
Vitamin B6	0.12 mg
Choline	8.01 mg
Folate	20.1 mcg
Vitamin A	141 mcg
Vitamin C	4.68 mg
Vitamin D	0.4 IU
Vitamin E	0.4 mg
Vitamin K	17 mcg
Minerals	
Calcium	122 mg
Copper	0.04 mg
Iron	1.54 mg
Magnesium	34.5 mg
Manganese	0.36 mg
Phosphorus	108 mg
Potassium	225 mg
Selenium	13.9 mcg
Sodium	148 mg
Zinc	2.16 mg

nutrition content estimated using the USDA database.

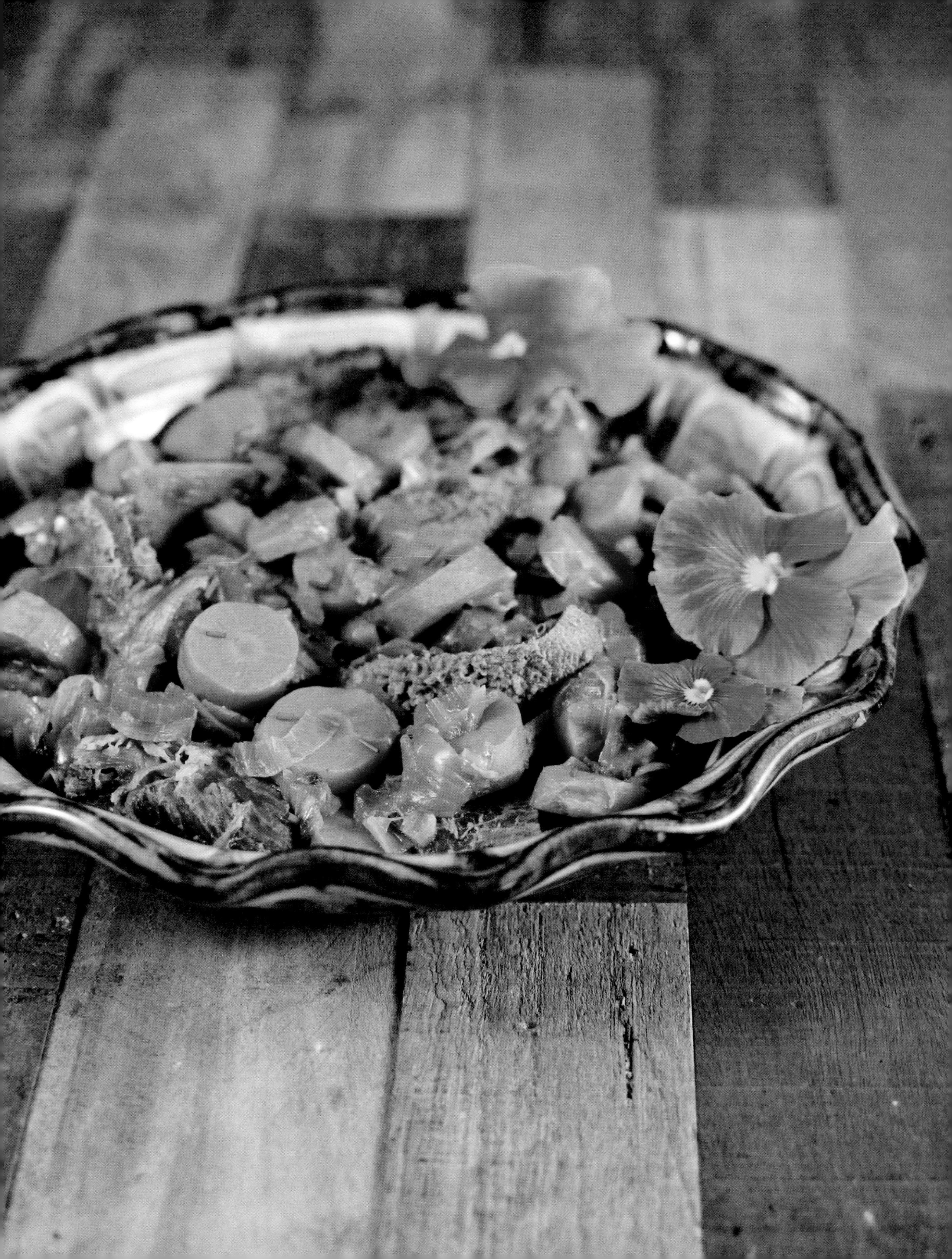

Rocky Mountain Oysters

Getting pork or lamb fries (a euphemism for testicles) to make this dish was a struggle, not because of a difficulty in finding a local meat farmer who requests fries from her meat processor, but because it was difficult to find a local farmer who didn't keep them all for herself! Testicle has a texture surprisingly similar to scallop, with a mild meaty flavor.

PREP TIME: 10 minutes
COOK TIME: 10 minutes
SERVINGS: 2 to 3

INGREDIENTS:

- 2 lamb or pork testicles (6 to 8 ounces total)
- ¼ cup tapioca starch or water chestnut flour
- ¼ teaspoon salt
- ¼ teaspoon ground turmeric
- Lard, for deep-frying
- Lemon wedges, for serving

SPECIAL EQUIPMENT

- Countertop deep-fryer or heavy-bottomed pot with an oil thermometer

1. Remove the outer membrane from each testicle (it should peel off easily) and cut the testicles into ⅜-inch-thick slices.
2. Combine the tapioca starch with the salt and turmeric in a shallow bowl.
3. Dry the testicle slices with paper towels, then dredge in the tapioca starch and salt mixture.
4. Heat the lard to 360°F in a countertop deep-fryer or heavy-bottomed pot over medium heat with a deep-fry thermometer attached to the side. Use enough lard to fill your deep-fryer to the fill line or to have 1½ inches of fat in the bottom of your pot.
5. Deep-fry the testicle slices in batches for 1 to 2 minutes, until golden brown.
6. Serve with lemon wedges.

TIPS:

Try making Tzatziki Sauce (page 258) for dip!

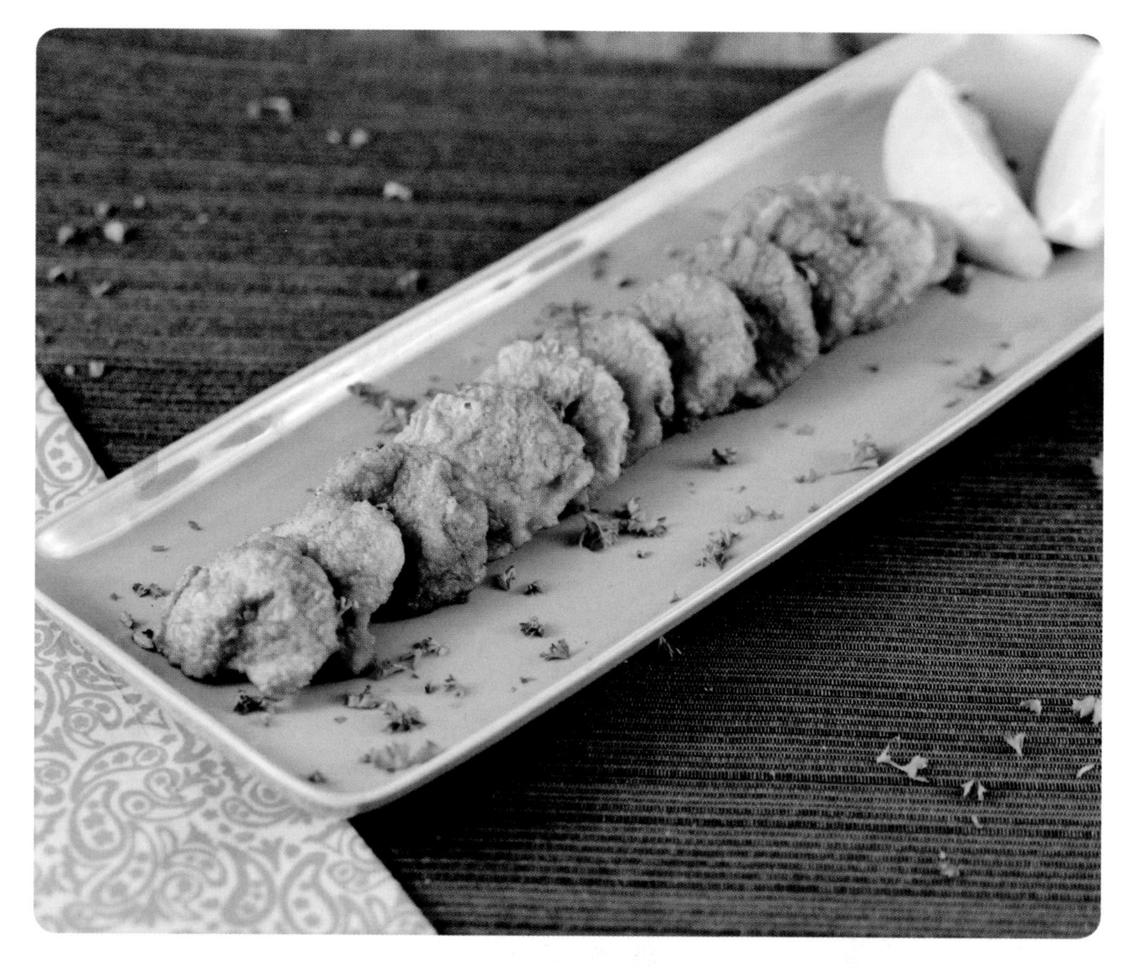

50/50/50 Burgers

This recipe is my absolute favorite way to sneak liver into my kids' and my husband's diet. The combination of a mild liver, like bison, lamb, or calf's, with ground beef and bacon means that you really can't taste even a hint of liver! These burgers are delicious however they're cooked—grilled, pan-fried, or oven-baked.

PREP TIME: 20 to 30 minutes
COOK TIME: 20 to 25 minutes
SERVINGS: 6 to 12

INGREDIENTS:

- 1 pound bison liver
- 1 pound bacon
- 1 pound ground beef
- 2 tablespoons good cooking fat or oil, such as tallow, lard, or coconut oil, for pan-frying

SPECIAL EQUIPMENT

- Meat grinder or food processor

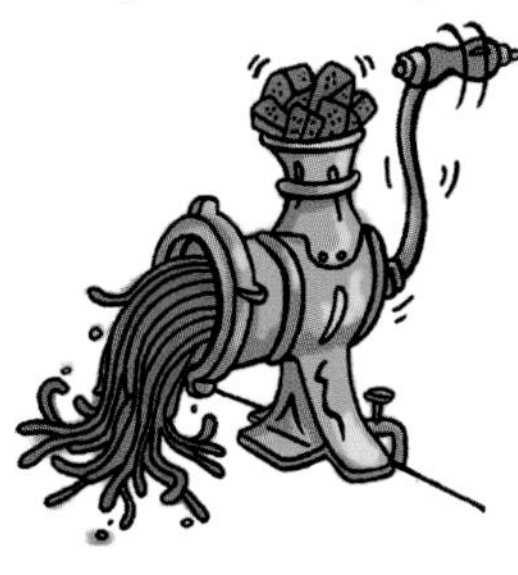

1. Grind the liver and bacon separately using a meat grinder or food processor.
2. In a large bowl, combine the ground liver and bacon with the ground beef. Form whatever size patties you want, typically 4 to 8 ounces each. (The liver makes the meat mixture a little sticky. If it's too sticky, try wetting your hands with cold water before forming the patties.)
3. To grill: Preheat a grill pan or a gas or charcoal grill to medium-high heat. Place the patties on the hot grill. Grill for 6 to 8 minutes per side, or until cooked to your liking.

   To pan-fry: Heat a couple tablespoons of cooking fat over medium-high heat. Place the patties in the hot pan. Cook for 8 to 12 minutes per side, or until cooked to your liking.

   To bake: Preheat the oven to 400°F. Place the patties on a deep-rimmed baking sheet or roasting pan. Bake for 18 to 22 minutes, or until cooked to your liking.
4. Let the burgers rest for 5 minutes before eating.

VARIATIONS:

Make these burgers even more nutrient dense by replacing the ground beef with ground beef heart!

You can use any liver you enjoy.

Serve with Guacamole (page 171) and grilled Portobello "Buns" (page 228) if you like!

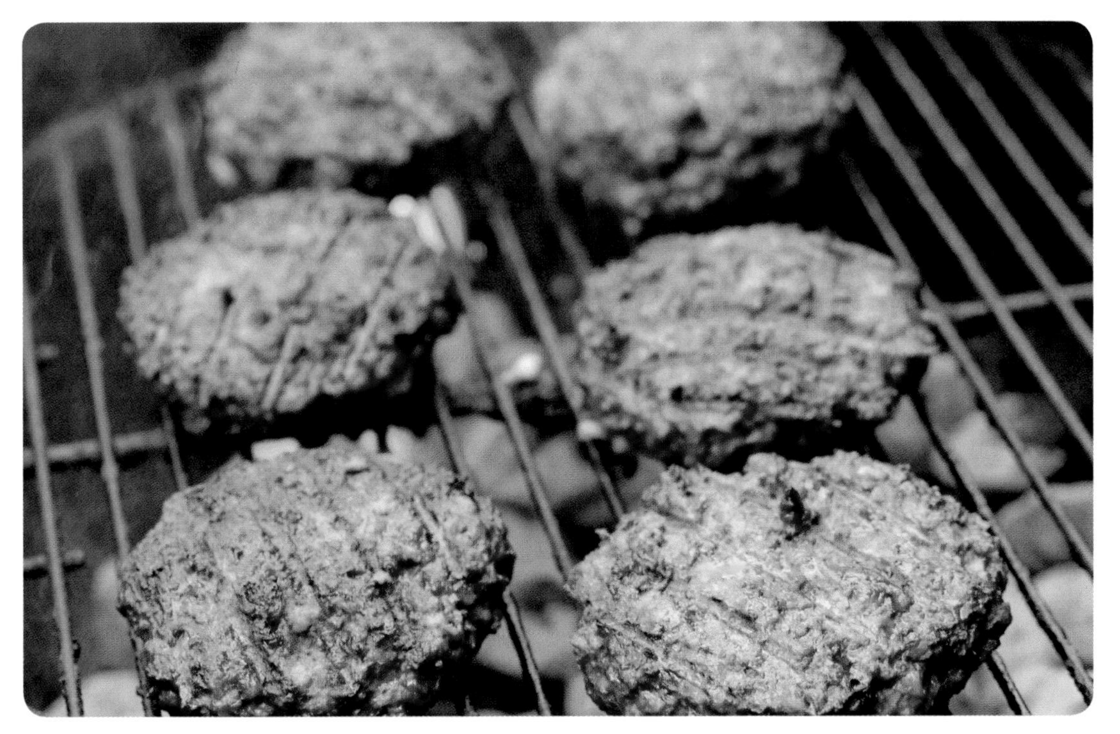

NUTRITION FACTS	
Serving Size	115 g
Recipe Yields	1374 g
Calories	**353**
Fats	**22.5 g**
MUFA	9.31 g
Omega-3	0.15 g
Omega-6	2.43 g
Saturated Fat	7.91 g
Carbohydrates	**2.59 g**
Fiber	0 g
Starch	1.95 g
Fructose	0 g
Glucose	0 g
Sucrose	0 g
Protein	**33.1 g**
Alanine	1.94 g
Arginine	2.1 g
Aspartic acid	3.06 g
Cystine	0.44 g
Glutamic acid	4.73 g
Glycine	1.86 g
Histidine	1.15 g
Isoleucine	1.53 g
Leucine	2.79 g
Lysine	2.76 g
Methionine	0.88 g
Phenylalanine	1.47 g
Proline	1.52 g
Serine	1.39 g
Threonine	1.38 g
Tryptophan	0.34 g
Tyrosine	1.22 g
Valine	1.77 g
Vitamins	
Vitamin B1	0.3 mg
Vitamin B12	28.2 mcg
Vitamin B2	1.46 mg
Vitamin B3	12.7 mg
Vitamin B5	3.35 mg
Vitamin B6	0.72 mg
Choline	226 mg
Folate	99.5mcg
Vitamin A	3590 mcg
Vitamin C	0.72 mg
Vitamin D	29.2 IU
Vitamin E	0.53 mg
Vitamin K	1.82 mcg
Minerals	
Calcium	16.3 mg
Copper	5.49 mg
Iron	3.83 mg
Magnesium	27.7 mg
Manganese	0.15 mg
Phosphorus	414 mg
Potassium	450 mg
Selenium	40.5 mcg
Sodium	701 mg
Zinc	5.48 mg

nutrition content estimated using the USDA database.

Honey-Garlic Roasted Pork Trotters

Rich in glycine because of all the connective tissue, trotters (yes, pig's feet) are a truly delightful meal when properly prepared. They are a traditional pub food in parts of Europe. A honey-garlic marinade marries them with the flavors of North American pub food. Save the bones for making broth when you're done!

PREP TIME: 20 minutes
COOK TIME: 2 hours, plus at least 6 hours marinating time
SERVINGS: 4 to 8

INGREDIENTS:

- ½ teaspoon salt
- 4 pounds pork trotters (approximately 4 pig's feet)
- ⅓ cup honey
- 1 teaspoon finely grated lemon zest
- ¼ cup fresh lemon juice
- 2 tablespoons coconut aminos
- 2 tablespoons apple cider vinegar
- 6 to 8 cloves garlic, crushed
- 1 teaspoon peeled and grated fresh ginger

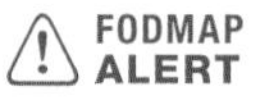

This recipe cannot be made low-FODMAP.

1. Fill a large stockpot approximately halfway with water, then add the salt. Bring to a boil over high heat.
2. Add the trotters. Return to a boil, then reduce the heat to a simmer and cover. Simmer for 1 hour.
3. Meanwhile, combine the honey, lemon zest and juice, coconut aminos, vinegar, garlic, and ginger in a small saucepan. Bring to a simmer over medium-high heat. Reduce the heat and continue to simmer uncovered for 5 minutes. Remove from the heat and let cool.
4. Remove the trotters from the pot, place in a baking pan or casserole dish, and let cool enough to handle. Score the meat with a sharp knife and cut into segments.
5. Place the trotters in a resealable plastic bag or nonreactive container and pour the marinade over them. Refrigerate for at least 6 hours and up to 24 hours, stirring once or twice to make sure the trotters are evenly coated with the marinade.
6. Preheat the oven to 350°F. Line a rimmed baking sheet with aluminum foil or a silicone mat.
7. Bake the trotters for 45 to 50 minutes, until golden brown.

TIPS:

Be prepared for sticky fingers! Eating trotters is very much like eating chicken wings. Although the texture of the meat is different, you'll be eating off the bone with your fingers. You can eat everything that is soft enough to chew!

VARIATIONS:

Instead of roasting the trotters in the oven, you can finish them on a preheated grill pan or medium-hot charcoal or gas grill. Grill for 10 to 12 minutes on each side.

Honey-Garlic Chicken Wings. This marinade is delicious with chicken wings! Instead of precooking the wings, simply add the raw wings to the marinade and marinate in the fridge for at least 4 hours (overnight is better). Then grill until cooked through (about 20 to 25 minutes) or roast at 400°F for 1 hour on a rimmed baking sheet lined with foil.

NUTRITION FACTS	
Serving Size	53 g
Recipe Yields	420 g
Calories	**126**
Fats	**6.66 g**
MUFA	2.93 g
Omega-3	0.01 g
Omega-6	0.53 g
Saturated Fat	2.35 g
Carbohydrates	**4.14 g**
Fiber	0.04 g
Starch	0.32 g
Fructose	1.77 g
Glucose	1.55 g
Sucrose	0.05 g
Protein	**11.9 g**
Alanine	0.69 g
Arginine	0.74 g
Aspartic acid	1.1 g
Cystine	0.15 g
Glutamic acid	1.86 g
Glycine	0.56 g
Histidine	0.47 g
Isoleucine	0.56 g
Leucine	0.95 g
Lysine	1.07 g
Methionine	0.31 g
Phenylalanine	0.47 g
Proline	0.48 g
Serine	0.49 g
Threonine	0.54 g
Tryptophan	0.15 g
Tyrosine	0.41 g
Valine	0.65 g
Vitamins	
Vitamin B1	0.27 mg
Vitamin B12	0.25 mcg
Vitamin B2	0.13 mg
Vitamin B3	2.23 mg
Vitamin B5	0.24 mg
Vitamin B6	0.17 mg
Choline	34.3 mg
Folate	4.01 mcg
Vitamin A	1.32 mcg
Vitamin C	1.25 mg
Vitamin D	18.9 IU
Vitamin E	0.19 mg
Vitamin K	0.04 mcg
Minerals	
Calcium	4.62 mg
Copper	0.01 mg
Iron	0.44 mg
Magnesium	10.1 mg
Manganese	0.02 mg
Phosphorus	95.5 mg
Potassium	160 mg
Selenium	17.8 mcg
Sodium	79.7 mg
Zinc	1.18 mg

nutrition content estimated using the USDA database.

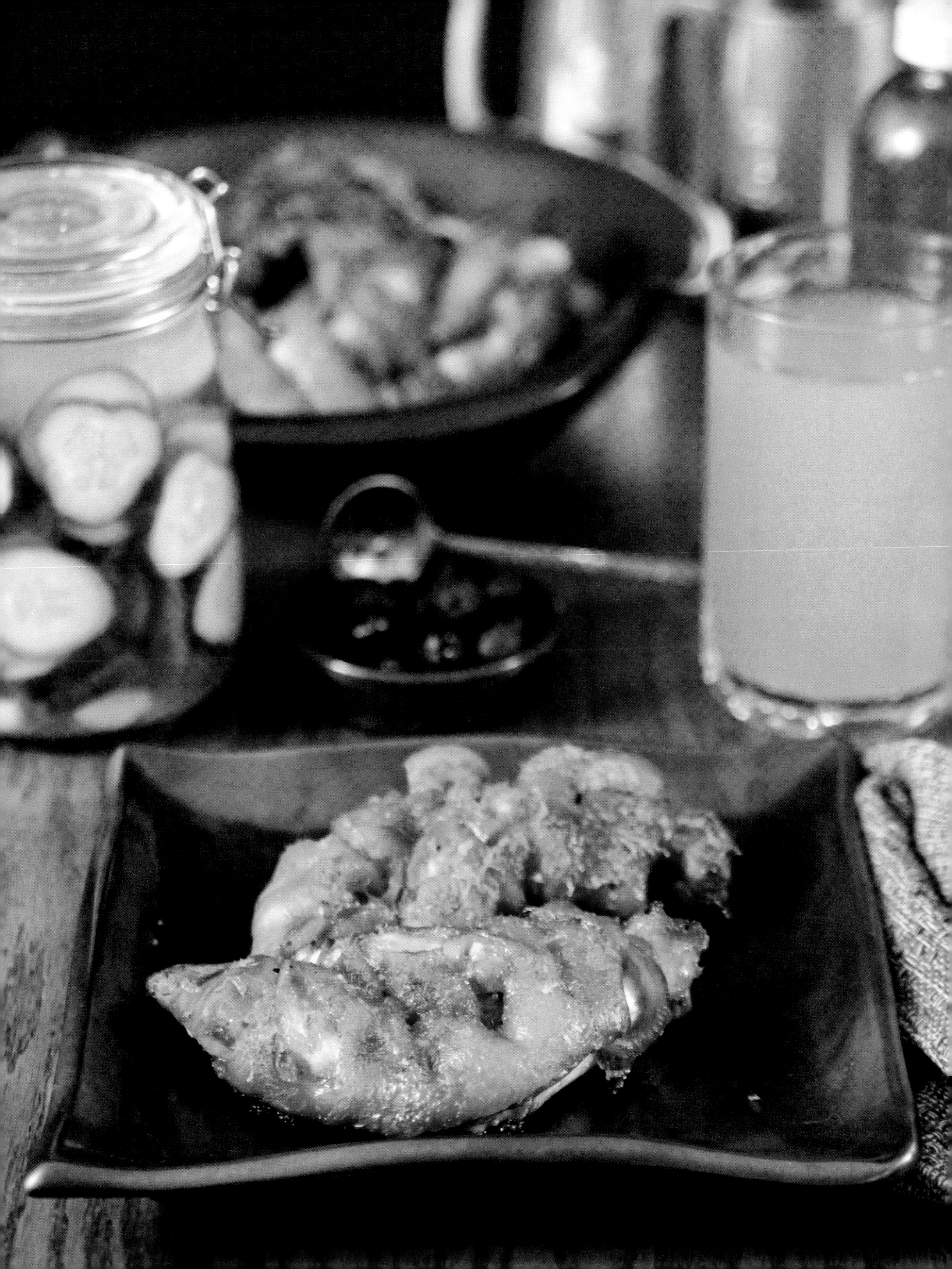

Chapter 11
Side Dishes

Vegetables do not need to be boring! This chapter is designed to show you the diversity of ways that a tremendous variety of vegetables can be cooked. You no longer have an excuse not to eat your greens!

Illustration by Rob Foster

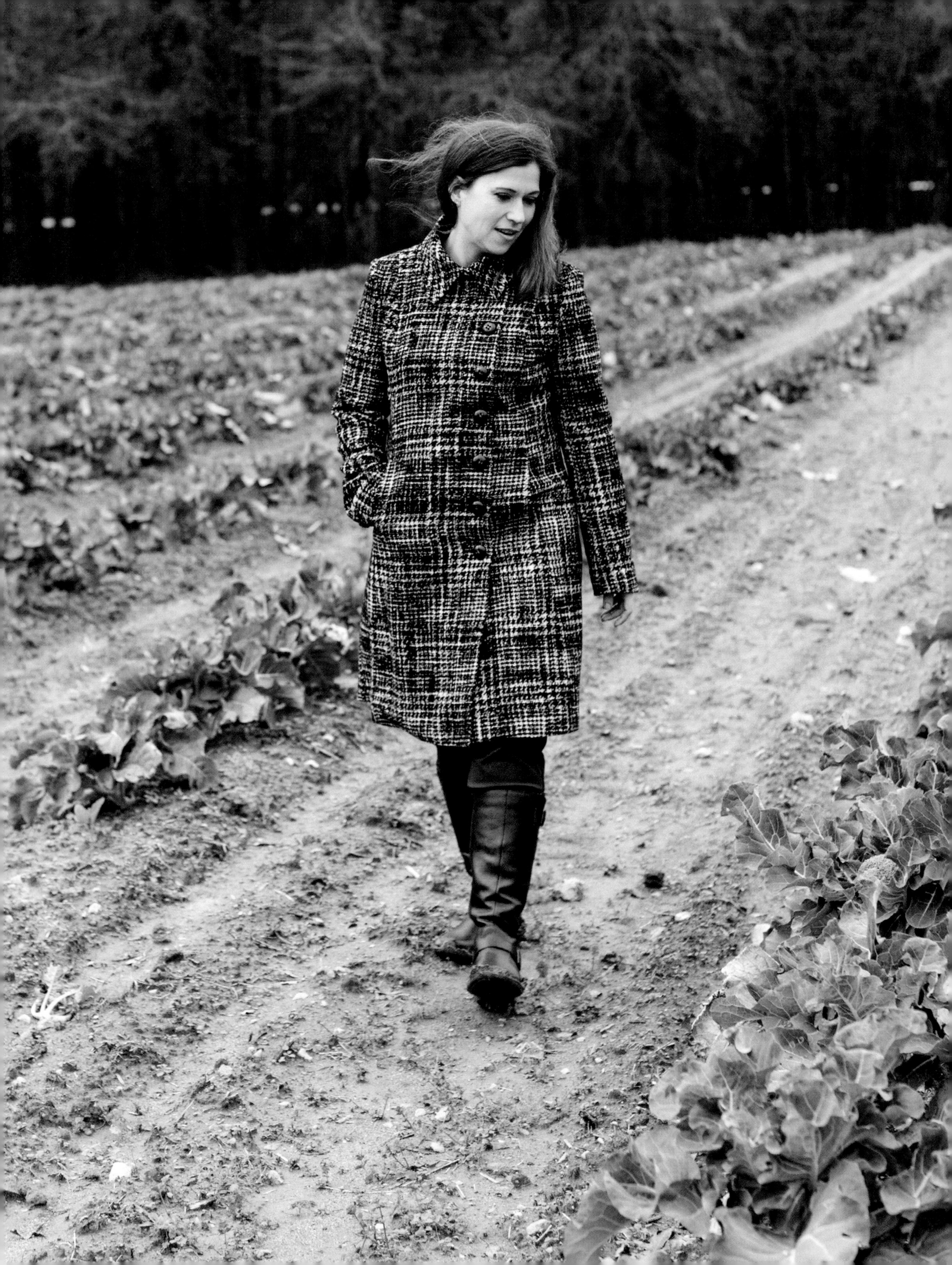

Cauliflower Mash

Cauliflower mash is the classic Paleo substitute for mashed potatoes. When done right, it is extremely similar in texture and flavor.

PREP TIME: 10 minutes
COOK TIME: 35 to 45 minutes
SERVINGS: 4

INGREDIENTS:

- 2 cups Bone Broth (chicken, page 110)
- 1 head cauliflower (about 2 pounds), cut into florets and the core cut into pieces
- 3 to 4 cloves garlic, whole
- 2 tablespoons duck fat, lard, or tallow
- ½ teaspoon salt or truffle salt
- 2 to 3 tablespoons chopped fresh parsley, chives, or a combination

1. Combine the broth and cauliflower in a stockpot. Cover and bring to a boil over high heat.
2. Reduce the heat to low and simmer until the cauliflower is very soft, approximately 30 to 40 minutes, depending on the size of the florets.
3. Add the garlic to the pot and simmer for 5 more minutes.
4. Drain, but reserve the liquid. Place the drained cauliflower, duck fat, and salt in a food processor and blend until you have a thick puree. (Or combine the ingredients in the stockpot and purée with an immersion blender.) Thin with the reserved liquid to the desired consistency.
5. Stir in the parsley and/or chives. Serve!

VARIATIONS:

Try replacing some of the cauliflower with turnips (Japanese turnips work best), celery root, cabbage hearts (maybe left over from making Sauerkraut, page 112), rutabaga, parsnips, Jerusalem artichokes, or white sweet potatoes. Whatever vegetable you are adding, peel (if necessary), cut into 1-inch cubes, and add to the pot with the cauliflower.

FODMAP ALERT

This recipe cannot be made low-FODMAP.

SPECIAL EQUIPMENT

- Food processor or immersion blender

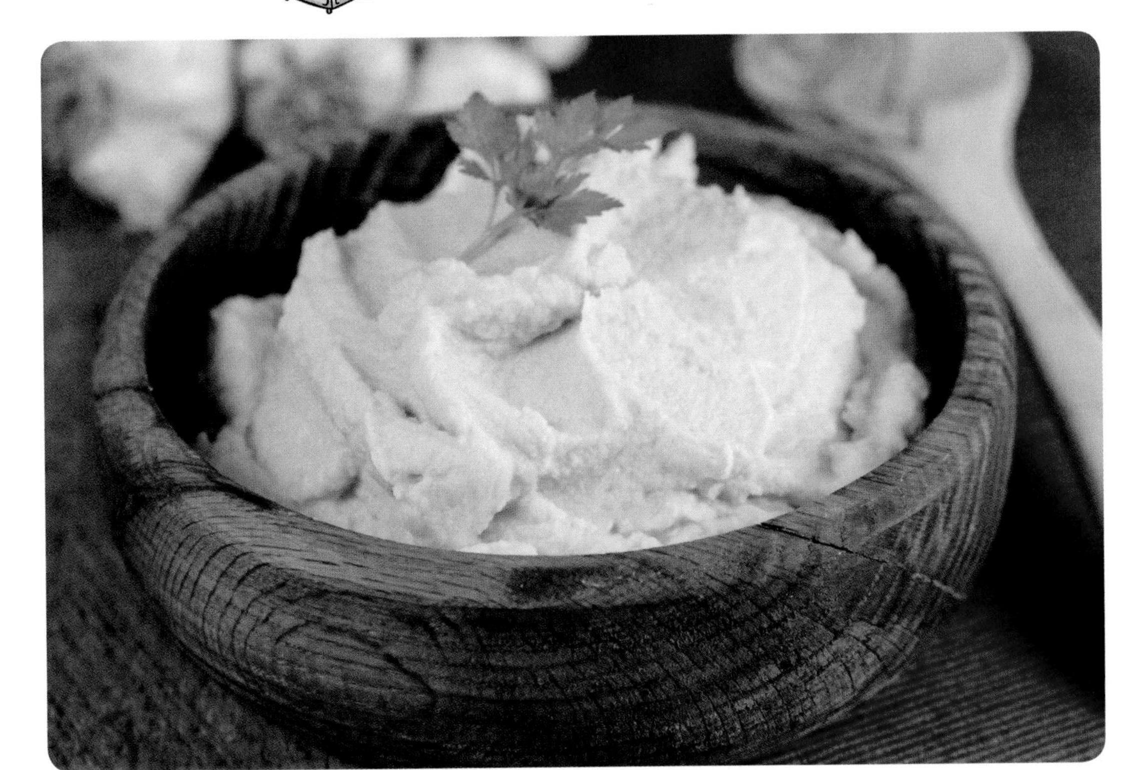

NUTRITION FACTS

Serving Size	148 g
Recipe Yields	591 g
Calories	**91.2**
Fats	**7.02 g**
MUFA	2.94 g
Omega-3	0.27 g
Omega-6	0.72 g
Saturated Fat	2.61 g
Carbohydrates	**6.03 g**
Fiber	2.97 g
Starch	0.72 g
Fructose	0 g
Glucose	0 g
Sucrose	0 g
Protein	**2.57 g**
Alanine	0.13 g
Arginine	0.13 g
Aspartic acid	0.28 g
Cystine	0.03 g
Glutamic acid	0.33 g
Glycine	0.08 g
Histidine	0.05 g
Isoleucine	0.09 g
Leucine	0.14 g
Lysine	0.13 g
Methionine	0.03 g
Phenylalanine	0.09 g
Proline	0.1 g
Serine	0.13 g
Threonine	0.09 g
Tryptophan	0.03 g
Tyrosine	0.05 g
Valine	0.12 g
Vitamins	
Vitamin B1	0.06 mg
Vitamin B12	<0.01 mcg
Vitamin B2	0.08 mg
Vitamin B3	0.58 mg
Vitamin B5	0.65 mg
Vitamin B6	0.24 mg
Choline	52.7 mg
Folate	57.6 mcg
Vitamin A	9.26 mcg
Vitamin C	58.3 mg
Vitamin D	6.54 IU
Vitamin E	0.15 mg
Vitamin K	48.4 mcg
Minerals	
Calcium	28.6 mg
Copper	0.03 mg
Iron	1.32 mg
Magnesium	12.8 mg
Manganese	0.21 mg
Phosphorus	44.8 mg
Potassium	203 mg
Selenium	1.13 mcg
Sodium	195 mg
Zinc	0.27 mg

nutrition content estimated using the USDA database.

Perfect Steamed Vegetables

It may not be the most exciting way to eat vegetables in the world, but steamed vegetables are an excellent staple, and sometimes a simpler flavor to the side of a more complex dish is exactly what's needed. And sometimes it's nice just to be able to cook up some food quickly and easily.

PREP TIME: 5 to 10 minutes
COOK TIME: 10 to 20 minutes
SERVINGS: variable

INGREDIENTS:

Vegetable of choice

SPECIAL EQUIPMENT

- Pot with steamer insert or steamer basket and lid

1. Fill a saucepot with enough water that it just barely reaches the bottom of a steamer insert or steamer basket.
2. Bring the water to a boil over high heat. Add the vegetables to the steamer insert or basket and cover with a loose-fitting lid. If using an insert, you can position the lid so that one side hangs over the insert just enough to let the steam escape.
3. Cook until the desired tenderness is reached, using the cooking times below as a guide.

COOKING TIMES:

Artichokes: 35 to 40 minutes for whole artichokes, 20 minutes for baby artichokes, 10 minutes for artichoke hearts

Asparagus: 4 minutes for thin spears; add an extra minute or two for thicker spears

Beets: 30 to 40 minutes for medium-sized whole beets or wedges of larger beets

Broccoli: 5 minutes for florets; add an extra minute or two if the florets are large

Brussels sprouts: 10 to 12 minutes for whole, 7 to 8 minutes if cut in half

Cabbage: 20 to 23 minutes for quartered, 8 to 10 minutes for shredded

Carrots: 8 minutes for ¼-inch-thick rounds

Cauliflower: 6 to 8 minutes for medium florets

Kohlrabi: 30 to 35 minutes for wedges

Leafy greens: 3 to 5 minutes, just until wilted

Turnips: 15 minutes for ¼-inch-thick slices

Winter squash: 5 to 10 minutes for 1-inch pieces

Zucchini and other summer squash: 8 to 10 minutes for ¼-inch-thick slices, 15 to 20 minutes for whole pattypan squash

---

VARIATIONS:

Want to add a little pizzazz? Add your favorite Handy-Dandy Spice Blend (page 108) to the vegetables before steaming. Alternately, drizzle your favorite Salad Dressing (page 126) over the top after steaming.

TIPS:

Adding 1 tablespoon lemon juice, white wine vinegar, or coconut water vinegar to the water under the steamer basket will help your vegetables retain nutrients.

Don't have a steamer insert or steamer basket? You can also "steam" vegetables by adding about ½ inch of salted water to a saucepot, adding the vegetables to the water once it comes to a boil (you can add lemon juice or vinegar here, too), and covering the pan with a lid.

If you use a microwave, cook times are typically a few minutes longer, depending on the wattage of your microwave. Simply rinse your vegetables and place them in a microwave-safe container with a vented or loose-fitting lid that you can leave open a little at one corner (and no additional water other than what clings to your veggies after rinsing).

If you plan on steaming frozen vegetables, the cook times are usually a bit shorter. Check the package for directions.

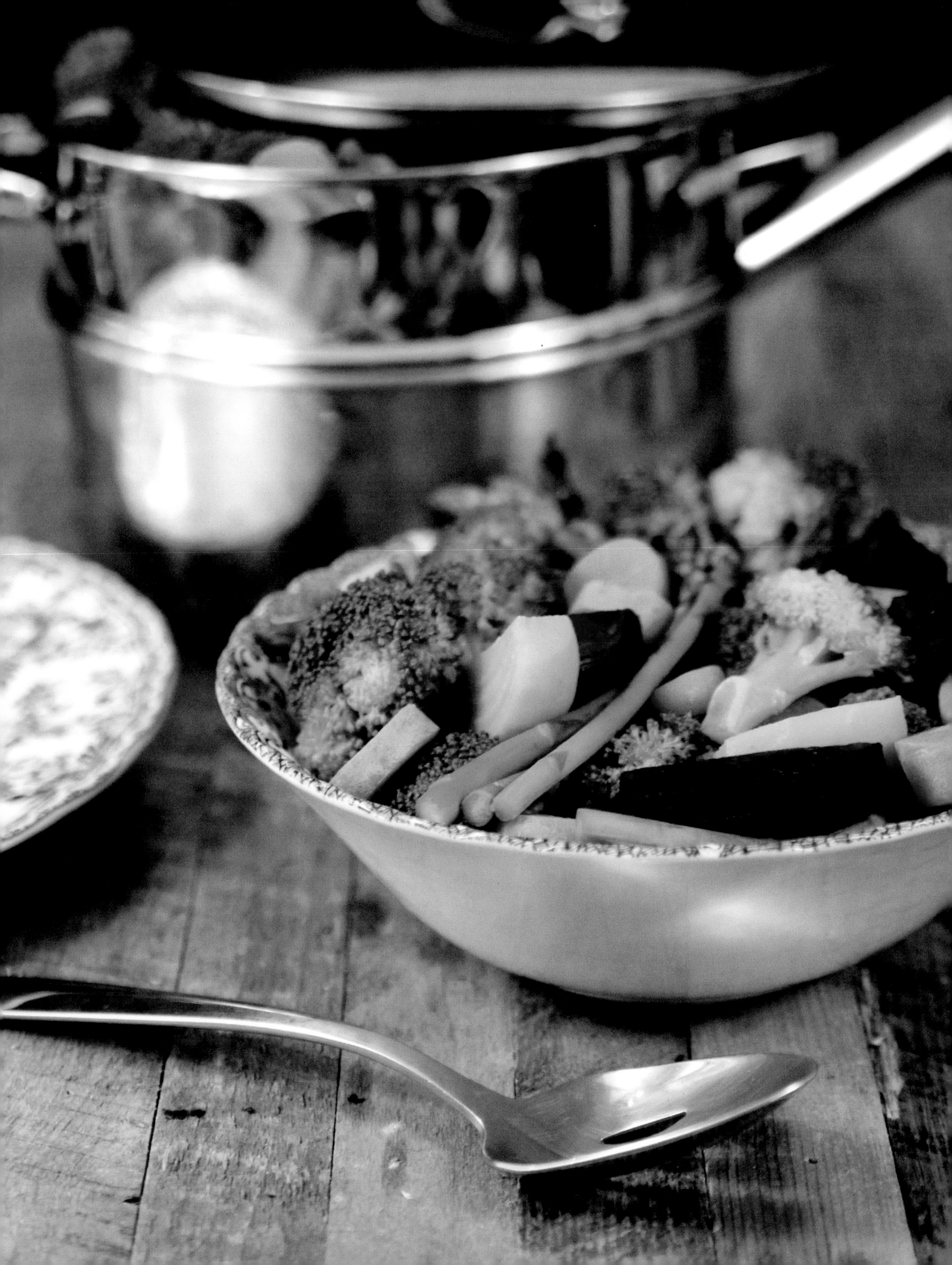

Cauliflower Rice—Three Ways

Cauliflower rice is a versatile side dish. Great with any meal that includes a sauce, it can easily be dressed up or down depending on what other flavors will be on your plate. Lemon-parsley cauliflower rice is a particularly good accompaniment to seafood. Asian-inspired cauliflower rice is particularly good with stir-fries and other Asian-inspired dishes. And plain? It goes with everything!

PREP TIME: 15 minutes
COOK TIME: 7 to 9 minutes
SERVINGS: 3 to 6

INGREDIENTS:

Plain:

- 1 small head cauliflower (about 2 pounds)
- 3 to 4 tablespoons avocado oil or other cooking fat
- ⅛ teaspoon salt

Lemon-Parsley:

- 1 small head cauliflower (about 2 pounds)
- 3 to 4 tablespoons coconut oil or other cooking fat
- 1 clove garlic, crushed
- 1 tablespoon finely grated lemon zest (about 1 lemon)
- 1 tablespoon fresh lemon juice
- ¼ cup chopped fresh parsley
- ⅛ teaspoon salt

Asian-Inspired:

- 1 small head cauliflower (about 2 pounds)
- 3 to 4 tablespoons coconut oil or other cooking fat
- 4 or 5 slices peeled fresh ginger (about 1 inch in diameter)
- 3 cloves garlic, crushed
- 1 tablespoon coconut water vinegar
- 1 tablespoon chopped fresh chives or good-quality dried chives
- ⅛ teaspoon salt

FODMAP ALERT

This recipe cannot be made low-FODMAP.

1. Core the cauliflower and place the florets in a food processor (you may have to do this in batches). Pulse until chopped to rice-grain size. Alternatively, you can grate the cauliflower with a box grater. Set aside.
2. Heat 3 tablespoons of the oil in a large skillet or wok over medium-high heat.
3. If making the Asian-inspired cauliflower rice, add the ginger slices to the oil and cook until fragrant and browned, 3 to 4 minutes. Remove the ginger slices and discard.
4. Add the cauliflower to the pan and cook, stirring frequently, until the cauliflower is cooked al dente, 6 to 8 minutes. If the rice starts sticking to the pan or the pan looks very dry, add an additional tablespoon of coconut oil. If making the lemon-parsley or Asian-inspired version, add the crushed garlic after the cauliflower has been cooking for 5 minutes.
5. Stir in the remaining ingredients and cook for 1 minute. Enjoy!

VARIATIONS:

You can add your favorite herbs to change up the flavor of cauliflower rice. Changing cooking fats also changes the flavor of the dish. Avocado oil has a more neutral taste. Lard, tallow, bacon fat, duck fat, coconut oil, and red palm oil all yield different-tasting (but all delicious) results.

SPECIAL EQUIPMENT

- Food processor or box grater
- Large skillet or wok

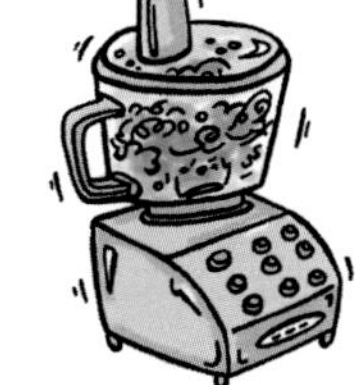

NUTRITION FACTS

Serving Size	55.3 g
Recipe Yields	332 g
Calories	**73**
Fats	**7.01 g**
MUFA	1.91 g
Omega-3	0.02 g
Omega-6	0.38 g
Saturated Fat	4.23 g
Carbohydrates	**2.68 g**
Fiber	0.98 g
Starch	0.79 g
Fructose	0.44 g
Glucose	0.42 g
Sucrose	0 g
Protein	**0.94 g**
Alanine	0.05 g
Arginine	0.04 g
Aspartic acid	0.09 g
Cystine	0.01 g
Glutamic acid	0.12 g
Glycine	0.04 g
Histidine	0.03 g
Isoleucine	0.04 g
Leucine	0.05 g
Lysine	0.1 g
Methionine	0.01 g
Phenylalanine	0.03 g
Proline	0.03 g
Serine	0.04 g
Threonine	0.04 g
Tryptophan	0.01 g
Tyrosine	0.02 g
Valine	0.06 g
Vitamins	
Vitamin B1	0.03 mg
Vitamin B12	0 mcg
Vitamin B2	0.03 mg
Vitamin B3	0.25 mg
Vitamin B5	0.31 mg
Vitamin B6	0.09 mg
Choline	20.1 mg
Folate	26.9 mcg
Vitamin A	3.95 mcg
Vitamin C	23.5 mg
Vitamin D	0 IU
Vitamin E	0.05 mg
Vitamin K	21.2 mcg
Minerals	
Calcium	13.1 mg
Copper	0.02 mg
Iron	0.39 mg
Magnesium	7.64 mg
Manganese	0.08 mg
Phosphorus	21.4 mg
Potassium	145 mg
Selenium	0.37 mcg
Sodium	35.4 mg
Zinc	0.14 mg

nutrition content estimated using the USDA database. values are based on an average of all variations.

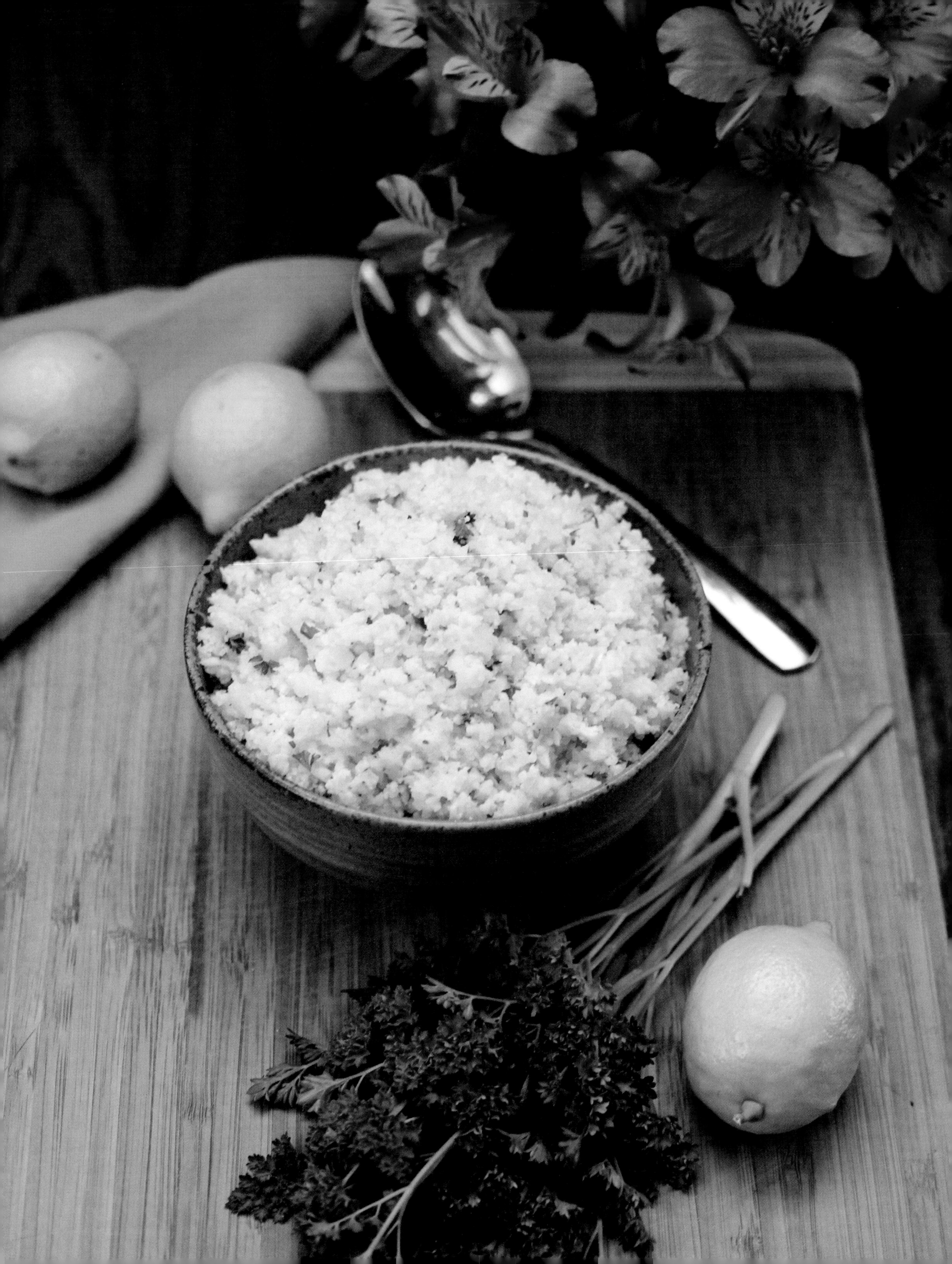

Braised Greens

Braising simply means cooking in both fat and liquid. It is a particularly nice and quick way to cook leafy greens (see page 160), especially those that can be bitter.

Any good cooking fat can be used to braise greens, and each will change the flavor slightly. Avocado oil has the most neutral flavor. Lard, bacon fat, coconut oil, duck fat, tallow, and red palm oil are all great options, too.

The easiest way to braise is to use water as your liquid. However, broth can contribute a wonderful flavor to your vegetables. Other liquids can also be used, including lemon juice (usually diluted in water), orange juice (delicious with garlic and ginger), vinegar (usually diluted in water), coconut aminos (usually combined with water or broth), and coconut milk (for more of a creamed vegetable end product).

The more tender the greens, the less time they take to braise. Very tender greens that might also be used as salad greens, like spinach, lamb's quarter, sorrel, mizuna, sweet potato greens, and celery leaves, cook very quickly—in as little as 3 to 4 minutes. Mustard greens, turnip greens, radish tops, carrot greens, baby collards, beet greens, kohlrabi greens, chard, and some more tender varieties of kale are more substantial and take longer to braise—5 to 10 minutes. The greens that take the longest to cook are those with the thickest and most substantial leaves, such as cabbage, kale, bok choy, broccoli leaves, cauliflower leaves, Brussels sprouts, and collards, which typically take 10 to 15 minutes to braise. The longer the cooking time, the more liquid is typically used.

As a general rule, the more tender the green, the more it will shrink as it cooks. So, for tender greens like spinach, you'll want to start out with more. If cooking a large amount of a tougher green, use 3 to 4 tablespoons of fat and be prepared to use as much as 2 cups of liquid.

PREP TIME: 5 to 10 minutes
COOK TIME: 3 to 15 minutes, depending on the type of greens
SERVINGS: 2 to 4

INGREDIENTS:

2 tablespoons cooking fat

4 to 12 cups chopped greens (less for substantial greens and more for tender greens)

1 tablespoon to 2 cups water or other braising liquid (see suggestions above)

Salt, to taste

SPECIAL EQUIPMENT

- Large skillet or wok

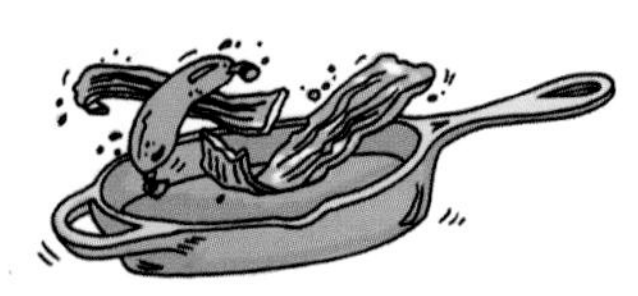

1. Heat the fat in a large skillet or wok over medium-high heat. Add the greens and 1 to 3 tablespoons of the liquid, adding less for tender greens and more for tougher greens. Stir relatively frequently. If the liquid evaporates before the greens are fully cooked, add a little more. For tender greens, you probably won't have to add more liquid. For tougher greens, you may need to add liquid several times during cooking.
2. When the greens are done to your liking, taste and season with salt if desired, then serve. Ideally, the greens will be done just as the liquid fully evaporates. Otherwise, you can serve the greens with tongs or a slotted spoon and leave the liquid in the pan.

VARIATIONS:

You can keep braised greens super simple, or you can play with adding herbs and other seasonings. Crushed garlic, grated ginger, and citrus zest should be added with the greens (if cooking very tender greens, you may even want to add garlic and ginger to the fat 2 to 3 minutes before adding the greens). Wood herbs like rosemary, thyme, and savory can also be added with the greens. Tender herbs like cilantro, parsley, tarragon, marjoram, basil, oregano, chives, and green onion can be added right at the end of the cooking time.

***Bacon-Braised Greens.** To braise in bacon, cut 4 to 6 strips of bacon into little pieces. Fully cook the bacon, then add the greens and braising liquid to the pan (the bacon fat is your cooking fat in this case). If you'd like to add onion, too, cook chopped onion with the bacon until soft and starting to brown (caramelize) before adding the greens and liquid.*

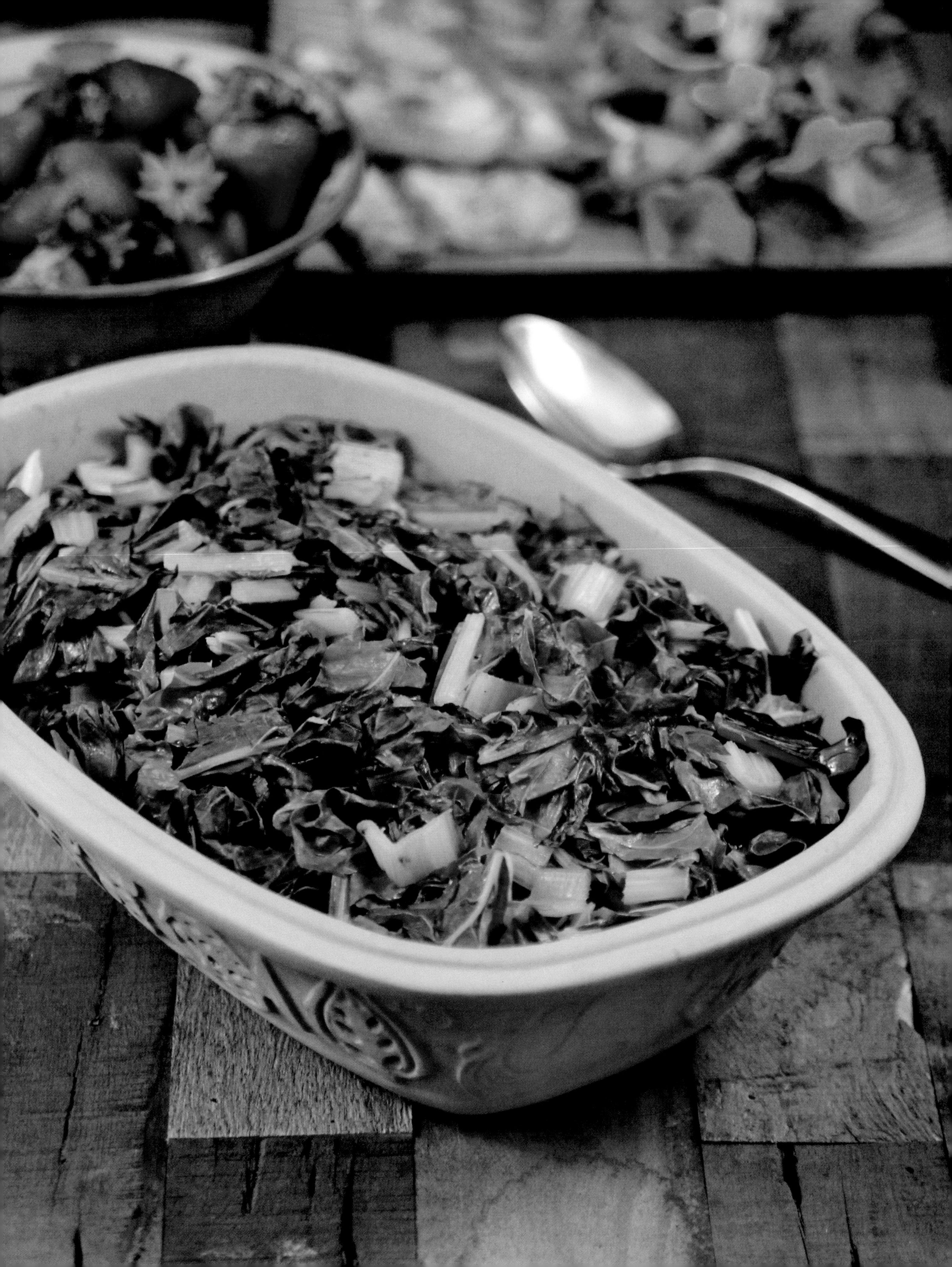

Roasted Broccoflower

This recipe can be made just as easily with broccoli or cauliflower or a mix of the two. You can also add your favorite herbs to change the flavor—thyme is particularly good, but tarragon, sage, rosemary, marjoram, and savory are all great options, too.

PREP TIME: 10 minutes
COOK TIME: 25 to 40 minutes
SERVINGS: 4 to 8

INGREDIENTS:

- 8 cups broccoflower florets and cubed stems (about 2 pounds)
- ¼ cup avocado oil
- 6 to 8 cloves garlic, crushed
- 1 tablespoon finely grated lemon zest (about 1 lemon)
- ¼ teaspoon salt or truffle salt
- ¼ cup chopped fresh parsley

1. Preheat the oven to 450°F.
2. In a casserole dish, toss the broccoflower florets and stems with the avocado oil, garlic, lemon zest, and salt.
3. Roast for 25 to 40 minutes, until the broccoflower is fully cooked (it depends on how big your florets are and how soft you like them), stirring once halfway through cooking.
4. Remove from the oven and toss with the fresh parsley. Serve!

VARIATIONS:

You can keep this recipe super simple for a quick weeknight side dish and roast your broccoflower with just avocado oil and salt.

Roasted Broccoli. *Can't find broccoflower? Broccoli, cauliflower, and Brussels sprouts can all be used in this recipe. Sliced carrots can be added, too.*

Asian-Inspired Roasted Cauliflower. *Try adding 2 to 3 tablespoons coconut aminos, switching out the garlic for grated fresh ginger, and omitting the lemon zest and parsley.*

FODMAP ALERT

This recipe cannot be made low-FODMAP.

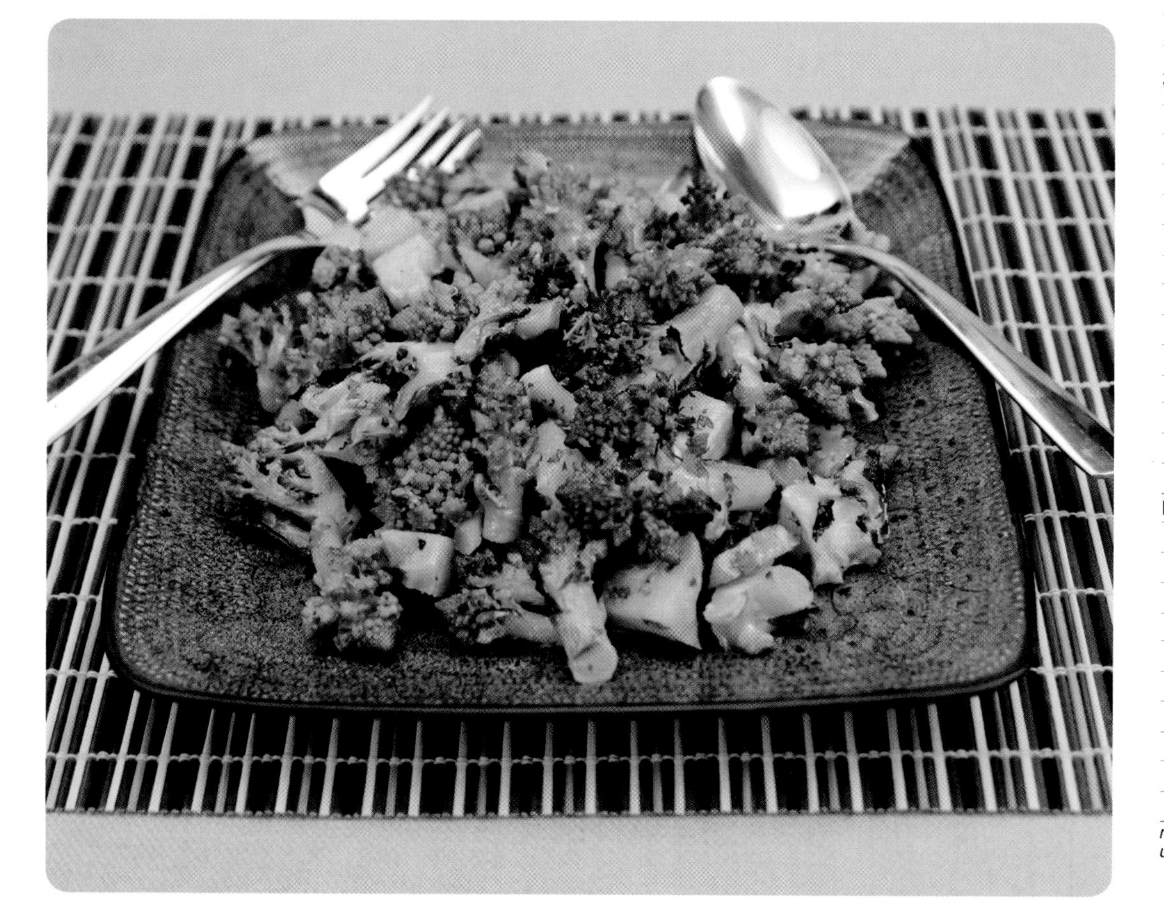

NUTRITION FACTS

Serving Size	103 g
Recipe Yields	823 g
Calories	**95.7**
Fats	**7.19 g**
MUFA	4.83 g
Omega-3	0.09 g
Omega-6	0.88 g
Saturated Fat	0.83 g
Carbohydrates	**7.03 g**
Fiber	2.56 g
Starch	2.86 g
Fructose	0.62 g
Glucose	0.45 g
Sucrose	0.09 g
Protein	**2.78 g**
Alanine	0.1 g
Arginine	0.19 g
Aspartic acid	0.31 g
Cystine	0.03 g
Glutamic acid	0.52 g
Glycine	0.09 g
Histidine	0.06 g
Isoleucine	0.08 g
Leucine	0.13 g
Lysine	0.13 g
Methionine	0.04 g
Phenylalanine	0.11 g
Proline	0.11 g
Serine	0.12 g
Threonine	0.09 g
Tryptophan	0.03 g
Tyrosine	0.05 g
Valine	0.12 g
Vitamins	
Vitamin B1	0.07 mg
Vitamin B12	0 mcg
Vitamin B2	0.11 mg
Vitamin B3	0.63 mg
Vitamin B5	0.55 mg
Vitamin B6	0.19 mg
Choline	17.9 mg
Folate	60.4 mcg
Vitamin A	36.2 mcg
Vitamin C	85.5 mg
Vitamin D	0 IU
Vitamin E	0.73 mg
Vitamin K	123 mcg
Minerals	
Calcium	50.9 mg
Copper	0.05 mg
Iron	1.01 mg
Magnesium	20.8 mg
Manganese	0.23 mg
Phosphorus	64.8 mg
Potassium	310 mg
Selenium	2.61 mcg
Sodium	63.7 mg
Zinc	0.42 mg

nutrition content estimated using the USDA database.

Garlicky Artichoke Hearts

Fresh artichoke is a completely different experience than canned. However, isolating the tender inner leaves and heart of the artichoke can be a fairly daunting task. Fortunately, it's getting easier and easier to find fresh or frozen artichoke hearts, which makes this a very fast side dish to whip together on a busy weeknight.

PREP TIME: 5 minutes
COOK TIME: 14 to 16 minutes
SERVINGS: 2 to 4

INGREDIENTS:

- 2 to 3 tablespoons bacon fat, lard, or duck fat
- 12 ounces fresh or frozen artichoke hearts
- 4 or 5 cloves garlic, crushed

FODMAP ALERT *Replace the garlic with green garlic or garlic scapes (green part only) or omit.*

1. Heat the bacon fat in a medium skillet over medium-high heat.
2. Add the artichokes (they can be added frozen). Cook, stirring occasionally, for 8 to 10 minutes, until they start to brown.
3. Add the garlic and cook for another 4 to 6 minutes, until the artichokes are tender and nicely browned.

TIPS:

To isolate the hearts from fresh artichokes, steam 5 or 6 artichokes following the directions on page 296. Let cool, then peel off the leaves, remove the choke with a paring knife, and cut the heart into quarters.

VARIATIONS:

Garlicky Baby Artichokes. *Baby artichokes, typically less than 2 inches in size, are so tender that you can eat the whole thing, even the choke! If you are lucky enough to find them, simmer whole for 10 minutes in salted water first. You can then cut them in half or leave them whole and sauté them.*

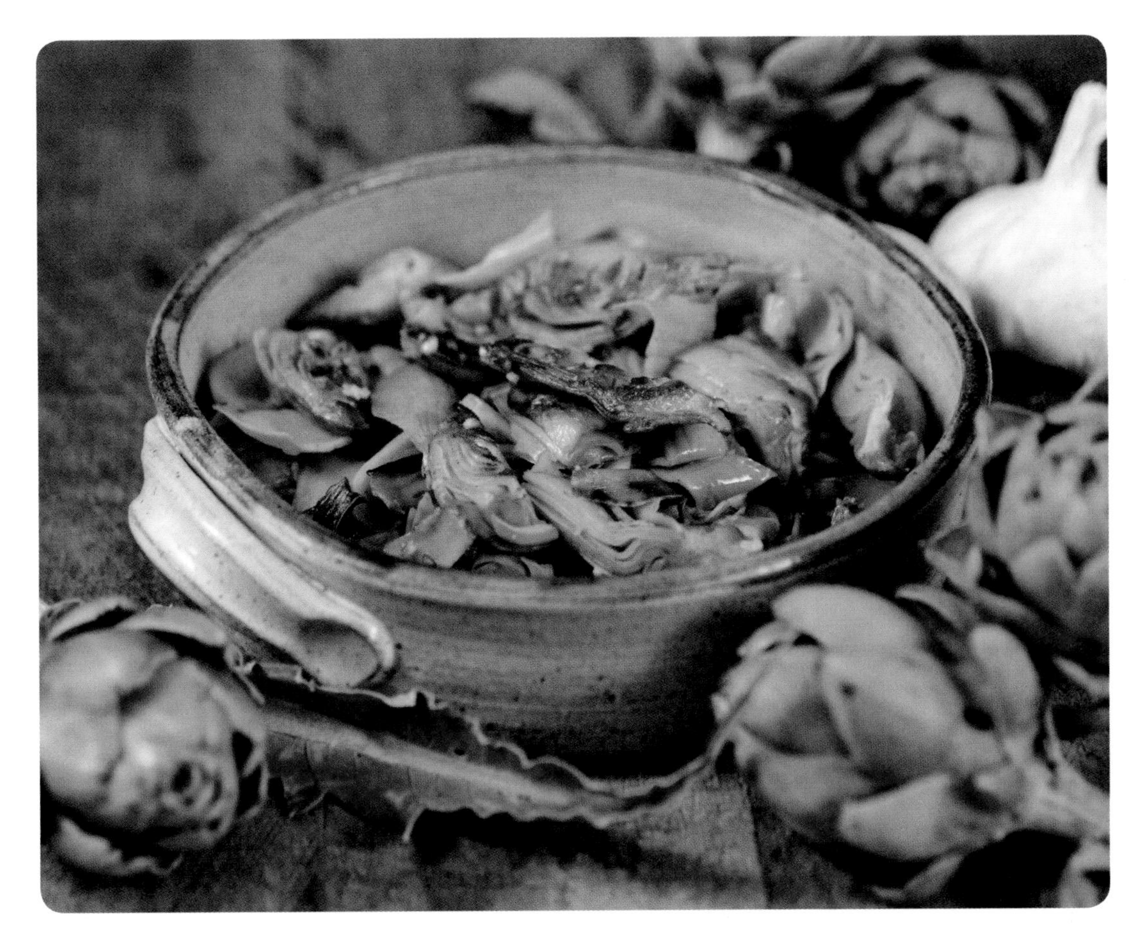

NUTRITION FACTS	
Serving Size	95 g
Recipe Yields	378 g
Calories	**93.9**
Fats	**6.47 g**
MUFA	2.91 g
Omega-3	0.08 g
Omega-6	0.71 g
Saturated Fat	2.56 g
Carbohydrates	**5.79 g**
Fiber	3.19 g
Starch	0.9 g
Fructose	0 g
Glucose	0 g
Sucrose	0 g
Protein	**3.32 g**
Alanine	<0.01 g
Arginine	0.02 g
Aspartic acid	0.01 g
Cystine	<0.01 g
Glutamic acid	0.02 g
Glycine	<0.01 g
Histidine	<0.01 g
Isoleucine	<0.01 g
Leucine	<0.01 g
Lysine	<0.01 g
Methionine	<0.01 g
Phenylalanine	<0.01 g
Proline	<0.01 g
Serine	<0.01 g
Threonine	<0.01 g
Tryptophan	<0.01 g
Tyrosine	<0.01 g
Valine	<0.01 g
Vitamins	
Vitamin B1	0.06 mg
Vitamin B12	0 mcg
Vitamin B2	0.06 mg
Vitamin B3	0.88 mg
Vitamin B5	0.31 mg
Vitamin B6	0.13 mg
Choline	3.44 mg
Folate	43.7 mcg
Vitamin A	0 mcg
Vitamin C	9.49 mg
Vitamin D	6.55 IU
Vitamin E	0.2 mg
Vitamin K	12.7 mcg
Minerals	
Calcium	8.59 mg
Copper	0.21 mg
Iron	1.15 mg
Magnesium	52.1 mg
Manganese	0.27 mg
Phosphorus	78.1 mg
Potassium	315 mg
Selenium	0.6 mcg
Sodium	91.5 mg
Zinc	0.46 mg

nutrition content estimated using the USDA database.

Balsamic-Roasted Beets

These beets are delicious right out of the oven or chilled as leftovers. Save the cooking liquid to make a vinaigrette!

PREP TIME: 10 minutes
COOK TIME: 45 minutes to 1 hour
SERVINGS: 4 to 8

INGREDIENTS:

6 to 8 medium beets, quartered

2 tablespoons balsamic vinegar

1 tablespoon extra-virgin coconut oil, melted

¼ teaspoon salt or truffle salt

1. Preheat the oven to 350°F. Lay a large piece of aluminum foil in a baking dish, lifting the sides to create an edge all the way around.
2. Combine the beets, vinegar, coconut oil, and salt. Pour into the foil. Fold the edges of the foil up and over the beets to make a pocket for the beets to cook in, sealing the edges closed. (Alternatively, you can use a greased baking dish with a lid.)
3. Bake for 45 minutes to 1 hour, until the beets are tender (it depends on the size of your beets).

VARIATIONS:

Beet, Pear, and Arugula Salad. *These beets are delicious chilled, sliced, and mixed with arugula, sliced pear, Toasted Coconut (page 160), and a simple vinaigrette made with the cooking liquid and extra-virgin olive oil!*

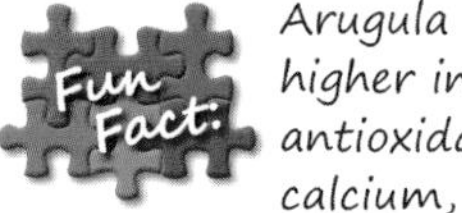

Arugula is higher in most antioxidants, calcium, magnesium, folate, and vitamin E than most other salad greens.

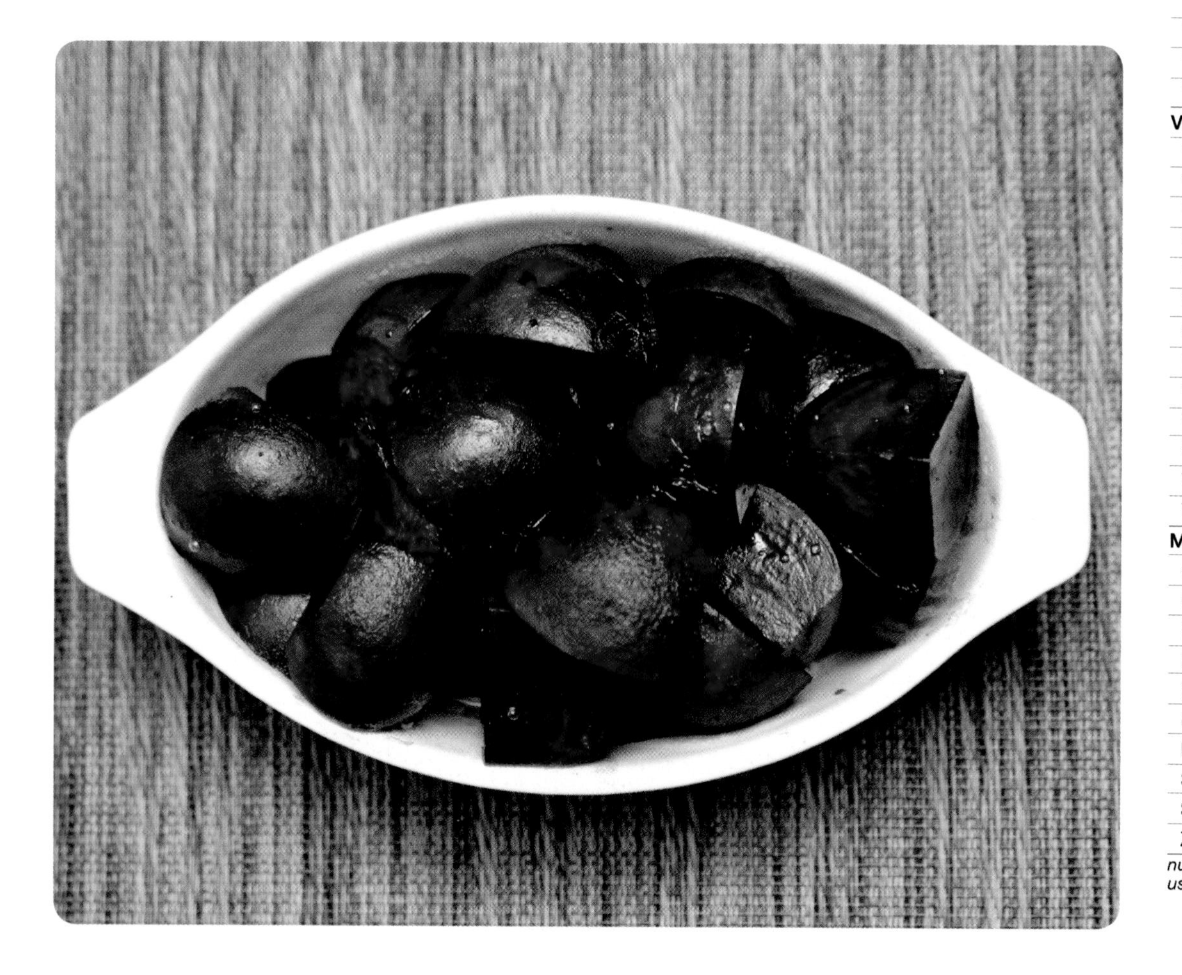

NUTRITION FACTS

Serving Size	67 g
Recipe Yields	539 g
Calories	**44.4**
Fats	**1.79 g**
MUFA	0.12 g
Omega-3	<0.01 g
Omega-6	0.06 g
Saturated Fat	1.48 g
Carbohydrates	**6.52 g**
Fiber	1.71 g
Starch	<0.01 g
Fructose	0.29 g
Glucose	0.3 g
Sucrose	0 g
Protein	**1 g**
Alanine	0.04 g
Arginine	0.03 g
Aspartic acid	0.07 g
Cystine	0.01 g
Glutamic acid	0.26 g
Glycine	0.02 g
Histidine	0.01 g
Isoleucine	0.03 g
Leucine	0.04 g
Lysine	0.04 g
Methionine	0.01 g
Phenylalanine	0.03 g
Proline	0.03 g
Serine	0.04 g
Threonine	0.03 g
Tryptophan	0.01 g
Tyrosine	0.02 g
Valine	0.03 g
Vitamins	
Vitamin B1	0.02 mg
Vitamin B12	0 mcg
Vitamin B2	0.02 mg
Vitamin B3	0.2 mg
Vitamin B5	0.09 mg
Vitamin B6	0.04 mg
Choline	3.67 mg
Folate	66.7 mcg
Vitamin A	1.22 mcg
Vitamin C	3 mg
Vitamin D	0 IU
Vitamin E	0.03 mg
Vitamin K	0.13 mcg
Minerals	
Calcium	11.2 mg
Copper	0.05 mg
Iron	0.71 mg
Magnesium	14.5 mg
Manganese	0.21 mg
Phosphorus	25.2 mg
Potassium	204 mg
Selenium	0.43 mcg
Sodium	80.5 mg
Zinc	0.22 mg

nutrition content estimated using the USDA database.

Wild Mushrooms and Tarragon

Really, you can use any mushroom or mix of mushrooms for this dish. It's amazing how a little tarragon, garlic, and lemon juice can completely transform mushrooms into something so delicious you'll want to make it again and again!

PREP TIME: 5 minutes
COOK TIME: 10 to 13 minutes
SERVINGS: 2 to 4

INGREDIENTS:

- 2 tablespoons lard, tallow, duck fat, or bacon fat
- 1½ pounds wild mushrooms
- 2 tablespoons chopped fresh tarragon
- 1 clove garlic, crushed
- 1 tablespoon fresh lemon juice
- ⅛ teaspoon salt

1. Heat the lard in a skillet over medium-high heat. Add the mushrooms and cook, stirring occasionally, until browned, 8 to 10 minutes. If the mushrooms are releasing a lot of water into the skillet and getting soupy, turn up the heat to keep the pan dry.
2. Add the tarragon, garlic, lemon juice, and salt and cook for 2 to 3 more minutes, stirring to incorporate. Serve!

TIPS:

Mushrooms with gills that run all the way down the stem, like chanterelle or oyster mushrooms, are stringy in texture, so they can be tough to slice with a knife. Instead, rip them apart with your fingers along the line of the gills.

FODMAP ALERT

This recipe cannot be made low-FODMAP.

NUTRITION FACTS	
Serving Size	182 g
Recipe Yields	729 g
Calories	**99.7**
Fats	**7.05 g**
MUFA	2.89 g
Omega-3	0.09 g
Omega-6	0.93 g
Saturated Fat	2.61 g
Carbohydrates	**6.5 g**
Fiber	1.79 g
Starch	0.86 g
Fructose	0.33 g
Glucose	2.55 g
Sucrose	0.02 g
Protein	**5.52 g**
Alanine	0.34 g
Arginine	0.14 g
Aspartic acid	0.34 g
Cystine	0.02 g
Glutamic acid	0.59 g
Glycine	0.16 g
Histidine	0.1 g
Isoleucine	0.13 g
Leucine	0.21 g
Lysine	0.18 g
Methionine	0.05 g
Phenylalanine	0.15 g
Proline	0.13 g
Serine	0.16 g
Threonine	0.18 g
Tryptophan	0.06 g
Tyrosine	0.08 g
Valine	0.4 g
Vitamins	
Vitamin B1	0.14 mg
Vitamin B12	0.07 mcg
Vitamin B2	0.7 mg
Vitamin B3	6.22 mg
Vitamin B5	2.55 mg
Vitamin B6	0.21 mg
Choline	33 mg
Folate	32.1 mcg
Vitamin A	1.89 mcg
Vitamin C	5.73 mg
Vitamin D	18.4 IU
Vitamin E	0.06 mg
Vitamin K	0.01 mcg
Minerals	
Calcium	17.3 mg
Copper	0.55 mg
Iron	1.34 mg
Magnesium	18.8 mg
Manganese	0.16 mg
Phosphorus	150 mg
Potassium	576 mg
Selenium	16 mcg
Sodium	41.3 mg
Zinc	0.94 mg

nutrition content estimated using the USDA database.

Easy Broiled Asparagus

With just three simple ingredients, you wouldn't expect this to be such an amazingly delicious side dish, but it truly is! Truffle salt is a magical ingredient and imparts an incredible earthiness to asparagus that just can't be described.

PREP TIME: 5 minutes
COOK TIME: 6 to 8 minutes
SERVINGS: 2 to 4

INGREDIENTS:

1 pound asparagus, tough ends of spears snapped off and discarded

2 tablespoons avocado oil

¼ teaspoon truffle salt

1. Position an oven rack 6 inches below the broiler. Preheat the broiler on high for 10 to 15 minutes. To make cleanup easier, line a rimmed baking sheet with aluminum foil.
2. Place the asparagus on the prepared baking sheet. Drizzle with the oil and sprinkle with the salt; toss to combine.
3. Broil for 6 to 8 minutes, until starting to brown.

VARIATIONS:

If you don't have truffle salt, regular pink or gray salt can be used instead.

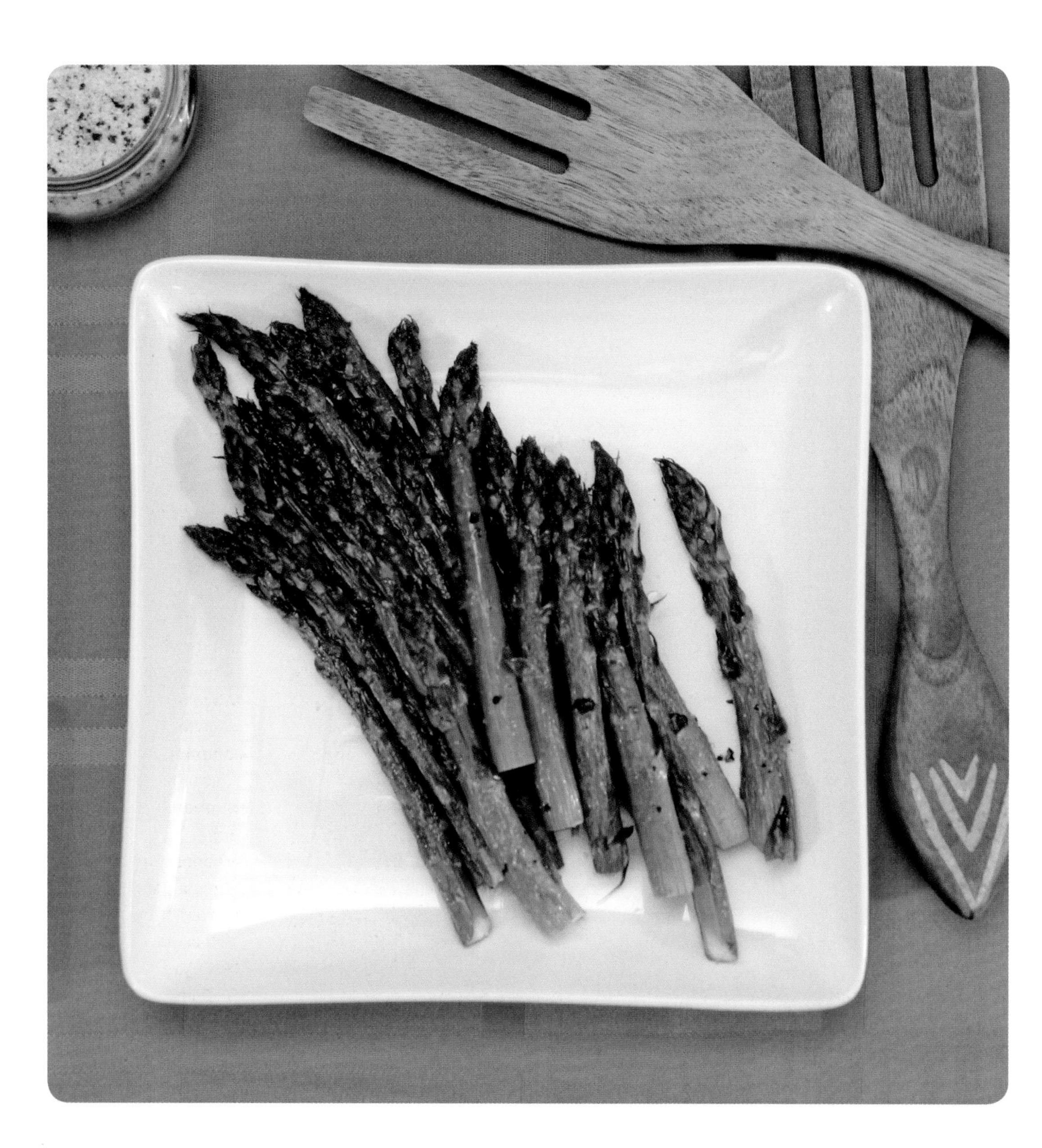

NUTRITION FACTS	
Serving Size	121 g
Recipe Yields	483 g
Calories	**87**
Fats	**7.26 g**
MUFA	4.95 g
Omega-3	0.1 g
Omega-6	0.97 g
Saturated Fat	0.87 g
Carbohydrates	**4.67 g**
Fiber	2.27 g
Starch	0.92 g
Fructose	0.9 g
Glucose	0.48 g
Sucrose	0.09 g
Protein	**2.73 g**
Alanine	0.14 g
Arginine	0.11 g
Aspartic acid	0.63 g
Cystine	0.04 g
Glutamic acid	0.29 g
Glycine	0.11 g
Histidine	0.06 g
Isoleucine	0.09 g
Leucine	0.16 g
Lysine	0.13 g
Methionine	0.04 g
Phenylalanine	0.09 g
Proline	0.09 g
Serine	0.13 g
Threonine	0.1 g
Tryptophan	0.03 g
Tyrosine	0.06 g
Valine	0.14 g
Vitamins	
Vitamin B1	0.18 mg
Vitamin B12	0 mcg
Vitamin B2	0.16 mg
Vitamin B3	1.23 mg
Vitamin B5	0.26 mg
Vitamin B6	0.09 mg
Choline	29.7 mg
Folate	169 mcg
Vitamin A	56.8 mcg
Vitamin C	8.75 mg
Vitamin D	0 IU
Vitamin E	1.7 mg
Vitamin K	57.5 mcg
Minerals	
Calcium	26.9 mg
Copper	0.19 mg
Iron	1.41 mg
Magnesium	15.9 mg
Manganese	0.17 mg
Phosphorus	61.4 mg
Potassium	257 mg
Selenium	6.93 mcg
Sodium	80.2 mg
Zinc	0.68 mg

nutrition content estimated using the USDA database.

Mashed Acorn Squash with Forty Cloves of Garlic

Just like its chicken recipe cousin, this recipe doesn't use exactly forty cloves of garlic—just a lot! Garlic becomes deliciously mild and sweet when the whole cloves are roasted. And the flavor is a delicious complement to baked winter squash (or anything, really!); with this cooking method, even the large amount of garlic used doesn't overwhelm the flavor of the squash. This recipe is also designed to highlight very high-quality extra-virgin olive oil, so go ahead and pull out the good stuff.

PREP TIME: 20 to 30 minutes
COOK TIME: 1 hour 15 minutes to 1 hour 30 minutes
SERVINGS: 6 to 8

INGREDIENTS:

- 2 large acorn squash (1½ pounds each)
- 3 to 4 heads garlic, peeled
- 1½ teaspoons avocado or coconut oil
- 1 teaspoon truffle salt
- 2 tablespoons extra-virgin olive oil

FODMAP ALERT *Acorn squash is delicious baked and mashed even without the garlic.*

1. Preheat the oven to 350°F.
2. Cut the acorn squash in half and remove the seeds. Place the halves cut side up on a rimmed baking sheet.
3. In a bowl, toss the garlic cloves with the avocado oil and distribute evenly among the 4 squash half middles. Sprinkle the squash halves with the truffle salt.
4. Roast for 1 hour 15 minutes to 1 hour 30 minutes, until the squash is soft.
5. Scoop out the squash and garlic and mash with a fork. Mix in the olive oil and serve.

VARIATIONS:

Instead of olive oil, you can use lard or duck fat. You can always use pink or gray salt in place of truffle salt if you prefer.

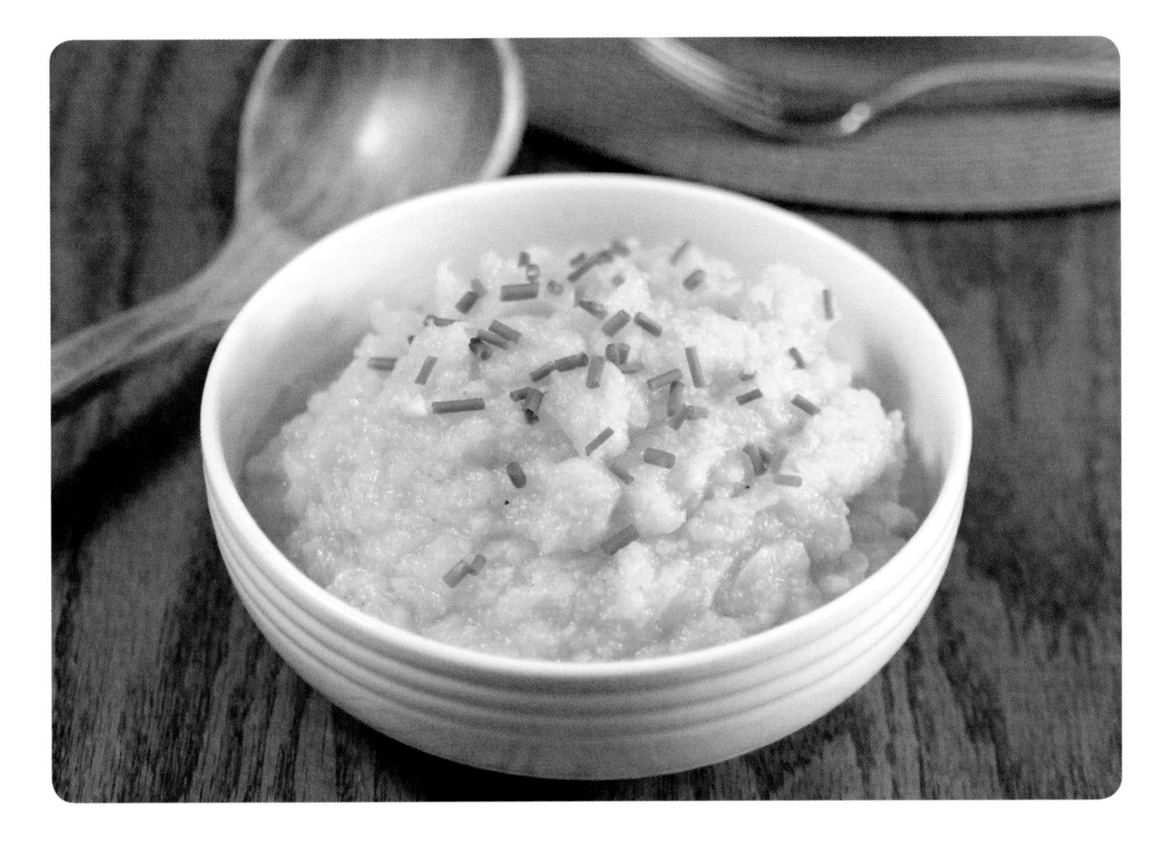

NUTRITION FACTS	
Serving Size	189 g
Recipe Yields	1508 g
Calories	**153**
Fats	**4.57 g**
MUFA	3.11 g
Omega-3	0.1 g
Omega-6	0.51 g
Saturated Fat	0.63 g
Carbohydrates	**29.3 g**
Fiber	7.79 g
Starch	4.05 g
Fructose	0 g
Glucose	g
Sucrose	g
Protein	**2.77 g**
Alanine	0.1 g
Arginine	0.19 g
Aspartic acid	0.27 g
Cystine	0.03 g
Glutamic acid	0.44 g
Glycine	0.1 g
Histidine	0.05 g
Isoleucine	0.1 g
Leucine	0.15 g
Lysine	0.11 g
Methionine	0.03 g
Phenylalanine	0.1 g
Proline	0.08 g
Serine	0.1 g
Threonine	0.08 g
Tryptophan	0.04 g
Tyrosine	0.08 g
Valine	0.12 g
Vitamins	
Vitamin B1	0.31 mg
Vitamin B12	0 mcg
Vitamin B2	0.04 mg
Vitamin B3	1.6 mg
Vitamin B5	0.94 mg
Vitamin B6	0.5 mg
Choline	3.15 mg
Folate	32.8 mcg
Vitamin A	35.8 mcg
Vitamin C	22.6 mg
Vitamin D	0 IU
Vitamin E	0.5 mg
Vitamin K	2.27 mcg
Minerals	
Calcium	101 mg
Copper	0.19 mg
Iron	2.59 mg
Magnesium	76.7 mg
Manganese	0.64 mg
Phosphorus	97.4 mg
Potassium	804 mg
Selenium	3.11 mcg
Sodium	138 mg
Zinc	0.45 mg

nutrition content estimated using the USDA database.

Roasted Butternut Squash

This simple savory squash pairs well with just about any dish.

PREP TIME: 15 minutes
COOK TIME: 30 to 35 minutes
SERVINGS: 4 to 6

INGREDIENTS:

2 pounds butternut squash

2 tablespoons extra-virgin coconut oil, lard, or duck fat, melted

2 teaspoons chopped fresh thyme leaves

¼ teaspoon salt

1. Preheat the oven to 425°F. Line a baking sheet with aluminum foil, parchment paper, or a silicone liner.
2. Pierce the squash once or twice with the tip of a knife, then microwave on high for 1 to 2 minutes. (This makes it easier to peel the squash but is not necessary if you don't have a microwave.) Peel the squash, cut in half lengthwise, and scoop out the seeds. Cut the squash into 1½-inch chunks.
3. In a large bowl, toss the squash with the oil, thyme, and salt. Spread out onto the prepared baking sheet.
4. Bake for 30 to 35 minutes, until slightly browned and tender. Shake the pan (or flip the squash chunks) every 10 minutes during baking.

VARIATIONS:

You can make this dish with any winter squash.

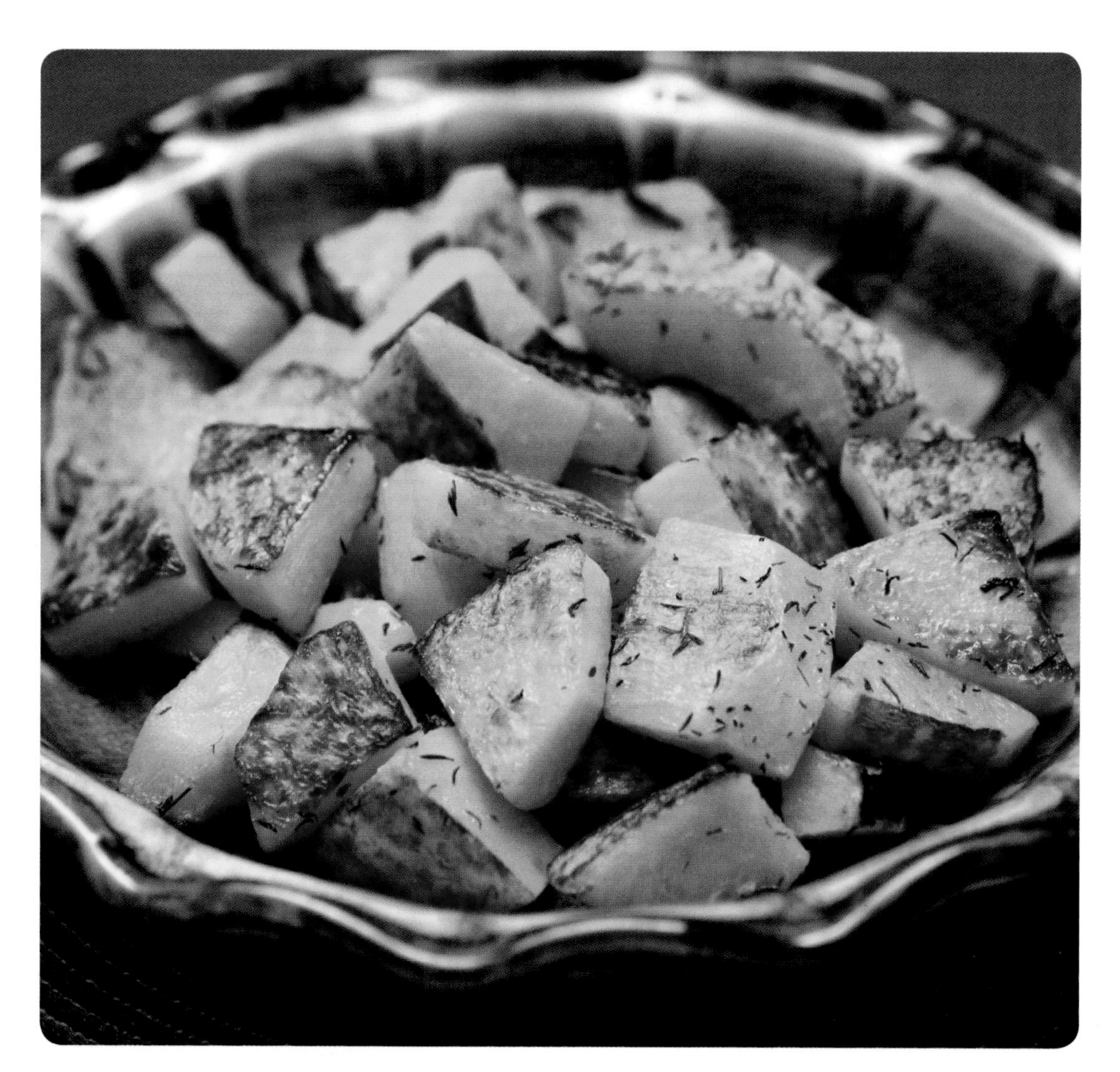

NUTRITION FACTS	
Serving Size	156 g
Recipe Yields	937 g
Calories	**99.7**
Fats	**4.67 g**
MUFA	0.27 g
Omega-3	0.04 g
Omega-6	0.1 g
Saturated Fat	3.95 g
Carbohydrates	**15.9 g**
Fiber	4.87 g
Starch	8.03 g
Fructose	0 g
Glucose	0 g
Sucrose	0 g
Protein	**1.37 g**
Alanine	0.06 g
Arginine	0.08 g
Aspartic acid	0.15 g
Cystine	0.01 g
Glutamic acid	0.24 g
Glycine	0.05 g
Histidine	0.03 g
Isoleucine	0.05 g
Leucine	0.08 g
Lysine	0.05 g
Methionine	0.02 g
Phenylalanine	0.05 g
Proline	0.05 g
Serine	0.05 g
Threonine	0.04 g
Tryptophan	0.02 g
Tyrosine	0.05 g
Valine	0.06 g
Vitamins	
Vitamin B1	0.11 mg
Vitamin B12	0 mcg
Vitamin B2	0.03 mg
Vitamin B3	1.47 mg
Vitamin B5	0.54 mg
Vitamin B6	0.19 mg
Choline	0.01 mg
Folate	28.8 mcg
Vitamin A	843 mcg
Vitamin C	23.2 mg
Vitamin D	0 IU
Vitamin E	1.95 mg
Vitamin K	1.53 mcg
Minerals	
Calcium	63.5 mg
Copper	0.1 mg
Iron	1.2 mg
Magnesium	44.2 mg
Manganese	0.26 mg
Phosphorus	41 mg
Potassium	432 mg
Selenium	0.75 mcg
Sodium	47.8 mg
Zinc	0.2 mg

nutrition content estimated using the USDA database.

Maple-Braised Butternut Squash

This sweeter treatment of squash is a delightful accompaniment to pork. While the syrup infuses the squash with maple flavor, only a fraction of the sugar is retained in the final dish.

PREP TIME: 15 minutes
COOK TIME: 18 to 22 minutes
SERVINGS: 4 to 8

INGREDIENTS:

- 2 pounds butternut squash
- 2 tablespoons extra-virgin coconut oil or lard
- ¼ cup Bone Broth (chicken, page 110)
- ¼ cup grade B maple syrup

1. Pierce the squash once or twice with the tip of a knife, then microwave on high for 1 to 2 minutes. (This makes it easier to peel the squash but is not necessary if you don't have a microwave.) Peel the squash, cut in half lengthwise, and scoop out the seeds. Cut the squash into 1½-inch chunks.
2. Heat the coconut oil in a large pot over medium-high heat. Once the oil is hot, add the broth and maple syrup. Add the squash and stir to coat.
3. Cover, reduce the heat to low, and simmer for 16 to 20 minutes, until the squash is soft and starting to absorb the liquid.
4. Drain and serve.

VARIATIONS:

You can make this dish with any winter squash.

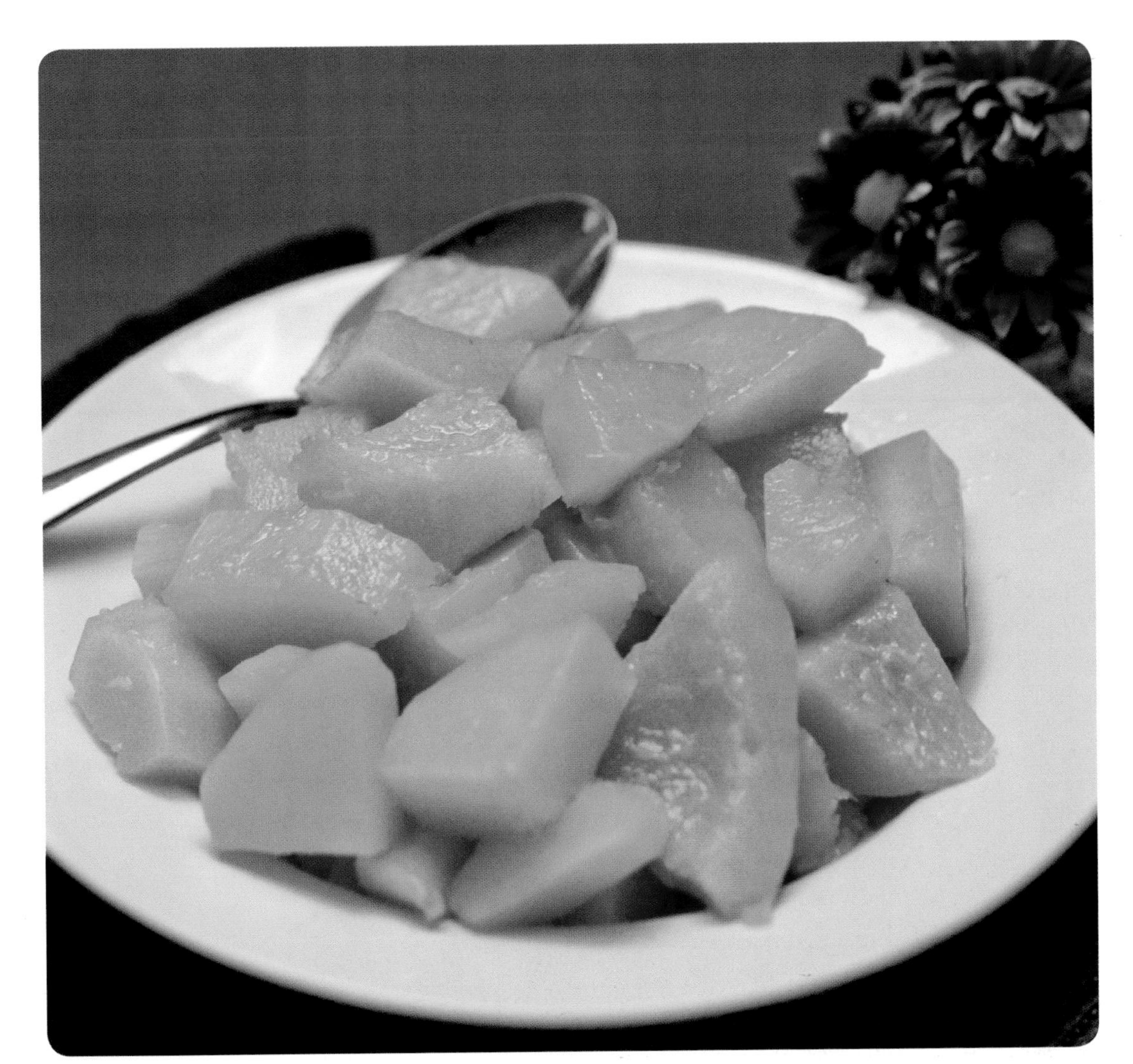

NUTRITION FACTS	
Serving Size	134 g
Recipe Yields	1074 g
Calories	**101**
Fats	**3.55 g**
MUFA	0.21 g
Omega-3	0.04 g
Omega-6	0.08 g
Saturated Fat	2.97 g
Carbohydrates	**18.5 g**
Fiber	3.62 g
Starch	6.02 g
Fructose	0.05 g
Glucose	0.16 g
Sucrose	5.73 g
Protein	**1.17 g**
Alanine	0.04 g
Arginine	0.06 g
Aspartic acid	0.11 g
Cystine	<0.01 g
Glutamic acid	0.18 g
Glycine	0.04 g
Histidine	0.02 g
Isoleucine	0.04 g
Leucine	0.06 g
Lysine	0.04 g
Methionine	0.01 g
Phenylalanine	0.04 g
Proline	0.04 g
Serine	0.04 g
Threonine	0.03 g
Tryptophan	0.01 g
Tyrosine	0.03 g
Valine	0.04 g
Vitamins	
Vitamin B1	0.09 mg
Vitamin B12	<0.01 mcg
Vitamin B2	0.15 mg
Vitamin B3	1.21 mg
Vitamin B5	0.41 mg
Vitamin B6	0.14 mg
Choline	0.87 mg
Folate	21.8 mcg
Vitamin A	632 mcg
Vitamin C	17.1 mg
Vitamin D	0 IU
Vitamin E	1.47 mg
Vitamin K	1.16 mcg
Minerals	
Calcium	58.7 mg
Copper	0.08 mg
Iron	0.71 mg
Magnesium	35 mg
Manganese	0.48 mg
Phosphorus	33 mg
Potassium	349 mg
Selenium	0.68 mcg
Sodium	29.9 mg
Zinc	0.3 mg

nutrition content estimated using the USDA database.

Mint Pesto Zucchini "Pasta"

Zucchini and mint are a match made in heaven. Given how well zucchini holds up when spiral-cut or julienned to form mock noodles, this seems like a perfect opportunity for a mint pesto pasta dish!

PREP TIME: 15 minutes, plus 1 hour to salt the zucchini
COOK TIME: 15 to 18 minutes
SERVINGS: 2 to 4

INGREDIENTS:

2 pounds zucchini (about 3 medium)

1 tablespoon salt

8 to 10 cloves garlic, unpeeled

2 tablespoons extra-virgin olive oil

2 tablespoons chopped fresh mint

2 to 3 tablespoons lard, coconut oil, or bacon fat

FODMAP ALERT *Replace the garlic with green garlic or garlic scapes (green part only).*

SPECIAL EQUIPMENT

- Spiral vegetable slicer or mandoline slicer
- Mini food processor or mortar and pestle
- Large skillet or wok

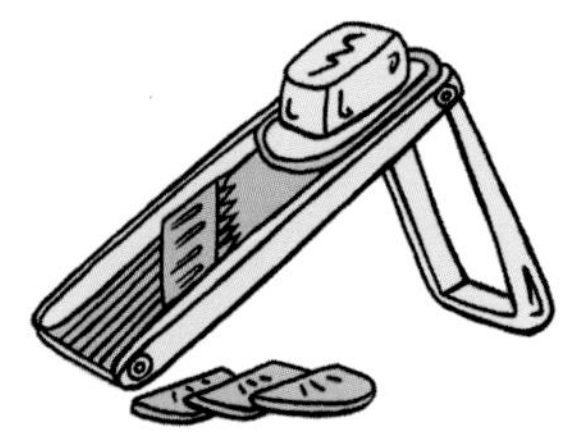

1. Slice the zucchini into long, thin noodles with a spiral vegetable slicer, mandoline slicer, or julienne peeler. (With some patience, you can also julienne long strips of zucchini with a knife.) Sprinkle liberally with the salt and place in a colander in the sink for 1 hour (this helps remove excess water so that the zucchini holds together better once cooked).
2. Meanwhile, make the mint pesto: Place the whole, unpeeled garlic cloves in a dry pan. Heat over medium-high heat, stirring or shaking the pan occasionally, until the papery peel of the garlic browns and starts to flake off, about 10 minutes.
3. Remove the garlic from the pan and let cool enough to handle. Remove the peel. Place the garlic, olive oil, and mint in a mini food processor and pulse until you get a pastelike texture, or grind the ingredients to a paste by hand using a mortar and pestle.
4. Rinse the zucchini noodles thoroughly. Drain and invert onto paper towels or a clean kitchen towel. Place another kitchen towel or paper towels on top and gently press to remove as much water as possible.
5. Heat the lard in a large skillet or wok over medium-high heat. Add the zucchini noodles once the pan is hot. Cook, stirring gently but frequently, until the zucchini is cooked al dente, 5 to 8 minutes. Keep the heat high enough that any liquid released by the zucchini is evaporating. If you a lot of liquid accumulates in the bottom of the pan, turn up the heat.
6. Remove from the heat and toss with the mint pesto. Serve.

TIPS:

This "pasta" is perfect with sliced grilled chicken or steak or grilled lamb chops. It's also a lovely side dish with fish.

VARIATIONS:

You can use the mint pesto sauce as a condiment for other dishes. It's especially good with lamb!

Traditional Pesto. *Using basil in place of the mint will give you a traditionally flavored pesto. Add 1 to 2 tablespoons nutritional yeast to mimic Parmesan cheese.*

Arugula Pesto. *Substitute fresh arugula or watercress for the mint for a peppery and refreshing arugula (or cress) pesto! This is a delicious condiment to serve with just about any meat or fish.*

Carrot Green Pesto. *Substitute the tender leaves from carrot greens, discarding the stems, for a delicious variation of traditional pesto.*

Zucchini Noodles. *If you want plain zucchini noodles to serve with other dishes, such as "Spaghetti" (page 224), simply follow the directions above and skip the pesto.*

NUTRITION FACTS

Serving Size	174 g
Recipe Yields	685 g
Calories	**152**
Fats	**13.6 g**
MUFA	7.82 g
Omega-3	0.21 g
Omega-6	1.37 g
Saturated Fat	3.57 g
Carbohydrates	**6.67 g**
Fiber	1.66 g
Starch	1.8 g
Fructose	2.03 g
Glucose	1.57 g
Sucrose	0.07 g
Protein	**2.19 g**
Alanine	0.1 g
Arginine	0.11 g
Aspartic acid	0.25 g
Cystine	0.02 g
Glutamic acid	0.24 g
Glycine	0.08 g
Histidine	0.05 g
Isoleucine	0.08 g
Leucine	0.12 g
Lysine	0.12 g
Methionine	0.03 g
Phenylalanine	0.08 g
Proline	0.06 g
Serine	0.08 g
Threonine	0.05 g
Tryptophan	0.02 g
Tyrosine	0.05 g
Valine	0.1 g
Vitamins	
Vitamin B1	0.08 mg
Vitamin B12	0 mcg
Vitamin B2	0.15 mg
Vitamin B3	0.72 mg
Vitamin B5	0.34 mg
Vitamin B6	0.31 mg
Choline	18.5 mg
Folate	36.3 mcg
Vitamin A	16.4 mcg
Vitamin C	28.4 mg
Vitamin D	6.52 IU
Vitamin E	1.19 mg
Vitamin K	10.5 mcg
Minerals	
Calcium	45 mg
Copper	0.1 mg
Iron	5.16 mg
Magnesium	28.6 mg
Manganese	0.37 mg
Phosphorus	65.6 mg
Potassium	438 mg
Selenium	1.16 mcg
Sodium	771 mg
Zinc	0.56 mg

nutrition content estimated using the USDA database.

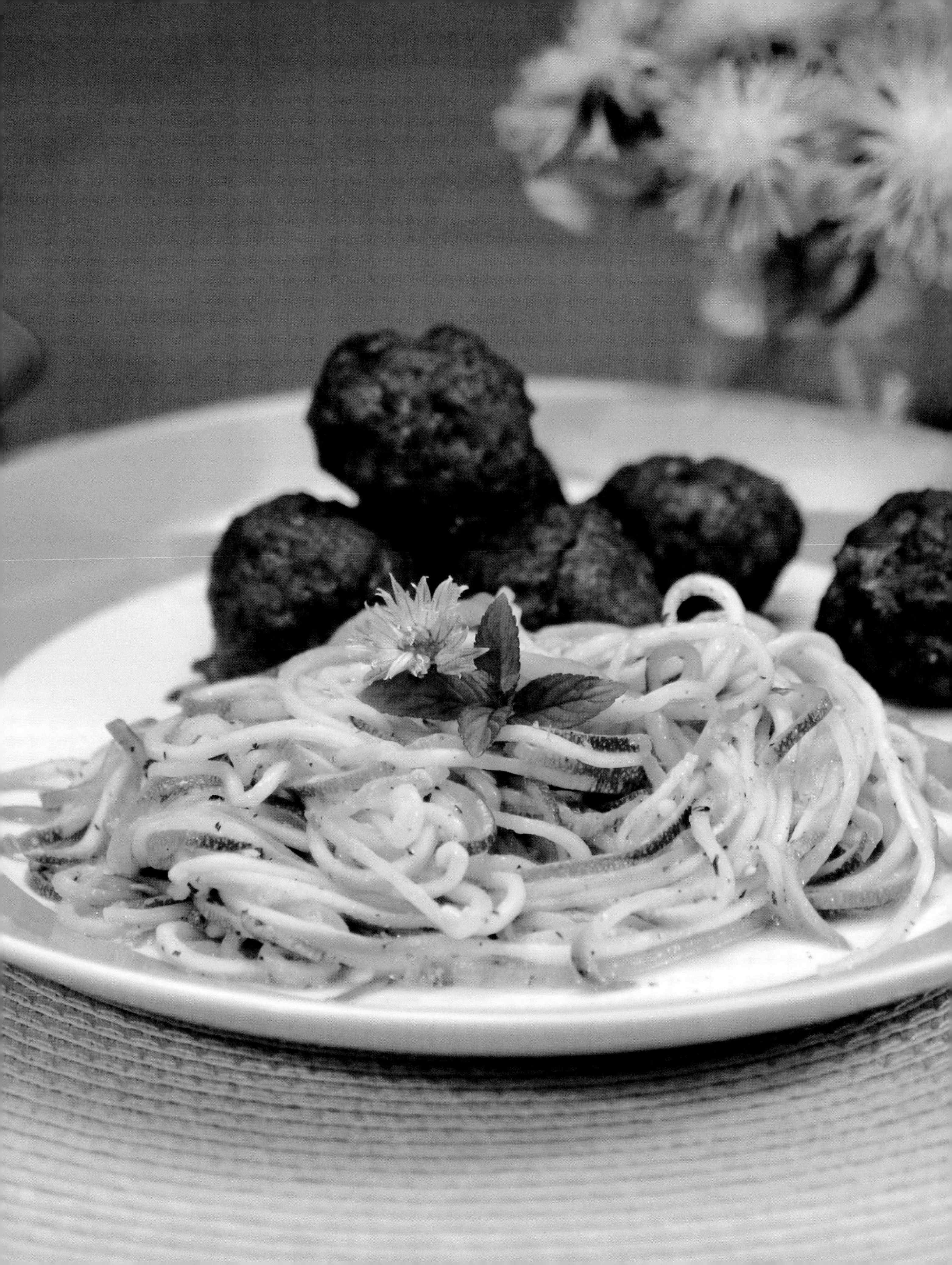

Fiddleheads

Fiddleheads were a staple of my childhood, and I relish them now when they are seasonally available in stores. They are actually baby ferns, picked before they unfurl their leaves, and a delicious, nutrient-dense green vegetable! Depending on where you live, you might also be able to find them frozen (they can be cooked directly from frozen without any modification of the recipe).

PREP TIME: 10 minutes
COOK TIME: 20 to 24 minutes
SERVINGS: 6

INGREDIENTS:

3 cups fresh fiddlehead ferns, ends trimmed

3 tablespoons coconut oil, lard, or bacon fat

1 clove garlic, minced

½ teaspoon salt or truffle salt

1 tablespoon fresh lemon juice

1. Bring a large pot of salted water to a boil. Cook the fiddleheads in the boiling water until barely tender, 7 to 10 minutes; drain. Alternatively, use a steamer insert or basket to steam the fiddleheads.
2. Heat the coconut oil in a large skillet over medium-high heat. Stir in the boiled fiddleheads, garlic, and salt (reduce or omit the salt if using bacon fat instead of coconut oil). Cook, stirring frequently, until the ferns are tinged lightly brown and tender, about 5 minutes. Remove from the heat, sprinkle with the lemon juice, and serve.

FODMAP ALERT *Replace the garlic with green garlic or garlic scapes (green part only) or omit.*

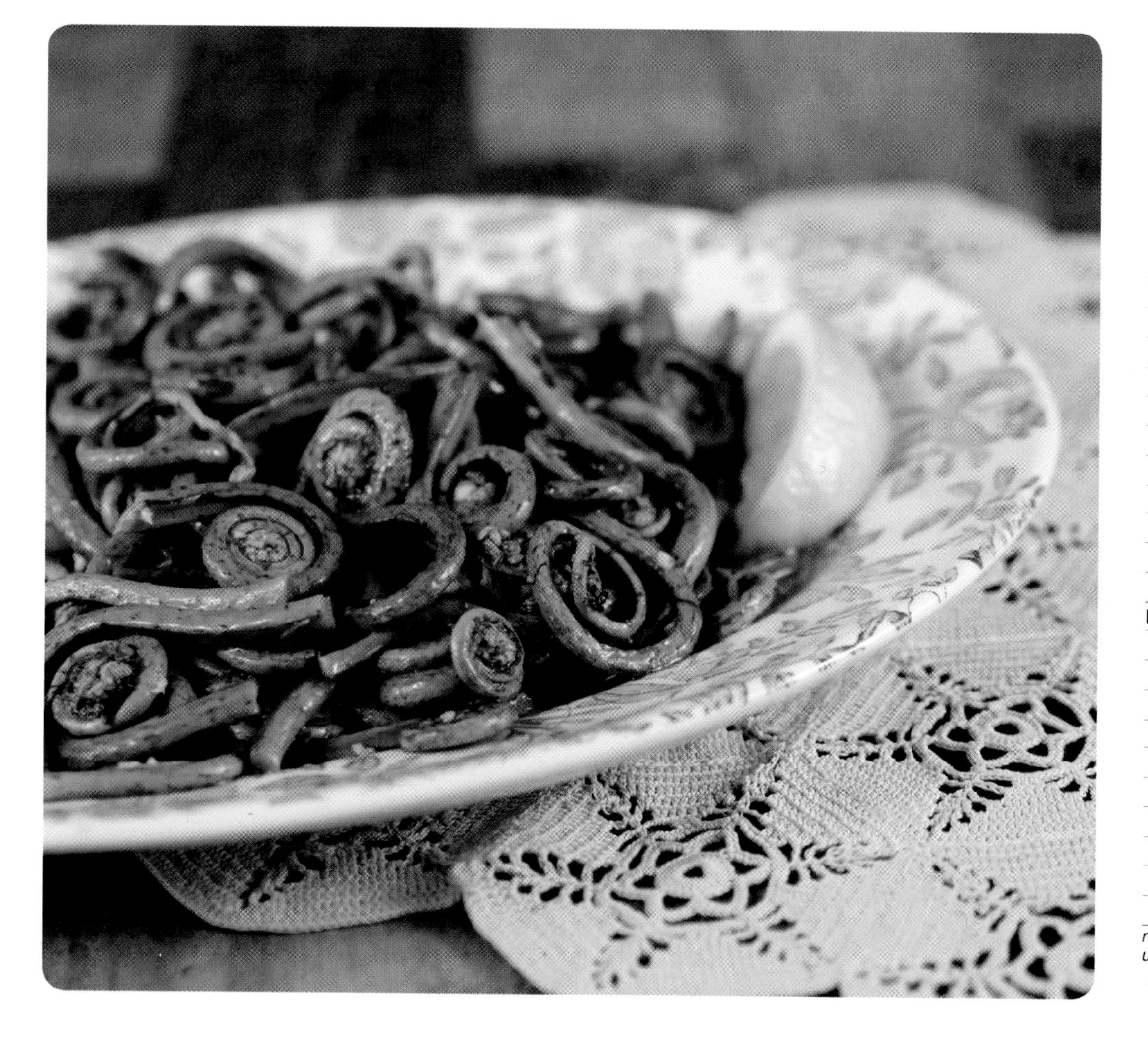

NUTRITION FACTS	
Serving Size	124 g
Recipe Yields	742 g
Calories	**98.7**
Fats	**7.28 g**
MUFA	0.4 g
Omega-3	<0.01 g
Omega-6	0.12 g
Saturated Fat	5.9 g
Carbohydrates	**6.64 g**
Fiber	0.02 g
Starch	0.25 g
Fructose	0.03 g
Glucose	0.03 g
Sucrose	0.01 g
Protein	**5.21 g**
Alanine	<0.01 g
Arginine	<0.01 g
Aspartic acid	<0.01 g
Cystine	<0.01 g
Glutamic acid	<0.01 g
Glycine	<0.01 g
Histidine	<0.01 g
Isoleucine	<0.01 g
Leucine	<0.01 g
Lysine	<0.01 g
Methionine	<0.01 g
Phenylalanine	<0.01 g
Proline	<0.01 g
Serine	<0.01 g
Threonine	<0.01 g
Tryptophan	<0.01 g
Tyrosine	<0.01 g
Valine	<0.01 g
Vitamins	
Vitamin B1	0.02 mg
Vitamin B12	0 mcg
Vitamin B2	0.24 mg
Vitamin B3	5.66 mg
Vitamin B5	<0.01 mg
Vitamin B6	<0.01 mg
Choline	0.27 mg
Folate	0.52 mcg
Vitamin A	206 mcg
Vitamin C	31.4 mg
Vitamin D	0 IU
Vitamin E	0.01 mg
Vitamin K	0.04 mcg
Minerals	
Calcium	37.9 mg
Copper	0.37 mg
Iron	1.5 mg
Magnesium	39 mg
Manganese	0.59 mg
Phosphorus	116 mg
Potassium	425 mg
Selenium	0.07 mcg
Sodium	197 mg
Zinc	0.95 mg

nutrition content estimated using the USDA database.

Roasted Sweet Potato

Use any variety of sweet potato you like for this dish, or a mix of varieties. If you are using smaller sweet potatoes, you can skip the peeling since the peel is typically fairly tender. Fingerling sweet potatoes can be left whole.

PREP TIME: 10 minutes
COOK TIME: 40 minutes
SERVINGS: 4 to 8

INGREDIENTS:

2 pounds sweet potatoes, peeled and cut into ½-inch-thick circles (or semicircles, if big around; you can also cut thick wedges to make sweet potato fries)

2 tablespoons extra-virgin coconut oil, melted

¼ teaspoon salt, to taste (optional)

1. Preheat the oven to 350°F. Line a rimmed baking sheet with aluminum foil or parchment paper, or use a silicone baking mat.
2. Place the sweet potato slices in a large bowl. Toss with the coconut oil and salt until evenly coated. Arrange the slices in a single layer on the prepared baking sheet.
3. Bake for 25 minutes, then remove from the oven and turn each slice over.
4. Bake for another 15 minutes. Enjoy!

VARIATIONS:

Spiced Sweet Potato. Sprinkle the sweet potato with 2 teaspoons ground cinnamon or 1 teaspoon ground mace for a spiced version.

FODMAP ALERT

This recipe cannot be made low-FODMAP.

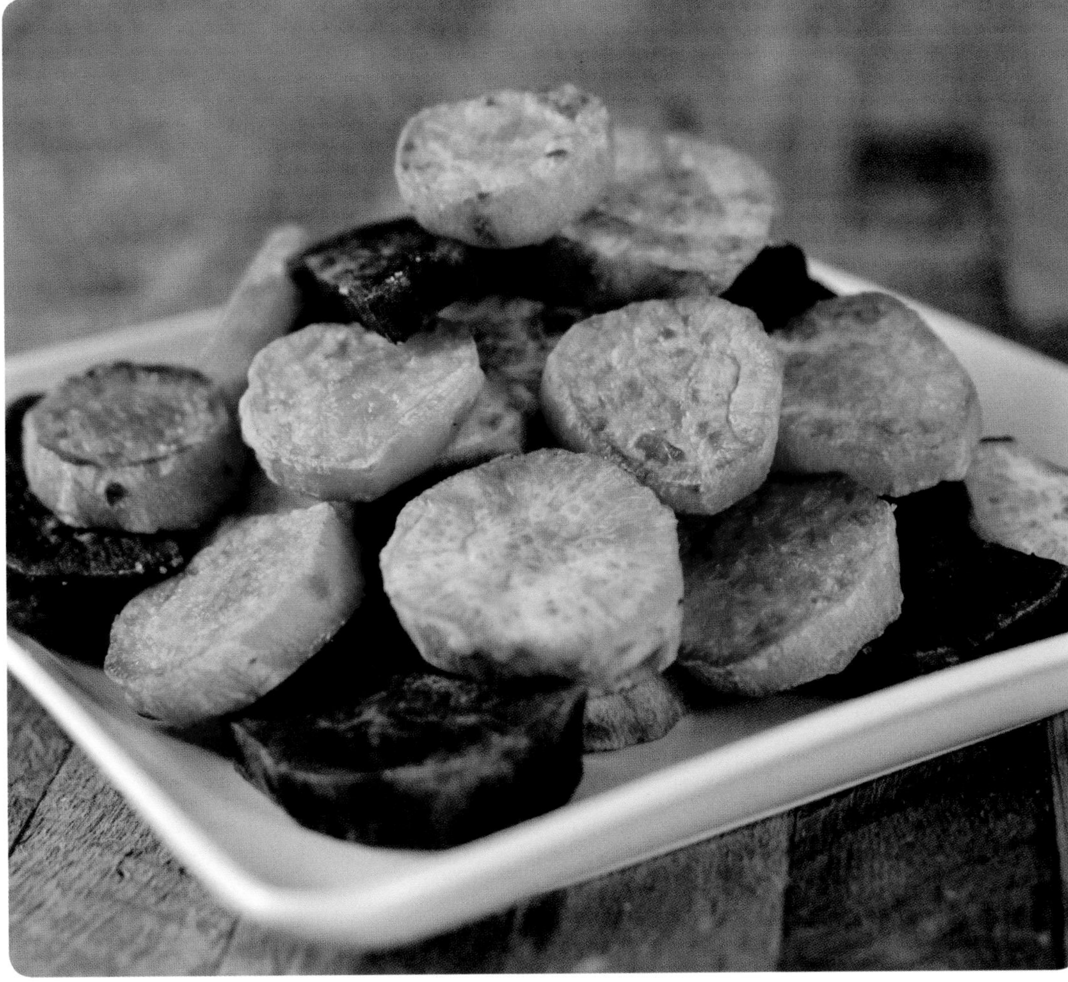

NUTRITION FACTS	
Serving Size	117 g
Recipe Yields	936 g
Calories	**131**
Fats	**3.57 g**
MUFA	0.2 g
Omega-3	<0.01 g
Omega-6	0.13 g
Saturated Fat	2.98 g
Carbohydrates	**23.5 g**
Fiber	3.74 g
Starch	8 g
Fructose	0.57 g
Glucose	0.65 g
Sucrose	2.59 g
Protein	**2.28 g**
Alanine	0.11 g
Arginine	0.08 g
Aspartic acid	0.55 g
Cystine	0.03 g
Glutamic acid	0.22 g
Glycine	0.09 g
Histidine	0.04 g
Isoleucine	0.08 g
Leucine	0.13 g
Lysine	0.1 g
Methionine	0.04 g
Phenylalanine	0.13 g
Proline	0.08 g
Serine	0.13 g
Threonine	0.12 g
Tryptophan	0.05 g
Tyrosine	0.05 g
Valine	0.12 g
Vitamins	
Vitamin B1	0.12 mg
Vitamin B12	0 mcg
Vitamin B2	0.12 mg
Vitamin B3	1.69 mg
Vitamin B5	1 mg
Vitamin B6	0.32 mg
Choline	14.9 mg
Folate	6.81 mcg
Vitamin A	1090 mcg
Vitamin C	22.2 mg
Vitamin D	0 IU
Vitamin E	0.81 mg
Vitamin K	2.63 mcg
Minerals	
Calcium	43.5 mg
Copper	0.18 mg
Iron	0.97 mg
Magnesium	30.6 mg
Manganese	0.56 mg
Phosphorus	61.3 mg
Potassium	540 mg
Selenium	0.23 mcg
Sodium	72.9 mg
Zinc	0.36 mg

nutrition content estimated using the USDA database.

Bacon-Braised Savoy Cabbage and Apple

There's something about the combination of cabbage, bacon, and apple that makes it the perfect accompaniment to pork. Of course, this side dish is also yummy with chicken, lamb, beef, fish . . . .

PREP TIME: 10 minutes
COOK TIME: 20 to 24 minutes
SERVINGS: 6

INGREDIENTS:

- 4 ounces bacon, chopped
- 1 head savoy cabbage, shredded or sliced into ⅜-inch-thick strips (12 to 14 cups)
- ½ cup Bone Broth (chicken, page 110)
- 1 apple, peeled, cored, and cut into ½-inch dice
- 1 tablespoon fresh lemon juice
- 4 cloves garlic, finely chopped
- ½ teaspoon grated fresh ginger
- ¼ teaspoon ground cinnamon

1. Add the bacon to a cold pan, then turn on the heat to medium-high. Cook, stirring occasionally, until the bacon is crisp, about 10 minutes.
2. Add the cabbage and broth. Cook until the cabbage has softened, stirring occasionally, 7 to 8 minutes.
3. Add the apple, lemon juice, garlic, ginger, and cinnamon. Cook for 4 to 5 more minutes.

TIPS:

Try cutting your bacon slices with scissors instead of a knife.

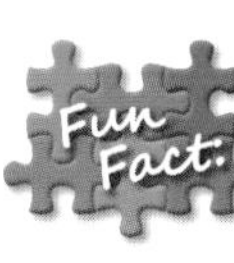

The best cooking apple varieties are Granny Smith, Fuji, and Rome Beauty because they hold their shape during cooking.

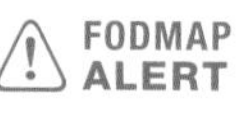

FODMAP ALERT

This recipe cannot be made low-FODMAP.

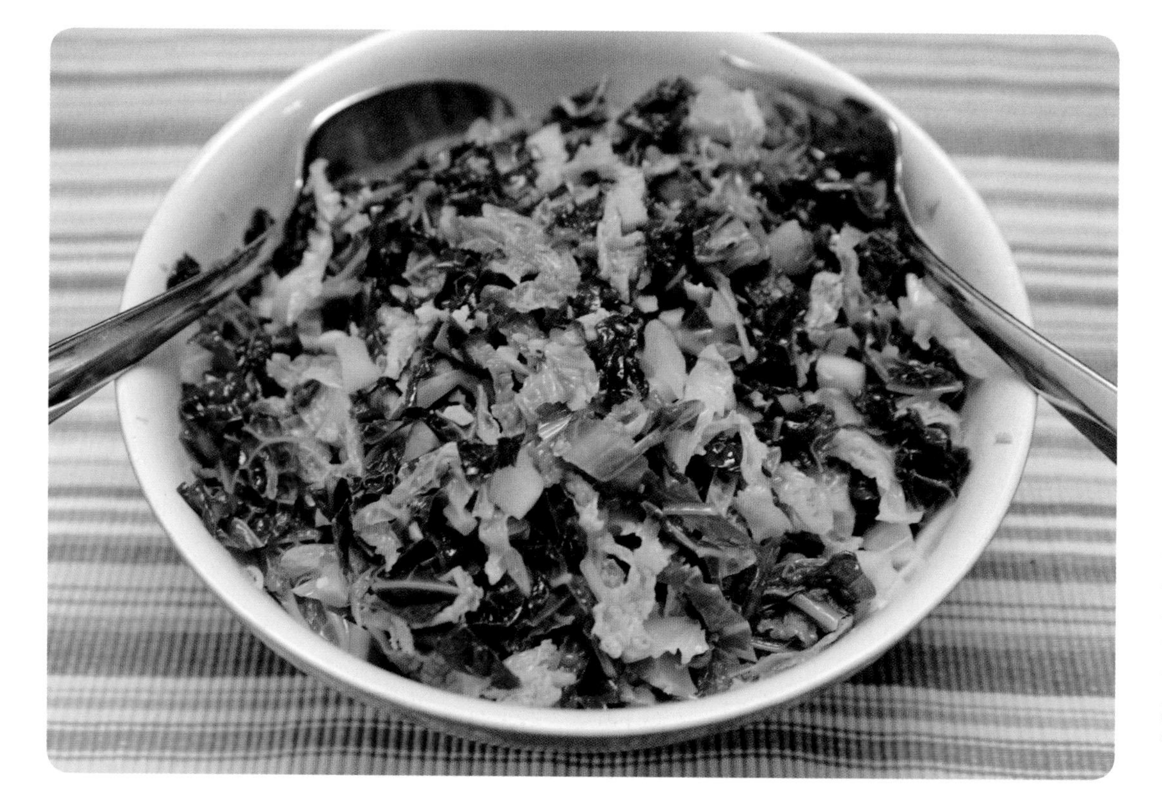

NUTRITION FACTS	
Serving Size	222 g
Recipe Yields	1333 g
Calories	**161**
Fats	**8.5 g**
MUFA	3.65 g
Omega-3	0.09 g
Omega-6	0.85 g
Saturated Fat	2.77 g
Carbohydrates	**13.5 g**
Fiber	4.24 g
Starch	1.27 g
Fructose	3.84 g
Glucose	3.42 g
Sucrose	0.35 g
Protein	**9.3 g**
Alanine	0.5 g
Arginine	0.56 g
Aspartic acid	0.85 g
Cystine	0.09 g
Glutamic acid	1.46 g
Glycine	0.53 g
Histidine	0.29 g
Isoleucine	0.37 g
Leucine	0.6 g
Lysine	0.64 g
Methionine	0.17 g
Phenylalanine	0.32 g
Proline	0.45 g
Serine	0.34 g
Threonine	0.32 g
Tryptophan	0.07 g
Tyrosine	0.24 g
Valine	0.43 g
Vitamins	
Vitamin B1	0.17 mg
Vitamin B12	0.24 mcg
Vitamin B2	0.12 mg
Vitamin B3	2.68 mg
Vitamin B5	0.55 mg
Vitamin B6	0.28 mg
Choline	42.1 mg
Folate	66.8 mcg
Vitamin A	10.4 mcg
Vitamin C	58 mg
Vitamin D	0 IU
Vitamin E	0.34 mg
Vitamin K	115 mcg
Minerals	
Calcium	74.7 mg
Copper	0.09 mg
Iron	1.1 mg
Magnesium	25.9 mg
Manganese	0.31 mg
Phosphorus	147 mg
Potassium	412 mg
Selenium	12 mcg
Sodium	506 mg
Zinc	0.97 mg

nutrition content estimated using the USDA database.

Whole Carrot "Tabouleh"

When you buy whole carrots with the greens attached, don't toss those greens! They make a wonderful pesto (page 310); they can also be added to salads (see page 160) or soups (see page 194) or used to make Braised Greens (page 300). They give this "tabouleh" a wonderful flavor and texture.

PREP TIME: 15 minutes
COOK TIME: none
SERVINGS: 2 to 3

INGREDIENTS:

- 3 to 4 large carrots, with greens attached (about 1½ pounds)
- 1½ teaspoons minced fresh mint
- 2 tablespoons raisins
- 2 tablespoons extra-virgin olive oil
- 2 tablespoons fresh lemon juice
- ½ teaspoon finely grated lemon zest
- Pinch of salt

SPECIAL EQUIPMENT

- Food processor

1. Cut the greens off the carrots. Remove the main stems (unless they are very tender) and finely chop the leaves. Cut the carrots into large chunks.
2. Place the carrots in a food processor fitted with an S-shaped blade. Process until couscous-sized, 30 seconds to 1 minute.
3. Toss the processed carrots with the chopped carrot leaves, mint, raisins, olive oil, lemon juice and zest, and salt. Serve!

TIPS:

You can make this salad up to 24 hours ahead and just give it a quick stir before serving. In fact, it tastes even better the next day.

Can't find carrots with the greens attached? Use parsley instead of carrot greens.

VARIATIONS:

For a slightly different flavor, try chopped dates or dried figs in place of the raisins. Chopped Honey-Candied Ginger (page 333) is also a fun addition.

Cauliflower "Rice" Tabouleh. *You can make this tabouleh with leftover Plain or Lemon-Parsley Cauliflower Rice (page 298), adding 2 to 4 tablespoons fresh parsley in place of the carrot greens (more if you are using the plain version, less if you are using the lemon parsley version).*

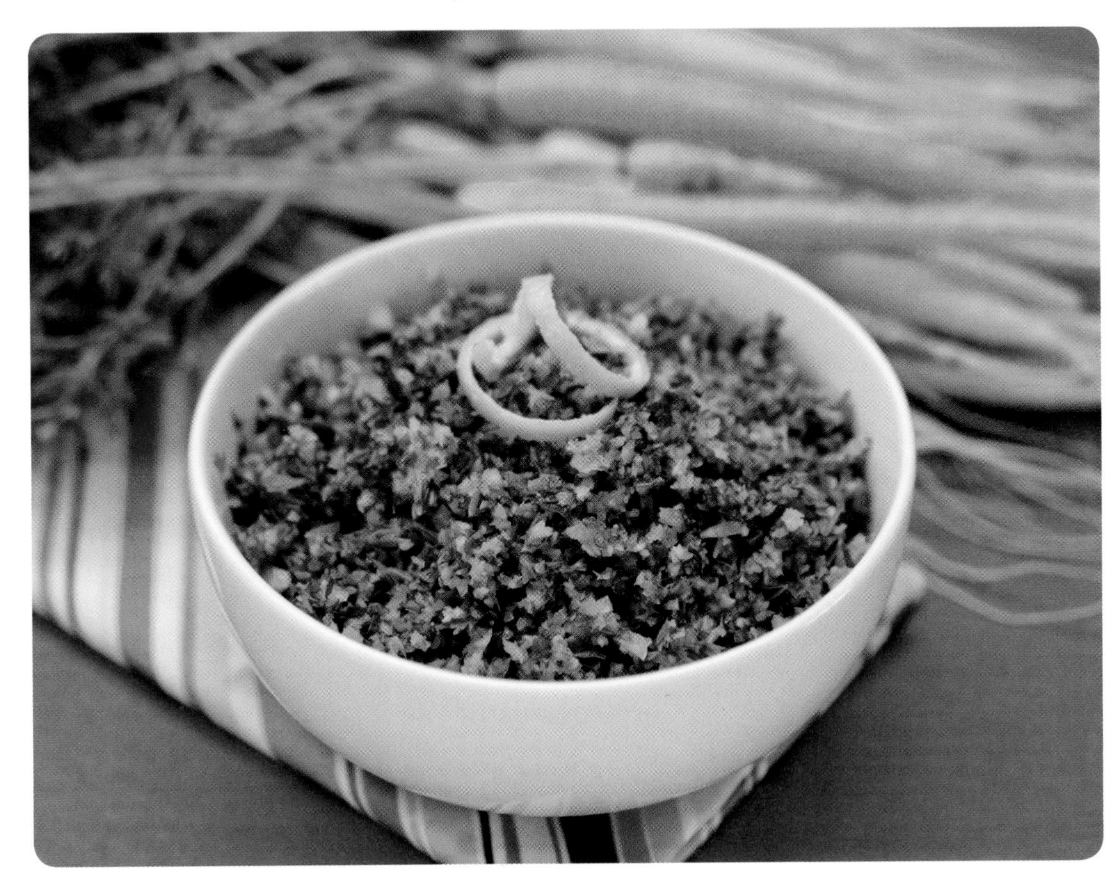

NUTRITION FACTS	
Serving Size	98 g
Recipe Yields	294 g
Calories	**130**
Fats	**9.22 g**
MUFA	6.58 g
Omega-3	0.07 g
Omega-6	0.96 g
Saturated Fat	1.28 g
Carbohydrates	**12.5 g**
Fiber	2.33 g
Starch	1.61 g
Fructose	2.3 g
Glucose	2.2 g
Sucrose	2.65 g
Protein	**0.91 g**
Alanine	0.09 g
Arginine	0.09 g
Aspartic acid	0.14 g
Cystine	0.06 g
Glutamic acid	0.27 g
Glycine	0.04 g
Histidine	0.03 g
Isoleucine	0.06 g
Leucine	0.08 g
Lysine	0.08 g
Methionine	0.02 g
Phenylalanine	0.05 g
Proline	0.05 g
Serine	0.04 g
Threonine	0.14 g
Tryptophan	0.01 g
Tyrosine	0.03 g
Valine	0.06 g
Vitamins	
Vitamin B1	0.06 mg
Vitamin B12	0 mcg
Vitamin B2	0.05 mg
Vitamin B3	0.77 mg
Vitamin B5	0.22 mg
Vitamin B6	0.12 mg
Choline	7.58 mg
Folate	16.4 mcg
Vitamin A	601 mcg
Vitamin C	8.83 mg
Vitamin D	0 IU
Vitamin E	1.79 mg
Vitamin K	15.1 mcg
Minerals	
Calcium	29.1 mg
Copper	0.05 mg
Iron	0.65 mg
Magnesium	11.4 mg
Manganese	0.13 mg
Phosphorus	32.3 mg
Potassium	290 mg
Selenium	0.12 mcg
Sodium	93.5 mg
Zinc	0.19 mg

nutrition content estimated using the USDA database.

Vegetable Terrine

A terrine is a great way to reinvent leftover vegetables and makes for a very pretty summer side dish, perfect for a barbecue or potluck.

PREP TIME: 1 hour
COOK TIME: 30 minutes
SERVINGS: 6 to 10

INGREDIENTS:

- 1 pound carrots, sliced into ¼-inch-thick rounds
- 3 to 6 tablespoons avocado oil
- 2 to 3 medium golden beets, sliced into ¼-inch-thick rounds
- 1 medium zucchini, sliced into ¼-inch-thick rounds
- 1 batch Easy Broiled Asparagus (page 306)
- 2 tablespoons gelatin
- 1 cup white wine
- 1 cup Bone Broth (chicken or pork, page 110)
- 2 sprigs fresh thyme
- Finely grated zest of 1 lemon
- Salt, to taste
- Coconut oil, for greasing the pan

1. Preheat the oven to 400°F. Prepare 3 rimmed baking sheets by lining them with parchment paper, aluminum foil, or silicone liners.
2. In a bowl, toss the sliced carrots with 1 to 2 tablespoons of the avocado oil to coat and place in a single layer on a baking sheet. Toss the sliced beets with 1 to 2 tablespoons of the avocado oil to coat and place in a single layer on the second baking sheet. Toss the sliced zucchini with 1 to 2 tablespoons of the avocado oil to coat and place in a single layer on the third baking sheet.
3. Roast the vegetables for 15 minutes, until soft and slightly browned on the bottom. Let cool completely.
4. In a small saucepan, sprinkle the gelatin over the cold broth and wine to bloom. Once the gelatin has absorbed the liquid and turned translucent, heat the gelatin mixture over medium-high heat, then reduce the heat to maintain a simmer. Simmer for 20 to 30 minutes to evaporate the alcohol.
5. Remove the saucepan from the heat and add the thyme and lemon zest. Taste and add salt if desired. Let cool for 10 to 15 minutes.
6. Grease a 9-by-5-inch loaf pan with coconut oil, line with wax paper, and grease the wax paper (or use a silicone pan or mold). Arrange the vegetables in the pan in layers, alternating colors. Pour the gelatin mixture over the top. Place in the refrigerator until fully set, 4 to 6 hours.
7. Invert onto a serving plate, slice, and enjoy!

VARIATIONS:

Don't be afraid to get creative with the vegetables. Grilled, broiled, or roasted vegetables give this dish the most flavor.

If you don't want to use wine, you can use kombucha, apple cider, or additional broth with a little fresh lemon juice instead.

NUTRITION FACTS	
Serving Size	186 g
Recipe Yields	1859 g
Calories	**104**
Fats	**4.76 g**
MUFA	3.01 g
Omega-3	0.11 g
Omega-6	0.68 g
Saturated Fat	0.6 g
Carbohydrates	**8.58 g**
Fiber	2.75 g
Starch	0.85 g
Fructose	0.57 g
Glucose	0.53 g
Sucrose	1.66 g
Protein	**4 g**
Alanine	0.25 g
Arginine	0.21 g
Aspartic acid	0.36 g
Cystine	0.06 g
Glutamic acid	0.6 g
Glycine	0.35 g
Histidine	0.06 g
Isoleucine	0.12 g
Leucine	0.16 g
Lysine	0.18 g
Methionine	0.04 g
Phenylalanine	0.1 g
Proline	0.28 g
Serine	0.13 g
Threonine	0.16 g
Tryptophan	0.02 g
Tyrosine	0.06 g
Valine	0.13 g
Vitamins	
Vitamin B1	0.08 mg
Vitamin B12	0.02 mcg
Vitamin B2	0.11 mg
Vitamin B3	1.43 mg
Vitamin B5	0.28 mg
Vitamin B6	0.13 mg
Choline	20.4 mg
Folate	95.2 mcg
Vitamin A	400 mcg
Vitamin C	21 mg
Vitamin D	0 IU
Vitamin E	0.92 mg
Vitamin K	43.3 mcg
Minerals	
Calcium	41 mg
Copper	0.14 mg
Iron	0.84 mg
Magnesium	20.8 mg
Manganese	0.25 mg
Phosphorus	64.9 mg
Potassium	373 mg
Selenium	2.73 mcg
Sodium	142 mg
Zinc	0.48 mg

nutrition content estimated using the USDA database.

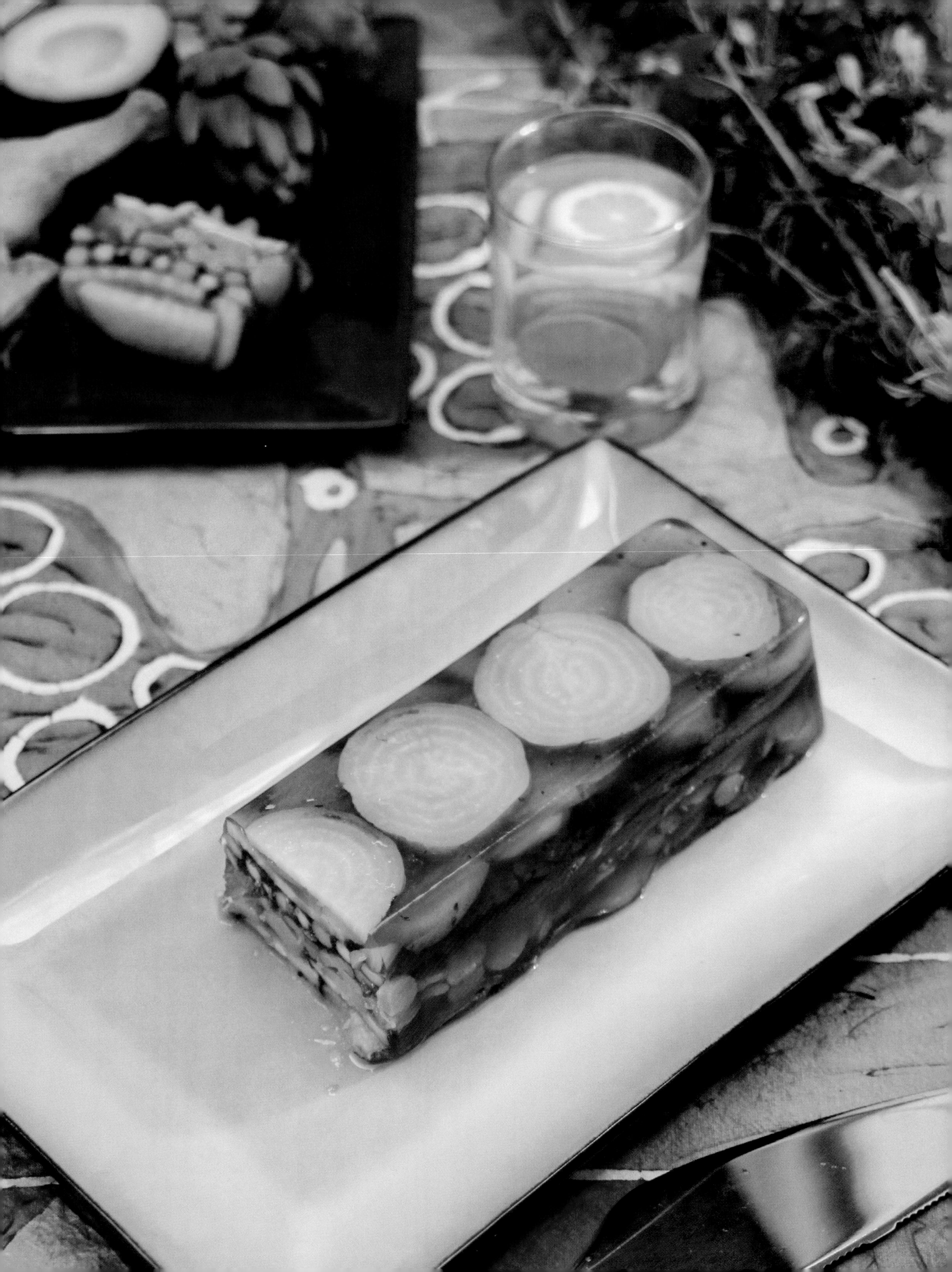

Kufu

Kufu is a tasty, traditional South American dish made with ripe plantains. It's a starchy and slightly sweet side that can be enjoyed with just about anything!

PREP TIME: 10 minutes
COOK TIME: 15 minutes
SERVINGS: 6 to 8

INGREDIENTS:

- 6 ounces bacon, chopped
- 1 medium onion, diced
- 4 cloves garlic, minced
- 3 ripe plantains (they should be mostly black), peeled and cut into 1-inch semicircles
- 2 cups Bone Broth (chicken or pork, page 110)

FODMAP ALERT
This recipe cannot be made low-FODMAP.

1. Add the bacon to a cold skillet, then turn on the heat to medium-high. Cook the bacon for 5 minutes, then add the onion and garlic, stirring occasionally. Continue cooking until the bacon is crisp and the onion is soft and caramelized, 8 to 10 minutes.
2. Meanwhile, place the plantains and broth in a saucepot and bring to a boil over high heat. Reduce the heat to maintain a simmer and cook until the plantains are tender when pierced with a knife, about 10 minutes.
3. Drain the plantains (reserving the cooking liquid) and mash with a fork or potato masher. Add the bacon mixture and all the grease from the pan and stir to incorporate. If you like a thinner mash, you can add some of the reserved cooking liquid.

VARIATIONS:

Mofongo. *When this dish is made with green plantains, it is called mofongo. Green plantains absorb a little more liquid, so increase the broth to 3 to 4 cups and cook for 20 minutes instead of 10.*

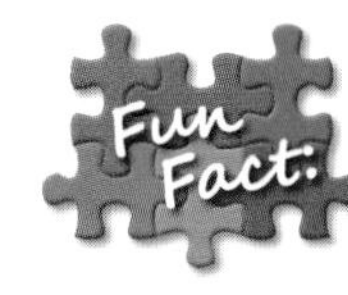

After chopping, mincing, crushing, or slicing garlic, let it rest for 10 minutes before cooking it. Doing so not only preserves but also heightens its nutrient availability.

NUTRITION FACTS	
Serving Size	110 g
Recipe Yields	877 g
Calories	**206**
Fats	**9.22 g**
MUFA	3.99 g
Omega-3	0.06 g
Omega-6	0.93 g
Saturated Fat	3.05 g
Carbohydrates	**23.6 g**
Fiber	1.82 g
Starch	10.8 g
Fructose	0.18 g
Glucose	0.27 g
Sucrose	0.44 g
Protein	**9.14 g**
Alanine	0.56 g
Arginine	0.63 g
Aspartic acid	0.86 g
Cystine	0.11 g
Glutamic acid	1.33 g
Glycine	0.61 g
Histidine	0.35 g
Isoleucine	0.41 g
Leucine	0.68 g
Lysine	0.73 g
Methionine	0.19 g
Phenylalanine	0.36 g
Proline	0.49 g
Serine	0.34 g
Threonine	0.35 g
Tryptophan	0.08 g
Tyrosine	0.28 g
Valine	0.47 g
Vitamins	
Vitamin B1	0.13 mg
Vitamin B12	0.27 mcg
Vitamin B2	0.1 mg
Vitamin B3	2.94 mg
Vitamin B5	0.45 mg
Vitamin B6	0.31 mg
Choline	36.8 mg
Folate	17.9 mcg
Vitamin A	40.1 mcg
Vitamin C	13.9 mg
Vitamin D	8.96 IU
Vitamin E	0.16 mg
Vitamin K	0.57 mcg
Minerals	
Calcium	10.5 mg
Copper	0.1 mg
Iron	0.78 mg
Magnesium	33.8 mg
Manganese	0.05 mg
Phosphorus	145 mg
Potassium	488 mg
Selenium	14.5 mcg
Sodium	498 mg
Zinc	0.89 mg

nutrition content estimated using the USDA database.

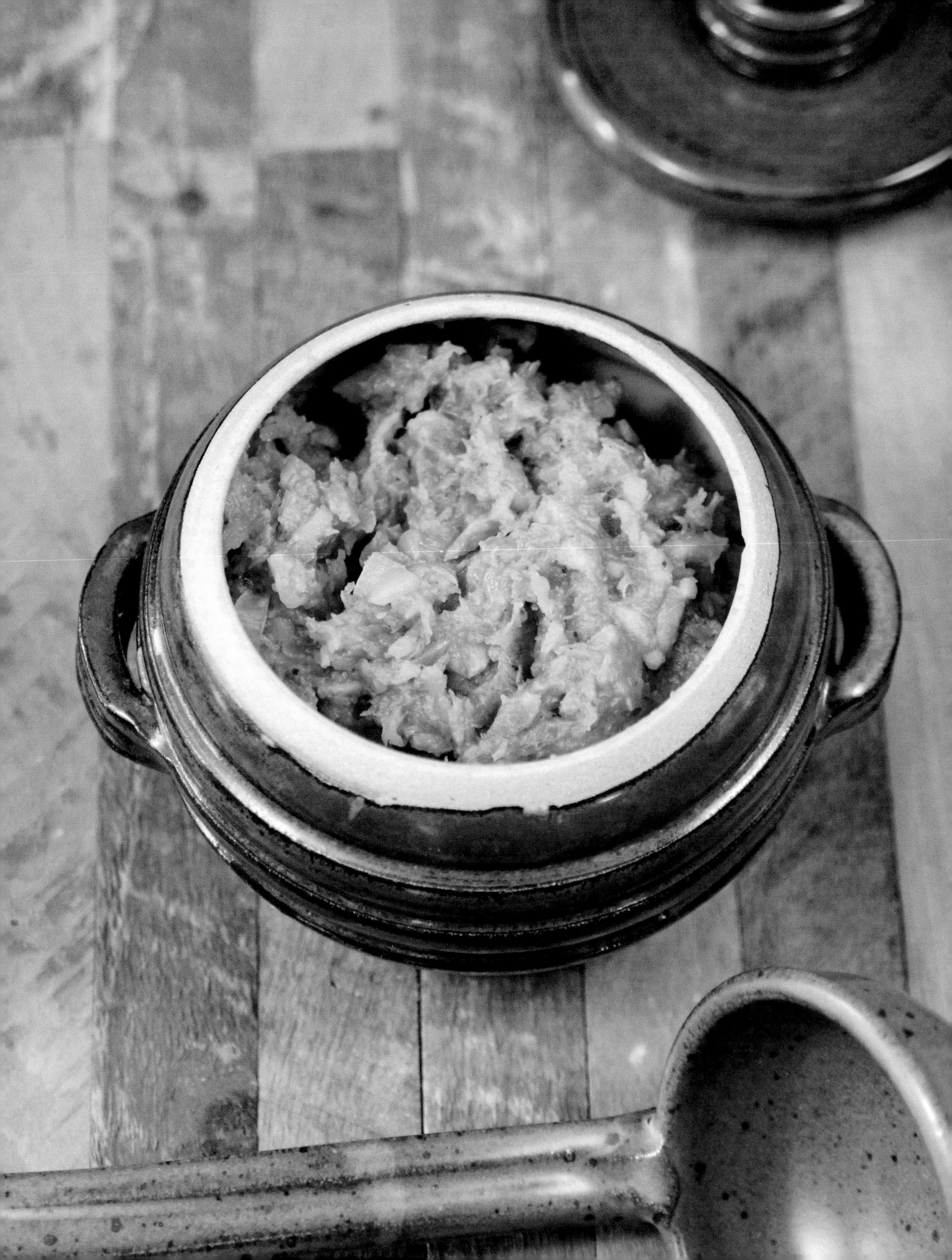

Savory Roasted Taro

Taro is one of the most delicious starchy tubers. This preparation minimizes its natural sliminess and creates an end product very reminiscent of roasted potatoes.

PREP TIME: 15 to 20 minutes
COOK TIME: 25 minutes
SERVINGS: 2 to 4

INGREDIENTS:

- 2 pounds fresh taro (8 to 10 small tubers)
- 3 tablespoons tallow, lard, or duck fat, melted
- 2 teaspoons dried savory
- 2 cloves garlic, crushed
- ½ teaspoon salt

FODMAP ALERT *Replace the garlic with green garlic or garlic scapes (green part only) or omit.*

SPECIAL EQUIPMENT

- Steamer basket or steamer insert

1. Place the whole unpeeled taro tubers in a steamer basket or steamer insert. Bring the water to a boil and steam for 10 to 15 minutes (depending on the size of the tubers) until you can pierce them easily with a knife but before they get too soft (think of the firmness of not-quite-cooked potatoes). Remove from the heat and let cool enough to handle.
2. Meanwhile, place an oven rack 6 to 8 inches from the broiler element, and preheat the broiler on high for 10 minutes.
3. Peel off the barklike skin of the taro with a paring knife (it should come off fairly easily). Cut the peeled taro into quarters or ½-inch-thick rounds and place in a large bowl. Pour the tallow, savory, garlic, and salt over the taro and toss to coat. Spread the taro on a rimmed baking sheet.
4. Broil for 10 minutes, flipping or stirring every 3 to 5 minutes, until browned and slightly crisp on the outside.

VARIATIONS:

Instead of savory, try using dried rosemary and thyme leaves.

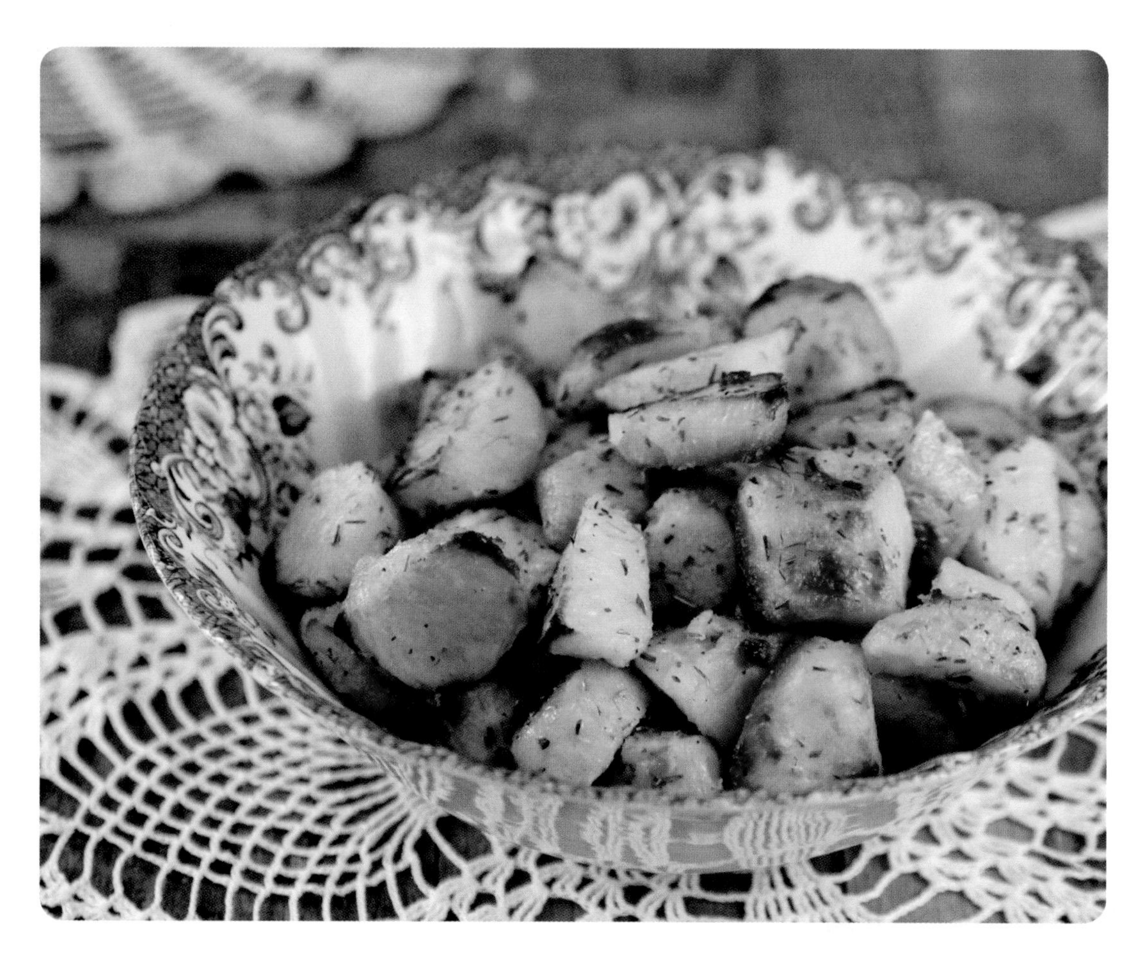

NUTRITION FACTS	
Serving Size	240 g
Recipe Yields	958 g
Calories	**414**
Fats	**9.93 g**
MUFA	4.36 g
Omega-3	0.13 g
Omega-6	1.06 g
Saturated Fat	3.85 g
Carbohydrates	**79.7 g**
Fiber	12 g
Starch	66.4 g
Fructose	0 g
Glucose	0 g
Sucrose	0 g
Protein	**1.33 g**
Alanine	0.06 g
Arginine	0.09 g
Aspartic acid	0.16 g
Cystine	0.03 g
Glutamic acid	0.15 g
Glycine	0.06 g
Histidine	0.03 g
Isoleucine	0.05 g
Leucine	0.09 g
Lysine	0.06 g
Methionine	0.02 g
Phenylalanine	0.07 g
Proline	0.05 g
Serine	0.08 g
Threonine	0.06 g
Tryptophan	0.02 g
Tyrosine	0.04 g
Valine	0.07 g
Vitamins	
Vitamin B1	0.25 mg
Vitamin B12	0 mcg
Vitamin B2	0.07 mg
Vitamin B3	1.2 mg
Vitamin B5	0.77 mg
Vitamin B6	0.78 mg
Choline	53.8 mg
Folate	45.3 mcg
Vitamin A	11.6 mcg
Vitamin C	12.2 mg
Vitamin D	9.82 IU
Vitamin E	6.73 mg
Vitamin K	2.75 mcg
Minerals	
Calcium	60 mg
Copper	0.47 mg
Iron	1.94 mg
Magnesium	71.4 mg
Manganese	1.09 mg
Phosphorus	176 mg
Potassium	1114 mg
Selenium	2.31 mcg
Sodium	328 mg
Zinc	0.67 mg

nutrition content estimated using the USDA database.

Bacon-Braised Brussels Sprouts

If you think you don't like Brussels sprouts, then this is the recipe to try. Braising reduces the bitterness that Brussels sprouts can achieve when boiled or steamed, and the combination of bacon and sprouts is wonderful!

PREP TIME: 5 to 10 minutes
COOK TIME: 30 to 40 minutes
SERVINGS: 2 to 4

INGREDIENTS:

6 ounces bacon, chopped

1 pound Brussels sprouts, cleaned and trimmed (cut in half if large)

2 tablespoons to 1 cup Bone Broth (chicken, beef, or pork, page 110)

1. Place the bacon in a cold skillet and turn on the heat to medium-high. Cook, stirring relatively frequently, until the bacon is mostly cooked and starting to brown, about 10 minutes.
2. Add the Brussels sprouts to the skillet with 2 tablespoons of the broth. Stir relatively frequently. As soon as the Brussels sprouts start to stick, add an additional 1 to 2 tablespoons of broth to the pan.
3. Keep adding a small amount of broth every time the Brussels sprouts start to stick, stirring relatively frequently.
4. Once the Brussels sprouts are cooked (15 to 25 minutes, depending on the size), stop adding broth. Just when they start to stick again, pour the bacon and sprouts into a serving dish and enjoy!

VARIATIONS:

Add 2 or 3 crushed garlic cloves and 2 tablespoons lemon juice 2 to 3 minutes before the sprouts are done.

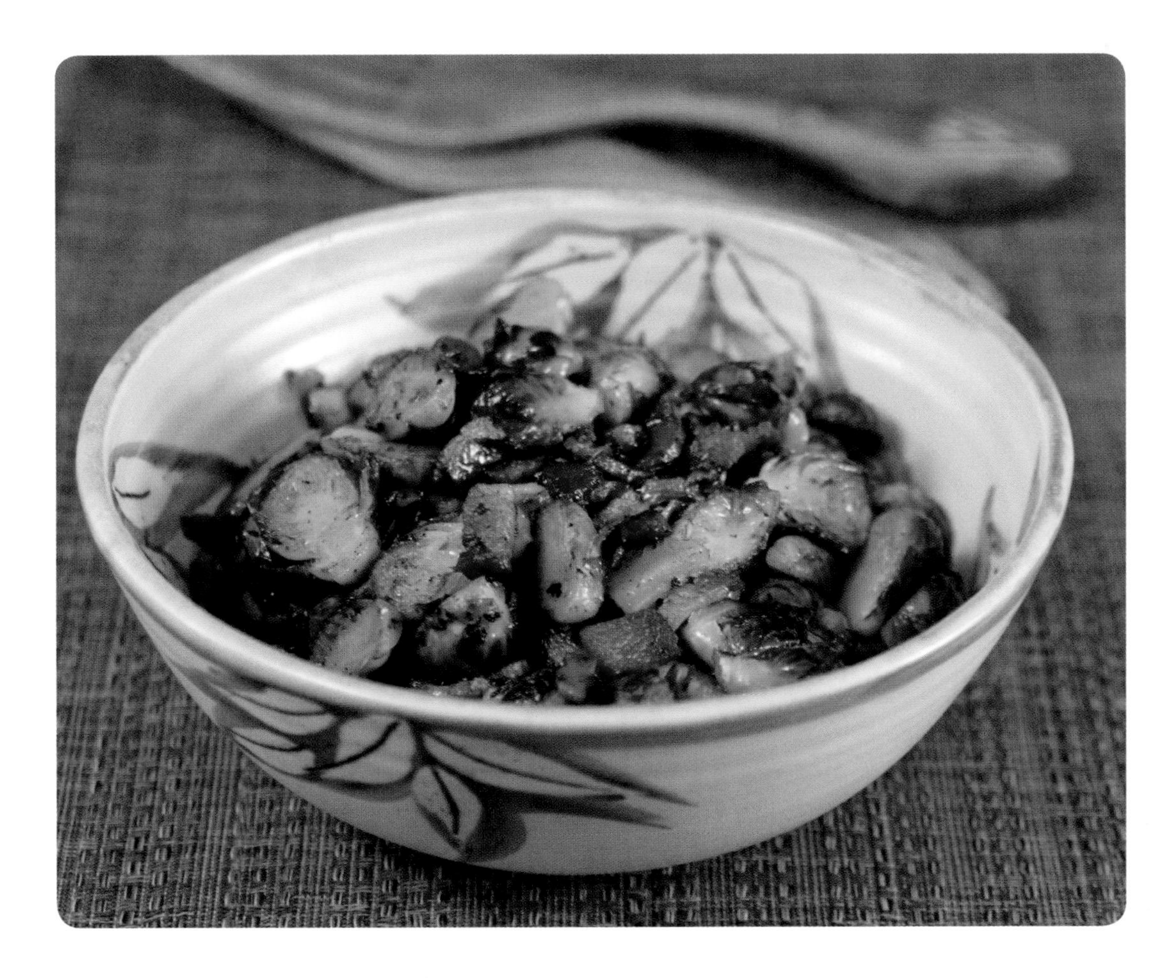

NUTRITION FACTS	
Serving Size	164 g
Recipe Yields	655 g
Calories	**275**
Fats	**19 g**
MUFA	8.17 g
Omega-3	0.29 g
Omega-6	1.92 g
Saturated Fat	6.16 g
Carbohydrates	**8.68 g**
Fiber	2.95 g
Starch	3.14 g
Fructose	0 g
Glucose	0 g
Sucrose	0 g
Protein	**18.2 g**
Alanine	0.97 g
Arginine	1.16 g
Aspartic acid	1.43 g
Cystine	0.19 g
Glutamic acid	2.24 g
Glycine	1.07 g
Histidine	0.64 g
Isoleucine	0.83 g
Leucine	1.31 g
Lysine	1.39 g
Methionine	0.37 g
Phenylalanine	0.69 g
Proline	0.83 g
Serine	0.58 g
Threonine	0.7 g
Tryptophan	0.16 g
Tyrosine	0.48 g
Valine	0.94 g
Vitamins	
Vitamin B1	0.27 mg
Vitamin B12	0.5 mcg
Vitamin B2	0.2 mg
Vitamin B3	5.23 mg
Vitamin B5	0.73 mg
Vitamin B6	0.33 mg
Choline	97 mg
Folate	69 mcg
Vitamin A	49 mcg
Vitamin C	70.4 mg
Vitamin D	0 IU
Vitamin E	0.63 mg
Vitamin K	159 mcg
Minerals	
Calcium	45.5 mg
Copper	0.17 mg
Iron	2 mg
Magnesium	35.6 mg
Manganese	0.27 mg
Phosphorus	279 mg
Potassium	591 mg
Selenium	26.9 mcg
Sodium	987 mg
Zinc	1.81 mg

nutrition content estimated using the USDA database.

Roasted Radishes

If you don't enjoy the peppery zing of raw radishes, then try them roasted! They lose that peppery flavor and instead have a delightful, almost potatolike taste.

PREP TIME: 5 to 10 minutes
COOK TIME: 20 to 25 minutes
SERVINGS: 3 to 4

INGREDIENTS:

1 pound radishes (about 3 bunches), trimmed and quartered

3 tablespoons lard, tallow, or duck fat, melted

¾ teaspoon salt

1. Preheat the oven to 375°F. Line a rimmed baking sheet with aluminum foil or a silicone liner for easier cleanup.
2. In a small bowl, toss the radishes with the melted fat.
3. Spread on the prepared baking sheet and sprinkle with the salt.
4. Roast for 20 to 25 minutes, until the radishes start to turn golden brown.

VARIATIONS:

Roasted Turnips. *Replace the radishes with turnips, peeled if waxed and cut into 1-inch chunks.*

Roasted Rutabaga. *Replace the radishes with rutabaga, peeled and cut into 1-inch chunks.*

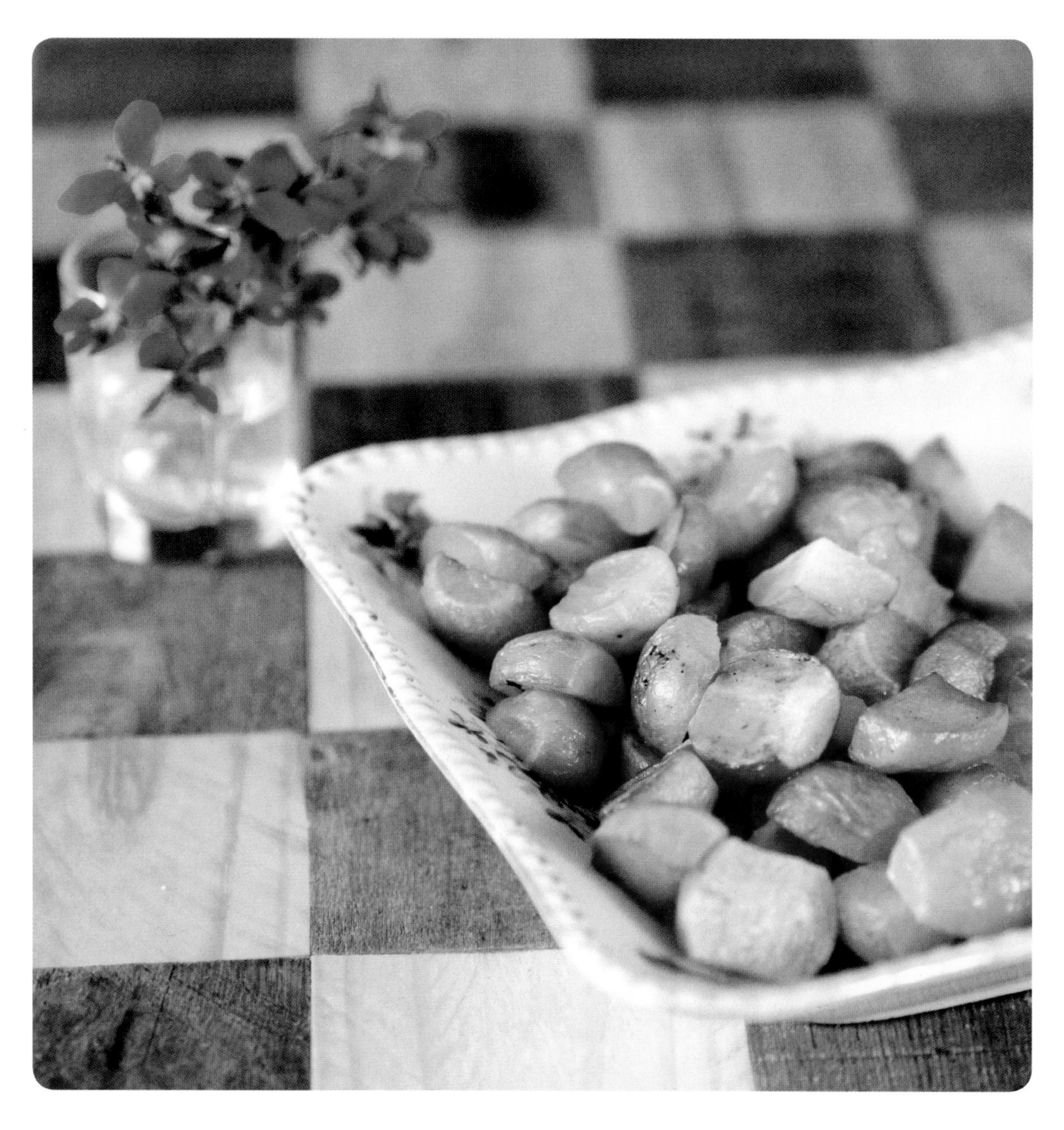

NUTRITION FACTS	
Serving Size	124 g
Recipe Yields	496 g
Calories	**105**
Fats	**9.7 g**
MUFA	4.34 g
Omega-3	0.13 g
Omega-6	1 g
Saturated Fat	3.8 g
Carbohydrates	**3.85 g**
Fiber	1.81 g
Starch	0 g
Fructose	0.8 g
Glucose	1.19 g
Sucrose	0.11 g
Protein	**0.77 g**
Alanine	0.03 g
Arginine	0.04 g
Aspartic acid	0.07 g
Cystine	0.01 g
Glutamic acid	0.18 g
Glycine	0.03 g
Histidine	0.01 g
Isoleucine	0.02 g
Leucine	0.04 g
Lysine	0.04 g
Methionine	0.01 g
Phenylalanine	0.04 g
Proline	0.02 g
Serine	0.03 g
Threonine	0.03 g
Tryptophan	0.01 g
Tyrosine	0.01 g
Valine	0.04 g
Vitamins	
Vitamin B1	0.01 mg
Vitamin B12	0 mcg
Vitamin B2	0.04 mg
Vitamin B3	0.29 mg
Vitamin B5	0.19 mg
Vitamin B6	0.08 mg
Choline	12.1 mg
Folate	28.3 mcg
Vitamin A	0 mcg
Vitamin C	16.8 mg
Vitamin D	9.78 IU
Vitamin E	0.06 mg
Vitamin K	1.47 mcg
Minerals	
Calcium	29.3 mg
Copper	0.06 mg
Iron	0.39 mg
Magnesium	11.4 mg
Manganese	0.08 mg
Phosphorus	22.7 mg
Potassium	264 mg
Selenium	0.7 mcg
Sodium	482 mg
Zinc	0.33 mg

nutrition content estimated using the USDA database.

French Fries

French fries get a bad rap for being unhealthy, but if you use nutrient-dense root vegetables or green plantains and a high-quality cooking fat that is kept below its smoke point and season with a mineral-rich unrefined salt, there's no reason why these fries can't be a staple in your home!

PREP TIME: 10 to 15 minutes
COOK TIME: 20 minutes
SERVINGS: 2 to 4

INGREDIENTS:

1 pound green plantains or starchy root vegetable (sweet potatoes, yam, lotus root, taro root, celery root, or parsnip; for yuca, see Tips)

Lard or other fat, for deep-frying

1 teaspoon pink or gray salt

1. Peel your root vegetables if they have a tough skin; otherwise, simply clean them. Cut the root vegetables into French fry–like strips (2 to 4 inches long and ½ inch thick), ½-inch-thick wedges, or ½-inch-thick rounds. Rinse and drain on paper towels.
2. Heat the lard to 360°F in a countertop deep-fryer or heavy-bottomed pot over medium heat with a deep-fry thermometer attached to the side. Use enough fat to fill your deep-fryer to the fill line or to have 2 inches of fat in the bottom of your pot.
3. Cook the vegetables in small batches so as to not overcrowd, for 3 to 7 minutes, until browned and crisp on the outside.
4. Allow to dry on a paper towel, tea towel, or newsprint-lined plate or rimmed baking sheet. Sprinkle with the salt while still warm.

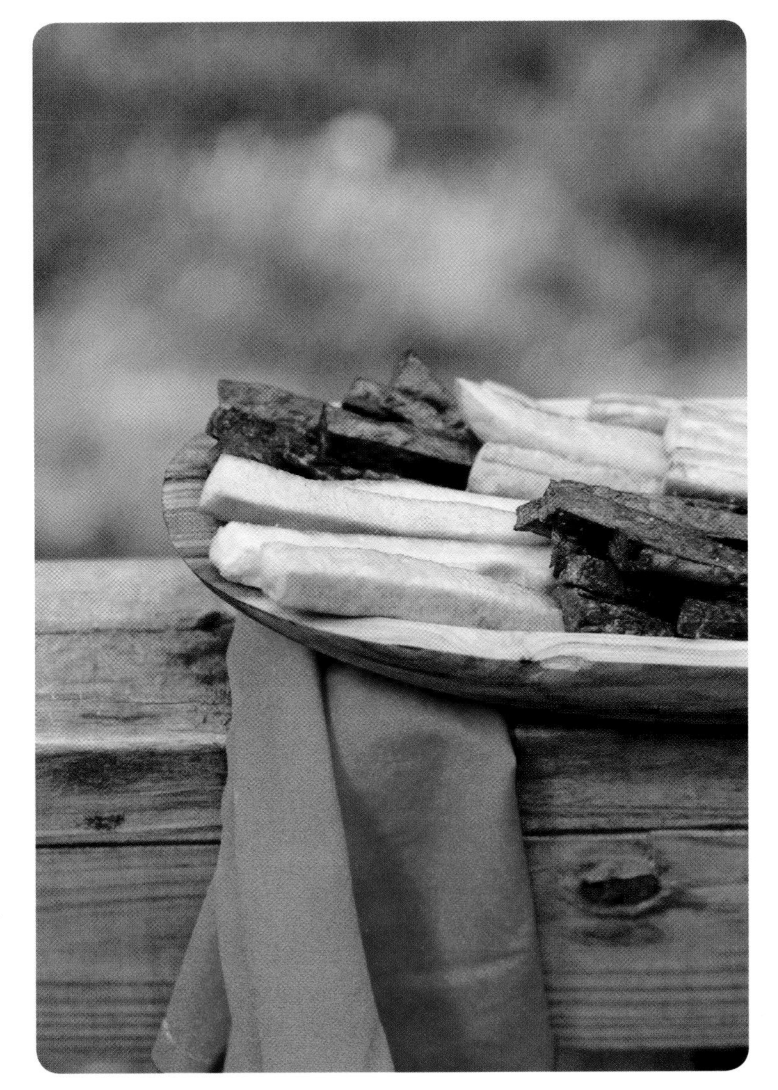

SPECIAL EQUIPMENT

- Countertop deep-fryer or heavy-bottomed pot with an oil thermometer

TIPS:

The best root vegetables for making French fries are those with a naturally low water content. Less starchy vegetables like rutabaga, turnips, carrots, and beets tend not to crisp up on the outside and are better left to other cooking methods. Even some varieties of sweet potato work better than others due to the water content.

If using yuca, a little extra prep work is required. Peel and cut into rectangular "fries," wedges, or rounds, then soak in water in the fridge for 24 hours; this reduces the cyanogenic glycoside content. Drain and rinse. Then boil in water for 10 minutes. Drain well and pat dry with paper towels before deep-frying.

If using more than one kind of root vegetable, cook the vegetables in separate batches, since different root vegetables require slightly different cooking times.

NUTRITION FACTS	
Serving Size	121 g
Recipe Yields	485 g
Calories	**196**
Fats	**6.8 g**
MUFA	2.92 g
Omega-3	0.09 g
Omega-6	0.7 g
Saturated Fat	2.66 g
Carbohydrates	**36.1 g**
Fiber	2.6 g
Starch	16.5 g
Fructose	0 g
Glucose	0 g
Sucrose	0 g
Protein	**1.47 g**
Alanine	0.06 g
Arginine	0.12 g
Aspartic acid	0.12 g
Cystine	0.02 g
Glutamic acid	0.13 g
Glycine	0.05 g
Histidine	0.07 g
Isoleucine	0.04 g
Leucine	0.07 g
Lysine	0.07 g
Methionine	0.02 g
Phenylalanine	0.05 g
Proline	0.06 g
Serine	0.05 g
Threonine	0.04 g
Tryptophan	0.02 g
Tyrosine	0.04 g
Valine	0.05 g
Vitamins	
Vitamin B1	0.06 mg
Vitamin B12	0 mcg
Vitamin B2	0.06 mg
Vitamin B3	0.78 mg
Vitamin B5	0.29 mg
Vitamin B6	0.34 mg
Choline	18.4 mg
Folate	24.9 mcg
Vitamin A	63.4 mcg
Vitamin C	20.8 mg
Vitamin D	6.51 IU
Vitamin E	0.2 mg
Vitamin K	0.79 mcg
Minerals	
Calcium	4.73 mg
Copper	0.09 mg
Iron	0.68 mg
Magnesium	42 mg
Manganese	0 mg
Phosphorus	38.5 mg
Potassium	564 mg
Selenium	1.71 mcg
Sodium	588 mg
Zinc	0.17 mg

nutrition content estimated using the USDA database. values vary based on ingredient selection.

Spiced Kabocha Squash

Kabocha squash is an Asian variety of winter squash that has become quite popular in American farmer's markets and natural food stores due to its thin skin, which makes it easier to prepare, and its delightful flavor. Kabocha can be green or orange (or green with orange patches). The orange squash is the fully ripe version, which tends to be a little sweeter and firmer and has a more distinct flavor. While I prefer orange kabocha squash for this recipe, it works equally well with green.

PREP TIME: 20 to 25 minutes
COOK TIME: 35 minutes
SERVINGS: 6 to 10

INGREDIENTS:

- 1 large orange or green kabocha squash (about 4 pounds)
- ¼ cup red palm oil, melted
- 1 tablespoon ground cinnamon
- 2 teaspoons ground ginger
- 2 teaspoons ground turmeric
- 1 teaspoon salt

1. Preheat the oven to 400°F. Line a rimmed baking sheet with aluminum foil or a silicone liner.
2. Cut the kabocha squash in half (this is a little easier if you slice off the stem first so that you have a spot to get your knife in). Scoop out the seeds. Cut the squash into wedges about 1 inch thick at the thickest part. You can either leave the peel on or peel it off with a paring knife—it's up to you.
3. Toss the squash wedges with the palm oil, spices, and salt and spread out onto the prepared baking sheet.
4. Roast for 30 to 35 minutes, flipping once at the 20-minute mark, until the squash is starting to turn golden brown and is cooked but still firm.

TIPS:

If you can't find red palm oil, you can easily substitute coconut oil or lard.

VARIATIONS:

You can use any winter squash in this recipe. Acorn and delicata are particularly good.

Roasted Winter Squash. *Want to keep it super simple? Try using coconut oil instead of palm oil and omit all the spices.*

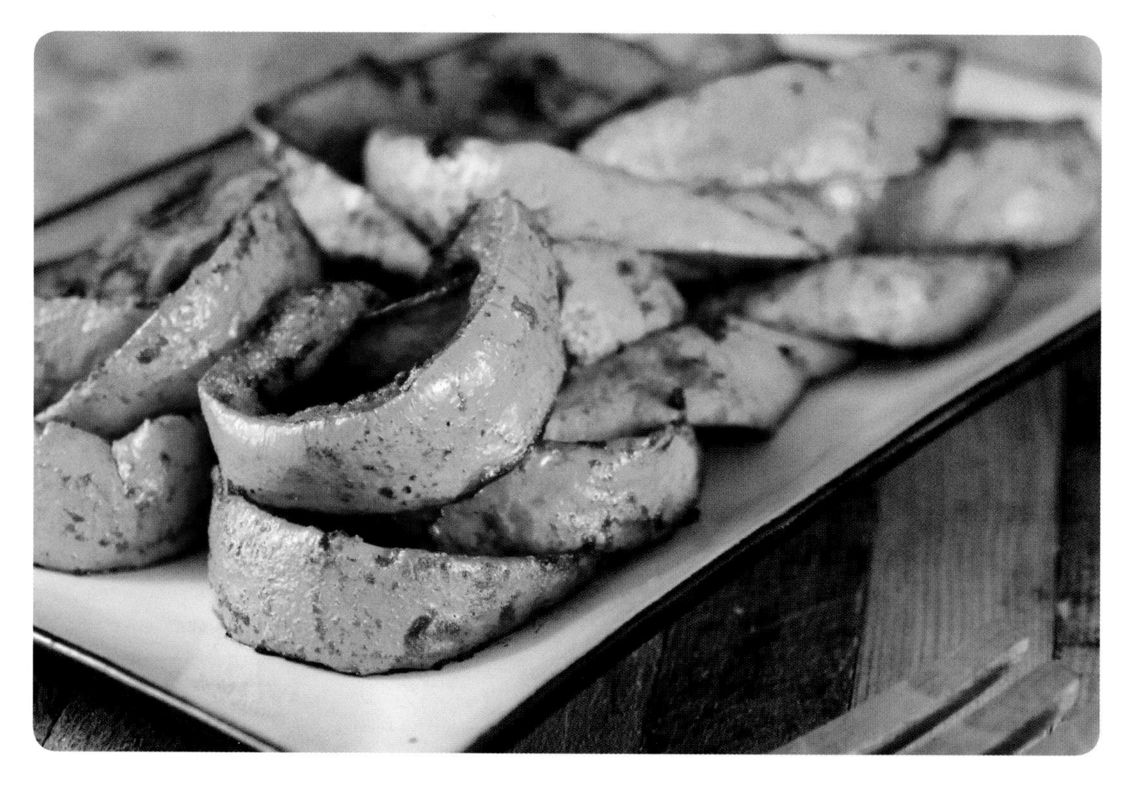

NUTRITION FACTS

Serving Size	189 g
Recipe Yields	485 g
Calories	**134**
Fats	**5.69 g**
MUFA	2.04 g
Omega-3	0.06 g
Omega-6	0.53 g
Saturated Fat	2.75 g
Carbohydrates	**22.4 g**
Fiber	4.19 g
Starch	14.2 g
Fructose	1.81 g
Glucose	1.81 g
Sucrose	0.41 g
Protein	**1.91 g**
Alanine	0.08 g
Arginine	0.11 g
Aspartic acid	0.2 g
Cystine	0.02 g
Glutamic acid	0.32 g
Glycine	0.07 g
Histidine	0.04 g
Isoleucine	0.07 g
Leucine	0.11 g
Lysine	0.07 g
Methionine	0.02 g
Phenylalanine	0.07 g
Proline	0.07 g
Serine	0.07 g
Threonine	0.06 g
Tryptophan	0.03 g
Tyrosine	0.06 g
Valine	0.08 g
Vitamins	
Vitamin B1	0.18 mg
Vitamin B12	0 mcg
Vitamin B2	0.04 mg
Vitamin B3	2.24 mg
Vitamin B5	0.73 mg
Vitamin B6	0.28 mg
Choline	0.47 mg
Folate	49.2 mcg
Vitamin A	965 mcg
Vitamin C	38.2 mg
Vitamin D	0 IU
Vitamin E	3.51 mg
Vitamin K	2.74 mcg
Minerals	
Calcium	96.6 mg
Copper	0.14 mg
Iron	1.59 mg
Magnesium	63.8 mg
Manganese	0.65 mg
Phosphorus	62.2 mg
Potassium	658 mg
Selenium	1.14 mcg
Sodium	241 mg
Zinc	0.32 mg

nutrition content estimated using the USDA database.

Roasted Parsnips

These parsnips are simple to prepare and taste amazing!

PREP TIME: 10 minutes
COOK TIME: 40 minutes
SERVINGS: 3 to 6

INGREDIENTS:

- 2 pounds parsnips, cut into ½-inch-wide rounds or ½-inch-thick wedges
- 3 tablespoons lard or duck fat, melted
- 1 tablespoon chopped fresh rosemary
- 1 tablespoon chopped fresh sage
- ¼ teaspoon salt or truffle salt

1. Preheat the oven to 350°F.
2. In a large bowl, toss the parsnips with the melted lard, herbs, and salt. Place in a single layer on a rimmed baking sheet.
3. Roast for 40 minutes, until golden brown, stirring at the 20-minute and 30-minute marks.

VARIATIONS:

You can also sauté the parsnips in a large skillet, although you may need a little extra lard.

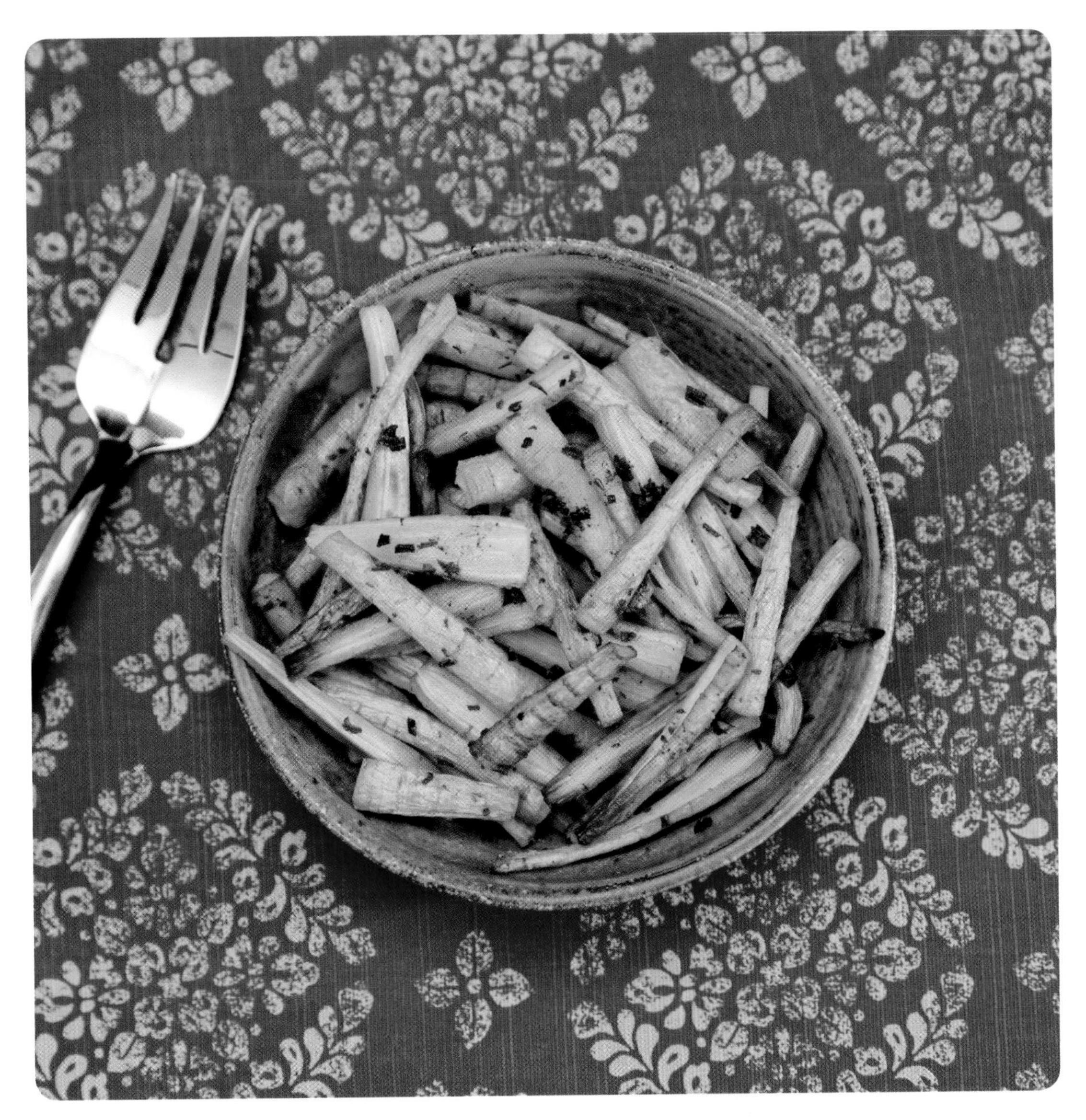

NUTRITION FACTS

Serving Size	158 g
Recipe Yields	949 g
Calories	**166**
Fats	**6.87 g**
MUFA	3.06 g
Omega-3	0.07 g
Omega-6	0.72 g
Saturated Fat	2.6 g
Carbohydrates	**25.8 g**
Fiber	5.52 g
Starch	13 g
Fructose	0 g
Glucose	0 g
Sucrose	0 g
Protein	**2.01 g**
Alanine	<0.01 g
Arginine	<0.01 g
Aspartic acid	<0.01 g
Cystine	<0.01 g
Glutamic acid	<0.01 g
Glycine	<0.01 g
Histidine	<0.01 g
Isoleucine	<0.01 g
Leucine	<0.01 g
Lysine	<0.01 g
Methionine	<0.01 g
Phenylalanine	<0.01 g
Proline	<0.01 g
Serine	<0.01 g
Threonine	<0.01 g
Tryptophan	<0.01 g
Tyrosine	<0.01 g
Valine	<0.01 g
Vitamins	
Vitamin B1	0.13 mg
Vitamin B12	0 mcg
Vitamin B2	0.08 mg
Vitamin B3	1.1 mg
Vitamin B5	0.89 mg
Vitamin B6	0.14 mg
Choline	44 mg
Folate	88.2 mcg
Vitamin A	0.76 mcg
Vitamin C	19.7 mg
Vitamin D	6.52 IU
Vitamin E	1.56 mg
Vitamin K	3.51 mcg
Minerals	
Calcium	59.2 mg
Copper	0.21 mg
Iron	1.18 mg
Magnesium	44.5 mg
Manganese	0.45 mg
Phosphorus	104 mg
Potassium	559 mg
Selenium	2.58 mcg
Sodium	57.9 mg
Zinc	0.41 mg

nutrition content estimated using the USDA database.

Russ' Flatbread

Sometimes there's a perfect recipe out there and it just can't be improved upon. This is one of those recipes. Russ Crandall of www.thedomesticman.com, the author of The Ancestral Table, *made a Paleo Approach–friendly version of his pizza crust for Stacy Toth and me when we were visiting. The result was such a delicious flatbread that I felt it absolutely must be included in this cookbook. It is reprinted here with Russ' permission.*

PREP TIME: 15 to 20 minutes
COOK TIME: 10 minutes
SERVINGS: 4 to 6

INGREDIENTS:

- 1½ cups tapioca starch
- ½ cup homemade Coconut Milk (page 116) or canned full-fat coconut milk
- 2 tablespoons coconut oil, avocado oil, or lard
- ½ teaspoon salt
- 3 tablespoons nutritional yeast
- 1 teaspoon dried rosemary, divided
- ½ teaspoon dried oregano leaves
- Olive oil, for drizzling
- Sea salt flakes or kosher salt for sprinkling

1. Place a pizza stone, cast-iron skillet, or heavy-duty baking sheet in the oven. Preheat the oven to 500°F.
2. Place the tapioca starch in a mixing bowl and set aside.
3. Place the coconut milk, oil, and salt in a small saucepan and set over medium heat. When the mixture is just about to come to a boil, pour it into the mixing bowl with the starch. Mix with a spoon until incorporated into the starch, then set aside for 5 minutes to cool.
4. Add the nutritional yeast, half of the rosemary, and the oregano to the dough, then knead together to incorporate everything. Carefully remove the hot pizza stone from the oven, then (again, carefully!) spread the dough over the stone, to about a ¼-inch thickness. Drizzle a little olive oil over the dough and sprinkle on the remaining rosemary.
5. Place in the oven and bake until crispy and firm to the touch, 8 to 10 minutes.
6. Drizzle with more olive oil and sprinkle with the sea salt flakes; slice and serve.

TIPS:

Serve beside your favorite saucy dish or enjoy plain with extra-virgin olive oil and balsamic vinegar!

FODMAP ALERT

If you do not tolerate coconut milk, skip this recipe.

SPECIAL EQUIPMENT

- Pizza stone, cast-iron skillet, or heavy-duty baking sheet

NUTRITION FACTS	
Serving Size	71 g
Recipe Yields	427 g
Calories	**229**
Fats	**8.66 g**
MUFA	0.44 g
Omega-3	<0.01 g
Omega-6	0.13 g
Saturated Fat	7.49 g
Carbohydrates	**36.2 g**
Fiber	1.04 g
Starch	34.6 g
Fructose	0.1 g
Glucose	0.19 g
Sucrose	0.89 g
Protein	**2.61 g**
Alanine	0.02 g
Arginine	0.07 g
Aspartic acid	0.04 g
Cystine	<0.01 g
Glutamic acid	0.1 g
Glycine	0.02 g
Histidine	0.01 g
Isoleucine	0.02 g
Leucine	0.03 g
Lysine	0.02 g
Methionine	<0.01 g
Phenylalanine	0.02 g
Proline	0.02 g
Serine	0.02 g
Threonine	0.02 g
Tryptophan	<0.01 g
Tyrosine	0.01 g
Valine	0.03 g
Vitamins	
Vitamin B1	2.11 mg
Vitamin B12	0.04 mcg
Vitamin B2	1.57 mg
Vitamin B3	11.6 mg
Vitamin B5	0.5 mg
Vitamin B6	0.01 mg
Choline	8.05 mg
Folate	345 mcg
Vitamin A	0.36 mcg
Vitamin C	0.3 mg
Vitamin D	0 IU
Vitamin E	0.05 mg
Vitamin K	0.54 mcg
Minerals	
Calcium	21.1 mg
Copper	0.07 mg
Iron	1.67 mg
Magnesium	25.9 mg
Manganese	0.22 mg
Phosphorus	30.3 mg
Potassium	237 mg
Selenium	2.79 mcg
Sodium	463 mg
Zinc	0.54 mg

nutrition content estimated using the USDA database.

Photo credit: Russ Crandall of www.thedomesticman.com

Root Vegetable Biscuits

These biscuits are inspired by Irish fadge, a traditional biscuit made with leftover potatoes, and are a handy way to use up leftover root vegetables. They are a wonderful special treat to enjoy beside soups and stews and are great for sopping up gravy! While these biscuits taste good right out of the oven, their texture is much better once they have cooled completely.

PREP TIME: 20 to 30 minutes, plus time to prepare the root vegetable mash
COOK TIME: 25 to 28 minutes
YIELD: 8 biscuits

INGREDIENTS:

- 1¼ cups mashed starchy root vegetable, such as Sweet Potato Mash (page 121) or mashed taro or yuca (about 1 pound, see Tips)
- 3 tablespoons lard or tallow, plus extra for brushing, melted
- ⅓ cup sifted coconut flour
- ⅔ cup tapioca starch
- ⅓ cup arrowroot powder
- 2 tablespoons chopped fresh chives
- ½ teaspoon salt
- ½ teaspoon cream of tartar
- ¼ teaspoon baking soda

SPECIAL EQUIPMENT

- Steamer basket (if using taro)

1. Preheat the oven to 400°F.
2. Combine the mashed root vegetable with the remaining ingredients to form a fairly stiff dough.
3. Pat the dough out to ¾ inch thick. Use a 2-inch biscuit cutter to cut into biscuits and transfer to a baking sheet. (You can also form biscuits by hand by rolling the dough into a ball, flattening it, and then shaping the edges.)
4. Brush the top of each biscuit with additional lard or tallow.
5. Bake for 25 to 28 minutes, until golden brown on top. Let cool and enjoy.

TIPS:

If you are using taro, place the whole taro tubers in a steamer basket. Bring the water to a boil and steam for 20 to 30 minutes, until the tubers slide right off a knife when pierced. Let cool. Remove the outer peel (it should come off easily once cooked). Mash the taro with a fork, wire potato masher, or immersion blender.

If using yuca, peel and cut the yuca into chunks. Soak in water in the fridge for 24 hours. Drain. Boil in water for at least 1 hour. Drain again. Mash with a fork or wire potato masher (don't use an immersion blender with yuca).

VARIATIONS:

Instead of chives, use parsley or your favorite herbs.

NUTRITION FACTS

Serving Size	86 g
Recipe Yields	684 g
Calories	**210**
Fats	**5.58 g**
MUFA	2.19 g
Omega-3	0.06 g
Omega-6	0.52 g
Saturated Fat	2.58 g
Carbohydrates	**38.5 g**
Fiber	4.9 g
Starch	28.4 g
Fructose	0.03 g
Glucose	0.06 g
Sucrose	0.3 g
Protein	**1.03 g**
Alanine	0.02 g
Arginine	0.03 g
Aspartic acid	0.04 g
Cystine	<0.01 g
Glutamic acid	0.05 g
Glycine	0.02 g
Histidine	<0.01 g
Isoleucine	0.01 g
Leucine	0.02 g
Lysine	0.02 g
Methionine	<0.01 g
Phenylalanine	0.02 g
Proline	0.01 g
Serine	0.02 g
Threonine	0.02 g
Tryptophan	<0.01 g
Tyrosine	0.01 g
Valine	0.02 g
Vitamins	
Vitamin B1	0.06 mg
Vitamin B12	0 mcg
Vitamin B2	0.02 mg
Vitamin B3	0.3 mg
Vitamin B5	0.22 mg
Vitamin B6	0.19 mg
Choline	14.8 mg
Folate	12.5 mcg
Vitamin A	3.93 mcg
Vitamin C	3.29 mg
Vitamin D	4.93 IU
Vitamin E	1.7 mg
Vitamin K	2.29 mcg
Minerals	
Calcium	16 mg
Copper	0.12 mg
Iron	0.77 mg
Magnesium	17.8 mg
Manganese	0.3 mg
Phosphorus	45 mg
Potassium	312 mg
Selenium	0.63 mcg
Sodium	206 mg
Zinc	0.18 mg

nutrition content estimated using the USDA database.

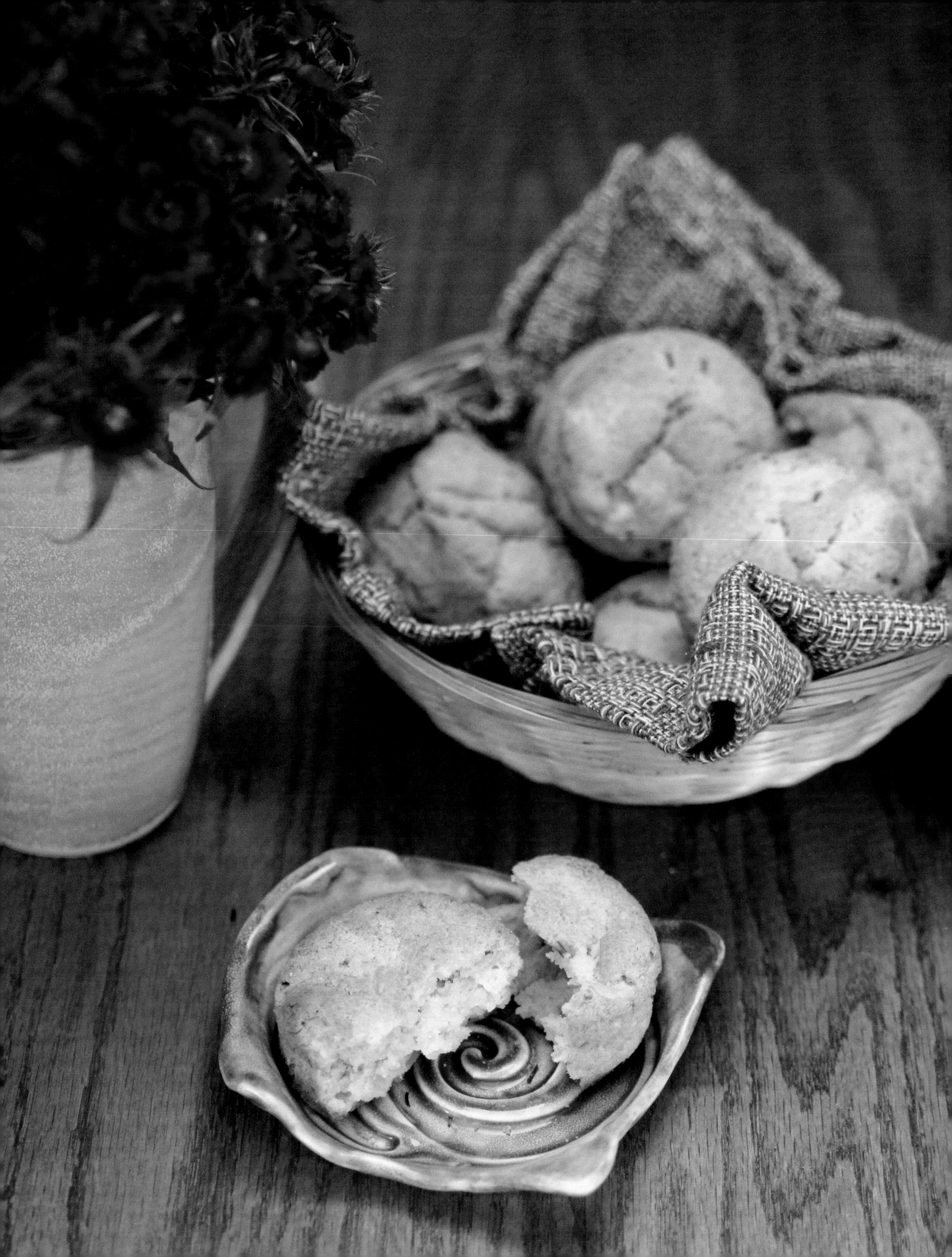

Chapter 12

Sweet Treats and Beverages

It may seem strange to include a chapter on treats, many with added sweeteners like honey, molasses, and muscovado sugar, after expounding on the detriments of a high-sugar diet for those with autoimmune disease. I've included this chapter for one very simple reason: We are still human.

It's critical that the Paleo Approach diet is sustainable for you. So how do you celebrate a birthday, anniversary, or job promotion? It is human nature to celebrate with special foods. While some may be happy celebrating with a prime rib or a massage, for others the sense of deprivation can be debilitating.

There are two types of recipes in this chapter. First, there are recipes that are really just dessertlike presentations of fresh fruit, with flavoring ingredients like fresh herbs and perhaps a trace of sweetener. These treats can be enjoyed frequently, as long as you are mindful of blood sugar regulation and your fructose intake. Second, there are recipes that include cooked alcohol and/or added sweeteners that should be reserved for special occasions. These recipes are designed to give you something special to eat that won't derail your efforts on birthdays and holidays. They can also be used prophylactically, when intense cravings for an old favorite threaten your ability to continue with the Paleo Approach. However, be mindful of other factors that may be contributing to those cravings, and make sure that you are addressing the root causes (like nutrient deficiency, chronic stress, inadequate sleep, or inactivity).

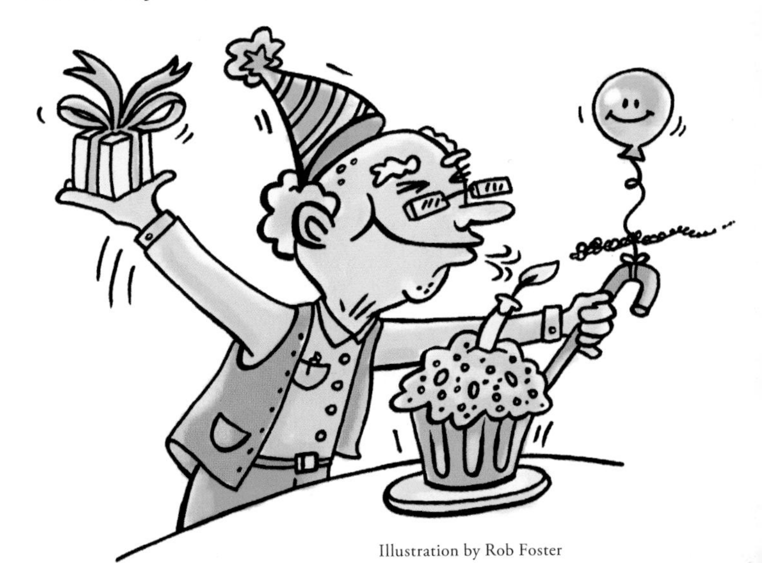

Illustration by Rob Foster

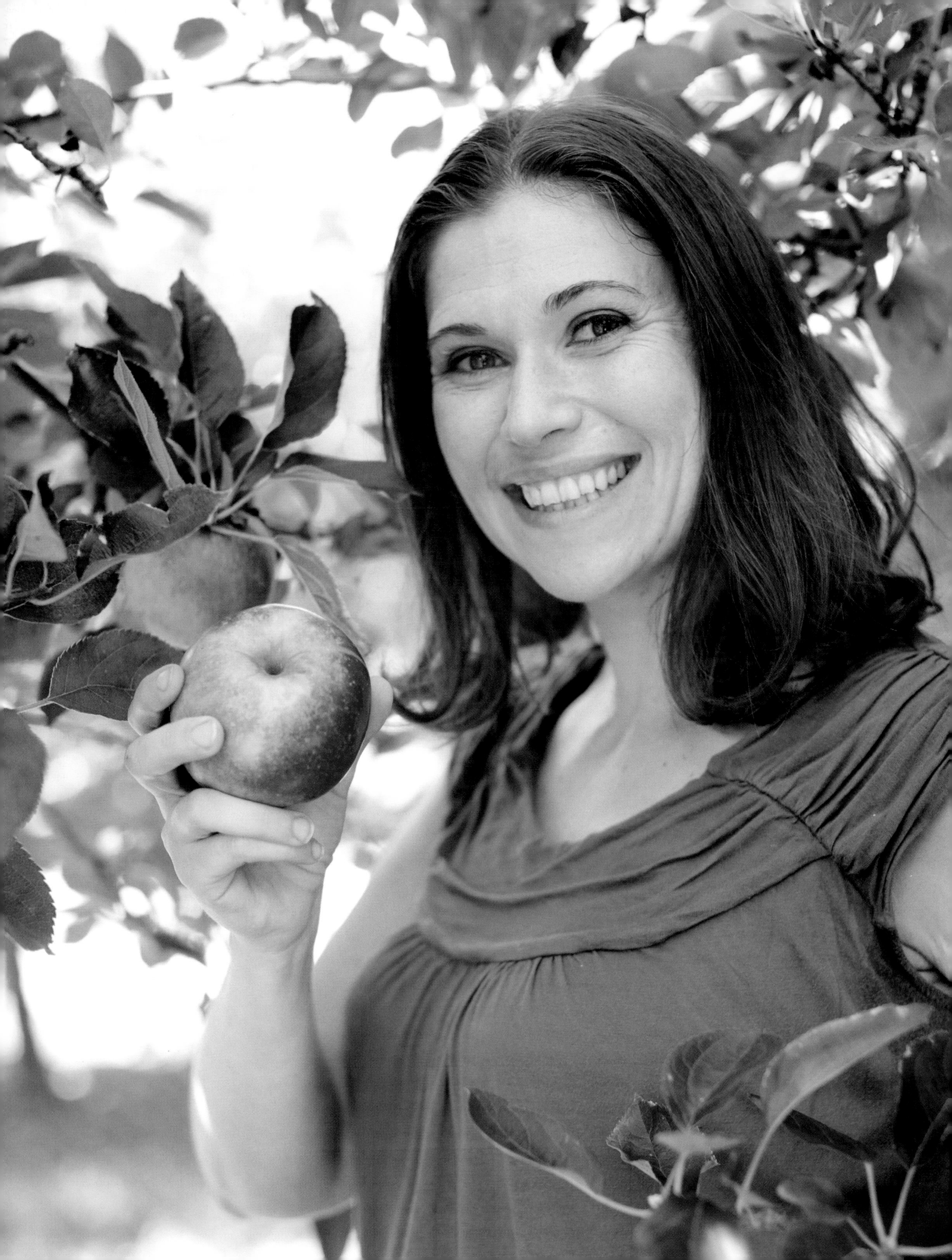

Honey-Candied Ginger

Candied ginger is a wonderful treat on its own, but it can also be chopped up and added to both sweet and savory dishes (especially when warm seasonings like cinnamon, mace, and turmeric are used). Try adding chopped candied ginger to ice cream or mixing it into fruit salad for a little extra zing.

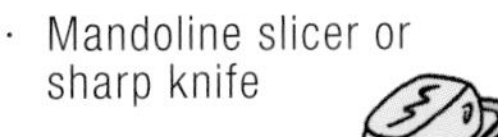

COOK TIME: 1 hour 15 minutes

SERVINGS: 10 to 20

INGREDIENTS:

½ pound fresh ginger
2 cups water
1¼ cups honey

FODMAP ALERT

This recipe cannot be made low-FODMAP.

SPECIAL EQUIPMENT

- Mandoline slicer or sharp knife

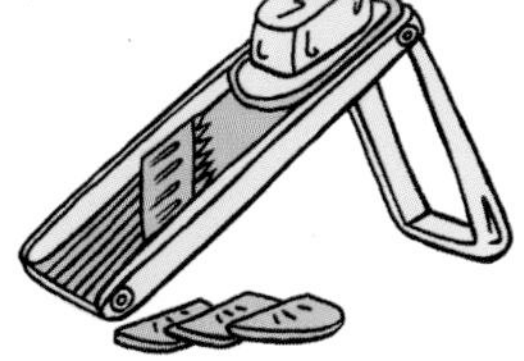

1. Peel the ginger and slice as thinly as possible (a mandoline slicer is helpful but not essential).
2. Bring the ginger and water to a boil in a pot over high heat. Cover and reduce to a simmer for 30 minutes, then uncover and continue to simmer for another 10 to 15 minutes, until tender. Make sure that the pot doesn't boil dry (add some water if it does).
3. Drain all but ¼ cup of the water from the pot. Add the honey to the pot. Simmer uncovered over low heat for another 30 to 40 minutes, until the ginger has turned darker in color and slightly translucent. Stir occasionally to make sure that it doesn't burn.
4. Remove from the heat. Store the candied ginger in the syrup in the fridge for up to several months.

VARIATIONS:

It's traditional to strain the ginger and roll it in sugar crystals. Doing so increases the sugar content of this candied ginger substantially, but is an option for a holiday treat.

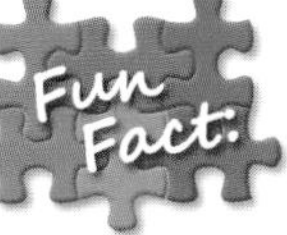

Beyond being a potent antiemetic and digestive aid, compounds in ginger have a variety of other beneficial properties, including antioxidant, anti-inflammatory, antiulcer, cardiotonic, antihypertensive, hypotensive, antihyperlipidemic, antimicrobial, and cancer prevention.

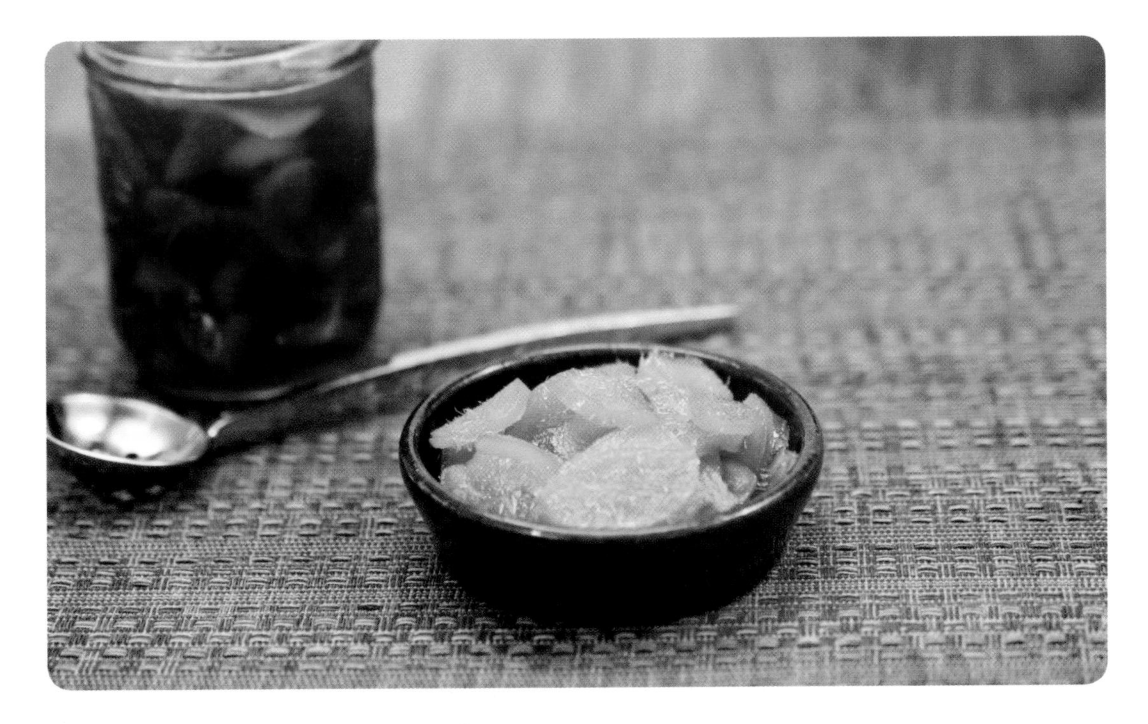

NUTRITION FACTS

Serving Size	16 g
Recipe Yields	312 g
Calories	**22.6**
Fats	**0.09 g**
MUFA	0.02 g
Omega-3	<0.01 g
Omega-6	0.01 g
Saturated Fat	0.02 g
Carbohydrates	**5.66 g**
Fiber	0.24 g
Starch	1.64 g
Fructose	1.78 g
Glucose	1.56 g
Sucrose	0.04 g
Protein	**0.23 g**
Alanine	<0.01 g
Arginine	<0.01 g
Aspartic acid	0.03 g
Cystine	<0.01 g
Glutamic acid	0.02 g
Glycine	<0.01 g
Histidine	<0.01 g
Isoleucine	<0.01 g
Leucine	<0.01 g
Lysine	<0.01 g
Methionine	<0.01 g
Phenylalanine	<0.01 g
Proline	<0.01 g
Serine	<0.01 g
Threonine	<0.01 g
Tryptophan	<0.01 g
Tyrosine	<0.01 g
Valine	<0.01 g
Vitamins	
Vitamin B1	<0.01 mg
Vitamin B12	0 mcg
Vitamin B2	<0.01 mg
Vitamin B3	0.09 mg
Vitamin B5	0.03 mg
Vitamin B6	0.02 mg
Choline	3.45 mg
Folate	1.37 mcg
Vitamin A	0 mcg
Vitamin C	0.6 mg
Vitamin D	0 IU
Vitamin E	0.03 mg
Vitamin K	0.01 mcg
Minerals	
Calcium	2.12 mg
Copper	0.03 mg
Iron	0.09 mg
Magnesium	5.1 mg
Manganese	0.03 mg
Phosphorus	4.13 mg
Potassium	50.6 mg
Selenium	0.12 mcg
Sodium	1.69 mg
Zinc	0.05 mg

nutrition content estimated using the USDA database.

Spa Water—Six Ways

Sometimes it's nice to spruce up some water. Adding a little flavor can do wonders. Four of these variations are classic spa water in the sense that they are made simply by adding aromatic fresh fruits and spices to cold water and refrigerating overnight before drinking. Two are technically iced herbal teas, but just as enjoyable!

PREP TIME: 5 to 10 minutes, plus up to 24 hours steeping time
COOK TIME: none
SERVINGS: 8 to 10

INGREDIENTS:

8 to 10 cups water

Orange-Mint

2 oranges, sliced
2 cups fresh mint

Classic Lime and Cucumber

3 limes, sliced
1 cucumber, sliced

Apple-Cinnamon

3 apples, sliced
1 stick cinnamon

Lemon-Grapefruit

3 lemons, sliced
1 grapefruit, sliced

Ginger-Lemon

2 thumbs ginger, sliced
1 lemon, sliced

Mint-Lemon

4 cups fresh mint
2 lemons, sliced

ORANGE-MINT, CLASSIC LIME AND CUCUMBER, APPLE-CINNAMON, LEMON-GRAPEFRUIT:

1. Place the flavoring ingredients and 8 to 10 cups of cold water in a pitcher. Refrigerate overnight and up to 24 hours.

GINGER-LEMON, MINT-LEMON:

1. Combine the flavoring ingredients in a teapot. Pour 4 cups of boiling hot water over the top to fill the pot.
2. Let cool completely. Pour the herbal tea through a sieve into a pitcher. Top off with 4 to 6 cups of cold water, depending on how concentrated you like the flavor.

TIPS:

If you are using organic citrus fruit, apples, cucumber, and ginger, there's no need to peel; in fact, the flavor is better if you leave the peel on.

VARIATIONS:

Variations are endless. Get creative!

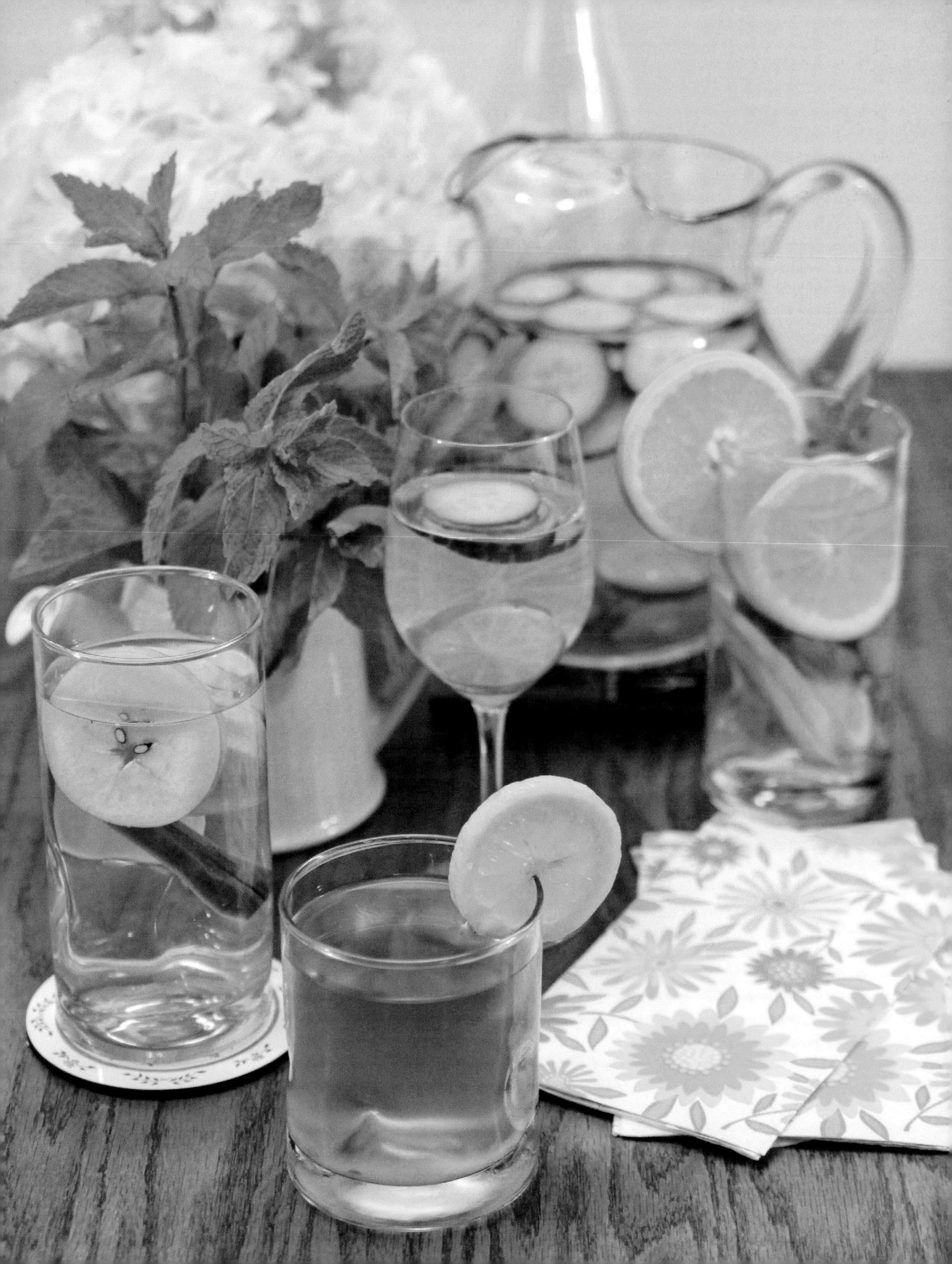

Fruit Salad

Fruit salad is the quintessential healthy dessert. When the only ingredients are fruit, there is no need to limit your consumption beyond paying attention to your fructose intake. Whatever your favorite combinations are for fruit salad, go ahead and enjoy it!

Here are some ideas for particularly delicious and unique flavor combinations. The amounts in the ingredients lists should be taken as a general guide only. Fruit salad is very forgiving; really, you can just toss a bunch of chopped fruit in a bowl and call it a day. Enjoy freshly made or chill to allow the flavors to blend first.

PREP TIME: 10 to 20 minutes

SERVINGS: 3 to 6

1. Combine the ingredients in a bowl and enjoy!

INGREDIENTS:

Thai-Inspired:

- 1 cup papaya chunks
- 1 cup mango chunks
- 1 cup pineapple chunks
- 1 cup thinly sliced starfruit (see Tips)
- 1 teaspoon finely chopped Honey-Candied Ginger (page 333)
- 1 teaspoon finely grated lime zest
- 1 to 2 tablespoons lime juice and/or strong-brewed, chilled jasmine tea

Tropical:

- 1 cup peeled, pitted, and halved lychee
- 1 cup pineapple chunks
- 1 cup orange segments (see Tips on page 242)
- 1 cup sliced banana (see Tips)
- 1 teaspoon finely grated lime zest
- 1 to 2 tablespoons fresh lime juice

Stone Fruits with Balsamic:

- 1 cup pitted and quartered apricots
- 1 cup pitted and halved cherries
- 1 cup sliced peaches or nectarines
- 1 to 2 tablespoons well-aged balsamic vinegar
- 1 teaspoon finely chopped fresh basil leaves

Red and Green:

- 1 cup watermelon chunks
- 1 cup strawberries
- 1 cup sliced kiwi
- 1 to 2 tablespoons fresh lemon juice
- 1 to 2 teaspoons finely chopped fresh mint leaves

FODMAP ALERT *Use only low-FODMAP fruits and keep portions small.*

TIPS:

Always cut starfruit crosswise to emphasize its star shape. Banana should always be added to fruit salad immediately before serving.

VARIATIONS:

Feel free to make any substitutions you want to reflect either your personal tastes or the availability of different fruits.

Try serving with coconut cream!

NUTRITION FACTS	
Serving Size	92.5 g
Recipe Yields	554 g
Calories	**46.9**
Fats	**0.25 g**
MUFA	0.05 g
Omega-3	0.02 g
Omega-6	0.06 g
Saturated Fat	0.03 g
Carbohydrates	**11.7 g**
Fiber	1.7 g
Starch	1.26 g
Fructose	2.58 g
Glucose	2.4 g
Sucrose	2.6 g
Protein	**0.79 g**
Alanine	0.04 g
Arginine	0.04 g
Aspartic acid	0.16 g
Cystine	0.01 g
Glutamic acid	0.1 g
Glycine	0.03 g
Histidine	0.02 g
Isoleucine	0.02 g
Leucine	0.04 g
Lysine	0.04 g
Methionine	0.01 g
Phenylalanine	0.02 g
Proline	0.04 g
Serine	0.04 g
Threonine	0.02 g
Tryptophan	0.01 g
Tyrosine	0.02 g
Valine	0.03 g
Vitamins	
Vitamin B1	0.03 mg
Vitamin B12	0 mcg
Vitamin B2	0.03 mg
Vitamin B3	0.42 mg
Vitamin B5	0.19 mg
Vitamin B6	0.08 mg
Choline	5.88 mg
Folate	17.7 mcg
Vitamin A	18.3 mcg
Vitamin C	36.3 mg
Vitamin D	0 IU
Vitamin E	0.36 mg
Vitamin K	4.46 mcg
Minerals	
Calcium	14.4 mg
Copper	0.08 mg
Iron	0.25 mg
Magnesium	12.1 mg
Manganese	0.21 mg
Phosphorus	17.2 mg
Potassium	175 mg
Selenium	0.3 mcg
Sodium	1.6 mg
Zinc	0.11 mg

nutrition content estimated using the USDA database. values are based on an average of all variations.

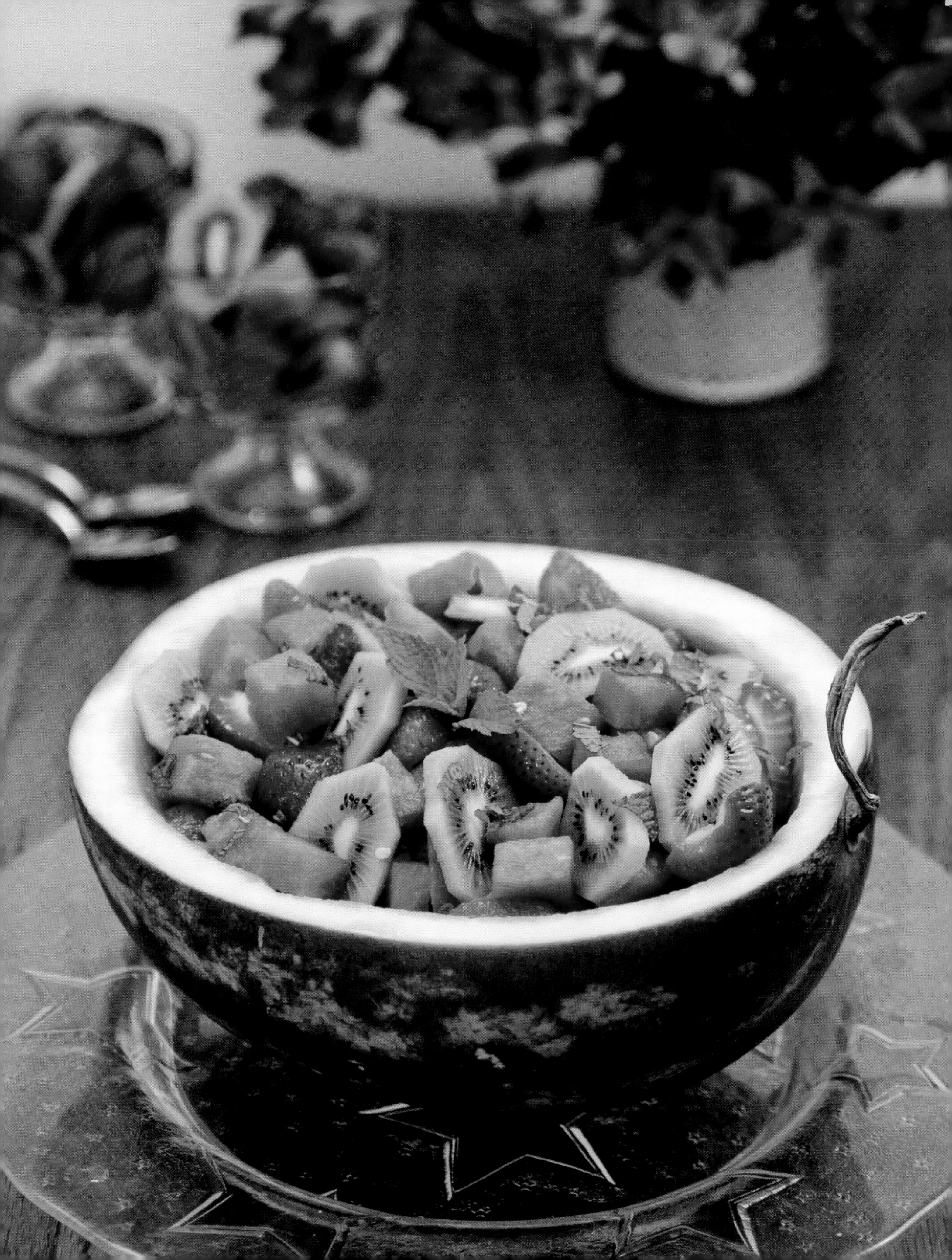

Strawberry Fro-Yo

An ice cream maker is a great investment and opens up many possibilities for guilt-free treats. Almost any fruit can be puréed, tossed into an ice cream maker, and turned into a wonderful treat in 10 to 15 minutes. This is a master recipe for frozen yogurt—make any flavor you like. If you are using tart fruit, you can add a tablespoon or two of honey for little sweetness.

PREP TIME: 20 minutes, plus at least 1 hour chilling time
COOK TIME: 10 to 15 minutes in an ice cream maker
YIELD: 1 quart

INGREDIENTS:

3 cups sliced fresh strawberries

1½ cups Coconut Milk Yogurt (page 118)

Honey, if needed

FODMAP ALERT

If you do not tolerate Coconut Milk Yogurt, skip this recipe.

SPECIAL EQUIPMENT

- Ice cream maker

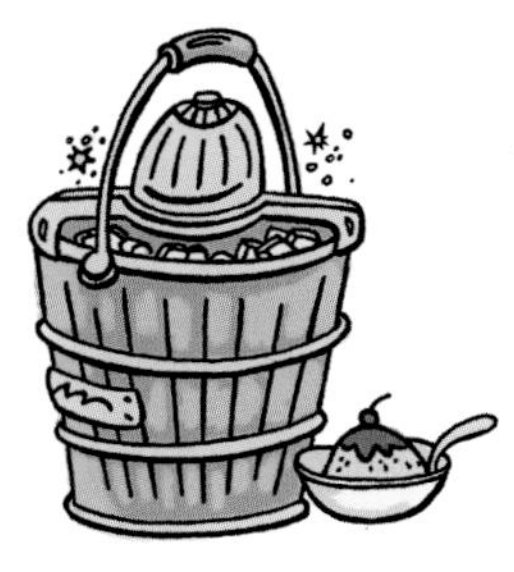

1. Combine the sliced strawberries and coconut milk yogurt in a blender or food processor. Blend until completely smooth. If your strawberries are not particularly sweet, you may wish to add 1 to 2 tablespoons of honey.
2. Chill the strawberry yogurt in the fridge for at least 1 hour.
3. Blend the chilled yogurt for 30 seconds, then place in an ice cream maker and churn following the manufacturer's directions. Enjoy! Store any leftovers in the soft zone of your freezer.

TIPS:

If you don't have an ice cream maker, you can make this fro-yo by putting the yogurt in a metal bowl in the freezer and whisking every 20 minutes or so for the 3 to 4 hours that it will take to harden. Alternatively, if you use frozen fruit with a high-powered blender, you can just pour your mixture into a container and freeze.

If using store-bought coconut milk yogurt or coconut milk kefir, add 1 to 2 teaspoons gelatin by blooming the gelatin in ½ cup of the blended yogurt and berry mixture, then gently heating on the stovetop or in the microwave until the gelatin dissolves (if you want to gauge using a thermometer and protect as many probiotic organisms as possible, gelatin dissolves at about 85°F). You can also skip the gelatin altogether if you want (it makes the fro-yo softer and more scoopable).

VARIATIONS:

You can make this frozen yogurt with any sweet fruit. Here are some other great combinations:

- *Vanilla-Mango Fro-Yo. Use peeled and seeded mango with 2 teaspoons vanilla extract or ½ teaspoon vanilla powder.*
- *Berry Fro-Yo. Other berries make great options. Use blackberries, blueberries, raspberries, cherries, or any combination.*
- *Straw-Nana Fro-Yo. Replace 1 cup of the strawberries with 1 cup sliced very ripe banana.*
- *Apricot-Ginger Fro-Yo. Replace the strawberries with fresh pitted apricot or peach and add 2 to 3 tablespoons chopped Honey-Candied Ginger (page 333) after blending the other ingredients.*

NUTRITION FACTS	
Serving Size	117 g
Recipe Yields	936 g
Calories	**148**
Fats	**12.7 g**
MUFA	0.56 g
Omega-3	0.04 g
Omega-6	0.19 g
Saturated Fat	11.1 g
Carbohydrates	**9.14 g**
Fiber	2.4 g
Starch	0.03 g
Fructose	2.24 g
Glucose	1.87 g
Sucrose	0.31 g
Protein	**2 g**
Alanine	0.12 g
Arginine	0.24 g
Aspartic acid	0.23 g
Cystine	0.03 g
Glutamic acid	0.37 g
Glycine	0.16 g
Histidine	0.04 g
Isoleucine	0.06 g
Leucine	0.12 g
Lysine	0.08 g
Methionine	0.03 g
Phenylalanine	0.08 g
Proline	0.12 g
Serine	0.09 g
Threonine	0.06 g
Tryptophan	0.02 g
Tyrosine	0.05 g
Valine	0.09 g
Vitamins	
Vitamin B1	0.03 mg
Vitamin B12	0 mcg
Vitamin B2	0.02 mg
Vitamin B3	0.64 mg
Vitamin B5	0.18 mg
Vitamin B6	0.05 mg
Choline	8.22 mg
Folate	23.5 mcg
Vitamin A	0.62 mcg
Vitamin C	38.1 mg
Vitamin D	0 IU
Vitamin E	0.26 mg
Vitamin K	1.42 mcg
Minerals	
Calcium	18.7 mg
Copper	0.18 mg
Iron	1.13 mg
Magnesium	27.7 mg
Manganese	0.72 mg
Phosphorus	67.7 mg
Potassium	234 mg
Selenium	3.69 mcg
Sodium	9.43 mg
Zinc	0.44 mg

nutrition content estimated using the USDA database.

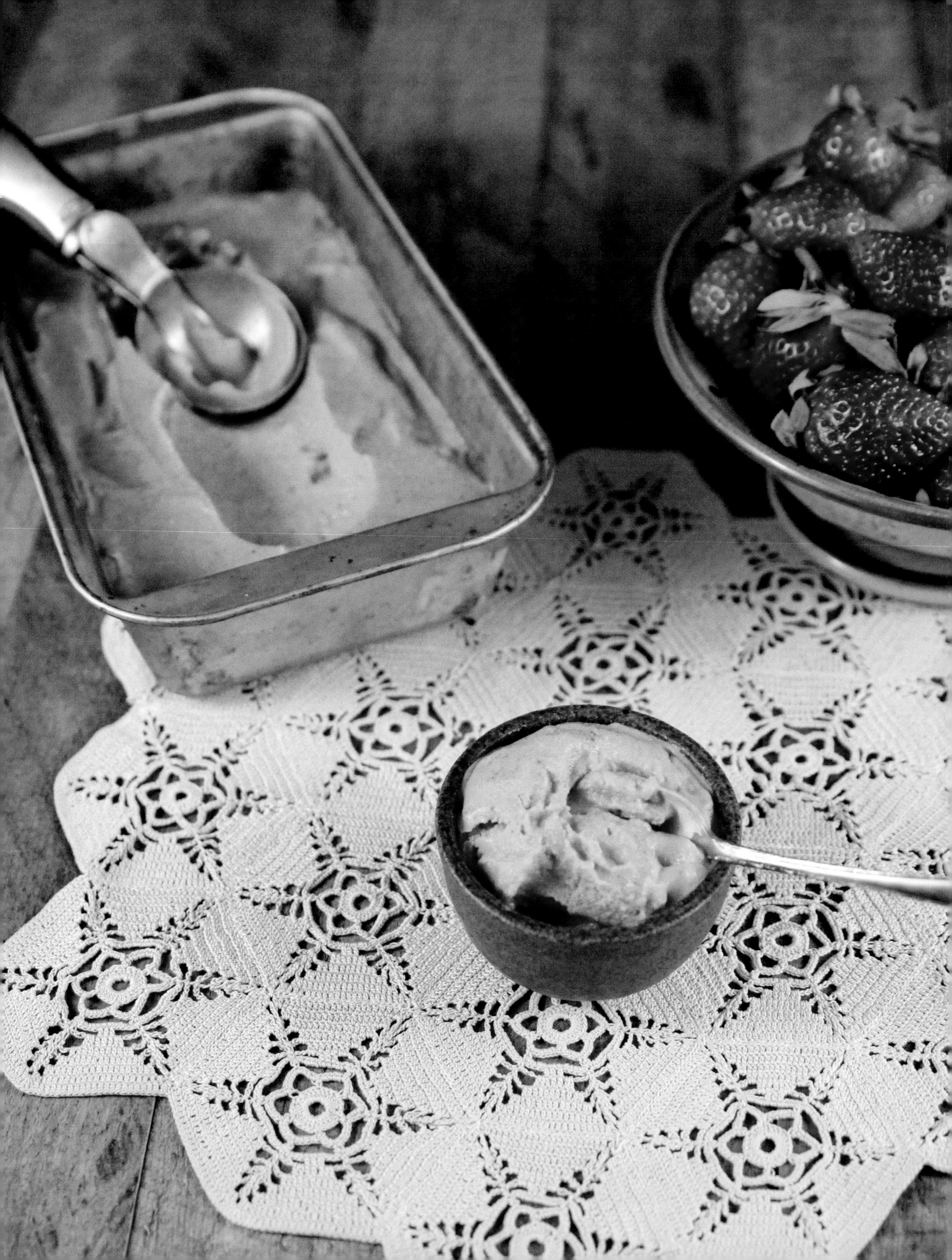

Honeydew Ice "Cream"

You can use any combination of fruit you like in this recipe to make your favorite flavor of ice "cream." Honeydew melon may sound like an odd choice, but it's remarkably delicious!

PREP TIME: 20 minutes, plus at least 2 hours chilling time
COOK TIME: 10 minutes, plus 10 to 15 minutes in an ice cream maker
YIELD: 1 quart

INGREDIENTS:

- 2 teaspoons gelatin
- 1¾ cups homemade Coconut Milk (page 116), full-fat canned coconut milk, or Coconut Cream (page 116)
- 2 tablespoons honey
- ⅛ teaspoon salt
- 3 cups chopped honeydew
- ½ teaspoon vanilla powder

⚠ **FODMAP ALERT** *Instead of honey, use 1 tablespoon evaporated cane juice dissolved into the coconut milk. If you do not tolerate coconut milk, skip this recipe.*

SPECIAL EQUIPMENT

- Blender or food processor
- Ice cream maker

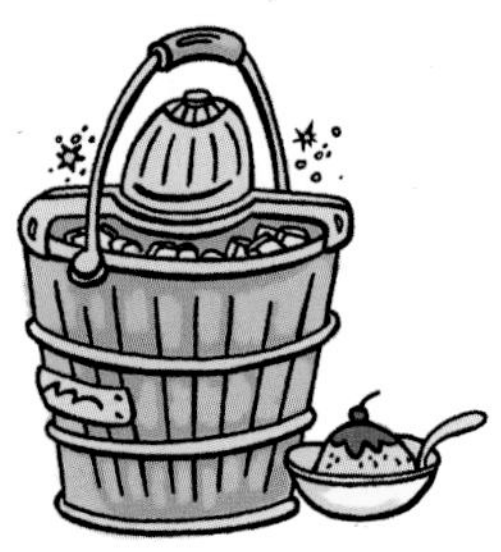

1. In a small saucepan, bloom the gelatin in the coconut milk by sprinkling the gelatin over the coconut milk and letting it sit until the gelatin has absorbed the liquid and looks translucent. Set the pan over medium heat and heat, stirring gently, until the gelatin has dissolved. Remove from the heat and let cool.
2. Combine the cooled milk with the rest of the ingredients in a blender or food processor. Blend until completely smooth.
3. Chill the mixture in the fridge for at least 2 hours.
4. Blend the chilled mixture for 30 seconds, then place in an ice cream maker and churn following the manufacturer's directions. Enjoy! Store any leftovers in the soft zone of the freezer.

TIPS:

If you don't have an ice cream maker, you can make this ice cream by putting the mix in a metal bowl in the freezer and whisking every 20 minutes or so until hardened to ice cream consistency, 3 to 4 hours.

VARIATIONS:

You can make this ice cream with any fruit. Here are some other great combinations:

- ***Mango-Lime Ice "Cream."*** *Instead of honeydew, use 2½ cups peeled, seeded, and chopped mango and ½ cup lime segments.*
- ***Pineapple-Lychee Ice "Cream."*** *Instead of honeydew, use 1½ cups peeled, cored, and chopped pineapple and 1½ cups peeled and pitted lychee.*
- ***Orangesicle Ice "Cream."*** *Instead of honeydew, use 3 cups orange segments (see Tips on page 242).*
- ***Berries 'n' Cream Ice "Cream."*** *Instead of honeydew, use strawberries, blackberries, blueberries, raspberries, cherries, or your favorite combination.*
- ***Melon Ice "Cream."*** *Replace the honeydew with watermelon, cantaloupe, or other melon.*
- ***Grilled Peach and Candied Ginger Ice "Cream."*** *Use grilled peaches instead of honeydew. Cut the peaches in half and pit them. Grill the peach halves for 3 to 4 minutes on each side. Add 2 to 3 tablespoons chopped Honey-Candied Ginger (page 333) after blending the other ingredients.*

NUTRITION FACTS

Serving Size	127 g
Recipe Yields	1017 g
Calories	**142**
Fats	**10.6 g**
MUFA	0.45 g
Omega-3	0.02 g
Omega-6	0.13 g
Saturated Fat	9.37 g
Carbohydrates	**12.2 g**
Fiber	0.58 g
Starch	<0.01 g
Fructose	4.26 g
Glucose	3.79 g
Sucrose	1.82 g
Protein	**1.9 g**
Alanine	0.13 g
Arginine	0.21 g
Aspartic acid	0.19 g
Cystine	0.02 g
Glutamic acid	0.39 g
Glycine	0.17 g
Histidine	0.03 g
Isoleucine	0.06 g
Leucine	0.1 g
Lysine	0.08 g
Methionine	0.03 g
Phenylalanine	0.07 g
Proline	0.13 g
Serine	0.08 g
Threonine	0.05 g
Tryptophan	0.02 g
Tyrosine	0.04 g
Valine	0.09 g

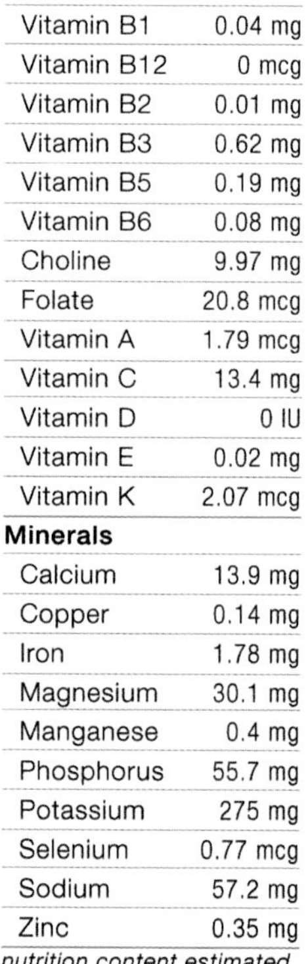

Vitamins	
Vitamin B1	0.04 mg
Vitamin B12	0 mcg
Vitamin B2	0.01 mg
Vitamin B3	0.62 mg
Vitamin B5	0.19 mg
Vitamin B6	0.08 mg
Choline	9.97 mg
Folate	20.8 mcg
Vitamin A	1.79 mcg
Vitamin C	13.4 mg
Vitamin D	0 IU
Vitamin E	0.02 mg
Vitamin K	2.07 mcg
Minerals	
Calcium	13.9 mg
Copper	0.14 mg
Iron	1.78 mg
Magnesium	30.1 mg
Manganese	0.4 mg
Phosphorus	55.7 mg
Potassium	275 mg
Selenium	0.77 mcg
Sodium	57.2 mg
Zinc	0.35 mg

nutrition content estimated using the USDA database.

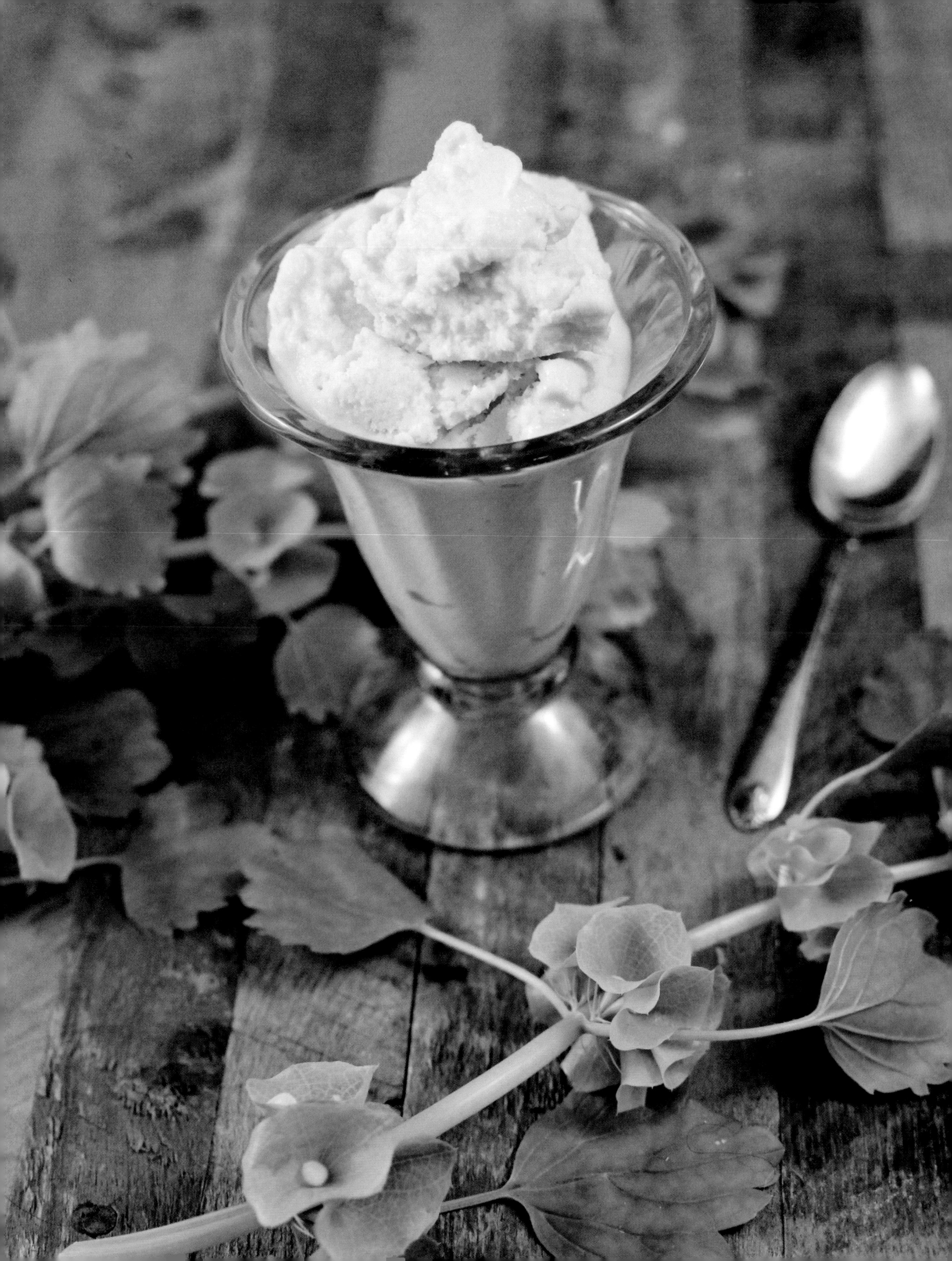

Berry Terrine

This is a magical way to transform simple berries into a decadent-feeling dessert that is healthy enough to be enjoyed daily.

PREP TIME: 30 minutes
COOK TIME: none
SERVINGS: 12

INGREDIENTS:

- 4 cups mixed berries
- ⅓ cup fresh mint leaves
- 2 tablespoons grated orange zest
- 1 tablespoon grated lemon zest (about 1 lemon)
- 1½ cups boiling water
- 2½ tablespoons gelatin
- ¾ cup cold water
- 1½ tablespoons honey (optional)
- 3 tablespoons fresh lemon juice

1. Grease 12 muffin cups (you can use a muffin pan with fun-shaped wells, like hearts or mini Bundt cakes) with coconut oil or line with silicone liners, or use a silicone muffin pan.
2. Fill each muffin cup with the berries.
3. Place the mint leaves, orange zest, and lemon zest in a teapot. Pour the hot water over the leaves and steep for 10 to 15 minutes.
4. Meanwhile, bloom the gelatin by sprinkling it over the cold water and waiting until the gelatin has absorbed the liquid and looks translucent.
5. Pour the mint tea through a sieve into the bloomed gelatin. Stir until the gelatin has dissolved. Let cool for 10 minutes. Add the honey and lemon juice, and stir to dissolve the honey.
6. Pour the mint tea gelatin mix over the berries to fill each well in the pan. Place in the refrigerator until set, 3 to 4 hours.

FODMAP ALERT *Omit the honey or use 2 teaspoons evaporated cane juice instead. Use only low-FODMAP berries.*

VARIATIONS:

With the exception of pineapple and papaya, which will stop the gelatin from setting, you can use just about any fruit for these terrines. Watermelon is an especially nice flavor with the minty gelatin. You can also use different herbal teas to change the flavor. Chamomile and lavender work especially well. Replace lemon juice with fresh orange juice and omit the honey for an orange-mint variation.

You can also make this terrine in a 9-by-5-inch loaf pan, tube pan, or large Bundt mold and slice into individual portions to serve.

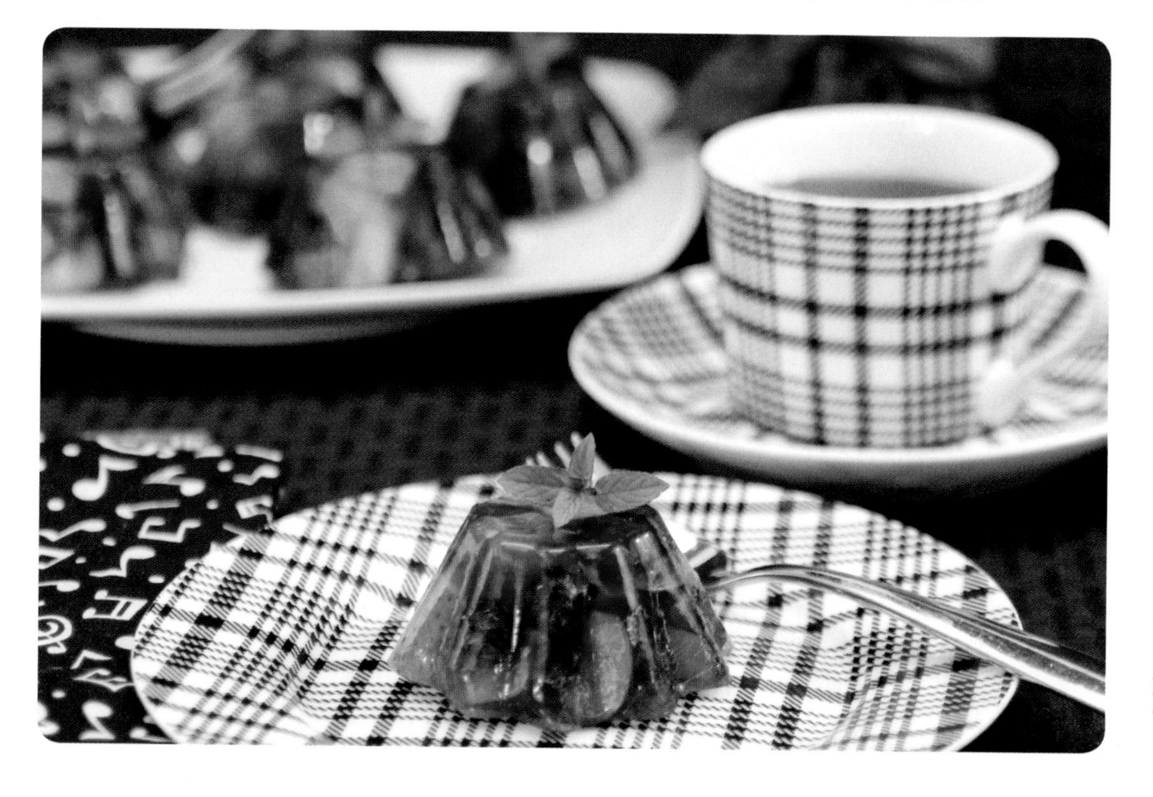

NUTRITION FACTS	
Serving Size	58 g
Recipe Yields	699 g
Calories	**37**
Fats	**0.22 g**
MUFA	0.03 g
Omega-3	0.04 g
Omega-6	0.07 g
Saturated Fat	0.01 g
Carbohydrates	**8.01 g**
Fiber	2.08 g
Starch	0.28 g
Fructose	2.59 g
Glucose	2.31 g
Sucrose	0.15 g
Protein	**1.77 g**
Alanine	0.13 g
Arginine	0.11 g
Aspartic acid	0.11 g
Cystine	<0.01 g
Glutamic acid	0.15 g
Glycine	0.29 g
Histidine	0.01 g
Isoleucine	0.02 g
Leucine	0.05 g
Lysine	0.06 g
Methionine	0.01 g
Phenylalanine	0.03 g
Proline	0.19 g
Serine	0.04 g
Threonine	0.03 g
Tryptophan	<0.01 g
Tyrosine	<0.01 g
Valine	0.04 g
Vitamins	
Vitamin B1	0.02 mg
Vitamin B12	0 mcg
Vitamin B2	0.02 mg
Vitamin B3	0.27 mg
Vitamin B5	0.12 mg
Vitamin B6	0.03 mg
Choline	4.65 mg
Folate	11.2 mcg
Vitamin A	3.09 mcg
Vitamin C	18.1 mg
Vitamin D	0 IU
Vitamin E	0.35 mg
Vitamin K	5.84 mcg
Minerals	
Calcium	13.4 mg
Copper	0.08 mg
Iron	0.3 mg
Magnesium	8.38 mg
Manganese	0.25 mg
Phosphorus	11.9 mg
Potassium	76 mg
Selenium	0.75 mcg
Sodium	3.66 mg
Zinc	0.16 mg

nutrition content estimated using the USDA database.

Gingerbread Ice "Cream"

This spicy ice "cream" has all the flavors of the holidays.

PREP TIME: 20 minutes, plus at least 2 hours chilling time
COOK TIME: 10 minutes, plus 10 to 15 minutes in an ice cream maker
YIELD: 1 quart

INGREDIENTS:

- 2 teaspoons gelatin
- 1¾ cups homemade Coconut Milk (page 116) or 1 (13½-ounce) can full-fat coconut milk
- 2 tablespoons grated fresh ginger
- 2 teaspoons ground cinnamon
- 1¾ cups pumpkin or other winter squash puree or sweet potato puree
- ¼ cup olive oil or avocado oil
- ⅓ cup blackstrap molasses
- 1 tablespoon honey
- ½ teaspoon vanilla powder
- ⅛ teaspoon salt

1. In a small saucepan, bloom the gelatin in the coconut milk by sprinkling the gelatin over the coconut milk and letting it sit until the gelatin has absorbed the liquid and turned translucent. Add the ginger and cinnamon to the pan and heat over medium heat, stirring gently, until the gelatin has dissolved. Remove from the heat and let cool.
2. Combine the cooled milk mixture with the rest of the ingredients in a blender or food processor. Blend until completely smooth.
3. Chill the mixture in the fridge for at least 2 hours.
4. Blend the chilled mixture for 30 seconds, then place in an ice cream maker and churn following the manufacturer's directions. Enjoy! Store any leftovers in the soft zone of your freezer.

TIPS:

If you don't have an ice cream maker, you can make this ice cream by putting the mixture in a metal bowl in the freezer and whisking every 20 minutes until it has hardened to ice cream consistency, 3 to 4 hours.

SPECIAL EQUIPMENT

- Blender or food processor
- Ice cream maker

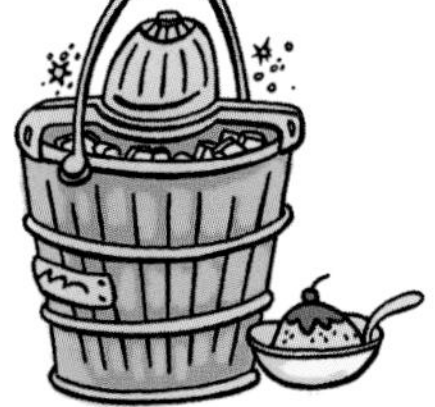

FODMAP ALERT *If you do not tolerate coconut milk, skip this recipe. Otherwise, use maple syrup instead of honey.*

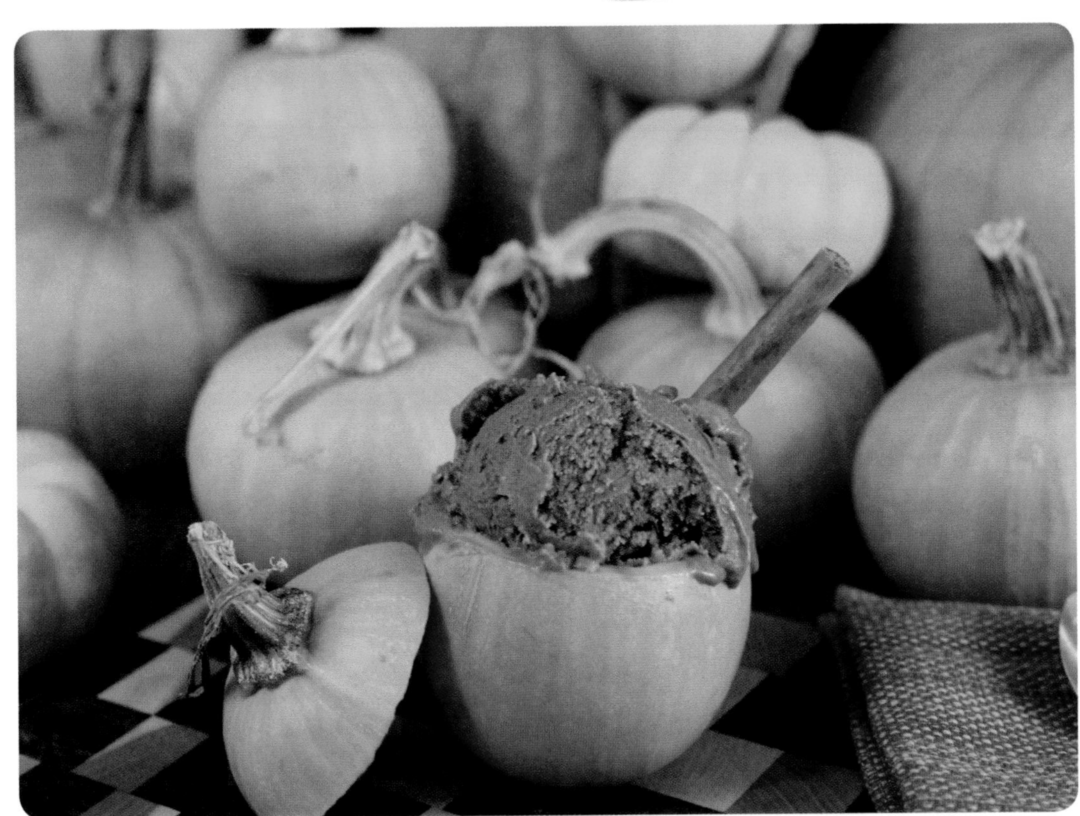

NUTRITION FACTS	
Serving Size	130 g
Recipe Yields	1036 g
Calories	**230**
Fats	**17.5 g**
MUFA	5.42 g
Omega-3	0.06 g
Omega-6	0.79 g
Saturated Fat	10.4 g
Carbohydrates	**19.3 g**
Fiber	1.94 g
Starch	1.4 g
Fructose	2.89 g
Glucose	2.63 g
Sucrose	4.16 g
Protein	**2.16 g**
Alanine	0.12 g
Arginine	0.24 g
Aspartic acid	0.2 g
Cystine	0.02 g
Glutamic acid	0.39 g
Glycine	0.18 g
Histidine	0.04 g
Isoleucine	0.07 g
Leucine	0.12 g
Lysine	0.1 g
Methionine	0.03 g
Phenylalanine	0.08 g
Proline	0.13 g
Serine	0.09 g
Threonine	0.06 g
Tryptophan	0.02 g
Tyrosine	0.06 g
Valine	0.1 g
Vitamins	
Vitamin B1	0.03 mg
Vitamin B12	0 mcg
Vitamin B2	0.03 mg
Vitamin B3	0.67 mg
Vitamin B5	0.41 mg
Vitamin B6	0.14 mg
Choline	12.2 mg
Folate	13.8 mcg
Vitamin A	419 mcg
Vitamin C	2.87 mg
Vitamin D	0 IU
Vitamin E	1.56 mg
Vitamin K	12.9 mcg
Minerals	
Calcium	59.3 mg
Copper	0.26 mg
Iron	3.26 mg
Magnesium	70.5 mg
Manganese	0.8 mg
Phosphorus	72.1 mg
Potassium	438 mg
Selenium	3 mcg
Sodium	32.1 mg
Zinc	0.43 mg

nutrition content estimated using the USDA database.

Orange and Banana Sorbet

This is my daughters' favorite summer dessert. With all the sweetness that ripe bananas provide, this sorbet needs no added sweeteners.

PREP TIME: 20 minutes, plus at least 2 hours chilling time
COOK TIME: 10 minutes, plus 10 to 15 minutes in an ice cream maker
SERVINGS: 4

INGREDIENTS:

- 2 teaspoons gelatin
- 4 oranges, segmented (see Tips)
- 2 overripe bananas
- 1 cup carrot juice

SPECIAL EQUIPMENT

- Blender or food processor
- Ice cream maker

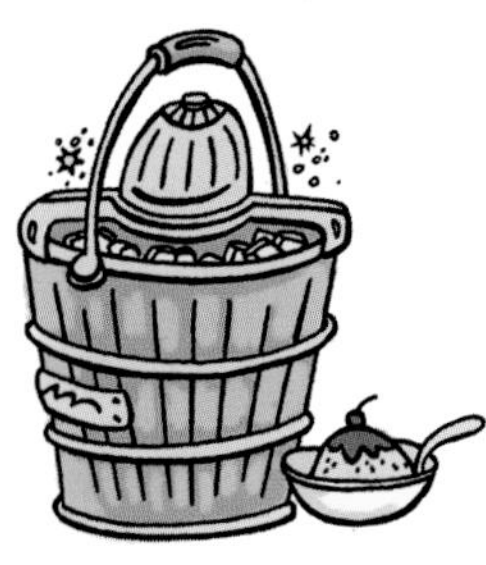

1. In a small saucepan, sprinkle the gelatin over the carrot juice to bloom. Once the gelatin has absorbed the liquid and turned translucent, set the saucepan over medium heat.
2. Heat, stirring gently, until the gelatin has dissolved. Remove from the heat and let cool.
3. Combine the cooled gelatin mixture with the rest of the ingredients in a blender or food processor. Blend until completely smooth.
4. Chill the puree in the fridge for at least 2 hours.
5. Blend the chilled puree for 30 seconds, then place in an ice cream maker and churn following the manufacturer's directions. Enjoy! Store any leftovers in the soft zone of your freezer.

TIPS:

If you have a powerful blender, you can skip segmenting the orange. Otherwise, see the Tips on page 242 for how to segment an orange.

This is a great way to use up overripe bananas. The riper they are, the sweeter this sorbet will be.

Banana-Orange Popsicles. *Instead of churning in an ice cream maker, pour into popsicle molds and freeze.*

NUTRITION FACTS

Serving Size	250 g
Recipe Yields	1001 g
Calories	**142**
Fats	**0.44 g**
MUFA	0.05 g
Omega-3	0.03 g
Omega-6	0.09 g
Saturated Fat	0.1 g
Carbohydrates	**34.3 g**
Fiber	5.08 g
Starch	3.17 g
Fructose	5.88 g
Glucose	5.92 g
Sucrose	8.59 g
Protein	**3.44 g**
Alanine	0.22 g
Arginine	0.22 g
Aspartic acid	0.37 g
Cystine	0.02 g
Glutamic acid	0.43 g
Glycine	0.39 g
Histidine	0.09 g
Isoleucine	0.09 g
Leucine	0.12 g
Lysine	0.16 g
Methionine	0.04 g
Phenylalanine	0.11 g
Proline	0.24 g
Serine	0.11 g
Threonine	0.08 g
Tryptophan	0.02 g
Tyrosine	0.04 g
Valine	0.13 g
Vitamins	
Vitamin B1	0.19 mg
Vitamin B12	0 mcg
Vitamin B2	0.13 mg
Vitamin B3	0.99 mg
Vitamin B5	0.66 mg
Vitamin B6	0.42 mg
Choline	23.1 mg
Folate	53.8 mcg
Vitamin A	580 mcg
Vitamin C	79.8 mg
Vitamin D	0 IU
Vitamin E	1.07 mg
Vitamin K	9.43 mcg
Minerals	
Calcium	70.1 mg
Copper	0.16 mg
Iron	0.57 mg
Magnesium	37.5 mg
Manganese	0.27 mg
Phosphorus	56.5 mg
Potassium	620 mg
Selenium	2.06 mcg
Sodium	41.8 mg
Zinc	0.29 mg

nutrition content estimated using the USDA database.

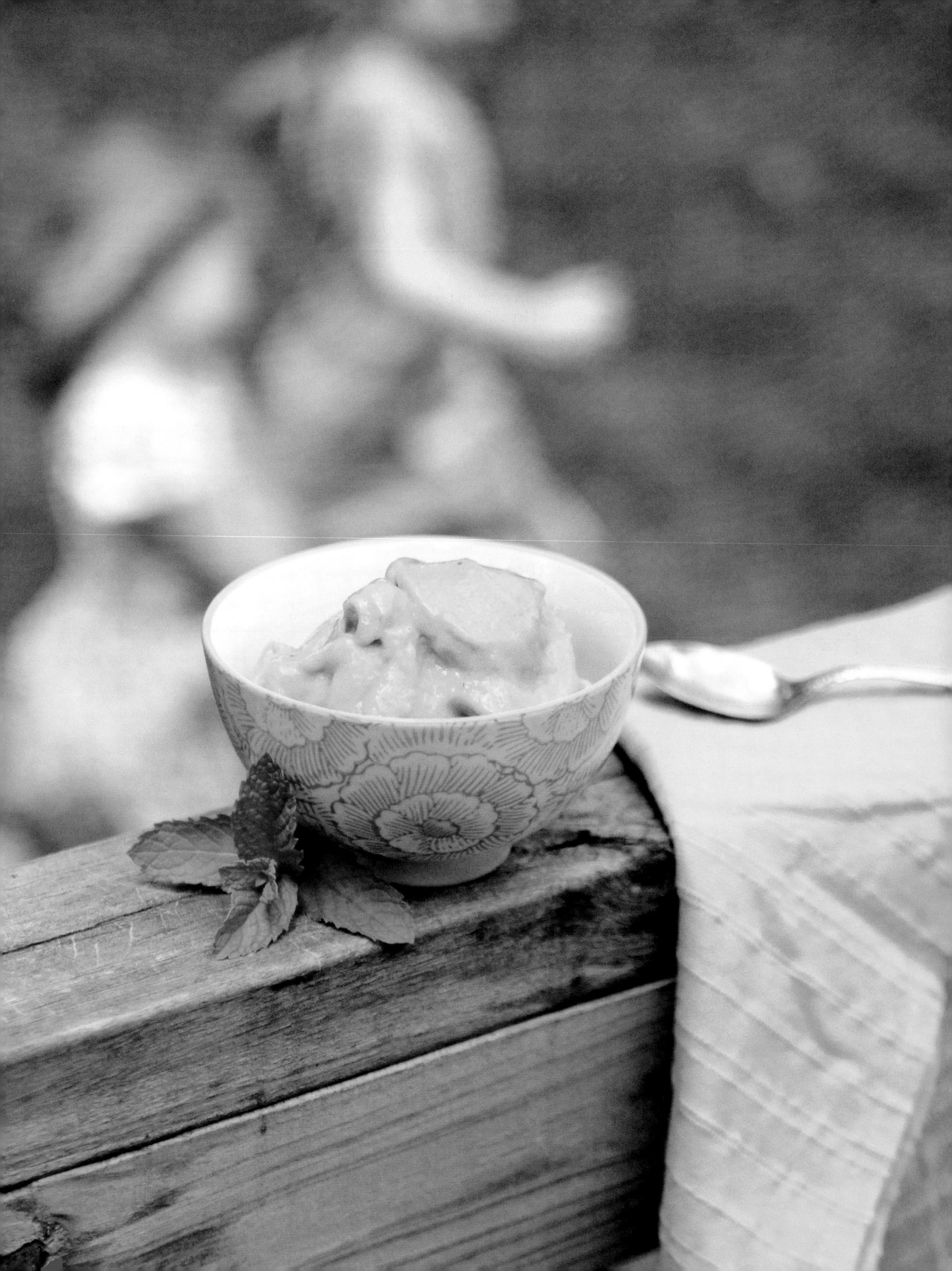

Mulled Wine and Pear Sorbet

This sorbet has a very grown-up flavor and is very refreshing.

PREP TIME: 20 minutes, plus at least 2 hours chilling time
COOK TIME: 15 to 20 minutes, plus 10 to 15 minutes in an ice cream maker
YIELD: 1 quart

INGREDIENTS:

- 2 teaspoons gelatin
- 2 cups red wine
- 1 cinnamon stick
- 2 whole mace avrils
- ½ teaspoon whole cloves
- ½ teaspoon grated fresh ginger
- 2 bay leaves
- Finely grated zest of 1 orange
- Finely grated zest of 1 lemon
- 3 pounds pears, peeled and cored

1. In a small saucepan, sprinkle the gelatin over the wine to bloom. Once the gelatin has turned translucent, add the cinnamon, mace, cloves, ginger, bay leaves, and orange and lemon zests and bring to a boil over medium heat.
2. Reduce the heat to maintain a simmer. Simmer uncovered for 15 to 20 minutes. Remove from the heat and let cool.
3. Pour the wine mixture through a strainer and discard the spices and zest. Put the pears in a blender or food processor along with the strained wine and blend until smooth.
4. Chill the puree in the fridge for at least 2 hours.
5. Blend the chilled puree for 30 seconds, then place in an ice cream maker and churn following the manufacturer's directions. Enjoy! Store any leftovers in the soft zone of your freezer.

TIPS:

If you don't have an ice cream maker, you can make this ice cream by putting the mix in a metal bowl in the freezer and whisking every 20 minutes or so until hardened to ice cream consistency, 3 to 4 hours.

VARIATIONS:

You can use apples in place of pears in this recipe.

You can also freeze the mixture in an ice cube tray, add the ice cubes to a blender, and turn this into a slushy drink using the blender's crush ice or margarita functions.

Mulled Wine. The long simmering cooks off most of the alcohol in the wine. If you like, you can enjoy the mulled wine as a hot beverage (omit the gelatin or leave it in for some extra glycine!) instead of adding the pears and turning it into sorbet.

FODMAP ALERT

This recipe cannot be made low-FODMAP.

SPECIAL EQUIPMENT

- Blender or food processor
- Ice cream maker

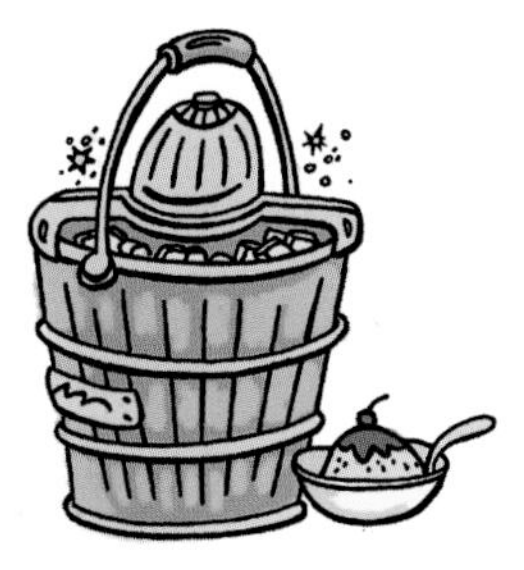

NUTRITION FACTS	
Serving Size	232 g
Recipe Yields	1855 g
Calories	**153**
Fats	**0.32 g**
MUFA	0.16 g
Omega-3	<0.01 g
Omega-6	0.17 g
Saturated Fat	0.06 g
Carbohydrates	**28.4 g**
Fiber	5.74 g
Starch	4.21 g
Fructose	11 g
Glucose	4.46 g
Sucrose	1.25 g
Protein	**1.23 g**
Alanine	0.07 g
Arginine	0.06 g
Aspartic acid	0.22 g
Cystine	<0.01 g
Glutamic acid	0.11 g
Glycine	0.14 g
Histidine	<0.01 g
Isoleucine	0.03 g
Leucine	0.05 g
Lysine	0.05 g
Methionine	<0.01 g
Phenylalanine	0.03 g
Proline	0.11 g
Serine	0.04 g
Threonine	0.03 g
Tryptophan	<0.01 g
Tyrosine	<0.01 g
Valine	0.04 g
Vitamins	
Vitamin B1	0.03 mg
Vitamin B12	0 mcg
Vitamin B2	0.07 mg
Vitamin B3	0.43 mg
Vitamin B5	0.12 mg
Vitamin B6	0.09 mg
Choline	12.7 mg
Folate	13.6 mcg
Vitamin A	2.68 mcg
Vitamin C	9.45 mg
Vitamin D	0 IU
Vitamin E	0.23 mg
Vitamin K	8.02 mcg
Minerals	
Calcium	28.9 mg
Copper	0.17 mg
Iron	0.75 mg
Magnesium	20.4 mg
Manganese	0.32 mg
Phosphorus	35.2 mg
Potassium	280 mg
Selenium	0.56 mcg
Sodium	5.84 mg
Zinc	0.28 mg

nutrition content estimated using the USDA database.

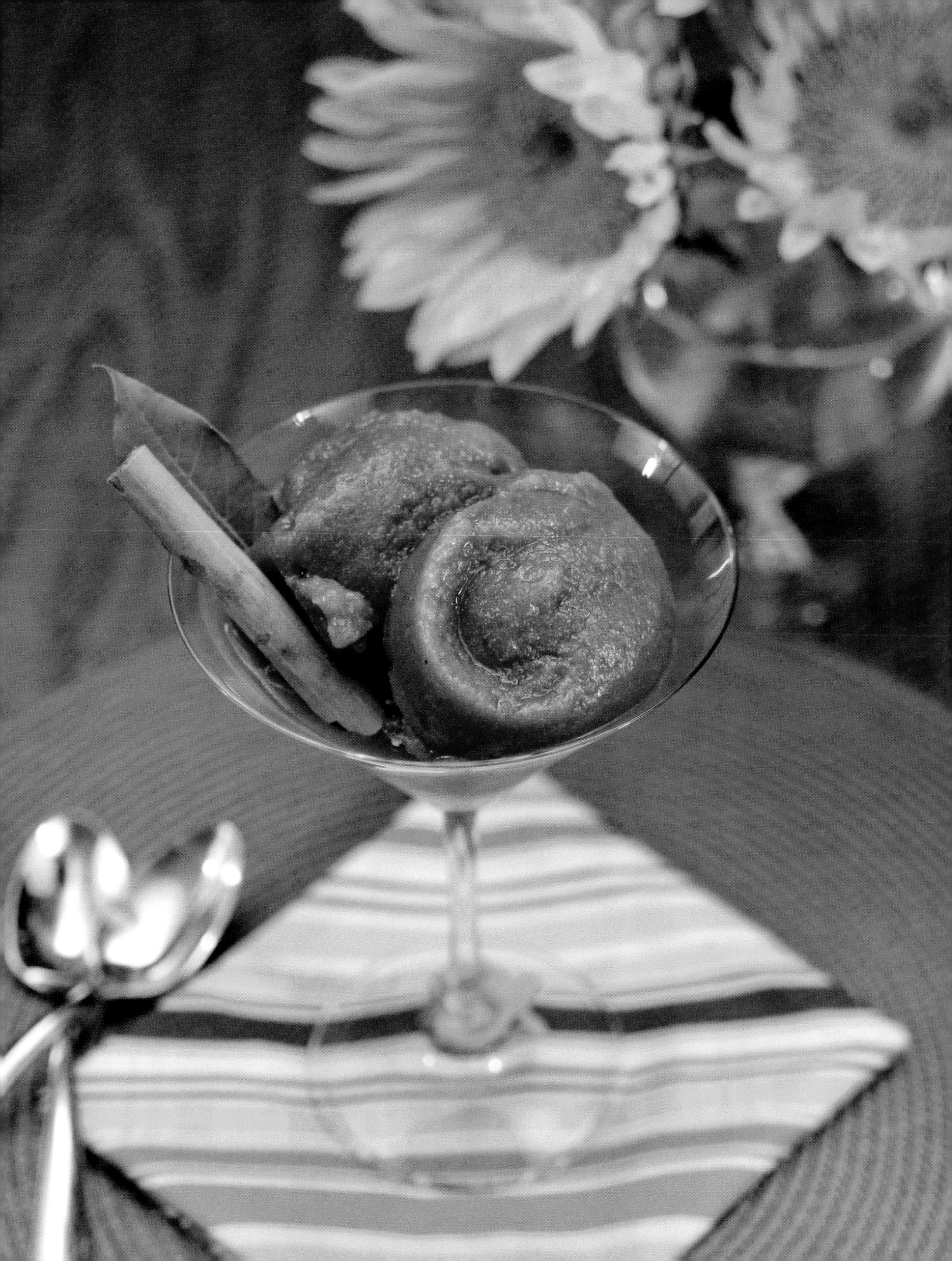

Banana Bread Squares

These banana bread squares could easily replace a muffin with your breakfast or be used as a lunchbox treat in an allergy-free school. You could also serve them with Coconut Whipped Topping (page 116) and enjoy them as a decadent dessert!

The riper the bananas, the sweeter this bread will be. Ideally, they should be covered in black spots and getting soft. If you have overripe bananas and aren't ready to make this bread, peel them and place them in a freezer bag until you are ready.

PREP TIME: 30 minutes, plus 2 hours for the gelatin to set
COOK TIME: 45 minutes
YIELD: 16 squares

INGREDIENTS:

- 2 tablespoons gelatin
- ¼ cup cool water
- ¼ cup boiling water
- ½ cup palm shortening, plus more for the pan
- 3 large overripe bananas, peeled
- 2 cups Plantain Flour (page 121)
- 1 tablespoon fresh lemon juice
- ½ teaspoon ground cinnamon
- ½ teaspoon salt
- 1 teaspoon baking soda

1. In a heat-safe measuring cup, bloom the gelatin by sprinkling it over the cool water. Stir, then let it sit for 3 to 4 minutes.
2. Add the boiling water to the gelatin mix. Stir until the gelatin has dissolved completely. (This may take several minutes. Let it sit after stirring initially, then stir every couple of minutes to check if the gelatin has dissolved.)
3. Refrigerate the gelatin until set, about 2 hours.
4. Preheat the oven to 350°F. Grease a 9-by-9-inch baking pan with palm shortening.
5. Combine the set gelatin and the remaining ingredients in a food processor. Process until completely smooth, at least 4 to 5 minutes, turning off the food processor to scrape the sides at least once.
6. Pour the batter into the prepared pan. Smooth out the top with a rubber spatula. Bake until the banana bread is golden brown and a toothpick inserted in the center comes out clean, about 45 minutes.
7. Let the bread cool for at least 10 minutes before inverting the pan. Cut into squares and enjoy!

FODMAP ALERT

This recipe cannot be made low-FODMAP.

SPECIAL EQUIPMENT

- Food processor

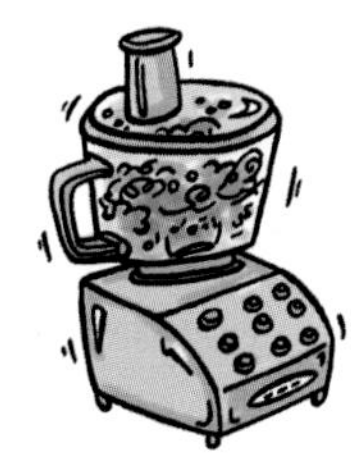

TIPS:

If you don't want to make your own plantain flour, it can be found in some ethnic grocery stores and online (it is sometimes called fufu flour). Check the ingredients, since plantain flour is sometimes combined with potato starch and other starches.

Like all baked goods that use plantains or plantain flour, these go stale quickly. Store in a resealable plastic bag with as much air pushed out as possible. Or, better yet, freeze any squares you don't plan to eat the same day you bake them (freeze on a baking sheet and then move to a freezer-safe container once frozen).

VARIATIONS:

This banana bread is also tasty with ½ teaspoon ground mace instead of cinnamon.

You can bake this bread in two 9-by-5-inch loaf pans, or make banana bread "pucks" (squat muffins, similar in dimension to hockey pucks) by baking in a muffin tin (in either case, reduce the baking time). However, if you try to bake it as a single, taller loaf of bread or as muffins, it will collapse.

NUTRITION FACTS	
Serving Size	58 g
Recipe Yields	931 g
Calories	**165**
Fats	**6.88 g**
MUFA	2.02 g
Omega-3	<0.01 g
Omega-6	0.05 g
Saturated Fat	4.48 g
Carbohydrates	**21.3 g**
Fiber	2.2 g
Starch	1.43 g
Fructose	1.24 g
Glucose	1.28 g
Sucrose	0.61 g
Protein	**5.52 g**
Alanine	0.08 g
Arginine	0.07 g
Aspartic acid	0.08 g
Cystine	<0.01 g
Glutamic acid	0.12 g
Glycine	0.18 g
Histidine	0.03 g
Isoleucine	0.02 g
Leucine	0.04 g
Lysine	0.04 g
Methionine	<0.01 g
Phenylalanine	0.03 g
Proline	0.11 g
Serine	0.03 g
Threonine	0.02 g
Tryptophan	<0.01 g
Tyrosine	<0.01 g
Valine	0.03 g
Vitamins	
Vitamin B1	<0.01 mg
Vitamin B12	0 mcg
Vitamin B2	0.02 mg
Vitamin B3	0.17 mg
Vitamin B5	0.09 mg
Vitamin B6	0.09 mg
Choline	2.88 mg
Folate	5.54 mcg
Vitamin A	0.77 mcg
Vitamin C	2.58 mg
Vitamin D	0 IU
Vitamin E	1.32 mg
Vitamin K	0.15 mcg
Minerals	
Calcium	2.98 mg
Copper	0.04 mg
Iron	0.27 mg
Magnesium	7.16 mg
Manganese	0.08 mg
Phosphorus	6.06 mg
Potassium	93.6 mg
Selenium	0.6 mcg
Sodium	112 mg
Zinc	0.04 mg

nutrition content estimated using the USDA database.

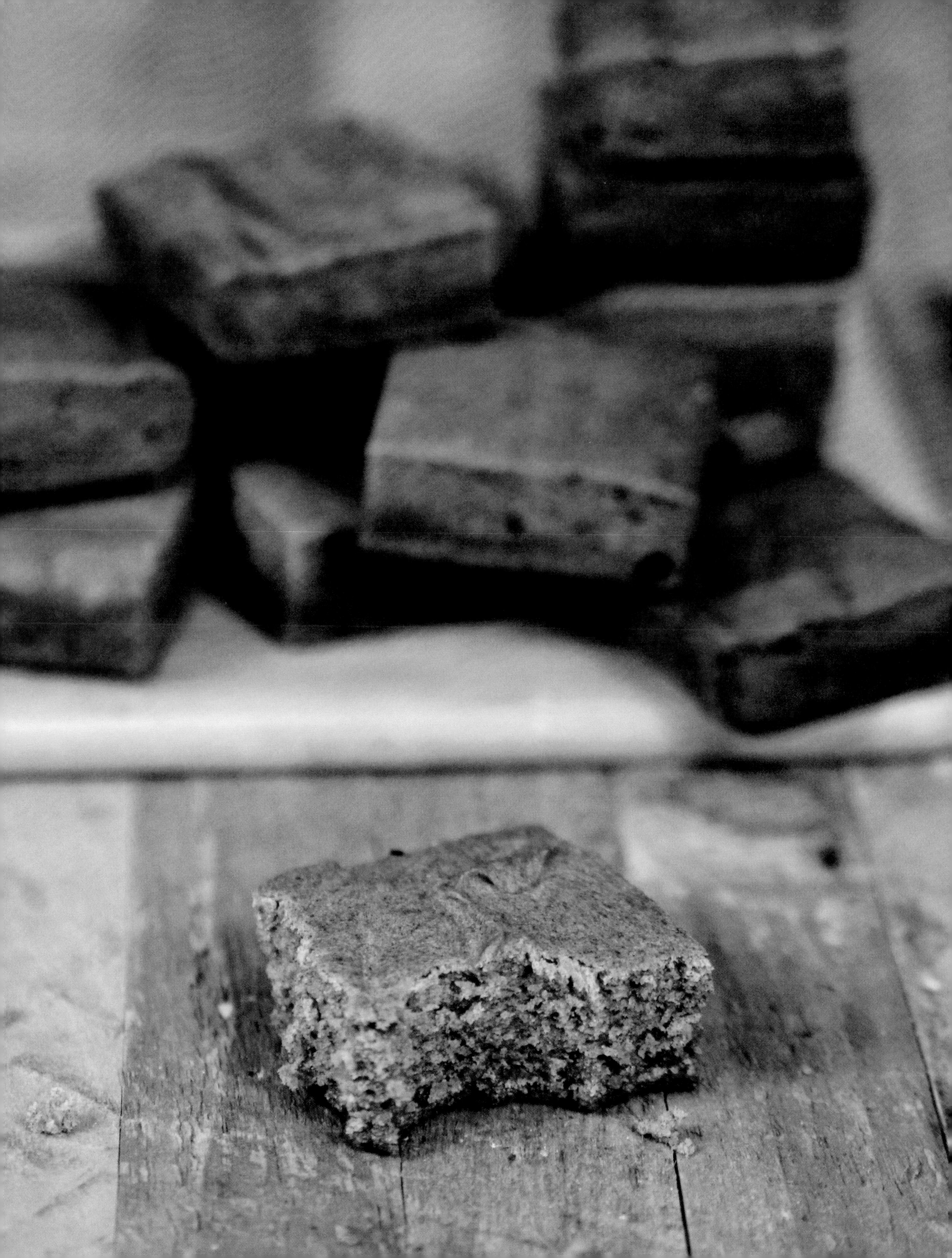

Apple Pie–Stuffed Apples

These apples are fun to eat and delicious. They make a great dessert but can also find a home on your dinner plate, especially when served beside pork roast or chops!

PREP TIME: 20 to 30 minutes
COOK TIME: 45 minutes to 1 hour
SERVINGS: 2

INGREDIENTS:

- 2 Fuji apples
- ½ teaspoon ground cinnamon
- ½ teaspoon finely grated lemon zest
- 1 tablespoon fresh lemon juice
- Pinch of salt

1. Preheat the oven to 375°F. Line a rimmed baking sheet with parchment paper, aluminum foil, or a silicone liner.
2. Make the apple "bowls" by cutting the top off each apple. Use an apple corer or sharp knife to core the apple, being careful not to cut all the way to the bottom. Use a melon baller to scoop out the most of the apple, leaving about ¼ inch of apple flesh so as not to rip the peel.
3. Roughly chop the scooped-out apple flesh and place it in a bowl. Toss the chopped apple with the cinnamon, lemon zest and juice, and salt. Stuff the apple "bowls" with the seasoned apple pieces.
4. Bake for 45 minutes to 1 hour, depending on the size of your apples, until the apples are soft and delicious!

FODMAP ALERT

This recipe cannot be made low-FODMAP.

SPECIAL EQUIPMENT

- Melon baller

TIPS:

Granny Smith apples are also great cooking apples. If you choose to use them, you will probably want to add some muscovado sugar to the apple pieces to cut through the tartness.

VARIATIONS:

If you want to keep this simple, just peel, core, and chop the apples, season, and cook in a baking dish. You can also double or triple the recipe and use it as the base for Apple Crisp (page 352).

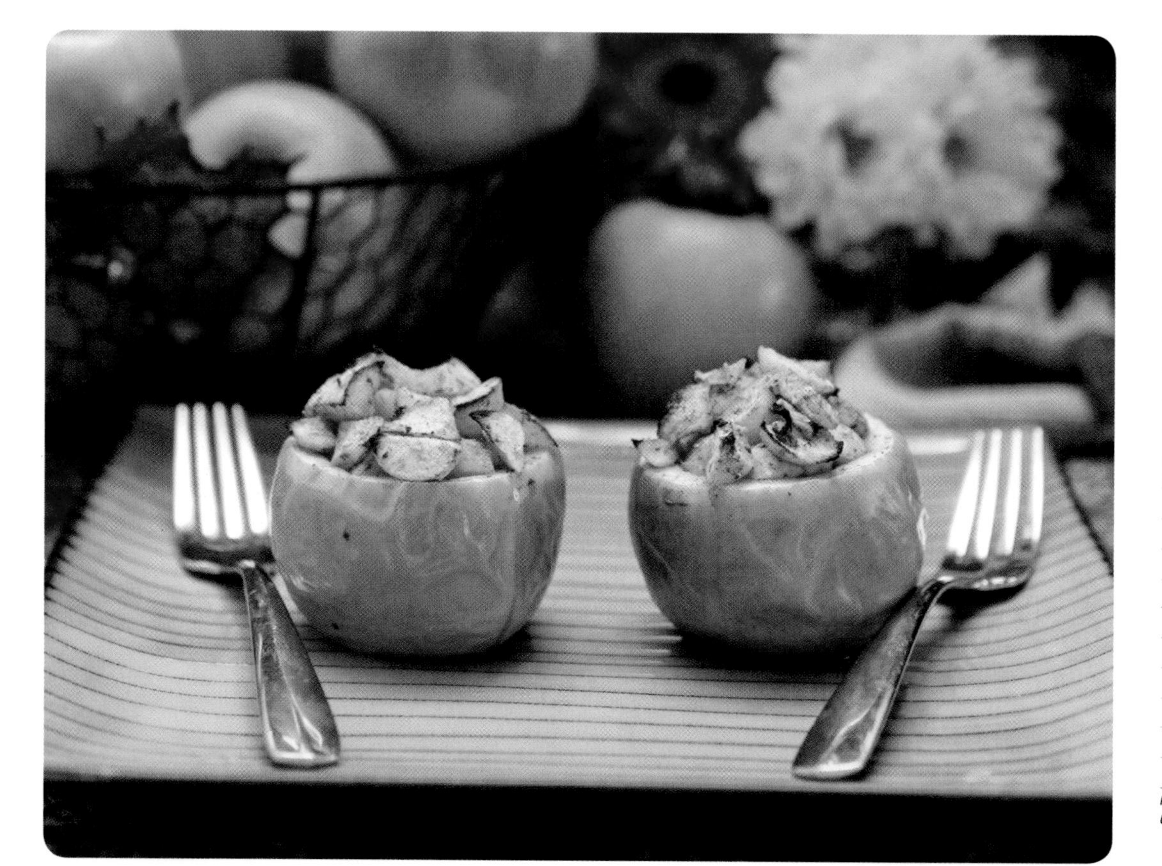

NUTRITION FACTS	
Serving Size	191 g
Recipe Yields	382 g
Calories	**98.1**
Fats	**0.34 g**
MUFA	0.01 g
Omega-3	0.02 g
Omega-6	0.08 g
Saturated Fat	0.06 g
Carbohydrates	**26.3 g**
Fiber	4.79 g
Starch	0.57 g
Fructose	10.8 g
Glucose	4.5 g
Sucrose	3.8 g
Protein	**0.53 g**
Alanine	0.02 g
Arginine	0.01 g
Aspartic acid	0.13 g
Cystine	<0.01 g
Glutamic acid	0.05 g
Glycine	0.02 g
Histidine	<0.01 g
Isoleucine	0.01 g
Leucine	0.03 g
Lysine	0.02 g
Methionine	<0.01 g
Phenylalanine	0.01 g
Proline	0.01 g
Serine	0.02 g
Threonine	0.01 g
Tryptophan	<0.01 g
Tyrosine	<0.01 g
Valine	0.02 g
Vitamins	
Vitamin B1	0.03 mg
Vitamin B12	0 mcg
Vitamin B2	0.05 mg
Vitamin B3	0.18 mg
Vitamin B5	0.12 mg
Vitamin B6	0.08 mg
Choline	6.69 mg
Folate	7.08 mcg
Vitamin A	5.57 mcg
Vitamin C	12 mg
Vitamin D	0 IU
Vitamin E	0.36 mg
Vitamin K	4.2 mcg
Minerals	
Calcium	19.3 mg
Copper	0.05 mg
Iron	0.66 mg
Magnesium	10 mg
Manganese	0.18 mg
Phosphorus	21.1 mg
Potassium	208 mg
Selenium	0.03 mcg
Sodium	66.1 mg
Zinc	0.09 mg

nutrition content estimated using the USDA database.

Parsnip Vanilla Custard

Pureed roasted parsnip gives this "custard" a wonderful texture, added sweetness, and a mildly nutty flavor.

PREP TIME: 40 minutes
COOK TIME: 40 minutes, plus 1 to 2 hours chilling time
SERVINGS: 6 to 8

INGREDIENTS:

- 1 pound parsnips
- 1 tablespoon extra-virgin coconut oil, melted
- 3⅓ cups homemade Coconut Milk (page 116) or 2 (13½-ounce) cans full-fat coconut milk
- 3 tablespoons vanilla extract
- 1 bay leaf
- 2 tablespoons honey

FODMAP ALERT *If you do not tolerate coconut milk, skip this recipe. Otherwise, use maple syrup instead of honey.*

SPECIAL EQUIPMENT

- Blender or immersion blender

1. Preheat the oven to 350°F.
2. Peel and chop the parsnips into large pieces and rub with coconut oil to coat. Place on a rimmed baking sheet and roast for 40 minutes, until soft and starting to brown.
3. Meanwhile, combine the coconut milk, vanilla, and bay leaf in a saucepot. Bring to a simmer over medium heat and simmer for 20 minutes.
4. Add the parsnips to the coconut milk, remove from the heat, remove and discard the bay leaf, and purée with an immersion blender (you can also use a countertop blender, being careful not to burn yourself). Let cool. Mix in the honey.
5. Refrigerate the parsnip puree until cold, 1 to 2 hours. Enjoy!

VARIATIONS:

Instead of vanilla extract, add 2 Madagascar vanilla beans to the coconut milk. After simmering, remove the vanilla beans, slice open, scrape out the seeds, and return to the coconut milk. Follow steps 4 and 5 as above.

This custard works well with other root vegetables, too! Try carrots with a little cinnamon or winter squash.

Frozen Custard. You can turn this into frozen custard by adding 2 teaspoons gelatin to the coconut milk (bloom in the cold coconut milk before heating) and then churning in an ice cream maker.

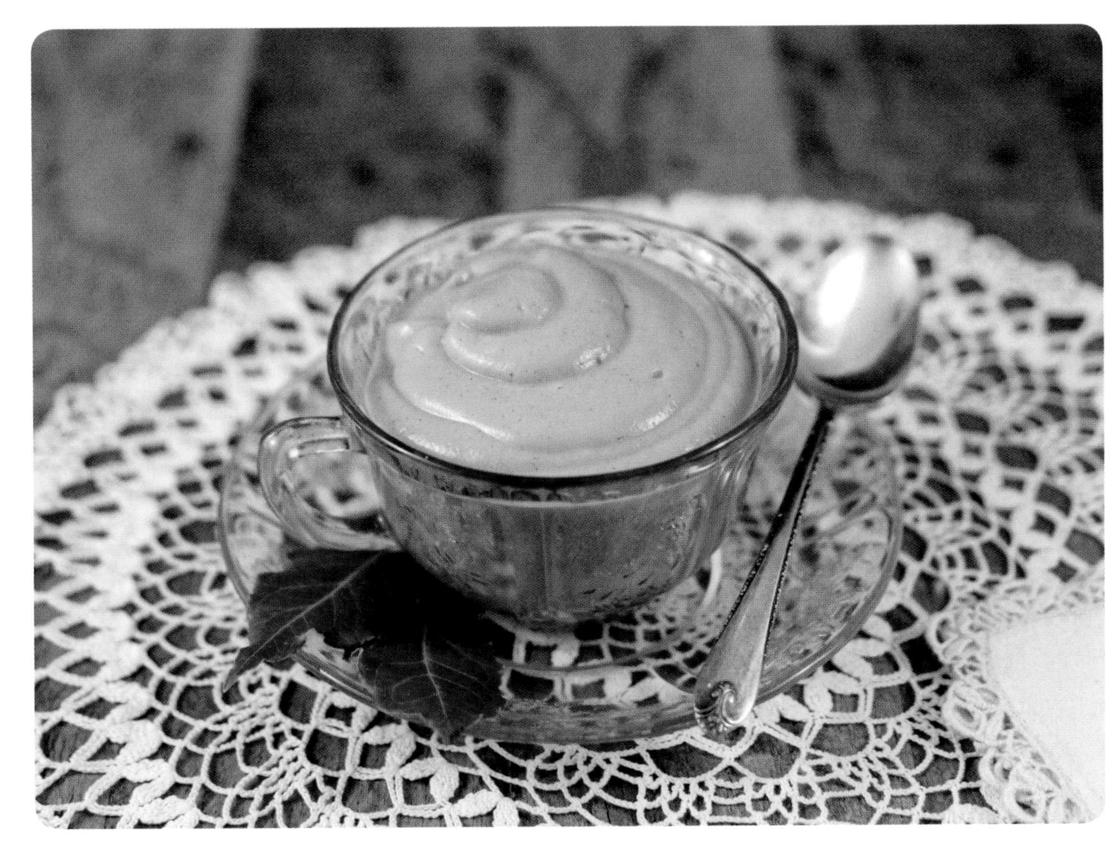

NUTRITION FACTS	
Serving Size	163 g
Recipe Yields	1303 g
Calories	**274**
Fats	**22 g**
MUFA	1.02 g
Omega-3	<0.01 g
Omega-6	0.28 g
Saturated Fat	19.3 g
Carbohydrates	**18 g**
Fiber	2.85 g
Starch	4.71 g
Fructose	2.15 g
Glucose	1.88 g
Sucrose	0.05 g
Protein	**2.62 g**
Alanine	0.1 g
Arginine	0.31 g
Aspartic acid	0.19 g
Cystine	0.04 g
Glutamic acid	0.44 g
Glycine	0.09 g
Histidine	0.04 g
Isoleucine	0.07 g
Leucine	0.14 g
Lysine	0.08 g
Methionine	0.04 g
Phenylalanine	0.1 g
Proline	0.08 g
Serine	0.1 g
Threonine	0.07 g
Tryptophan	0.02 g
Tyrosine	0.06 g
Valine	0.12 g
Vitamins	
Vitamin B1	0.07 mg
Vitamin B12	0 mcg
Vitamin B2	0.04 mg
Vitamin B3	1.03 mg
Vitamin B5	0.5 mg
Vitamin B6	0.08 mg
Choline	8.26 mg
Folate	51.7 mcg
Vitamin A	0.7 mcg
Vitamin C	10.7 mg
Vitamin D	0 IU
Vitamin E	0.85 mg
Vitamin K	12.8 mcg
Minerals	
Calcium	40.1 mg
Copper	0.28 mg
Iron	3.57 mg
Magnesium	60.7 mg
Manganese	1.07 mg
Phosphorus	131 mg
Potassium	431 mg
Selenium	1.07 mcg
Sodium	18.6 mg
Zinc	0.89 mg

nutrition content estimated using the USDA database.

Blueberry Crisp

The secret to this blueberry crisp is to cook down half of the blueberries until they are the thickness of jam. The sweeter your blueberries, the sweeter your crisp will be.

PREP TIME: 30 minutes
COOK TIME: 1 hour
SERVINGS: 6 to 10

INGREDIENTS:

Topping:

1 batch Plantain Crackers (page 149)

2 tablespoons muscovado sugar

1½ tablespoons extra-virgin coconut oil, melted

½ teaspoon ground cinnamon

¼ teaspoon ground mace

Blueberry Base:

24 ounces blueberries (about 5 cups), fresh or frozen

2 tablespoons arrowroot powder

1 Granny Smith apple, peeled and grated

Finely grated zest of 1 lemon

Juice of 1 lemon

Pinch of salt

FODMAP ALERT

This recipe cannot be made low-FODMAP.

SPECIAL EQUIPMENT

- Food processor

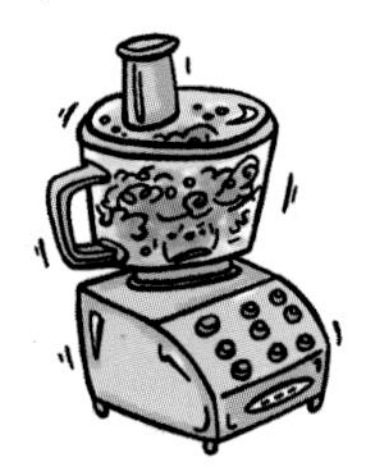

1. Make the topping: Place the plantain crackers in a food processor and process until they are fine crumbs. Combine with the sugar, coconut oil, cinnamon, and mace. Refrigerate for at least 1 hour.
2. Make the base: Heat 2½ cups of the blueberries in a saucepan over medium heat. Cook, stirring frequently, until thick, 20 to 25 minutes. Remove from the heat and let cool.
3. Combine the cooked blueberries with the remaining ingredients for the base in a bowl. Stir to fully mix. Place in a pie pan, casserole dish, or individual ramekins (about 8).
4. Preheat the oven to 425°F.
5. Use a knife or spoon to break up the crisp topping (you want to keep some larger chunks) and distribute it evenly over the surface of the blueberry base.
6. Bake for 25 to 30 minutes, until bubbling and browned on top (bake for 15 to 20 minutes if using individual ramekins).
7. Enjoy warm or chilled.

TIPS:

When you make Plantain Crackers for this recipe, omit or halve the salt.

If you like a really crunchy crisp, you can process your Plantain Crackers a little less to leave some slightly bigger pieces.

VARIATIONS:

If you don't want to make Plantain Crackers for the crumble, you can use store-bought plantain chips instead.

Apple Crisp. Make a double batch of the Apple Pie–Stuffed Apples recipe on page 350 to use as the base (core, peel, and chop the whole apples instead of coring and scooping out the middle) and top with the crisp topping.

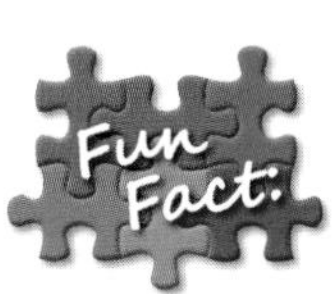

Most berries have more antioxidants when cooked.

NUTRITION FACTS	
Serving Size	145 g
Recipe Yields	1453 g
Calories	**222**
Fats	**13.3 g**
MUFA	0.8 g
Omega-3	0.05 g
Omega-6	0.32 g
Saturated Fat	11.3 g
Carbohydrates	**28.5 g**
Fiber	3.1 g
Starch	5.48 g
Fructose	4.5 g
Glucose	3.8 g
Sucrose	3.2 g
Protein	**1.05 g**
Alanine	0.04 g
Arginine	0.07 g
Aspartic acid	0.09 g
Cystine	0.01 g
Glutamic acid	0.11 g
Glycine	0.04 g
Histidine	0.03 g
Isoleucine	0.03 g
Leucine	0.05 g
Lysine	0.03 g
Methionine	0.01 g
Phenylalanine	0.03 g
Proline	0.04 g
Serine	0.03 g
Threonine	0.03 g
Tryptophan	<0.01 g
Tyrosine	0.02 g
Valine	0.04 g
Vitamins	
Vitamin B1	0.05 mg
Vitamin B12	0 mcg
Vitamin B2	0.05 mg
Vitamin B3	0.55 mg
Vitamin B5	0.2 mg
Vitamin B6	0.15 mg
Choline	9.86 mg
Folate	13.7 mcg
Vitamin A	22.7 mcg
Vitamin C	16.6 mg
Vitamin D	0 IU
Vitamin E	0.49 mg
Vitamin K	13.9 mcg
Minerals	
Calcium	10.4 mg
Copper	0.08 mg
Iron	0.85 mg
Magnesium	18.8 mg
Manganese	0.27 mg
Phosphorus	23 mg
Potassium	260 mg
Selenium	0.62 mcg
Sodium	66.6 mg
Zinc	0.18 mg

nutrition content estimated using the USDA database.

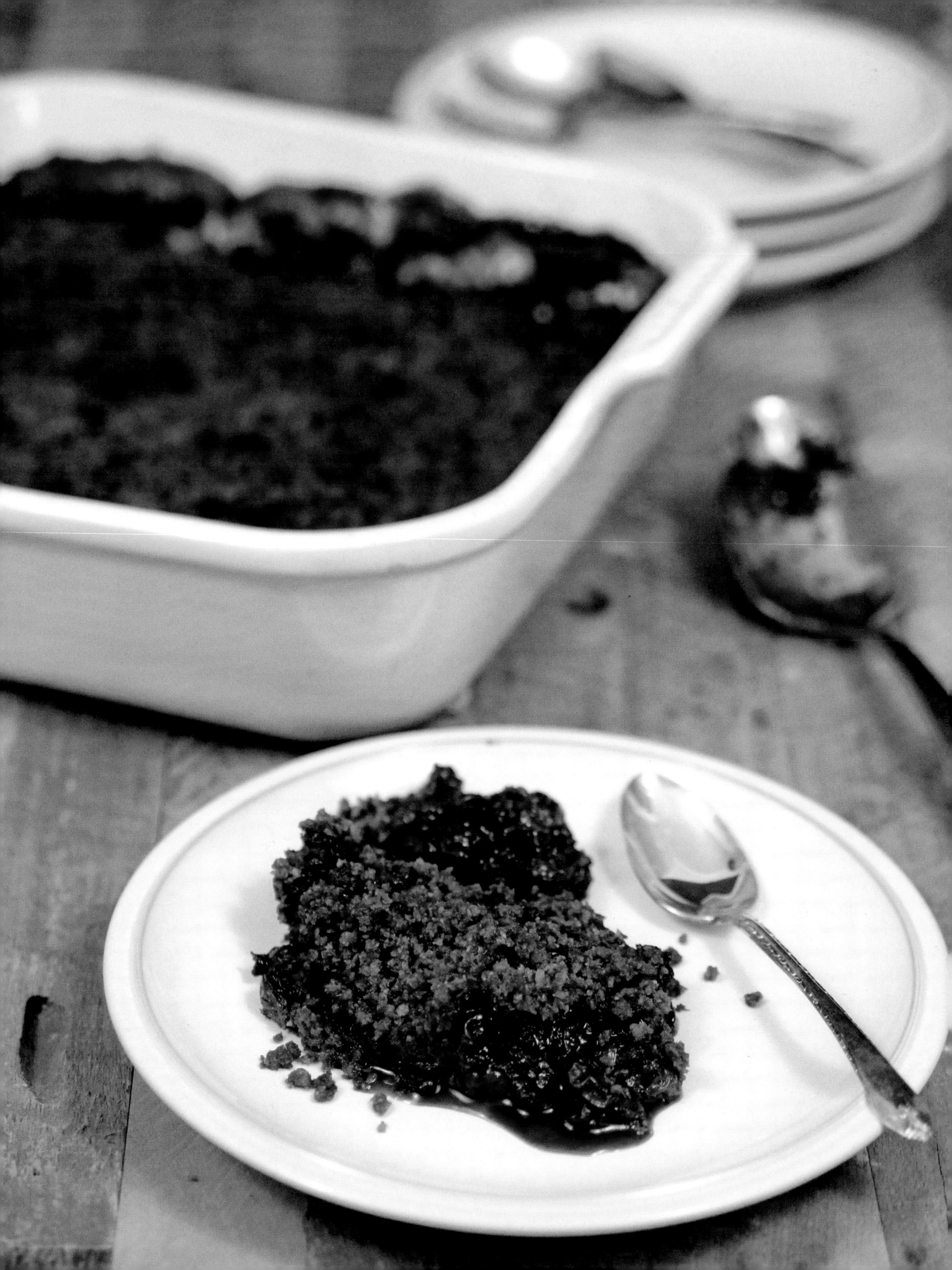

Piña Colada Popsicles

The tropical flavor combination of pineapple and coconut is so refreshing. Simmering dark rum removes most of the alcohol, but the flavor it contributes is still wonderful. Alcohol-free rum extract can be used as a substitute, or the rum can be omitted altogether.

This recipe makes 10 (3-ounce) popsicles and can easily be scaled up or down to accommodate your popsicle molds.

PREP TIME: 10 minutes
COOK TIME: 20 minutes, plus 4 to 6 hours freezing time
YIELD: 10 popsicles

INGREDIENTS:

- 1 cup dark rum (optional)
- 2 cups fresh pineapple chunks (about 1 small pineapple)
- 1¼ cups Coconut Cream (page 116)

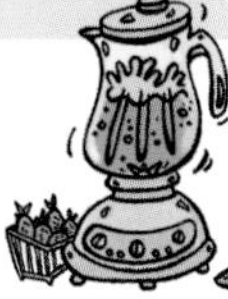

SPECIAL EQUIPMENT

- Blender or food processor
- Popsicle molds

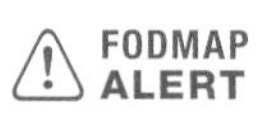

FODMAP ALERT

If you do not tolerate coconut milk or cream, skip this recipe.

1. If using rum, place in a small saucepan and bring to a simmer over medium-high heat. Reduce the heat to maintain a rapid simmer for 20 minutes, until you can't smell alcohol in the vapors and the volume has decreased by about three-quarters.
2. Combine the pineapple, coconut cream, and reduced rum in a blender or food processor. Blend until completely smooth, about 2 minutes.
3. Pour into popsicle molds and place in the freezer until completely frozen, 4 to 6 hours.

VARIATIONS:

Piña Colada Cocktail. Instead of making popsicles, you can pour some of the piña colada mixture into a blender along with some ice and purée to make a sweet and refreshing dessert drink. Don't forget a little paper umbrella!

You can also churn this mixture in an ice cream maker for piña colada ice cream. For smoother ice cream, add 2 teaspoons gelatin to the coconut cream, then heat to dissolve before blending with the other ingredients.

If you are making your popsicles without rum, try adding 1 teaspoon finely grated lime zest.

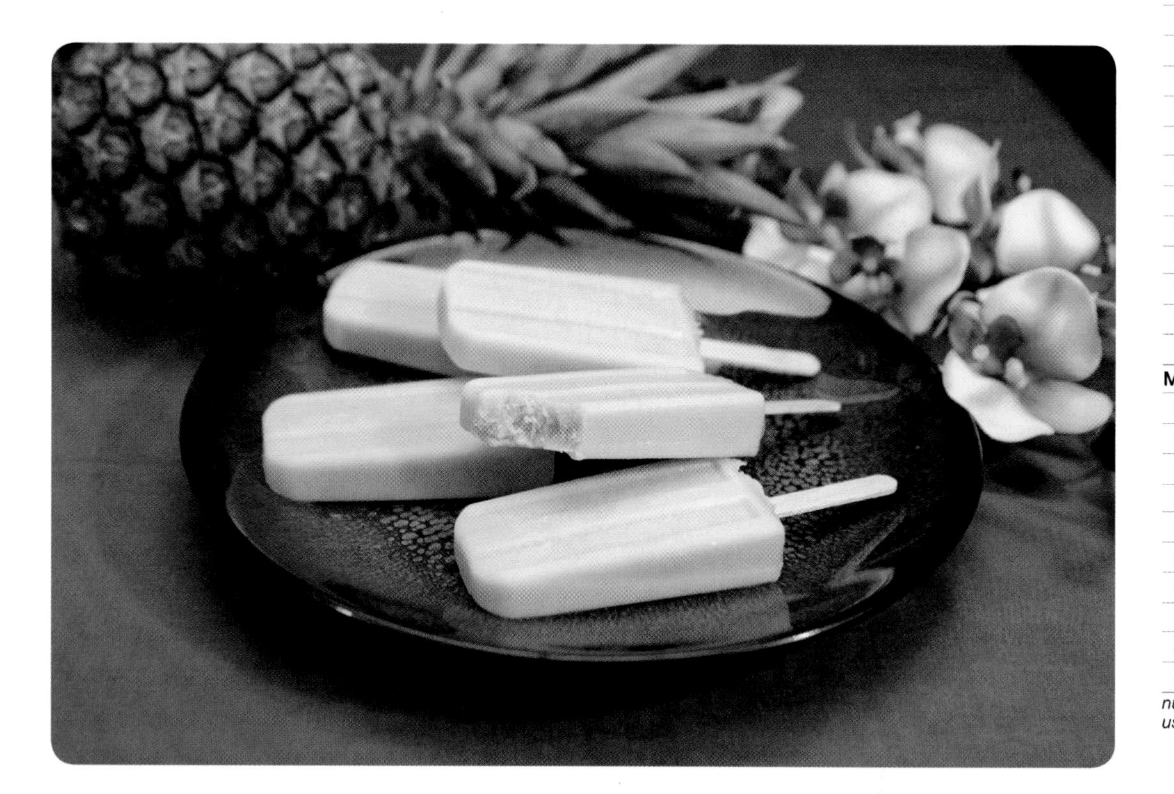

NUTRITION FACTS	
Serving Size	61 g
Recipe Yields	613 g
Calories	**71.9**
Fats	**6.04 g**
MUFA	0.26 g
Omega-3	<0.01 g
Omega-6	0.07 g
Saturated Fat	5.32 g
Carbohydrates	**5.1 g**
Fiber	0.46 g
Starch	0.61 g
Fructose	0.7 g
Glucose	0.57 g
Sucrose	1.97 g
Protein	**0.75 g**
Alanine	0.04 g
Arginine	0.1 g
Aspartic acid	0.1 g
Cystine	0.02 g
Glutamic acid	0.16 g
Glycine	0.03 g
Histidine	0.02 g
Isoleucine	0.03 g
Leucine	0.05 g
Lysine	0.03 g
Methionine	0.01 g
Phenylalanine	0.04 g
Proline	0.03 g
Serine	0.04 g
Threonine	0.03 g
Tryptophan	<0.01 g
Tyrosine	0.02 g
Valine	0.04 g
Vitamins	
Vitamin B1	0.03 mg
Vitamin B12	0 mcg
Vitamin B2	0.01 mg
Vitamin B3	0.34 mg
Vitamin B5	0.11 mg
Vitamin B6	0.04 mg
Choline	4.2 mg
Folate	9.85 mcg
Vitamin A	0.99 mcg
Vitamin C	16 mg
Vitamin D	0 IU
Vitamin E	<0.01 mg
Vitamin K	0.23 mcg
Minerals	
Calcium	9.34 mg
Copper	0.1 mg
Iron	1.02 mg
Magnesium	16.9 mg
Manganese	0.52 mg
Phosphorus	29.6 mg
Potassium	97.7 mg
Selenium	0.03 mcg
Sodium	3.99 mg
Zinc	0.2 mg

nutrition content estimated using the USDA database.

Olive Oil Ice "Cream"

Olive oil ice "cream" is one of the most amazingly decadent and delicious ice cream flavors you will ever try. This recipe is meant to be made with very high-quality olive oil, so you also get the benefit of the extremely high polyphenol content. Top this ice cream with a thick aged balsamic vinegar and prepare yourself for a life-changing dessert experience that also happens to be full of antioxidants!

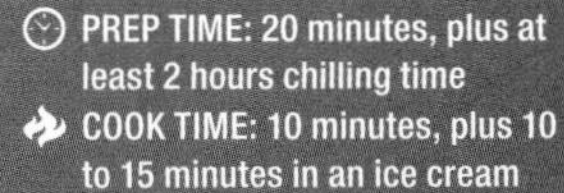

PREP TIME: 20 minutes, plus at least 2 hours chilling time
COOK TIME: 10 minutes, plus 10 to 15 minutes in an ice cream maker
YIELD: 1 quart

INGREDIENTS:

- 1¾ cups homemade Coconut Milk or Coconut Cream (page 116) or 1 (13½-ounce) can full-fat coconut milk
- 1 tablespoon gelatin
- ⅔ cup high-quality extra-virgin olive oil
- ¼ cup honey
- ¼ teaspoon salt
- ⅛ teaspoon vanilla powder or ½ teaspoon vanilla extract

FODMAP ALERT

This recipe cannot be made low-FODMAP.

SPECIAL EQUIPMENT

- Blender or food processor
- Ice cream maker

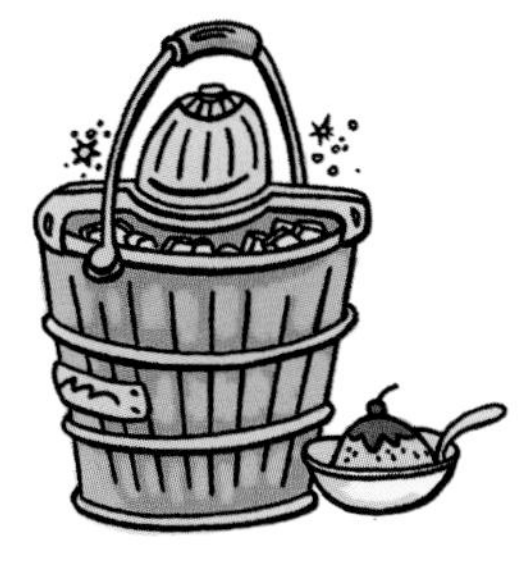

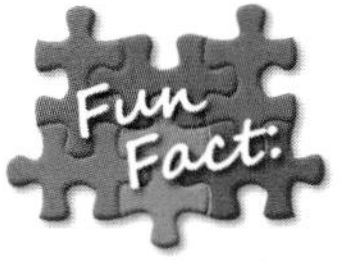

High-quality fresh olive oil is very high in antioxidant polyphenols, which give it a peppery taste. You know you have good-quality olive oil if, when you take a sip, you feel a peppery heat at the back of your throat.

1. In a small saucepan, sprinkle the gelatin over the coconut milk to bloom. Let it sit until the gelatin has absorbed some of the liquid and turned translucent. Place the pan over medium heat, stirring gently, until the gelatin has dissolved. Remove from the heat and let cool.
2. Combine the cooled milk and gelatin mixture with the rest of the ingredients in a blender or food processor. Blend until completely smooth.
3. Chill the mixture in the fridge for at least 2 hours.
4. Blend the chilled mixture for 30 seconds. Then place in an ice cream maker and churn following the manufacturer's directions. Enjoy! Store any leftovers in the soft zone of your freezer.

TIPS:

If you don't have an ice cream maker, you can make this ice cream by freezing it most of the way in a freezer-safe container, putting it back in the blender or food processor and puréeing for 1 minute, and then freezing until solid.

Don't be tempted to use olive oil ice "cream" with another dessert for "à la mode." While absolutely sublime with balsamic vinegar, it doesn't pair well with most other desserts.

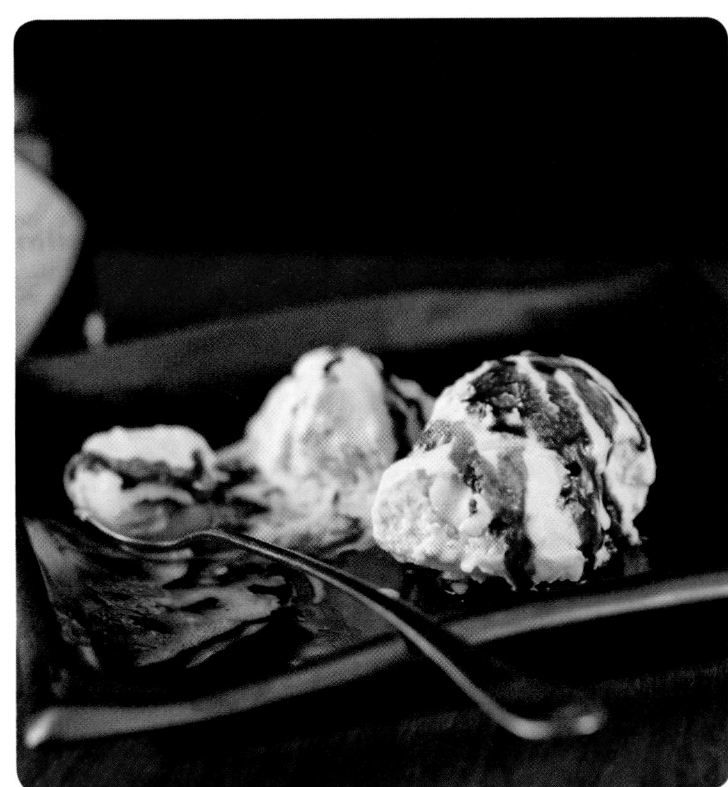

NUTRITION FACTS

Serving Size	79 g
Recipe Yields	634 g
Calories	**292**
Fats	**28.6 g**
MUFA	13.6 g
Omega-3	0.14 g
Omega-6	1.88 g
Saturated Fat	11.8 g
Carbohydrates	**10.1 g**
Fiber	0.02 g
Starch	<0.01 g
Fructose	4.32 g
Glucose	3.78 g
Sucrose	0.09 g
Protein	**1.77 g**
Alanine	0.12 g
Arginine	0.22 g
Aspartic acid	0.15 g
Cystine	0.02 g
Glutamic acid	0.31 g
Glycine	0.21 g
Histidine	0.03 g
Isoleucine	0.05 g
Leucine	0.1 g
Lysine	0.07 g
Methionine	0.02 g
Phenylalanine	0.07 g
Proline	0.16 g
Serine	0.07 g
Threonine	0.05 g
Tryptophan	0.01 g
Tyrosine	0.03 g
Valine	0.08 g
Vitamins	
Vitamin B1	0.01 mg
Vitamin B12	0 mcg
Vitamin B2	<0.01 mg
Vitamin B3	0.33 mg
Vitamin B5	0.08 mg
Vitamin B6	0.02 mg
Choline	4.81 mg
Folate	7.37 mcg
Vitamin A	0 mcg
Vitamin C	0.55 mg
Vitamin D	0 IU
Vitamin E	2.59 mg
Vitamin K	10.9 mcg
Minerals	
Calcium	10.5 mg
Copper	0.13 mg
Iron	1.97 mg
Magnesium	23.1 mg
Manganese	0.39 mg
Phosphorus	48.1 mg
Potassium	115 mg
Selenium	0.43 mcg
Sodium	40.9 mg
Zinc	0.3 mg

nutrition content estimated using the USDA database.

Carob Brownie Bites

Carob is a wonderful substitute for chocolate. While carob is technically a legume, carob powder is made from the pod of the bean and not the bean itself.

PREP TIME: 20 minutes
COOK TIME: 9 to 10 minutes
YIELD: 12 to 16 cookies

INGREDIENTS:

- 1 large green plantain
- ¼ cup palm shortening
- 2 tablespoons extra-virgin coconut oil
- 2 tablespoons molasses
- ½ cup carob powder
- 2 tablespoons tapioca flour
- 2 tablespoons arrowroot powder
- 2 teaspoons vanilla extract
- ⅛ teaspoon baking soda
- Pinch of salt
- Pinch of ground cinnamon

1. Preheat the oven to 350°F.
2. Peel the green plantain (see page 57). Place the plantain, palm shortening, coconut oil, and molasses in a food processor and process for 2 to 3 minutes, until it is a smooth puree.
3. Add the remaining ingredients and process until combined.
4. Using your hands, roll the dough into 1½-inch balls and place on a baking sheet. Use your palm or the bottom of a glass to flatten the dough balls to ½ inch thick.
5. Bake for 9 to 10 minutes, until the balls are just starting to brown on the bottom and edges. Let cool and enjoy.

VARIATIONS:

These bites can be made with either tapioca or arrowroot powder if you have a sensitivity to (or can't source) one or the other. Simply use a full 4 tablespoons of one or the other. When made with arrowroot, the texture is a little denser and chewier. Made with tapioca, the texture is a little airier and more cakey.

NUTRITION FACTS	
Serving Size	29 g
Recipe Yields	456 g
Calories	**98.7**
Fats	**5.24 g**
MUFA	1.13 g
Omega-3	<0.01 g
Omega-6	0.06 g
Saturated Fat	3.78 g
Carbohydrates	**12.7 g**
Fiber	1.3 g
Starch	2.63 g
Fructose	0.33 g
Glucose	0.3 g
Sucrose	0.75 g
Protein	**0.64 g**
Alanine	<0.01 g
Arginine	0.01 g
Aspartic acid	0.01 g
Cystine	<0.01 g
Glutamic acid	0.01 g
Glycine	<0.01 g
Histidine	<0.01 g
Isoleucine	<0.01 g
Leucine	<0.01 g
Lysine	<0.01 g
Methionine	<0.01 g
Phenylalanine	<0.01 g
Proline	<0.01 g
Serine	<0.01 g
Threonine	<0.01 g
Tryptophan	<0.01 g
Tyrosine	<0.01 g
Valine	<0.01 g
Vitamins	
Vitamin B1	<0.01 mg
Vitamin B12	0 mcg
Vitamin B2	<0.01 mg
Vitamin B3	0.1 mg
Vitamin B5	0.05 mg
Vitamin B6	0.05 mg
Choline	1.88 mg
Folate	2.65 mcg
Vitamin A	6.38 mcg
Vitamin C	2.09 mg
Vitamin D	0 IU
Vitamin E	0.68 mg
Vitamin K	0.09 mcg
Minerals	
Calcium	6.73 mg
Copper	0.02 mg
Iron	0.25 mg
Magnesium	10.5 mg
Manganese	0.05 mg
Phosphorus	4.8 mg
Potassium	95.4 mg
Selenium	0.62 mcg
Sodium	22.1 mg
Zinc	0.03 mg

nutrition content estimated using the USDA database.

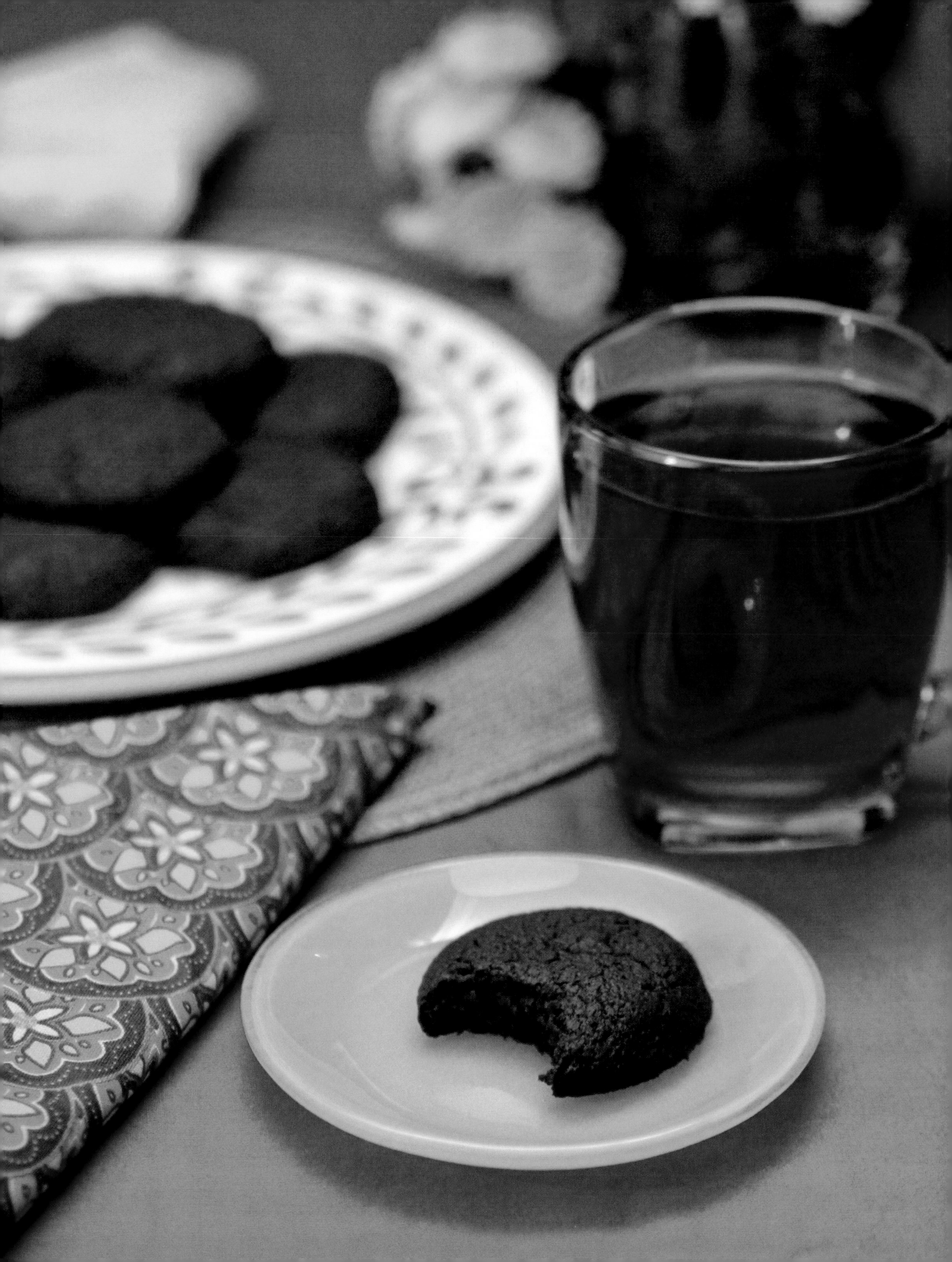

Maple Shortbread Cookies

Shortbread cookies, often called "sandies" or "meltaways," were a holiday staple of my childhood. In fact, my family prided itself on having the "shortest" shortbread. This version of my favorite cookie literally melts in your mouth.

PREP TIME: 20 minutes, plus 1 to 2 hours chilling time
COOK TIME: 20 to 25 minutes
YIELD: 20 cookies

INGREDIENTS:

- ½ cup maple sugar
- 1 cup palm shortening
- 1 cup arrowroot powder
- ⅔ cup sifted coconut flour

FODMAP ALERT

This recipe cannot be made low-FODMAP.

1. Preheat the oven to 300°F. Line a baking sheet with parchment paper, aluminum foil, or a silicone liner.
2. Place the maple sugar in a spice grinder or blender and blend until it is a fine powder. Measure ½ cup after blending.
3. Combine the ingredients in a bowl and mix to form a sticky dough. You can drop balls of dough onto the baking sheet and flatten with your fingers or the back of a spoon (if the dough is just too sticky, refrigerate for 20 minutes). Alternatively, you can chill the dough completely in the fridge (1 to 2 hours), pat it out to ½ inch thick, and cut it into shapes with a knife or cookie cutters. As the dough warms up, it gets sticky and harder to work with, so you may need to stick it back into the fridge periodically to firm up again.
4. Bake for 20 to 25 minutes (depending on the size of your cookies) until they turn a light golden brown. Let cool completely on the baking sheet before moving to a serving plate.

TIPS:

These cookies are very fragile, so handle with care. They will fall apart more easily if undercooked.

Always measure coconut flour after sifting.

VARIATIONS:

You can substitute evaporated cane juice for the maple sugar. You can also substitute lard for half of the palm shortening. However, if you substitute more than that, the cookies will be too crumbly and won't hold together at all.

NUTRITION FACTS	
Serving Size	31 g
Recipe Yields	615 g
Calories	**174**
Fats	**12.1 g**
MUFA	3.25 g
Omega-3	<0.01 g
Omega-6	0.06 g
Saturated Fat	8.32 g
Carbohydrates	**15.4 g**
Fiber	3.02 g
Starch	1.12 g
Fructose	0 g
Glucose	0 g
Sucrose	0 g
Protein	**1.15 g**
Alanine	<0.01 g
Arginine	<0.01 g
Aspartic acid	<0.01 g
Cystine	<0.01 g
Glutamic acid	<0.01 g
Glycine	<0.01 g
Histidine	<0.01 g
Isoleucine	<0.01 g
Leucine	<0.01 g
Lysine	<0.01 g
Methionine	<0.01 g
Phenylalanine	<0.01 g
Proline	<0.01 g
Serine	<0.01 g
Threonine	<0.01 g
Tryptophan	<0.01 g
Tyrosine	<0.01 g
Valine	<0.01 g
Vitamins	
Vitamin B1	<0.01 mg
Vitamin B12	0 mcg
Vitamin B2	<0.01 mg
Vitamin B3	<0.01 mg
Vitamin B5	0.01 mg
Vitamin B6	<0.01 mg
Choline	0.12 mg
Folate	0.45 mcg
Vitamin A	0 mcg
Vitamin C	0 mg
Vitamin D	0 IU
Vitamin E	2.09 mg
Vitamin K	0 mcg
Minerals	
Calcium	7.72 mg
Copper	<0.01 mg
Iron	0.32 mg
Magnesium	1.28 mg
Manganese	0.28 mg
Phosphorus	0.49 mg
Potassium	16.4 mg
Selenium	0.05 mcg
Sodium	17.6 mg
Zinc	0.35 mg

nutrition content estimated using the USDA database.

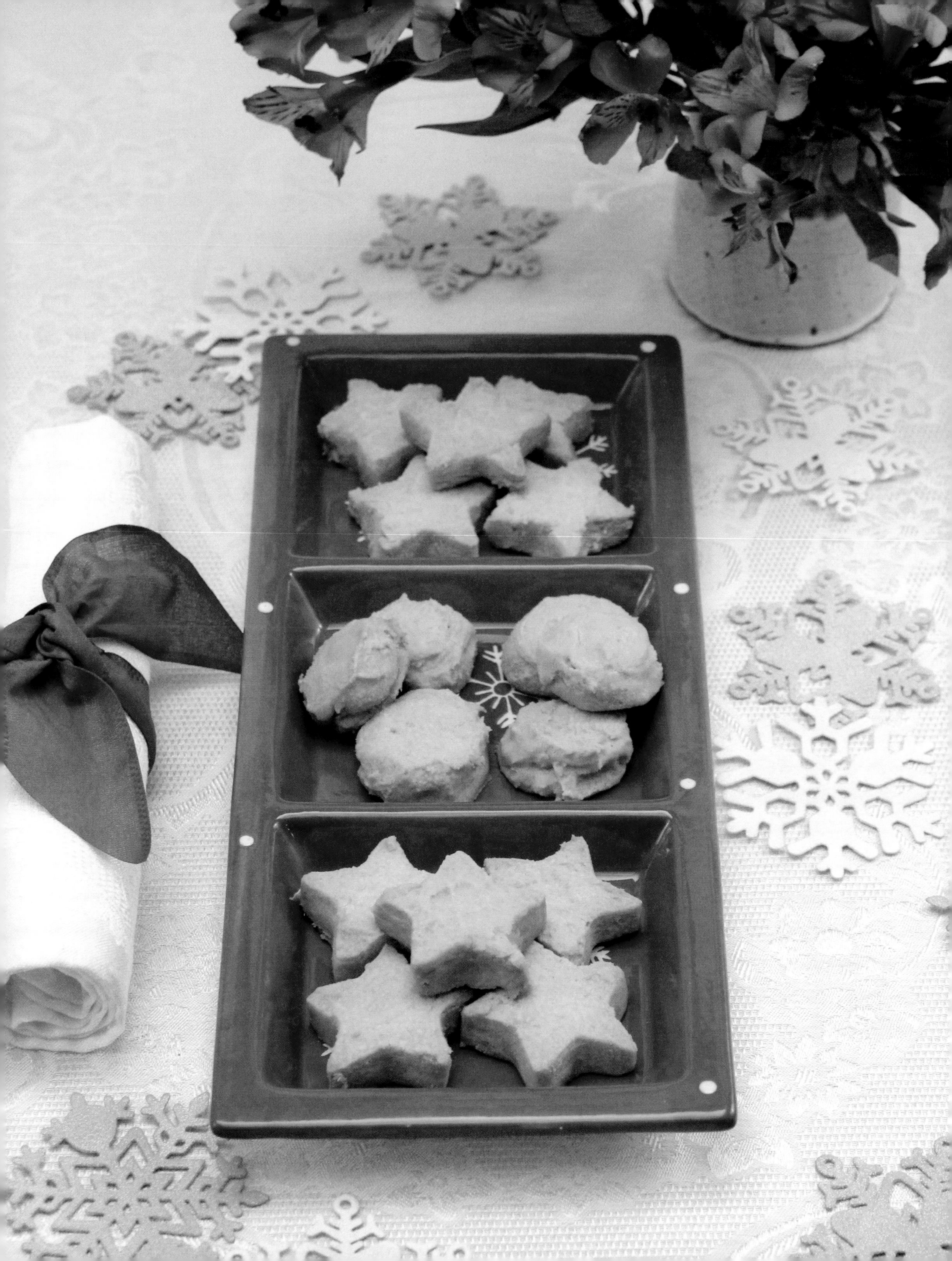

Carob Ganache Mini Tortes

Need a decadent chocolate fix or a beautiful but simple dessert to serve company? This recipe definitely fits the bill. The combination of carob powder, vanilla, coconut, and cinnamon is surprisingly similar to chocolate. This ganache is beautiful when chilled in a silicone mold and inverted onto a plate. However, you can also keep it simple and pour into individual ramekins or even a big serving bowl and just spoon out individual servings when you're ready.

PREP TIME: 5 minutes, plus 3 to 4 hours chilling time
COOK TIME: 5 minutes
SERVINGS: 2 to 4

INGREDIENTS:

- ⅔ cup homemade Coconut Milk (page 116) or canned full-fat coconut milk
- ⅓ cup extra-virgin coconut oil
- 2 tablespoons vanilla extract or 1½ teaspoons vanilla powder
- ⅓ cup carob powder
- Dash of ground cinnamon

FODMAP ALERT *If you do not tolerate coconut milk, skip this recipe.*

SPECIAL EQUIPMENT

- Blender or food processor
- Ramekins, silicone molds, or serving dish

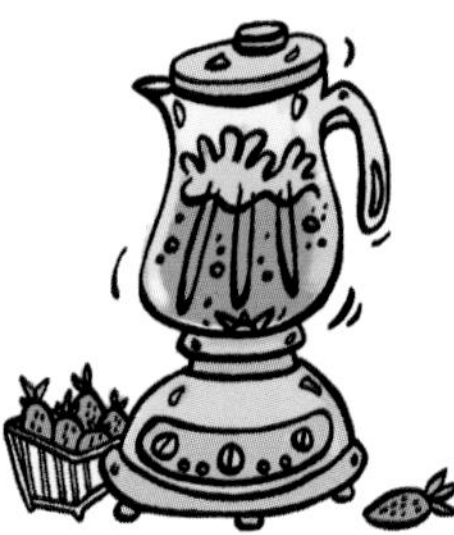

1. Bring the coconut milk, coconut oil, and vanilla to a low simmer in a small saucepan over medium-low heat. If using vanilla extract, let simmer for 5 to 10 minutes, stirring frequently, to burn off the majority of the alcohol (if using vanilla powder, skip the simmering and simply heat to melt the coconut oil).
2. Pour the coconut milk mixture into a blender or food processor. Add the carob and cinnamon and blend for 30 seconds to 1 minute to thoroughly combine.
3. Pour into individual ramekins, silicone molds, or a large serving bowl. Chill until set, 3 to 4 hours.
4. Enjoy plain or serve with berries.

TIPS:

Simmering the vanilla in the coconut milk burns off only about half of the alcohol. If you know that you are very sensitive to alcohol, use vanilla powder or omit the vanilla.

VARIATIONS:

Mint "Chocolate" Ganache Torte. *Instead of using cinnamon, add a few drops of peppermint oil.*

Rum-Ball Ganache Torte. *Heat 4 tablespoons dark rum and simmer until 2 tablespoons are left. Use in place of the vanilla.*

"Chocolate" Mousse. *Increase the amount of coconut milk to 1 cup. Pour into individual ramekins or a large serving bowl to chill (the mousse does not work in silicone molds).*

NUTRITION FACTS	
Serving Size	81 g
Recipe Yields	325 g
Calories	**308**
Fats	**26 g**
MUFA	1.38 g
Omega-3	<0.01 g
Omega-6	0.41 g
Saturated Fat	22.6 g
Carbohydrates	**15.7 g**
Fiber	2.55 g
Starch	2.53 g
Fructose	<0.01 g
Glucose	<0.01 g
Sucrose	<0.01 g
Protein	**2.02 g**
Alanine	0.04 g
Arginine	0.13 g
Aspartic acid	0.07 g
Cystine	0.02 g
Glutamic acid	0.17 g
Glycine	0.04 g
Histidine	0.02 g
Isoleucine	0.03 g
Leucine	0.06 g
Lysine	0.03 g
Methionine	0.01 g
Phenylalanine	0.04 g
Proline	0.03 g
Serine	0.04 g
Threonine	0.03 g
Tryptophan	<0.01 g
Tyrosine	0.02 g
Valine	0.05 g
Vitamins	
Vitamin B1	<0.01 mg
Vitamin B12	0 mcg
Vitamin B2	<0.01 mg
Vitamin B3	0.27 mg
Vitamin B5	0.06 mg
Vitamin B6	0.01 mg
Choline	3.27 mg
Folate	5.29 mcg
Vitamin A	0.01 mcg
Vitamin C	0.38 mg
Vitamin D	0 IU
Vitamin E	0.02 mg
Vitamin K	0.11 mcg
Minerals	
Calcium	8.31 mg
Copper	0.09 mg
Iron	1.27 mg
Magnesium	18.2 mg
Manganese	0.32 mg
Phosphorus	36.7 mg
Potassium	92.9 mg
Selenium	<0.01 mcg
Sodium	11.8 mg
Zinc	0.22 mg

nutrition content estimated using the USDA database.

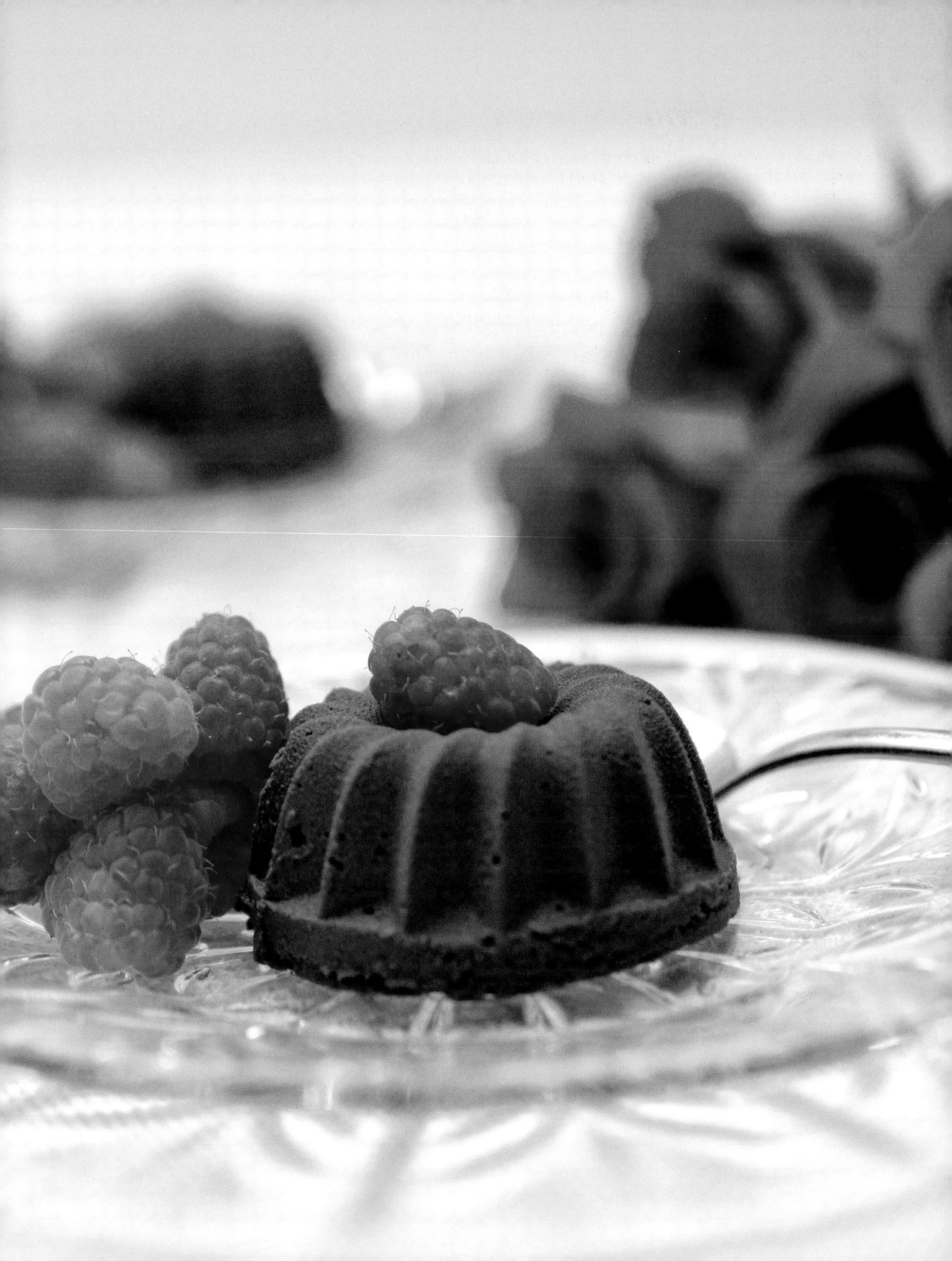

Applesauce Spice Cake with Caramel Sauce

While this simple spice cake could easily replace a muffin with your breakfast, the addition of caramel sauce (which can be enjoyed warm or at room temperature) turns it into a truly decadent dessert.

PREP TIME: 30 minutes, plus 2 hours for the gelatin to set
COOK TIME: 1 to 1½ hours
SERVINGS: 12 to 16

INGREDIENTS:

Caramel Sauce:

- 1 cup Coconut Cream (page 116)
- 1 cup honey
- Pinch of salt

Cake:

- 2 tablespoons gelatin
- ¼ cup fresh orange juice
- ¼ cup boiling water
- ⅓ cup palm shortening, plus more for greasing the pan (if not using silicone bakeware)
- 1¼ cups arrowroot powder, plus more for greasing the pan (if not using silicone bakeware)
- 2 cups Applesauce (page 122)
- 1½ cups Plantain Flour (page 121)
- 1 tablespoon finely grated orange zest
- 1½ teaspoons baking soda
- 1 teaspoon ground cinnamon
- 1 teaspoon ground mace
- ½ teaspoon ground ginger
- ½ teaspoon salt
- ¼ teaspoon ground cloves

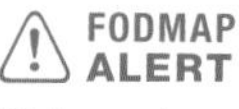

This recipe cannot be made low-FODMAP.

SPECIAL EQUIPMENT

- Candy thermometer
- Silicone tube pan or Bundt pan
- Food processor

CARAMEL SAUCE:

1. Combine the coconut cream, honey, and salt in a saucepan. Attach a candy thermometer to the side of the pot.
2. Slowly heat over medium-low heat, stirring occasionally to ensure that it's heating evenly, until the caramel reaches 230°F (this should take about 30 minutes and can be done while the cake is baking).
3. Pour the caramel sauce into a mason jar, serving cup, or pitcher and set aside. The caramel sauce can be enjoyed warmed or at room temperature and can be stored for up to several months in the refrigerator. (Warm it before serving.)

CAKE:

1. Bloom the gelatin by sprinkling it over the orange juice in a heatproof measuring cup. Stir, then let it sit for 3 to 4 minutes.
2. Add the boiling water to the orange juice and gelatin mixture. Stir until the gelatin has completely dissolved. (This may take several minutes. Let it sit after stirring initially, then stir every couple of minutes to check if the gelatin has dissolved.)
3. Refrigerate the gelatin until set, about 2 hours.
4. Preheat the oven to 350°F. A silicone tube or Bundt pan is preferred. Otherwise, thoroughly grease and "flour" a regular tube pan or Bundt pan with palm shortening and arrowroot powder.
5. Combine the set gelatin and the remaining cake ingredients in a food processor. Process until completely smooth, at least 4 to 5 minutes, turning off the food processor to scrape the sides at least once.
6. Pour the batter into the tube or Bundt pan. Smooth out the top with a rubber spatula. Bake for 1 hour, until a toothpick inserted in the middle comes out clean.
7. Let the cake cool for at least 20 minutes before inverting the pan. Serve with the caramel sauce.

TIPS:

This recipe is very precise chemistry, so follow the directions and measure the ingredients carefully. This cake is naturally fairly squat; doubling the recipe will not make it taller. Like all baked goods that use plantains or plantain flour, it goes stale quickly. Store covered in plastic wrap and reheat leftovers slightly before eating. Or, better yet, freeze any portions you don't plan to eat the same day you bake them.

VARIATIONS:

Add some chopped Honey-Candied Ginger (page 333) to the caramel sauce for a little zing. As an alternative to the caramel sauce, you can serve this cake with Coconut Whipped Topping (page 116) or eat it plain.

The caramel sauce can also be made with maple syrup or half honey and half maple syrup.

NUTRITION FACTS	
Serving Size	102 g
Recipe Yields	1634 g
Calories	**246**
Fats	**7.59 g**
MUFA	1.47 g
Omega-3	<0.01 g
Omega-6	0.07 g
Saturated Fat	5.63 g
Carbohydrates	**42.4 g**
Fiber	2.01 g
Starch	0.41 g
Fructose	10.5 g
Glucose	8.27 g
Sucrose	0.53 g
Protein	**4.6 g**
Alanine	0.09 g
Arginine	0.11 g
Aspartic acid	0.1 g
Cystine	<0.01 g
Glutamic acid	0.16 g
Glycine	0.19 g
Histidine	0.01 g
Isoleucine	0.03 g
Leucine	0.05 g
Lysine	0.05 g
Methionine	0.01 g
Phenylalanine	0.04 g
Proline	0.14 g
Serine	0.04 g
Threonine	0.03 g
Tryptophan	<0.01 g
Tyrosine	0.02 g
Valine	0.04 g
Vitamins	
Vitamin B1	0.02 mg
Vitamin B12	0 mcg
Vitamin B2	0.02 mg
Vitamin B3	0.17 mg
Vitamin B5	0.07 mg
Vitamin B6	0.02 mg
Choline	2.96 mg
Folate	5.65 mcg
Vitamin A	0.84 mcg
Vitamin C	3.02 mg
Vitamin D	0 IU
Vitamin E	0.91 mg
Vitamin K	0.25 mcg
Minerals	
Calcium	13.3 mg
Copper	0.08 mg
Iron	0.96 mg
Magnesium	9.34 mg
Manganese	0.25 mg
Phosphorus	17.8 mg
Potassium	78 mg
Selenium	0.66 mcg
Sodium	163 mg
Zinc	0.15 mg

nutrition content estimated using the USDA database.

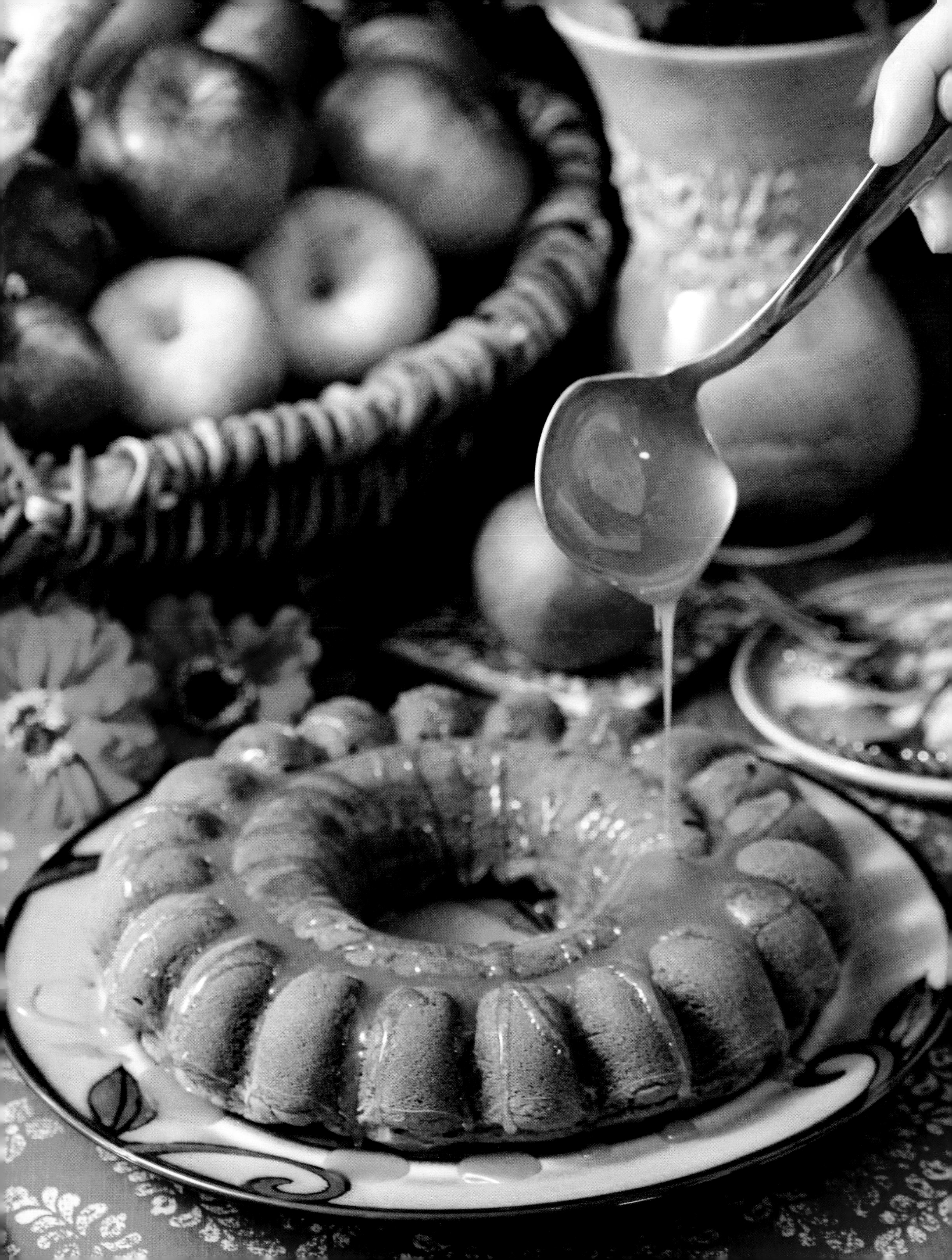

Carob Layer Cake

Need an actual birthday cake that doesn't contain any gut-irritating or pro-inflammatory ingredients? Well, here you go!

As a word of caution, this cake is very rich and dense. A typical serving size is half or less than what you would normally expect from a layer cake. For this reason, the recipe yields one cake layer and enough frosting for only one layer—think brownie. If you want a layer cake but don't want a cake that will serve so many people, you can make one layer in a square pan and then cut it in half for a rectangular-shaped two-layer cake, or make a semicircle using a round cake pan. Alternatively, you can freeze any leftovers.

If you want a two-layer or three-layer cake, you will have to multiply the recipe accordingly. You may have to process the ingredients for each layer separately unless you have a very large food processor.

Leftovers should be kept in the refrigerator or freezer, but if you are eating leftover cake, it is far tastier at room temperature. Let your slice come to room temperature before eating, or warm it up in the microwave.

You can also skip the frosting and serve with berries and Coconut Whipped Topping (page 116).

PREP TIME: 20 minutes, plus 2 hours for the gelatin to set and time for the cake to cool
COOK TIME: 35 to 40 minutes
SERVINGS: 1 (1-layer) cake makes 6 to 8 servings, 1 (2-layer) cake makes 12 to 16 servings, 1 (3-layer) cake makes 20 to 24 servings

INGREDIENTS:

Carob Frosting (for 1 layer):

- 1 cup palm shortening
- ½ cup carob powder, sifted
- ½ teaspoon vanilla extract
- Dash of ground cinnamon

Cake (1 Layer):

- 2 tablespoons gelatin
- ⅓ cup cool water
- ⅓ cup boiling water
- ½ cup palm shortening, plus more for the pan (if not using silicone bakeware)
- Arrowroot powder, for the pan (if not using silicone bakeware)
- 2 large plantains (about 1½ cups puréed)
- ¾ cup carob powder
- 2 tablespoons blackstrap molasses
- 2 tablespoons vanilla extract
- ¾ teaspoon baking soda
- ½ teaspoon salt

FROSTING:

1. Mix all the frosting ingredients together using a wire whisk or mixer until light and fluffy. Cover with plastic wrap and leave at room temperature until you are ready to frost your cake.

CAKE:

1. In a small bowl, sprinkle the gelatin over the cool water and let sit for 3 to 4 minutes to bloom. Add the boiling water and stir until the gelatin has completely dissolved. Refrigerate until completely set, about 2 hours.
2. Preheat the oven to 350°F. Have a silicone or regular 8- or 9-inch round or 8-inch-square cake pan out and ready to use. If not using silicone bakeware, prepare the pan by following the Tip on the opposite page.
3. Peel the plantains and place in a food processor. Process for 1 to 2 minutes.
4. Add the set gelatin and remaining ingredients to the food processor. Process for 4 to 5 minutes (or longer if your food processor is not particularly powerful) until a completely smooth cake batter is formed.
5. Pour the batter into the silicone or prepared regular cake pan. Smooth the top with a rubber spatula to make sure it's even.
6. Repeat steps 1 through 5 for each layer if you are making more than one.
7. Bake for 35 to 40 minutes, until a toothpick inserted in the middle comes out clean (or with small dry crumbs on it).
8. If using silicone bakeware, let the cake cool completely in the pan. If using regular bakeware, let the cake cool for at least 15 minutes before removing from the pan. Finish cooling on a wire rack.
9. Frost the cake as you normally would. Serve at room temperature.

NUTRITION FACTS	
Serving Size	152 g
Recipe Yields	1216 g
Calories	**560**
Fats	**41.1 g**
MUFA	12.1 g
Omega-3	0.01 g
Omega-6	0.23 g
Saturated Fat	26.8 g
Carbohydrates	**44.5 g**
Fiber	5.78 g
Starch	11.3 g
Fructose	0.64 g
Glucose	0.6 g
Sucrose	1.47 g
Protein	**4.45 g**
Alanine	0.16 g
Arginine	0.16 g
Aspartic acid	0.14 g
Cystine	<0.01 g
Glutamic acid	0.21 g
Glycine	0.35 g
Histidine	0.04 g
Isoleucine	0.04 g
Leucine	0.07 g
Lysine	0.09 g
Methionine	0.02 g
Phenylalanine	0.05 g
Proline	0.24 g
Serine	0.06 g
Threonine	0.04 g
Tryptophan	<0.01 g
Tyrosine	0.02 g
Valine	0.06 g
Vitamins	
Vitamin B1	0.03 mg
Vitamin B12	0 mcg
Vitamin B2	0.03 mg
Vitamin B3	0.37 mg
Vitamin B5	0.16 mg
Vitamin B6	0.17 mg
Choline	7.38 mg
Folate	10.4 mcg
Vitamin A	25.1 mcg
Vitamin C	8.24 mg
Vitamin D	0 IU
Vitamin E	7.83 mg
Vitamin K	0.33 mcg
Minerals	
Calcium	14.7 mg
Copper	0.1 mg
Iron	0.91 mg
Magnesium	29.7 mg
Manganese	0.09 mg
Phosphorus	17.7 mg
Potassium	304 mg
Selenium	2.25 mcg
Sodium	202 mg
Zinc	0.09 mg

nutrition content estimated using the USDA database.

SPECIAL EQUIPMENT

- 8- or 9-inch-round or 8-inch-square silicone cake pan(s)
- Food processor

⚠ **FODMAP ALERT** *This cake is probably too carbohydrate-dense to be well tolerated by those with FODMAP intolerance.*

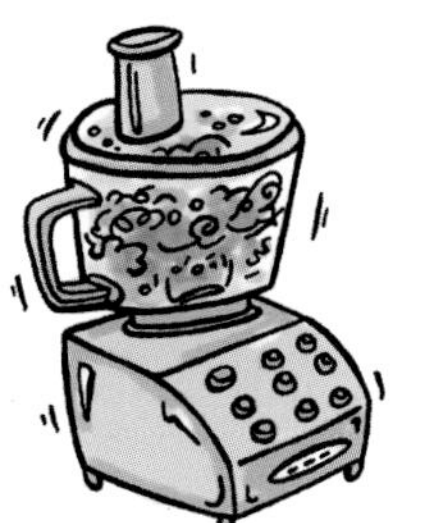

TIPS:

If you don't have silicone bakeware, you can use traditional cake pans. Cut a circle (or square if using square pans) of wax paper that exactly lines the bottom of the pan. Grease the pan with palm shortening, then place the wax paper over the top of the grease. Grease the wax paper, then "flour" the cake pan with arrowroot powder.

This cake recipe uses very precise chemistry. Follow the directions and measure your ingredients carefully!

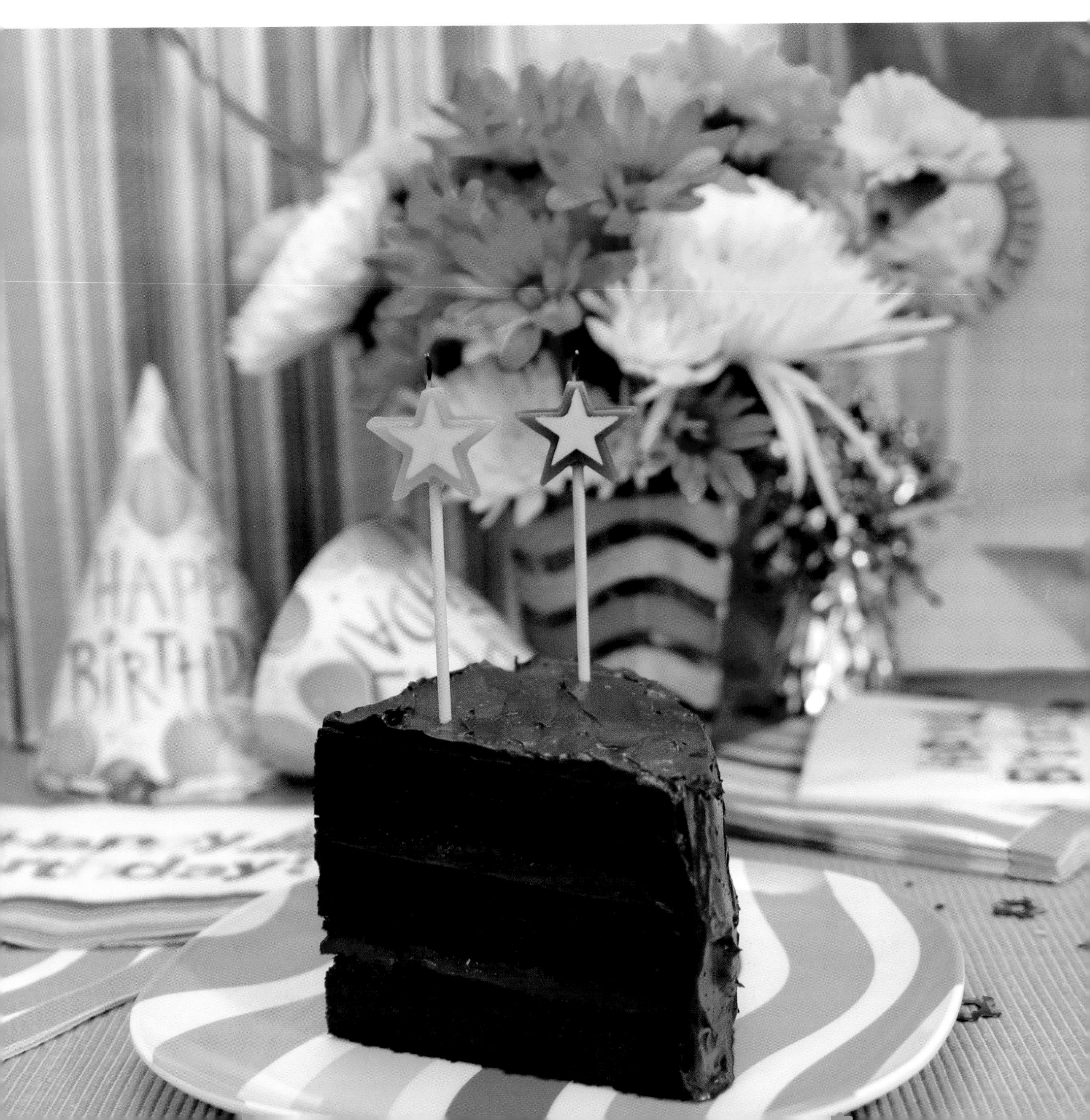

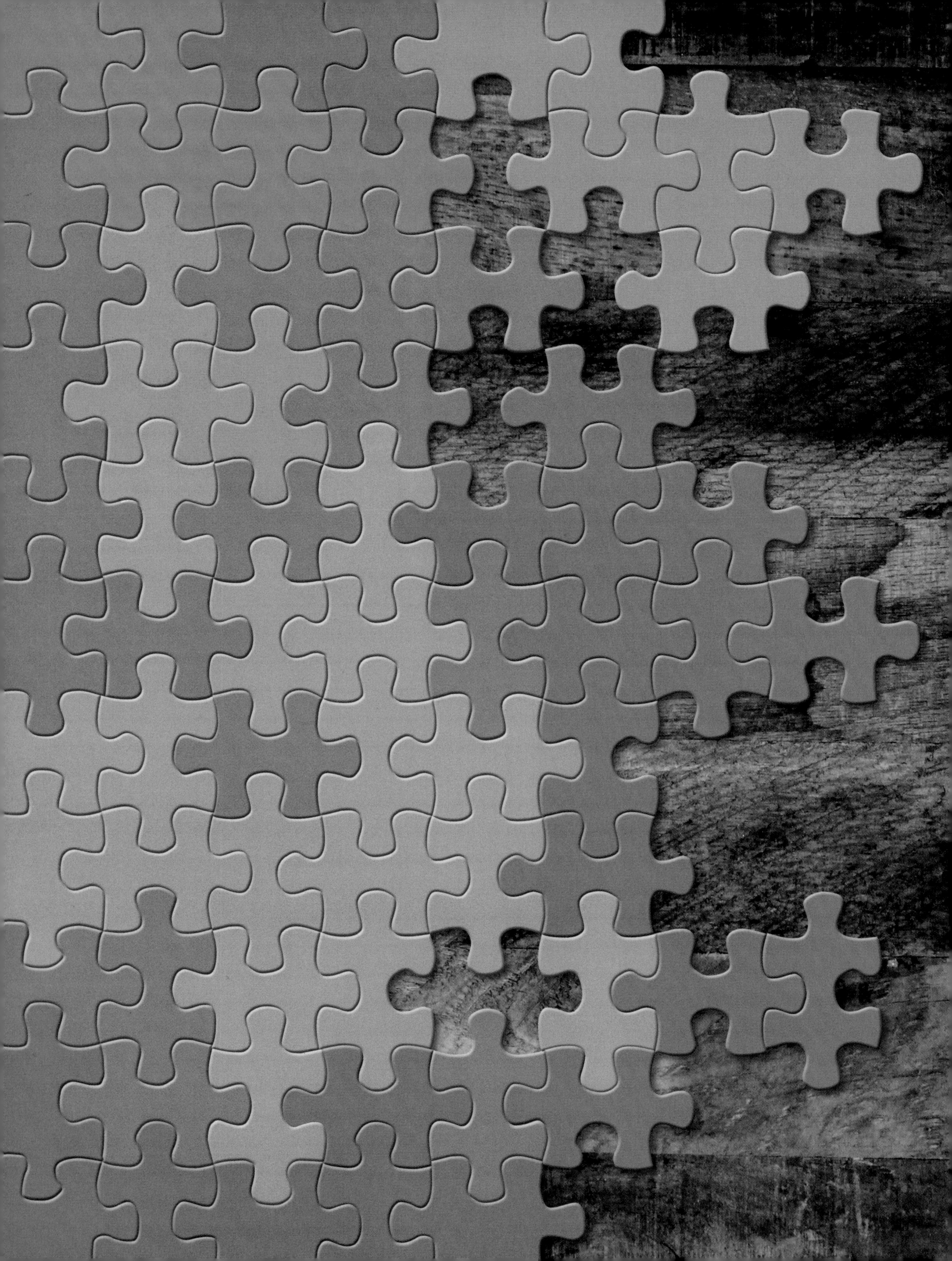

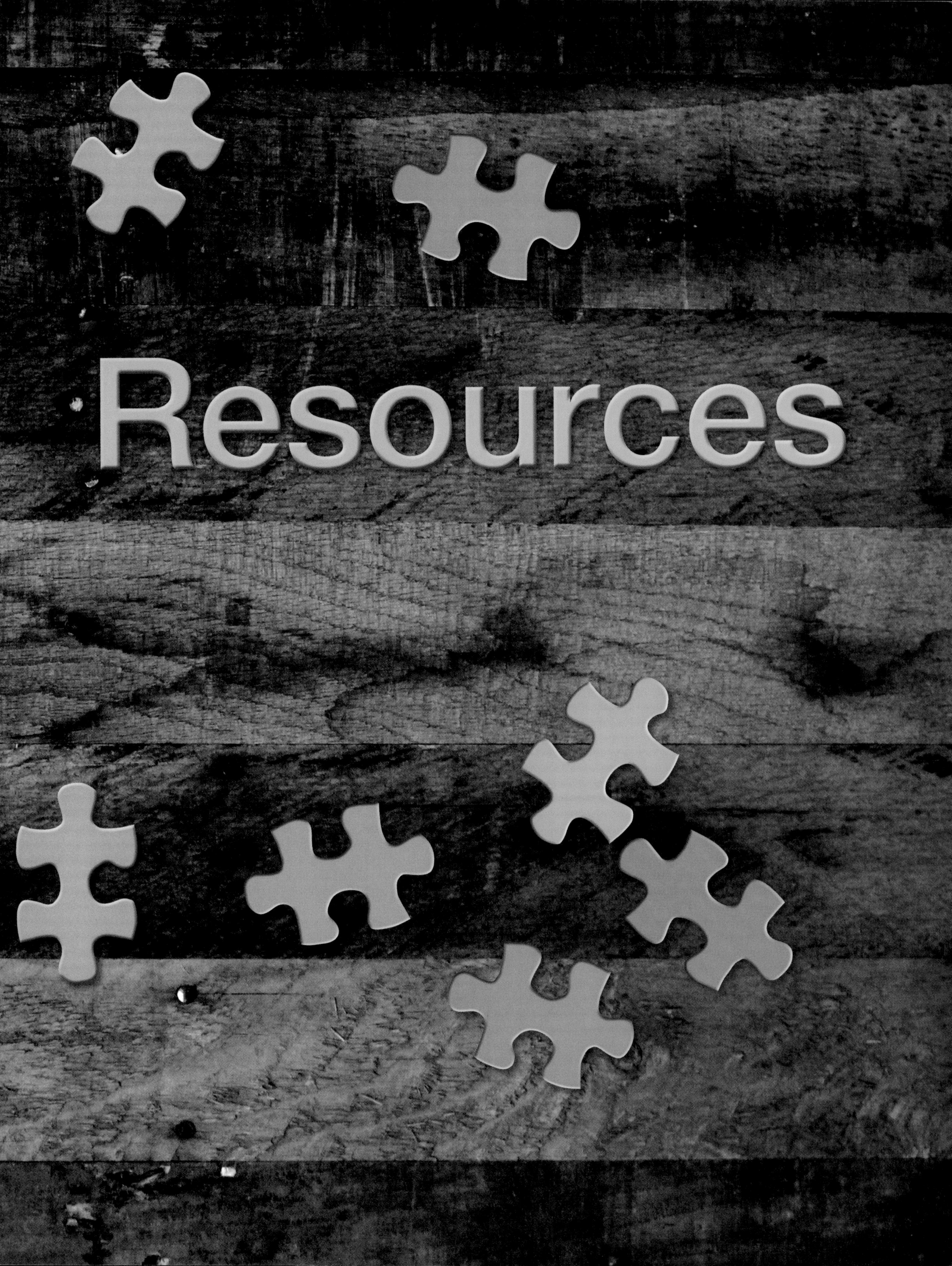
Resources

Reading Labels

Trying to figure out whether a product is Paleo Approach friendly? It helps to know the many aliases that some pervasive foods go by.

☒ Gluten in Foods

Avoiding gluten can take some effort. Ingredients derived from wheat and other gluten-containing grains are found in a vast array of packaged and manufactured foods, but also in some ingredients not normally considered to be processed foods. The following list includes some of these hidden—and not-so-hidden—sources of gluten.

- Asian rice paper
- atta flour
- bacon (check ingredients)
- barley
- barley grass
- barley malt
- beer (unless gluten-free)
- bleached or unbleached flour
- bran
- bread flour
- breading
- brewer's yeast
- bulgur
- coating mixes
- communion wafers
- condiments
- couscous
- croutons
- dinkle (spelt)
- durum
- einkorn
- emmer (durum wheat)
- farina
- farro (called emmer wheat except in Italy)
- food starch
- French fries
- fu (a dried form of gluten)
- gliadin
- glue used on some envelopes, stamps, and labels
- gluten peptides
- glutenin
- graham
- gravies
- hydrolyzed wheat gluten
- hydrolyzed wheat protein
- ice cream (may contain flour as an anticrystallizing agent)
- imitation fish
- kamut
- lunch meats
- maida (Indian wheat flour)
- malt
- malt vinegar
- marinades
- matzah (aka matso)
- medications (prescription or over the counter)
- mir (a wheat and rye cross)
- nutritional and herbal supplements
- oats
- panko (bread crumbs)
- pilafs (containing orzo)
- prepared foods
- processed cereals (often contain barley malt)
- rye
- salad dressings
- sauces
- seitan
- self-basting poultry
- semolina
- soup bases and bouillon
- soy or rice drinks (barley malt or malt enzymes may be used during manufacturing)
- soy sauce (unless wheat-free)
- spelt
- spice mixes (often contain wheat as an anticaking agent, filler, or thickening agent)
- starch
- stuffings
- syrups
- thickeners
- triticale
- wheat
- wheat bran
- wheat germ
- wheat grass
- wheat starch

Common Sources of Gluten/Wheat Contamination:

- art supplies: paint, clay, glue, and play dough (can be transferred to the mouth if hands aren't washed)
- flour dust
- foods sold in bulk (often contaminated by scoops used in other bins and by flour dust)
- grills, pans, cutting boards, utensils, toasters and other appliances, and oils that have been used for preparing foods containing gluten
- household products (may be transferred to the lips and ingested)
- knives (double-dipping knives into food spreads after spreading on bread can leave gluten-containing crumbs)
- millet, white rice flour, buckwheat flour, sorghum flour, and soy flour (commonly contaminated)
- personal care products, especially shampoos (may be transferred to the lips and ingested)
- powder coating inside rubber gloves (may be derived from wheat)
- waxes or resins on fruits and vegetables

☒ Gluten Cross-Reactors

Some foods have a higher likelihood of cross-reacting with gluten, meaning that the antibodies your body makes against gluten recognize similar proteins in these foods, so your body sees these foods and gluten as being one and the same. While gluten sensitivity doesn't automatically mean that you are sensitive to all or any of these foods, it's prudent to be cautious of them:

- brewer's/baker's/nutritional yeast
- corn
- dairy proteins (casein, casomorphin, butyrophilin, whey)
- instant coffee
- millet
- oats
- potatoes
- rice
- sorghum

☒ Corn in Foods

Ingredients derived from corn can be found in the vast majority of packaged and manufactured foods. If you are very sensitive to corn-derived products, avoiding these pervasive ingredients can be overwhelming. However, avoiding processed foods in general will make a huge difference. You may or may not need to go to the extent of avoiding all traces of corn-derived ingredients (in medications, for example); however, being aware of where corn exposure may be sneaking into your life will help you identify whether it is a problem. The following list includes some hidden—and not-so-hidden—sources of corn.

Ingredients Derived from Corn

- acetic acid
- alcohol
- alpha tocopherol
- artificial flavorings
- artificial sweeteners
- ascorbates
- ascorbic acid
- aspartame
- astaxanthin
- baking powder
- barley malt
- bleached flour
- blended sugar
- brown sugar
- calcium citrate
- calcium fumarate
- calcium gluconate
- calcium lactate
- calcium magnesium acetate (CMA)
- calcium stearate
- calcium stearoyl lactylate
- caramel and caramel color
- carboxymethylcellulose sodium
- cellulose, microcrystalline
- cellulose, powdered
- cetearyl glucoside
- choline chloride
- citric acid
- citrus cloud emulsion (CCS)
- cocoglycerides
- confectioners' sugar
- corn oil
- corn sweetener
- corn sugar
- corn syrup
- corn syrup solids
- cornmeal
- cornstarch
- crosscarmellose sodium
- crystalline dextrose
- crystalline fructose
- cyclodextrin
- datum (dough conditioner)
- decyl glucoside
- decyl polyglucose
- dextrin
- dextrose (also found in IV solutions)
- dextrose anything (such as monohydrate or anhydrous)
- d-Gluconic acid
- distilled white vinegar
- drying agent
- erythorbic acid
- erythritol
- ethanol
- Ethocel 20
- ethylcellulose
- ethyl acetate
- ethyl alcohol
- ethyl lactate
- ethyl maltol
- ethylene
- Fibersol-2
- flavorings
- food starch
- fructose
- fruit juice concentrate
- fumaric acid
- germ/germ meal
- gluconate
- gluconic acid
- glucono delta-lactone
- gluconolactone
- glucosamine
- glucose
- glucose syrup (also found in IV solutions)
- glutamate
- gluten
- gluten feed/meal
- glycerides
- glycerin
- glycerol
- golden syrup
- grits
- hominy
- honey
- hydrolyzed corn
- hydrolyzed corn protein
- hydrolyzed vegetable protein
- hydroxypropyl methylcellulose
- hydroxypropyl methylcellulose phthalate (HPMCP)
- inositol
- invert syrup or sugar
- lactate
- lactic acid
- lauryl glucoside
- lecithin
- linoleic acid
- lysine
- magnesium fumarate
- maize
- malic acid
- malonic acid
- malt syrup from corn
- malt, malt extract
- maltitol
- maltodextrin
- maltol
- maltose
- mannitol
- margarine
- methyl gluceth
- methyl glucose
- methyl glucoside
- methylcellulose
- modified cellulose gum
- modified cornstarch
- modified food starch
- molasses (corn syrup may be present; check label)
- mono- and diglycerides
- monosodium glutamate (MSG)
- monostearate
- natural flavorings
- olestra/Olean
- polenta
- polydextrose
- polylactic acid (PLA)
- polysorbates (e.g., Polysorbate 80)
- polyvinyl acetate
- potassium citrate
- potassium fumarate
- potassium gluconate
- powdered sugar
- pregelatinized starch
- propionic acid
- propylene glycol
- saccharin
- salt (iodized)
- semolina (unless from wheat)
- simethicone
- sodium carboxymethylcellulose
- sodium citrate
- sodium erythorbate
- sodium fumarate
- sodium lactate
- sodium starch glycolate
- sodium stearoyl fumarate
- sorbate
- sorbic acid
- sorbitan
- sorbitan monooleate
- sorbitan trioleate
- sorbitol
- sorghum (syrup and/or grain may be mixed with corn)
- Splenda (artificial sweetener)
- starch
- stearic acid
- stearoyls
- Sucralose (artificial sweetener)
- sucrose
- sugar
- talc
- threonine
- tocopherol (vitamin E)
- treacle
- triethyl citrate
- unmodified starch
- vanilla, natural flavoring
- vanilla, pure or extract
- vanillin
- vinegar, distilled white
- vinyl acetate
- vitamin C
- vitamin E
- vitamin supplements
- xanthan gum
- xylitol
- yeast
- zea mays
- zein

☒ Soy in Foods

Soy is another ingredient that has permeated the food supply. Soy lecithin and soy protein are especially common ingredients to find in packaged goods. The following list includes foods that are derived from soy:

- bean curd
- bean sprouts
- chocolate (soy lecithin may be used in manufacturing)
- edamame (fresh soybeans)
- hydrolyzed soy protein (HSP)
- kinako
- miso (fermented soybean paste)
- mono- and diglycerides
- monosodium glutamate (MSG)
- natto
- nimame
- okara
- shoyu
- soy albumin
- soy cheese
- soy fiber
- soy flour
- soy grits
- soy ice cream
- soy lecithin
- soy meal
- soy nuts
- soy pasta
- soy protein (concentrate, hydrolyzed, isolate)
- soy sauce
- soy sprouts
- soy yogurt
- soya
- soybean (curds, granules)
- soybean oil
- soymilk
- tamari
- tempeh
- teriyaki sauce
- textured vegetable protein (TVP)
- tofu (dofu, kori-dofu)
- yuba

Potentially Cross-Contaminated Foods Must Be Labeled:

- "may contain soy"
- "produced on shared equipment with soy"
- "produced in a facility that also processes soy"

Products That Commonly Contain Soy

- Asian cuisine (Chinese, Korean, Japanese, Thai)
- baked goods
- baking mixes
- bouillon cubes
- candy
- cereal
- chicken (raw or cooked) processed with chicken broth
- chicken broth
- deli meats
- energy bars
- imitation dairy foods, such as soymilk, vegan cheese, and vegan ice cream
- infant formula
- margarine
- mayonnaise
- meat products with fillers; for example, burgers and sausages
- nutrition bars
- nutrition supplements (vitamins)
- peanut butter and peanut butter substitutes
- protein powders
- sauces, gravies, and soups
- smoothies
- vegetable broth
- vegetarian meat substitutes (veggie burgers, imitation chicken patties, imitation lunch meats, imitation bacon bits)
- waxes or horticultural oils on fruits

☒ Sugar in Foods

When you are reading food labels, it is helpful to know how to decipher which ingredients are sugar. While most of them are refined, some are unrefined (which typically means that the sugar retains some minerals). It is also common for manufactured products to contain more than one form of sugar. The following ingredients are all forms of sugar:

- agave
- agave nectar
- barley malt
- barley malt syrup
- beet sugar
- brown rice syrup
- brown sugar
- cane crystals
- cane juice
- cane sugar
- caramel
- coconut sugar
- corn sweetener
- corn syrup
- corn syrup solids
- crystalline fructose
- date sugar
- dehydrated cane juice
- demerara sugar
- dextrin
- dextrose
- diastatic malt
- evaporated cane juice
- fructose
- fruit juice
- fruit juice concentrate
- galactose
- glucose
- glucose solids
- golden syrup
- high-fructose corn syrup
- honey
- inulin
- invert sugar
- jaggery
- lactose
- malt syrup
- maltodextrin
- maltose
- maple syrup
- molasses
- monk fruit (luo han guo)
- muscovado sugar
- palm sugar
- panela
- panocha
- rapadura
- raw cane sugar
- raw sugar
- refined sugar
- rice bran syrup
- rice syrup
- saccharose
- sorghum
- sorghum syrup
- sucanat
- sucrose
- syrup
- treacle
- turbinado sugar
- yacon syrup

☒ Dairy in Foods

Dairy ingredients are more and more commonly used in manufactured and prepackaged foods. The following ingredients found on a label indicate the presence of milk protein.

- milk — acidophilus milk, buttermilk, buttermilk blend, buttermilk solids, cultured milk, condensed milk, dried milk, dry milk solids (DMS), evaporated milk, fat-free milk, fully cream milk powder, goat's milk, Lactaid milk, lactose-free milk, low-fat milk, malted milk, milk derivative, milk powder, milk protein, milk solids, milk solid pastes, nonfat dry milk, nonfat milk, nonfat milk solids, pasteurized milk, powdered milk, sheep's milk, skim milk, skim milk powder, sour milk, sour milk solids, sweet cream buttermilk powder, sweetened condensed milk, sweetened condensed skim milk, whole milk, 1% milk, 2% milk
- butter — artificial butter, artificial butter flavor, butter extract, butter fat, butter flavored oil, butter solids, dairy butter, natural butter, natural butter flavor, whipped butter
- casein & caseinates — ammonium caseinate, calcium caseinate, hydrolyzed casein, iron caseinate magnesium caseinate, potassium caseinate, sodium caseinate, zinc caseinate
- cheese — cheese flavor (artificial and natural), cheese food, cottage cheese, cream cheese, imitation cheese, vegetarian cheeses with casein
- cream, whipped cream
- curds
- custard
- dairy product solids
- galactose
- ghee (cultured ghee may be OK)
- half & half
- hydrolysates — casein hydrolysate, milk protein hydrolysate, protein hydrolysate, whey hydrolysate, whey protein hydrolysate
- ice cream, ice milk, sherbet
- lactalbumin, lactalbumin phosphate
- lactate solids
- lactic yeast
- lactitol monohydrate
- lactoglobulin
- lactose
- lactulose
- milk fat, anhydrous milk fat
- nisin preparation
- nougat
- pudding
- quark
- recaldent
- rennet, rennet casein
- Simplesse (fat replacer)
- sour cream, sour cream solids, imitation sour cream
- whey — acid whey, cured whey, delactosed whey, demineralized whey, hydrolyzed whey, powdered whey, reduced mineral whey, sweet dairy whey, whey powder, whey protein, whey protein concentrate, whey solids
- yogurt (regular or frozen), yogurt powder

May contain milk:

- caramel flavoring
- flavoring
- high-protein flour
- lactic acid
- lactic acid starter culture
- natural flavoring

"Nondairy" products may contain casein. Foods covered by the FDA labeling laws that contain milk must be labeled "contains milk"; however, prescription and over-the-counter medications are exempt.

Recipe Top Ten

Are you deficient in a specific micronutrient? Instead of choosing which recipe to make based on what was on sale or your mood, you can choose one of the recipes highest per serving in the specific micronutrient that you need more of!

Remember that many nutrient deficiencies (and excesses!) actually indicate deficiencies in synergistic nutrients required for absorption or utilization. This is why taking vitamin C can help if you are iron deficient; why vitamin D deficiency so often goes hand-in-hand with B-vitamin deficiencies and zinc deficiency; and why iodine excess can be a consequence of selenium deficiency.

The great news is that when you focus on getting your nutrients from whole foods, you typically get all the synergistic nutrients you need, too.

Use these Top Ten lists of recipes highest in each micronutrient for a whole food–based approach to restoring normal and balanced micronutrient levels. Also note the frequent flyers (hello, organ meat!). Looking at which recipes repeatedly make the Top Ten list is a great way to emphasize the major tenets of the Paleo Approach summarized on page 48!

Vitamins

	Vitamin A (RAE)
1	Liver and Onions (page 281)
2	Hidden Liver Meatloaf (page 272)
3	50/50/50 Burgers (page 289)
4	Bacon and Bison Liver Pâté with Fresh Fig Jam (page 152)
5	Hidden Offal Swedish Meatballs (page 282)
6	Superfood Smoothie (page 141)
7	Roasted Sweet Potato (page 313)
8	Sweet Potato Linguine with Bolognese Sauce (page 226)
9	Spiced Kabocha Squash (page 324)
10	Carrot-Ginger Soup (page 189)

	Vitamin C
1	"Cream" of Broccoli Soup (page 183)
2	Bacon-Braised Whitefish and Brussels (page 254)
3	Superfood Smoothie (page 141)
4	Kale Chips (page 166)
5	Pork Pad Thai (page 234)
6	Beef Heart "Chow Mein" (page 278)
7	Garden Salad (page 160)
8	Roasted Broccoflower (page 302)
9	Orange and Banana Sorbet (page 344)
10	Lemon and Thyme Broiled Salmon with Blood Orange Salsa (page 242)

	Vitamin D
1	Asian-Inspired Salmon en Papillote (page 262)
2	Simple Baked Whitefish (page 244)
3	Baked Whole Fish (page 240)
4	Scalloped Hake and Oysters (page 248)
5	Seafood and Leek Soup (page 190)
6	Salmon with Maitre D' "Butter" (page 245)
7	Pan-Fried Sardines (page 252)
8	Sardine Salad (page 163)
9	Lemon and Thyme Broiled Salmon with Blood Orange Salsa (page 242)
10	BBQ Pork Ribs (page 216)

	Vitamin E
1	Savory Roasted Taro (page 320)
2	Seafood and Leek Soup (page 190)
3	Sardine Salad (page 163)
4	"Cream" of Broccoli Soup (page 183)
5	Guacamole (page 171)
6	Garden Green Vichyssoise (page 188)
7	Spiced Kabocha Squash (page 324)
8	Taro Hash (page 138)
9	Superfood Smoothie (page 141)
10	Deep-Fried Whole Shrimp with Cocktail Sauce (page 256)

These Top Ten lists are based on data available from the USDA database. They are not calorie adjusted and instead represent nutrient content per serving.

Vitamin K
1 Kale Chips (page 166)
2 Bacon-Braised Whitefish and Brussels (page 254)
3 Superfood Smoothie (page 141)
4 Garden Salad (page 160)
5 Smoked Salmon and Roe Endive Boats (page 174)
6 Oxtail-Braised Greens (page 284)
7 "Cream" of Broccoli Soup (page 183)
8 Bacon-Braised Brussels Sprouts (page 321)
9 Seafood and Leek Soup (page 190)
10 Braised Greens (page 300)

Vitamin B_1
1 Russ' Flatbread (page 326)
2 Pork Pie–Stuffed Acorn Squash (page 231)
3 Tarragon Roasted Pork (page 208)
4 BBQ Pork Ribs (page 216)
5 Braised Pork Chops with Apple and Fennel (page 220)
6 Lemon and Thyme Broiled Pork Chops (page 230)
7 Pork Pad Thai (page 234)
8 Garlic-Roasted Pork Shoulder (page 214)
9 Hidden Liver Meatloaf (page 272)
10 Honey-Garlic Roasted Pork Trotters (page 290)

Vitamin B_2
1 Liver and Onions (page 281)
2 Steak and Kidney Pot Pie (page 274)
3 Fried Kidney with Kumquat and Cranberry Chutney (page 268)
4 Hidden Liver Meatloaf (page 272)
5 Beef Heart "Chow Mein" (page 278)
6 Stuffed Heart Roast (page 276)
7 Hidden Offal Swedish Meatballs (page 282)
8 Russ' Flatbread (page 326)
9 Beef Heart Borscht (page 192)
10 50/50/50 Burgers (page 289)

Vitamin B_3
1 Liver and Onions (page 281)
2 Whole Turkey with Mofongo Stuffing (page 210)
3 Seafood and Leek Soup (page 190)
4 BBQ Pork Ribs (page 216)
5 Roasted Chicken (page 209)
6 Oxtail and Pearl Onion Soup (page 191)
7 Bacon-Apple Chicken Burgers with Maple-Cranberry Sauce (page 222)
8 Hidden Liver Meatloaf (page 272)
9 "Spaghetti" (page 224)
10 Tarragon Roasted Pork (page 208)

Vitamin B_5
1 Liver and Onions (page 281)
2 Hidden Liver Meatloaf (page 272)
3 Lobster Bisque (page 186)
4 50/50/50 Burgers (page 289)
5 Hidden Offal Swedish Meatballs (page 282)
6 "Spaghetti" (page 224)
7 Beef Heart "Chow Mein" (page 278)
8 Stuffed Heart Roast (page 276)
9 BBQ Pork Ribs (page 216)
10 Steak and Kidney Pot Pie (page 274)

Vitamin B_6
1 Whole Turkey with Mofongo Stuffing (page 210)
2 Liver and Onions (page 281)
3 Seafood and Leek Soup (page 190)
4 Tarragon Roasted Pork (page 208)
5 Salmon with Maitre D' "Butter" (page 245)
6 Beef Heart "Chow Mein" (page 278)
7 Pork Pie–Stuffed Acorn Squash (page 231)
8 Hidden Liver Meatloaf (page 272)
9 Oxtail and Pearl Onion Soup (page 191)
10 Pomegranate Molasses-Glazed Salmon (page 239)

Vitamin B_9 (Folate)
1 Russ' Flatbread (page 326)
2 Liver and Onions (page 281)
3 Superfood Smoothie (page 141)
4 Beef Heart "Chow Mein" (page 278)
5 Seafood and Leek Soup (page 190)
6 Kale Chips (page 166)
7 Garden Salad (page 160)
8 Easy Broiled Asparagus (page 306)
9 Hidden Liver Meatloaf (page 272)
10 "Cream" of Broccoli Soup (page 183)

Vitamin B_{12}
1 Liver and Onions (page 281)
2 Hidden Liver Meatloaf (page 272)
3 50/50/50 Burgers (page 289)
4 Hidden Offal Swedish Meatballs (page 282)
5 Steak and Kidney Pot Pie (page 274)
6 Bacon and Bison Liver Pâté with Fresh Fig Jam (page 152)
7 Fried Kidney with Kumquat and Cranberry Chutney (page 268)
8 Beef Heart "Chow Mein" (page 278)
9 Oysters on the Half Shell (page 263)
10 Stuffed Heart Roast (page 276)

These Top Ten lists are based on data available from the USDA database. They are not calorie adjusted and instead represent nutrient content per serving.

Minerals

	Choline
1	Steak and Kidney Pot Pie (page 274)
2	Liver and Onions (page 281)
3	Fried Kidney with Kumquat and Cranberry Chutney (page 268)
4	Beef Heart "Chow Mein" (page 278)
5	Hidden Liver Meatloaf (page 272)
6	Stuffed Heart Roast (page 276)
7	Hidden Offal Swedish Meatballs (page 282)
8	Beef Heart Borscht (page 192)
9	Seafood and Leek Soup (page 190)
10	Beef Tongue with Celery Root and Fennel Slaw (page 270)

	Calcium
1	Sardine Salad (page 163)
2	Beef Heart "Chow Mein" (page 278)
3	Deep-Fried Fish Heads (page 285)
4	Pan-Fried Sardines (page 252)
5	Seafood and Leek Soup (page 190)
6	Lobster Bisque (page 186)
7	Kale Chips (page 166)
8	"Spaghetti" (page 224)
9	Superfood Smoothie (page 141)
10	Bacon-Braised Whitefish and Brussels (page 254)

	Copper
1	Liver and Onions (page 281)
2	Hidden Liver Meatloaf (page 272)
3	50/50/50 Burgers (page 289)
4	Hidden Offal Swedish Meatballs (page 282)
5	Bacon and Bison Liver Pâté with Fresh Fig Jam (page 152)
6	Lobster Bisque (page 186)
7	Calamari with Tzatziki Sauce (page 258)
8	Superfood Smoothie (page 141)
9	Kale Chips (page 166)
10	Oysters on the Half Shell (page 263)

	Iron
1	Beef Heart "Chow Mein" (page 278)
2	Seafood and Leek Soup (page 190)
3	Stuffed Heart Roast (page 276)
4	Beef Heart Borscht (page 192)
5	Steak and Kidney Pot Pie (page 274)
6	Rabbit and Wild Mushroom Stew (page 200)
7	Liver and Onions (page 281)
8	Hidden Offal Swedish Meatballs (page 282)
9	Hidden Liver Meatloaf (page 272)
10	"Spaghetti" (page 224)

	Magnesium
1	Lobster Bisque (page 186)
2	Seafood and Leek Soup (page 190)
3	Pork Pie–Stuffed Acorn Squash (page 231)
4	Superfood Smoothie (page 141)
5	Beef Heart "Chow Mein" (page 278)
6	Pork Pad Thai (page 234)
7	Bacon-Braised Whitefish and Brussels (page 254)
8	"Spaghetti" (page 224)
9	Sardine Salad (page 163)
10	Sweet Potato Linguine with Bolognese Sauce (page 226)

	Manganese
1	Seafood and Leek Soup (page 190)
2	Superfood Smoothie (page 141)
3	Lobster Bisque (page 186)
4	Savory Roasted Taro (page 320)
5	Sweet Potato Linguine with Bolognese Sauce (page 226)
6	Coconut Cream, Milk, and Whipped Topping (page 116)
7	Coconut Milk Yogurt (page 118)
8	Bacon-Apple Chicken Burgers with Maple-Cranberry Sauce (page 222)
9	New England Clam Chowder (page 196)
10	Kale Chips (page 166)

	Phosphorous
1	Seafood and Leek Soup (page 190)
2	Bacon-Braised Whitefish and Brussels (page 254)
3	Liver and Onions (page 281)
4	Sardine Salad (page 163)
5	Lobster Bisque (page 186)
6	Beef Heart "Chow Mein" (page 278)
7	Pan-Fried Sardines (page 252)
8	Bacon-Apple Chicken Burgers with Maple-Cranberry Sauce (page 222)
9	Steak and Kidney Pot Pie (page 274)
10	Hidden Liver Meatloaf (page 272)

	Potassium
1	Seafood and Leek Soup (page 190)
2	Pork Pie–Stuffed Acorn Squash (page 231)
3	Beef Heart "Chow Mein" (page 278)
4	Pork Pad Thai (page 234)
5	Superfood Smoothie (page 141)
6	Bacon-Apple Chicken Burgers with Maple-Cranberry Sauce (page 222)
7	Vegetable Soup with Chicken Sausage (page 194)
8	Sweet Potato Linguine with Bolognese Sauce (page 226)
9	Bacon-Braised Whitefish and Brussels (page 254)
10	"Spaghetti" (page 224)

These Top Ten lists are based on data available from the USDA database. They are not calorie adjusted and instead represent nutrient content per serving.

	Selenium
1	Lobster Bisque (page 186)
2	Steak and Kidney Pot Pie (page 274)
3	Fried Kidney with Kumquat and Cranberry Chutney (page 268)
4	Seafood and Leek Soup (page 190)
5	Oysters on the Half Shell (page 263)
6	BBQ Pork Ribs (page 216)
7	Scalloped Hake and Oysters (page 248)
8	Braised Pork Chops with Apple and Fennel (page 220)
9	Lemon and Thyme Broiled Pork Chops (page 230)
10	Pork Pie–Stuffed Acorn Squash (page 231)

	Zinc
1	Oysters on the Half Shell (page 263)
2	Scalloped Hake and Oysters (page 248)
3	Lobster Bisque (page 186)
4	"Spaghetti" (page 224)
5	Leg of Lamb with Mint Vinegar (page 206)
6	Rustic Bison Pot Roast (page 212)
7	Beef Cheek and Daikon Radish Stew (page 198)
8	Hidden Liver Meatloaf (page 272)
9	Oxtail and Pearl Onion Soup (page 191)
10	Sweet Potato Linguine with Bolognese Sauce (page 226)

Other

	Fiber
1	Savory Roasted Taro (page 320)
2	"Cream" of Broccoli Soup (page 183)
3	Superfood Smoothie (page 141)
4	Pork Pie–Stuffed Acorn Squash (page 231)
5	Guacamole (page 171)
6	Garden Green Vichyssoise (page 188)
7	Beef Heart "Chow Mein" (page 278)
8	Mashed Acorn Squash with Forty Cloves of Garlic (page 307)
9	"Spaghetti" (page 224)
10	Seafood and Leek Soup (page 190)

	Omega-3 Polyunsaturated Fatty Acids
1	Bacon-Braised Whitefish and Brussels (page 254)
2	Salmon with Maitre D' "Butter" (page 245)
3	Pomegranate Molasses–Glazed Salmon (page 239)
4	Seafood and Leek Soup (page 190)
5	Scalloped Hake and Oysters (page 248)
6	Sardine Salad (page 163)
7	Pan-Fried Sardines (page 252)
8	Lemon and Thyme Broiled Salmon with Blood Orange Salsa (page 242)
9	Simple Baked Whitefish (page 244)
10	Teriyaki-Poached Trout (page 250)

	Glycine
1	Pork Rinds (page 167)
2	Roasted Chicken (page 209)
3	Lobster Bisque (page 186)
4	Seafood and Leek Soup (page 190)
5	Beef Cheek and Daikon Radish Stew (page 198)
6	Hidden Liver Meatloaf (page 272)
7	Whole Turkey with Mofongo Stuffing (page 210)
8	Bacon-Apple Chicken Burgers with Maple-Cranberry Sauce (page 222)
9	"Spaghetti" (page 224)
10	Rabbit and Wild Mushroom Stew (page 200)

	Tryptophan
1	Pork Pad Thai (page 234)
2	Sausage (any variety) (page 132)
3	Rabbit and Wild Mushroom Stew (page 200)
4	Pork Pie–Stuffed Acorn Squash (page 231)
5	BBQ Pork Ribs (page 216)
6	Roasted Chicken (page 209)
7	Leg of Lamb with Mint Vinegar (page 206)
8	Lobster Bisque (page 186)
9	Seafood and Leek Soup (page 190)
10	Whole Turkey with Mofongo Stuffing (page 210)

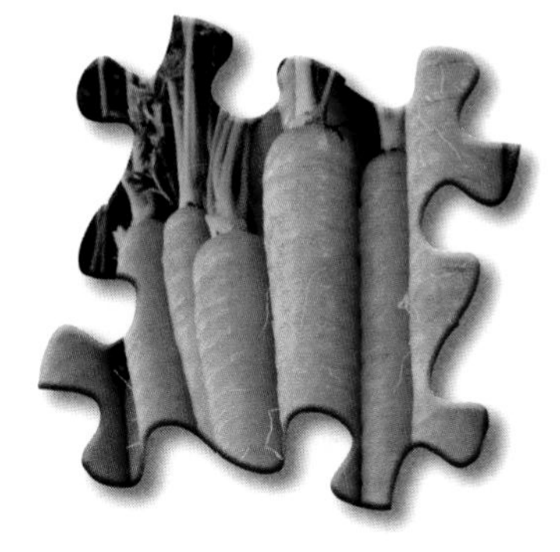

These Top Ten lists are based on data available from the USDA database. They are not calorie adjusted and instead represent nutrient content per serving.

Alphabetical Yes-No-Maybe So

Having trouble finding a food in any of the food lists? Search for it here alphabetically to determine whether the food in question is Paleo Approach friendly!

YES. Go ahead and eat it unless you're allergic or have a sensitivity to it.

NO. Don't eat it for now. Refer to *The Paleo Approach* for information on if and when it might be reintroduced.

MAYBE. This food might be tolerated. If you aren't sure, leave it out of your diet for now. (These foods are not included in the recipes in this book.) Refer to *The Paleo Approach* for more information.

MODERATION. This food is okay to eat, but there are some compelling reasons to keep portions small. Refer to *The Paleo Approach* for more information.

A

Food	YES	NO	MAYBE	MODERATION
abalone	✓			
abiu	✓			
abusgata	✓			
açaí	✓			
acerola	✓			
acesulfame potassium		✓		
ackee	✓			
acrylamide		✓		
adzuki beans		✓		
African moringa	✓			
agar agar	✓			
agave		✓		
agave nectar		✓		
agave worm	✓			
alcohol		✓		
allspice			✓	
almonds		✓		
amanatsu	✓			
amaranth		✓		
amaranth greens	✓			
ambarella	✓			
anchovy	✓			
anchovy paste (check ingredients)	✓			
anemone	✓			
anise seed			✓	
annatto seed			✓	
ant	✓			
antelope	✓			
aonori	✓			
apple	✓			
apple cider vinegar	✓			
apricot	✓			
arame	✓			
Arctic char	✓			
arracacha	✓			
arrowroot	✓			
arrowroot powder	✓			
artichoke	✓			
artificial flavors		✓		
artificial food color		✓		
arugula	✓			
asafetida (check ingredients)	✓			
ashwagandha		✓		
asparagus	✓			
aspartame		✓		
Atlantic croaker	✓			
autolyzed protein		✓		
avocado	✓			
avocado oil	✓			

B

Food	YES	NO	MAYBE	MODERATION
babaco	✓			
bacon	✓			
baking soda	✓			
balm	✓			
balsamic vinegar	✓			
bamboo shoot	✓			
bamboo worm	✓			
banana	✓			
barcheek goby	✓			
barley		✓		
barley malt		✓		
barley malt syrup		✓		
basil leaf	✓			
bass	✓			
bay leaf	✓			
bear	✓			
bearberry	✓			
beaver	✓			
bee larvae	✓			

Food	YES	NO	MAYBE	MODERATION
beech mushroom	✓			
beef	✓			
beefsteak leaves	✓			
beet and other vegetable kvasses (check ingredients)	✓			
beet greens	✓			
beet root	✓			
beet sugar		✓		
bell pepper		✓		
bilberry	✓			
biriba	✓			
bison	✓			
bitter gourd	✓			
bitter melon	✓			
black beans		✓		
black caraway			✓	
black cumin			✓	
black tea				✓
black-eyed peas		✓		
blackberry	✓			
blood orange	✓			
blueberry	✓			
boar	✓			
bok choy	✓			
boletus	✓			
bonito	✓			
bonito flakes	✓			
borage greens	✓			
Brazil nuts		✓		
bream				✓
brill	✓			
brisling	✓			
broad beans		✓		
broadleaf arrowhead	✓			
broccoli	✓			
broccoli rabe	✓			
brominated vegetable oil		✓		
brown rice syrup		✓		
brown sugar		✓		
Brussels sprouts	✓			
buckwheat		✓		
Buddha's hand	✓			
buffalo	✓			
burdock	✓			
butter		✓		
butter beans		✓		
butter oil		✓		
butterfly kingfish	✓			

Food	YES	NO	MAYBE	MODERATION
buttermilk		✓		
button mushroom	✓			

C

Food	YES	NO	MAYBE	MODERATION
cabbage	✓			
calendula	✓			
calico beans		✓		
cam sành	✓			
camas	✓			
camel	✓			
camucamu	✓			
canary melon	✓			
cane crystals		✓		
cane juice		✓		
cane sugar		✓		
canistel	✓			
canna	✓			
cannellini beans		✓		
canola leaves	✓			
canola oil		✓		
cantaloupe	✓			
cape gooseberries		✓		
capers	✓			
capsicums		✓		
carambola	✓			
caramel		✓		
caraway			✓	
carbonated water	✓			
cardamom			✓	
cardoon	✓			
caribou	✓			
carnation	✓			
carob powder	✓			
carola	✓			
carp	✓			
carrageenan		✓		
carrot	✓			
carrot greens	✓			
carrot powder	✓			
casaba	✓			
cashews		✓		
cassava	✓			
cat's-ear	✓			
catfish	✓			
cauliflower	✓			
caviar (check ingredients)	✓			
cayenne pepper		✓		
celeriac	✓			
celery	✓			

YES. Go ahead and eat it unless you're allergic or have a sensitivity to it.

NO. Don't eat it for now. Refer to *The Paleo Approach* for information on if and when it might be reintroduced.

MAYBE. This food might be tolerated. If you aren't sure, leave it out of your diet for now. (These foods are not included in the recipes in this book.) Refer to *The Paleo Approach* for more information.

MODERATION. This food is okay to eat, but there are some compelling reasons to keep portions small. Refer to *The Paleo Approach* for more information.

Food	YES	NO	MAYBE	MODERATION
celery seed			✓	
cellulose gum		✓		
celtuce	✓			
centipede	✓			
ceriman	✓			
Ceylon spinach	✓			
chamomile	✓			
chanterelle	✓			
Charentais	✓			
chayote	✓			
cheese		✓		
cherimoya	✓			
cherries	✓			
chervil	✓			
chestnuts		✓		
chia		✓		
chicken	✓			
chickpeas		✓		
chickweed	✓			
chicory	✓			
chili pepper flakes		✓		
chili peppers		✓		
chili powder		✓		
Chinese artichoke	✓			
Chinese broccoli	✓			
Chinese mallow	✓			
chives	✓			
chokeberry	✓			
chokecherry	✓			
Christmas melon	✓			
chrysanthemum leaves	✓			
chuck roast	✓			
cicada	✓			
cilantro	✓			
cinnamon	✓			
citron	✓			
clams	✓			
clementine	✓			
cloudberry	✓			
clover	✓			
cloves	✓			

Food	YES	NO	MAYBE	MODERATION
cockles	✓			
cockroach	✓			
coco plum	✓			
coconut				✓
coconut aminos	✓			
coconut butter				✓
coconut cream	✓			
coconut cream concentrate				✓
coconut flour				✓
coconut milk (emulsifier-free)	✓			
coconut milk kefir (check ingredients)	✓			
coconut milk yogurt (check ingredients)	✓			
coconut oil	✓			
coconut sugar			✓	
coconut water	✓			
coconut water vinegar	✓			
cod	✓			
coffee (not daily)			✓	
collagen supplements	✓			
collard greens	✓			
common dab	✓			
conch	✓			
conger	✓			
coriander leaf	✓			
coriander seed			✓	
corn		✓		
corn oil		✓		
corn sweetener		✓		
corn syrup		✓		
corn syrup solids		✓		
cottage cheese		✓		
cottonseed oil		✓		
crab	✓			
crabapple	✓			
cranberry	✓			
crappie	✓			
crawfish	✓			
cream		✓		
cream of tartar	✓			
creamed coconut				✓
Crenshaw melon	✓			

	Food	YES	NO	MAYBE	MODERATION
	cress	✓			
	cricket	✓			
	crimini	✓			
	croaker	✓			
	crocodile	✓			
	crowberry	✓			
	crystalline fructose		✓		
	cucumber	✓			
	cultured grass-fed ghee			✓	
	cumin seed			✓	
	curds		✓		
	currant	✓			
	curry leaves	✓			
	curry powder		✓		
	custard apple	✓			
	cuttlefish	✓			
D	dabberlocks	✓			
	daikon	✓			
	dairy protein isolates		✓		
	dandelion	✓			
	date	✓			
	date sugar				✓
	deer	✓			
	dehydrated cane juice				✓
	demerara sugar		✓		
	derishi	✓			
	dextrin		✓		
	dextrose		✓		
	diastatic malt		✓		
	dill seed			✓	
	dill weed	✓			
	dove	✓			
	dragonfly	✓			
	dragonfruit	✓			
	dried fruit				✓
	drum	✓			
	duck	✓			
	dulse	✓			
	dung beetle	✓			
	durian	✓			
	durum		✓		
E	earthnut pea	✓			
	earthworm	✓			
	edamame		✓		
	edible flowers	✓			
	eel	✓			
	egg white		✓		

	Food	YES	NO	MAYBE	MODERATION
	egg yolk			✓	
	eggplant		✓		
	einkorn		✓		
	elderberry	✓			
	elephant foot yam	✓			
	elephant garlic	✓			
	elk	✓			
	emu	✓			
	emulsifiers (carrageenan, cellulose gum, guar gum, lecithin, xanthan gum)		✓		
	endive	✓			
	enokitake	✓			
	Ensete	✓			
	erythritol		✓		
	evaporated cane juice				✓
F	falberry	✓			
	fat hen	✓			
	fava beans		✓		
	fennel	✓			
	fennel leaf	✓			
	fennel seed			✓	
	fenugreek			✓	
	fenugreek leaves	✓			
	fera	✓			
	fernandina	✓			
	fiddlehead	✓			
	field blewit	✓			
	fig	✓			
	filefish	✓			
	fish sauce (check ingredients)	✓			
	flaxseed		✓		
	Florence fennel	✓			
	fluted pumpkin leaves	✓			
	fly pupae	✓			
	fonio		✓		
	frog	✓			
	fructose (added)		✓		
	fructose (naturally occurring)				✓
	fruit juice		✓		
	fruit juice concentrate		✓		
G	galactose		✓		
	galangal	✓			
	Galia melon	✓			
	gambooge	✓			
	gar	✓			
	garbanzo beans		✓		
	garden huckleberries		✓		
	garlic	✓			

YES. Go ahead and eat it unless you're allergic or have a sensitivity to it.

NO. Don't eat it for now. Refer to *The Paleo Approach* for information on if and when it might be reintroduced.

MAYBE. This food might be tolerated. If you aren't sure, leave it out of your diet for now. (These foods are not included in the recipes in this book.) Refer to *The Paleo Approach* for more information.

MODERATION. This food is okay to eat, but there are some compelling reasons to keep portions small. Refer to *The Paleo Approach* for more information.

Food	YES	NO	MAYBE	MODERATION
gelatin	✓			
ghee			✓	
ginger	✓			
gladiolas	✓			
glucose		✓		
glucose solids		✓		
goat	✓			
goji berries		✓		
golden syrup		✓		
Good King Henry	✓			
goose	✓			
gooseberries	✓			
granadilla	✓			
grapefruit	✓			
grapes	✓			
grasshopper	✓			
Great Northern beans	✓			
greater plantain	✓			
green banana flour	✓			
green beans			✓	
green tea				✓
greengage	✓			
ground cherries		✓		
grouse	✓			
guanabana	✓			
guar gum		✓		
guava	✓			
guavaberry	✓			
guinea hen	✓			
gypsy mushroom	✓			

H

Food	YES	NO	MAYBE	MODERATION
hackberry	✓			
haddock	✓			
hake	✓			
halibut	✓			
Hamburg parsley	✓			
hare	✓			
hawthorn	✓			
hazelnuts		✓		
heavy cream		✓		
hedgehog mushroom	✓			
hemp seed		✓		
herring	✓			
hibiscus	✓			
high-fructose corn syrup		✓		
high-glycemic-load foods (if not explicitly eliminated)				✓
hijiki	✓			
honey				✓
honeydew	✓			
honeysuckle	✓			
horned melon	✓			
hornworm	✓			
horse	✓			
horseradish	✓			
horseradish sauce (check ingredients)	✓			
hot peppers		✓		
huckleberry	✓			
hydrolyzed vegetable protein		✓		

I

Food	YES	NO	MAYBE	MODERATION
ice cream		✓		
ilama	✓			
inulin		✓		
invert sugar		✓		
Italian beans		✓		
ivy gourd	✓			

J

Food	YES	NO	MAYBE	MODERATION
jackfruit	✓			
jaggery				✓
jellyfish	✓			
Jerusalem artichoke	✓			
jicama	✓			
Job's tears		✓		
John Dory	✓			
jujube	✓			
june bug	✓			
juniper			✓	

K

Food	YES	NO	MAYBE	MODERATION
kaffir lime	✓			
kai-lan	✓			
kale	✓			
kamut		✓		
kangaroo	✓			
karonda	✓			
kefir (coconut milk) (check ingredients)	✓			
kefir (dairy)		✓		
kefir (water) (check ingredients)	✓			

Food	YES	NO	MAYBE	MODERATION
key lime	✓			
kidney beans		✓		
king mackerel	✓			
king trumpet mushroom	✓			
kinnow	✓			
kiwi	✓			
kiyomi	✓			
kohlrabi	✓			
kohlrabi greens	✓			
komatsuna	✓			
kombu	✓			
kombucha (check ingredients)	✓			
konjac	✓			
korlan	✓			
kudzu	✓			
kumquat	✓			
kurrat	✓			
kuzu starch	✓			
kvass (check ingredients)	✓			

L

Food	YES	NO	MAYBE	MODERATION
lactofermented condiments (check ingredients)			✓	
lactofermented fruits (check ingredients)			✓	
lactofermented vegetables (check ingredients)			✓	
lactose		✓		
Lagos bologi	✓			
lamb	✓			
lamb's lettuce	✓			
lamprey	✓			
land cress	✓			
lavender	✓			
laver	✓			
lecithin		✓		
leek	✓			
lemon	✓			
lemon balm	✓			
lentils		✓		
lettuce	✓			
lima beans		✓		
lime	✓			
limetta	✓			
limpets	✓			
ling	✓			
lingonberry	✓			
lion's mane mushroom	✓			
lips	✓			
lizard's tail	✓			
loach	✓			
lobster	✓			
locust	✓			
loganberry	✓			
longan	✓			
loofa	✓			
loquat	✓			
lotus root	✓			
lychee	✓			

M

Food	YES	NO	MAYBE	MODERATION
macadamia nut oil			✓	
macadamia nuts		✓		
mace	✓			
mackerel	✓			
mahi mahi	✓			
maitake	✓			
malt syrup		✓		
maltodextrin		✓		
maltose		✓		
mamey sapote	✓			
mandarin	✓			
mango	✓			
mangosteen	✓			
manioc	✓			
mannitol		✓		
maple sugar				✓
maple syrup				✓
marigold	✓			
marjoram leaf	✓			
marlin	✓			
mashua	✓			
matsutake	✓			
maypop	✓			
mealworm	✓			
medlar	✓			
melokhia	✓			
melon pear	✓			
mesquite flour		✓		
Meyer lemon	✓			
milk		✓		
milkfish	✓			
millet		✓		
mineral water	✓			
minnow	✓			
mizuna	✓			
moderate-glycemic-load vegetables and fruits				✓
molasses				✓
monk fruit (luo han guo)		✓		
monkfish		✓		
monosodium glutamate (MSG)		✓		

YES. Go ahead and eat it unless you're allergic or have a sensitivity to it.

NO. Don't eat it for now. Refer to *The Paleo Approach* for information on if and when it might be reintroduced.

MAYBE. This food might be tolerated. If you aren't sure, leave it out of your diet for now. (These foods are not included in the recipes in this book.) Refer to *The Paleo Approach* for more information.

MODERATION. This food is okay to eat, but there are some compelling reasons to keep portions small. Refer to *The Paleo Approach* for more information.

Food	YES	NO	MAYBE	MODERATION
moose	✓			
morel	✓			
mozuku	✓			
mulberry	✓			
mullet				✓
mung beans		✓		
muscadines	✓			
muscovado sugar				✓
mushrooms	✓			
muskmelon	✓			
mussels	✓			
mustard greens	✓			
mustard seed			✓	
mutton	✓			

N

Food	YES	NO	MAYBE	MODERATION
nance	✓			
nannyberry	✓			
napa cabbage	✓			
naranjilla		✓		
nasturtiums	✓			
natural flavors		✓		
navy beans		✓		
nectarine	✓			
neotame		✓		
net melon	✓			
New Zealand spinach	✓			
nitrates or nitrites (naturally occurring are OK)		✓		
nopal	✓			
nori	✓			
nutmeg			✓	
nutritional yeast	✓			

O

Food	YES	NO	MAYBE	MODERATION
oak mushroom	✓			
oats		✓		
octopus	✓			
ogen melon	✓			
ogonori	✓			
okra	✓			
olestra		✓		
olive oil	✓			
olives	✓			
omega-6 polyunsaturated fat–rich foods				✓
onion	✓			
orache	✓			
orange	✓			
orangelo	✓			
Oregon grape	✓			
oregano leaf	✓			
oroblanco	✓			
ostrich	✓			
oyster	✓			
oyster mushroom	✓			

P

Food	YES	NO	MAYBE	MODERATION
palm kernel oil		✓		
palm nectar			✓	
palm oil (look for ethically and sustainably sourced)	✓			
palm shortening (look for ethically and sustainably sourced)	✓			
palm sugar			✓	
pandora	✓			
panela		✓		
panocha		✓		
pansies	✓			
papaya	✓			
paprika		✓		
parsley	✓			
parsnip	✓			
partridge	✓			
passion fruit	✓			
pawpaw	✓			
pea			✓	
pea leaves	✓			
peach	✓			
peanut butter fruit	✓			
peanut oil		✓		
peanuts		✓		
pear	✓			
pearl onion	✓			
pecans		✓		
pepino		✓		
pepino melon	✓			
pepper (black, green, pink, or white)			✓	
pepper (red)		✓		
peppermint	✓			
perch	✓			
periwinkle	✓			

Food	YES	NO	MAYBE	MODERATION
Persian melon	✓			
persimmon	✓			
pheasant	✓			
phosphoric acid		✓		
pigeon	✓			
pignut	✓			
pilchard	✓			
pimento		✓		
pine nuts		✓		
pineapple	✓			
pinto beans		✓		
pistachios		✓		
plaice	✓			
plantain	✓			
plantain flour (check ingredients)	✓			
plum	✓			
poke	✓			
pollock	✓			
pomegranate	✓			
pomegranate molasses				✓
pomelo	✓			
pompia	✓			
ponkan	✓			
poppy seeds		✓		
pork	✓			
portobello	✓			
potato		✓		
potato onion	✓			
prairie turnip	✓			
prawns	✓			
propylene glycol		✓		
Prussian asparagus	✓			
primrose	✓			
pulasan	✓			
pumpkin	✓			
pumpkin powder	✓			
pumpkin seed		✓		
pumpkin sprouts	✓			
Q				
quail	✓			
quince	✓			
quinoa		✓		
R				
rabbit	✓			
radicchio	✓			
radish	✓			
radish sprouts	✓			
rambutan	✓			
ramp	✓			

Food	YES	NO	MAYBE	MODERATION
rangpur	✓			
rapadura		✓		
rapeseed oil		✓		
raspberry	✓			
raw cane sugar		✓		
raw sugar		✓		
red palm oil	✓			
red pepper		✓		
red wine vinegar	✓			
refined sugar		✓		
rhubarb (stems only)	✓			
riberry	✓			
rice		✓		
rice bran syrup		✓		
rice syrup		✓		
roe (check ingredients)	✓			
rose apple	✓			
rose hip	✓			
rosemary	✓			
rowan	✓			
Russian caraway			✓	
Russian melon	✓			
rutabaga	✓			
rye		✓		
S				
saccharose		✓		
safflower oil		✓		
saffron	✓			
saffron milk cap	✓			
safou	✓			
sage	✓			
sago worm	✓			
sailfish	✓			
salak	✓			
salmon	✓			
salmonberry	✓			
salo	✓			
salsify	✓			
salt				✓
samphire	✓			
santol	✓			
sardine	✓			
sauerkraut (check ingredients)	✓			
saury	✓			
savory leaf	✓			
scallion	✓			
scallop	✓			
scarlet runner beans			✓	

YES. Go ahead and eat it unless you're allergic or have a sensitivity to it.

NO. Don't eat it for now. Refer to *The Paleo Approach* for information on if and when it might be reintroduced.

MAYBE. This food might be tolerated. If you aren't sure, leave it out of your diet for now. (These foods are not included in the recipes in this book.) Refer to *The Paleo Approach* for more information.

MODERATION. This food is okay to eat, but there are some compelling reasons to keep portions small. Refer to *The Paleo Approach* for more information.

Food	YES	NO	MAYBE	MODERATION
saccharin		✓		
scented geranium	✓			
scorzonera	✓			
sculpit	✓			
sea beet	✓			
sea buckthorn	✓			
sea cucumber	✓			
sea grape	✓			
sea kale	✓			
sea lettuce	✓			
sea lion	✓			
sea squirt	✓			
sea urchin	✓			
sea vegetable powder (or salt)	✓			
seafood	✓			
seal	✓			
semolina		✓		
service tree	✓			
serviceberry	✓			
sesame seed		✓		
shad	✓			
shallot	✓			
shark				✓
sharlyn	✓			
sheepshead	✓			
shiitake	✓			
shimeji	✓			
shipova	✓			
shonan gold	✓			
shrimp	✓			
silkworm	✓			
silverside	✓			
skirret	✓			
smelt	✓			
smooth-tailed trevally	✓			
snail	✓			
snake	✓			
snakehead	✓			
snapper	✓			
snow fungus	✓			
snow pea			✓	

Food	YES	NO	MAYBE	MODERATION
soda water	✓			
sole	✓			
sorbitol		✓		
sorghum		✓		
sorghum syrup		✓		
sorrel	✓			
sour cream		✓		
soursop	✓			
soybean oil		✓		
soybeans		✓		
spa water (homemade)	✓			
Sparassis crispa	✓			
sparkling water	✓			
spearmint	✓			
spelt		✓		
spinach	✓			
spinach powder	✓			
spring onion	✓			
spring water	✓			
squash	✓			
squash blossoms	✓			
squid	✓			
star anise			✓	
star apple	✓			
starfish	✓			
starfruit	✓			
stevia		✓		
straw mushroom	✓			
strawberry	✓			
strawberry tree	✓			
stridolo	✓			
strutto	✓			
sucanat		✓		
sucralose		✓		
sucrose		✓		
sudachi	✓			
sugar apple	✓			
sugar snap pea			✓	
sumac			✓	
summer purslane	✓			
summer squash	✓			

Food	YES	NO	MAYBE	MODERATION
sunflower oil		✓		
sunflower seed		✓		
sunflower sprouts	✓			
swede	✓			
sweet melon	✓			
sweet pepper		✓		
sweet potato	✓			
sweet potato flour, powder, or starch	✓			
sweet potato greens	✓			
sweet tooth fungus	✓			
Swiss chard	✓			
swordfish				✓
syrup		✓		

T

Food	YES	NO	MAYBE	MODERATION
tamarillo		✓		
tamarind	✓			
tangelo	✓			
tangerine	✓			
tangor	✓			
tapioca	✓			
tapioca flour, powder, or starch	✓			
taro	✓			
tarpon	✓			
tarragon	✓			
tatsoi	✓			
tea, green or black				✓
tea, herbal	✓			
teff	✓			
tempeh	✓			
textured vegetable protein	✓			
thimbleberry	✓			
thyme	✓			
ti	✓			
tiger nut	✓			
tilapia	✓			
tilefish	✓			
tinda	✓			
tofu		✓		
tomatillo		✓		
tomato		✓		
trans fats (partially hydrogenated vegetable oil, hydrogenated oil)		✓		
treacle		✓		
tree ear fungus	✓			
tree onion	✓			
triticale		✓		
trout	✓			
truffle	✓			
truffle oil (made with extra-virgin olive oil; check ingredients)	✓			
truffle salt (check ingredients)	✓			
tub gurnard	✓			
tuna	✓			
turbinado sugar		✓		
turbot	✓			
turkey	✓			
turmeric	✓			
turnip	✓			
turnip greens	✓			
turtle	✓			

U

Food	YES	NO	MAYBE	MODERATION
ugli	✓			
ugni	✓			
ulluco	✓			
umeboshi paste	✓			
umeboshi plums	✓			
unrefined cane sugar				✓
Uzbek melon	✓			

V

Food	YES	NO	MAYBE	MODERATION
vanilla bean			✓	
vanilla extract (if alcohol will be cooked off)	✓			
vanilla powder (check ingredients)	✓			
vegetable kvass (check ingredients)	✓			
vegetable juices and smoothies				✓
vegetable powder (pumpkin, sweet potato, spinach, etc.)	✓			

W

Food	YES	NO	MAYBE	MODERATION
wakame	✓			
walleye	✓			
walnut oil			✓	
walnuts		✓		
wampee	✓			
wasabi	✓			
water	✓			
water caltrop	✓			
water chestnut	✓			
water chestnut flour	✓			
water kefir	✓			
water spinach	✓			
watercress	✓			
watermelon	✓			
West Indian gherkin	✓			
whale				✓
wheat (all varieties)		✓		
whelk	✓			
whey		✓		
whey protein isolate		✓		
whipping cream		✓		
white wine vinegar	✓			
whiting	✓			
wild leek	✓			

YES. Go ahead and eat it unless you're allergic or have a sensitivity to it.

NO. Don't eat it for now. Refer to *The Paleo Approach* for information on if and when it might be reintroduced.

MAYBE. This food might be tolerated. If you aren't sure, leave it out of your diet for now. (These foods are not included in the recipes in this book.) Refer to *The Paleo Approach* for more information.

MODERATION. This food is okay to eat, but there are some compelling reasons to keep portions small. Refer to *The Paleo Approach* for more information.

Food	YES	NO	MAYBE	MODERATION
wild rice		✓		
wild-fermented condiments (check ingredients)	✓			
wild-fermented fruits (check ingredients)	✓			
wild-fermented vegetables (check ingredients)	✓			
wine (for drinking)		✓		
wine (for cooking; if alcohol will be cooked off)				✓
wineberry	✓			
winter melon	✓			
winter mushroom	✓			
winter squash	✓			
winter purslane	✓			
wolfberries		✓		

	Food	YES	NO	MAYBE	MODERATION
X	xanthan gum		✓		
	xylitol		✓		
Y	yacón	✓			
	yacon syrup		✓		
	yam	✓			
	yeast (brewer's, baker's, nutritional)	✓			
	yeast extract		✓		
	yogurt		✓		
	yuca	✓			
Z	yuzu	✓			
	zucchini	✓			

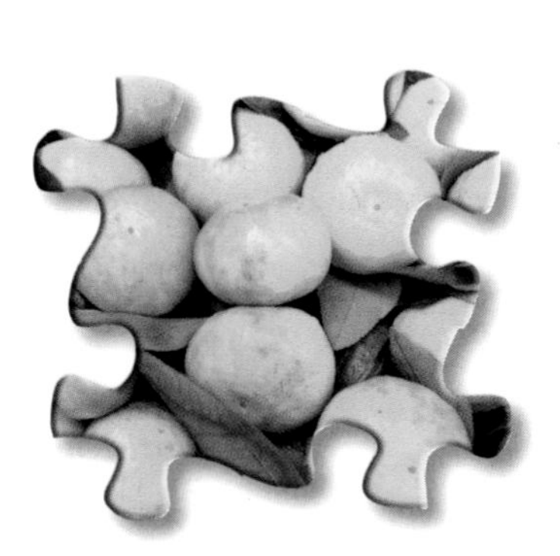

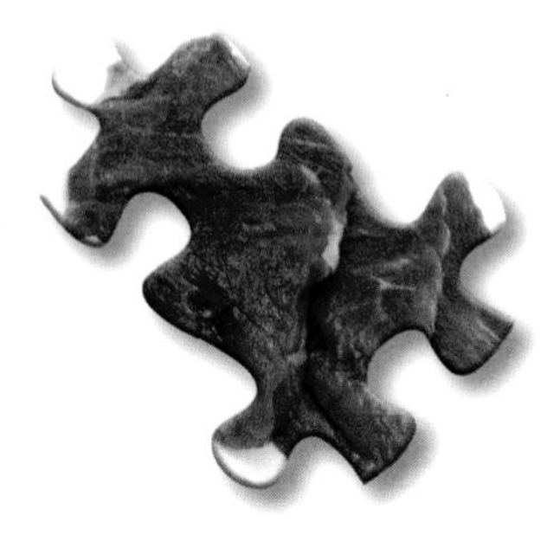

Selenium Health Benefit Values of Fish and Shellfish

The selenium health benefit value (Se-HBV) is essentially a measure of the ratio of selenium to methylmercury in each type of fish. This is important because selenium counteracts the negative effects of mercury (this is discussed in more detail in *The Paleo Approach*). If the number is greater than zero, the fish contains more selenium than mercury and is safe to consume. If the number is less than zero, the fish contains a higher level of mercury than selenium and should be avoided.

Fresh Fish and Shellfish	Se-HBV
albacore	45.4
anchovy	8.0
anglerfish	6.0
bigeye	48.6
blue marlin	34.1
blue shark	–1.0
blue whiting	1.0
bluefish	2.5
cat shark	–12.0
Chilean sea bass	7.0
clam	87.0
cod	11.5
common sole	25.0
croaker	10.5
cuttlefish	17.0
escolar	8.3
European hake	7.0
European sea bass	1.0
flounder	5.3
gilt-head bream	–1.0
grouper	3.4
hake	8.0
mackerel	73.0
mahi mahi	78.4
mako shark	–11.1
megrim	7.0
mussel	>1000
opah	5.9
orange roughy	2.3
pangasius	>1000
perch	3.0
porgy	24.0
red mullet	0.0
red snapper	8.8
salmon (Norway)	>1000
salmon (USA)	10.1
sardine	74.0
scad	36.0
scallop	0.5
shrimp (large; USA)	13.3
shrimp (small; USA)	4.4
shrimp (Spain)	1.0
sickle pomfret	44.4
skipjack	232.7
spearfish	71.0
squid	>1000
striped marlin	118.3
swordfish (Spain)	13.0
swordfish (USA)	–0.1
thresher shark	2.5
tuna (Spain)	21.0
tuna (USA)	4.9
wahoo	76.2
walleye pollock	0.9
whiting	62.5
yellowfin (USA, Atlantic)	2.0
yellowfin (USA, Pacific)	201.7

Canned Fish and Shellfish	Se-HBV
anchovy	45.0
clam	>1000
cockle	2.0
frigate	>1000
mackerel	45.0
mussel	>1000
octopus	>1000
sardine	>1000
small sardine	>1000
squid	>1000
tuna (albacore)	>1000
tuna (gourmet)	43.8
tuna (light)	20.4
tuna (white)	5.7

Frozen Seafood	Se-HBV
cod	>1000
common sole	>1000
hake	7
prawn	96
shrimp	3
squid	>1000

Scientists are just starting to understand the variability of the selenium health benefit value within a species of fish or shellfish and why some types of fish naturally have higher values than others. (Variability is due to the type of fish, size/age of the fish, geographic location and migration routes, and exact diet of the fish.) Also note that selenium levels have not been measured in several species known to contain high mercury, like tilefish and king mackerel. However, the take-home message is that most fish have positive selenium health benefit values, reflecting higher selenium than mercury levels, and therefore are safe to consume.

Data compiled from:

Burger, J., and Gochfeld, M., *Selenium and mercury molar ratios in commercial fish from New Jersey and Illinois: variation within species and relevance to risk communication.* Food Chem Toxicol. 2013;57:235–45

Kaneko, J.J., and Ralston, N.V. *Selenium and mercury in pelagic fish in the central north Pacific near Hawaii.* Biol Trace Elem Res. 2007;119(3):242–54

Olmedo P., et al., *Determination of essential elements (copper, manganese, selenium and zinc) in fish and shellfish samples. Risk and nutritional assessment and mercury-selenium balance.* Food Chem Toxicol. 2013;62C:299–307

Recipe Index

Kitchen Staples

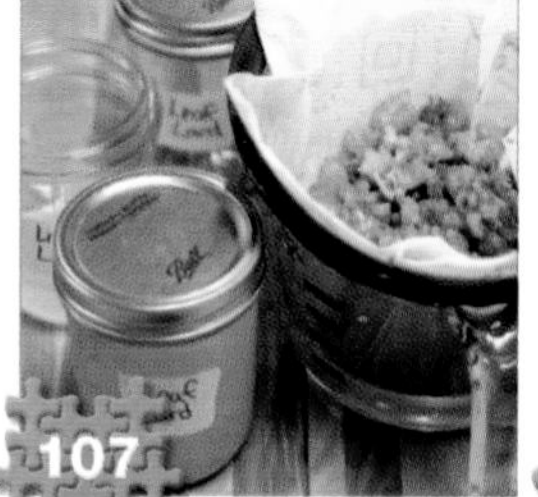
107 Tallow and Lard

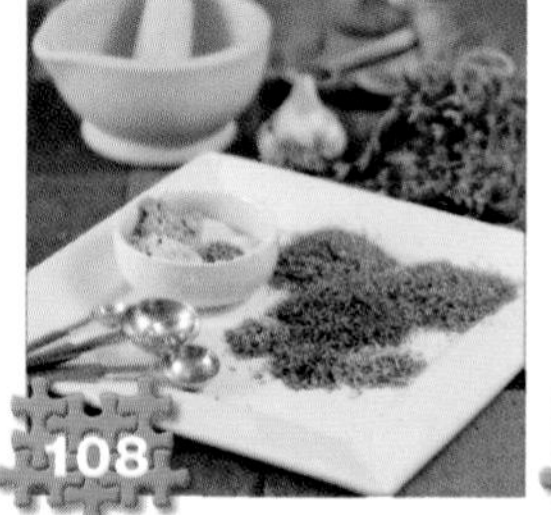
108 Handy-Dandy Spice Blends

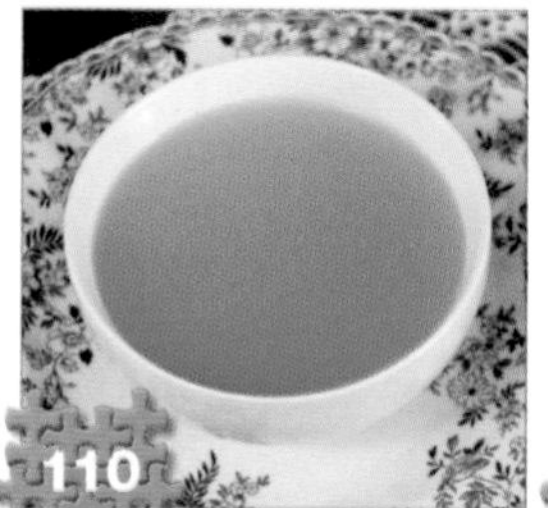
110 Bone Broth

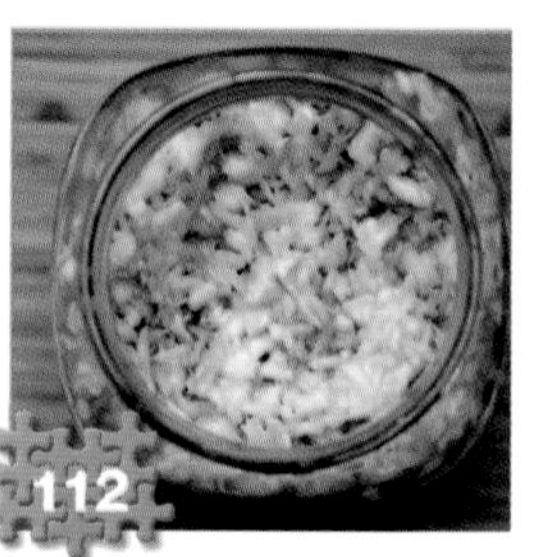
112 Sauerkraut

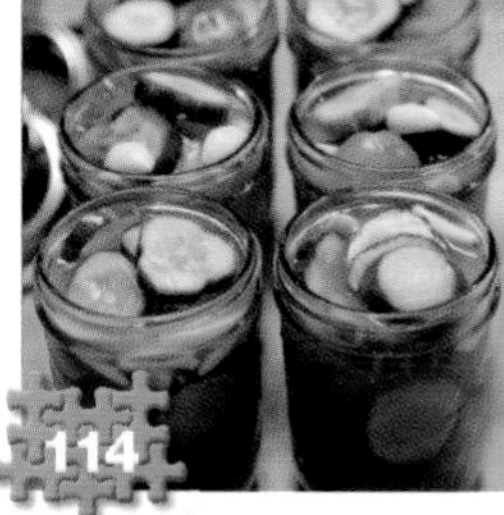
114 Green Tea and Garlic Pickles

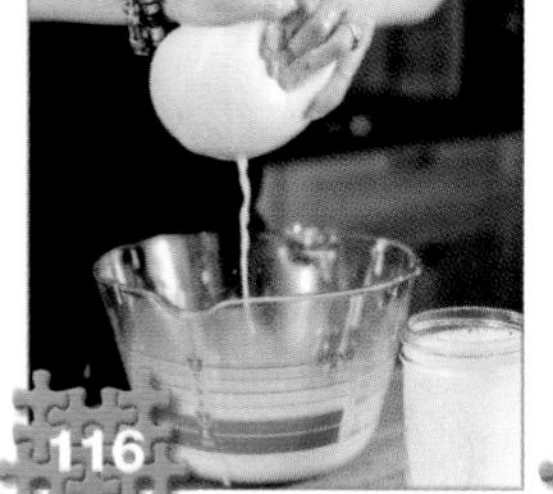
116 Coconut Milk, Cream, and Whipped Topping

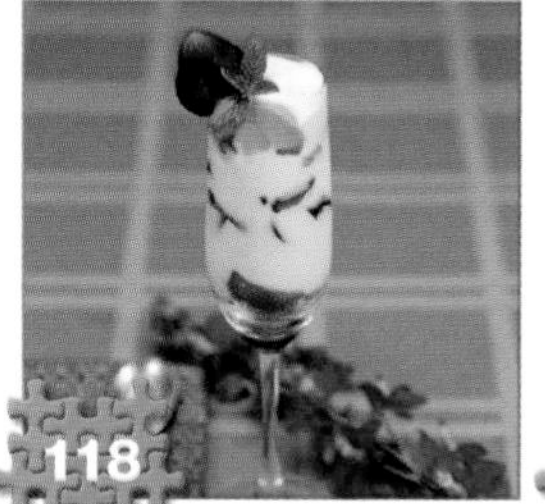
118 Coconut Milk Yogurt

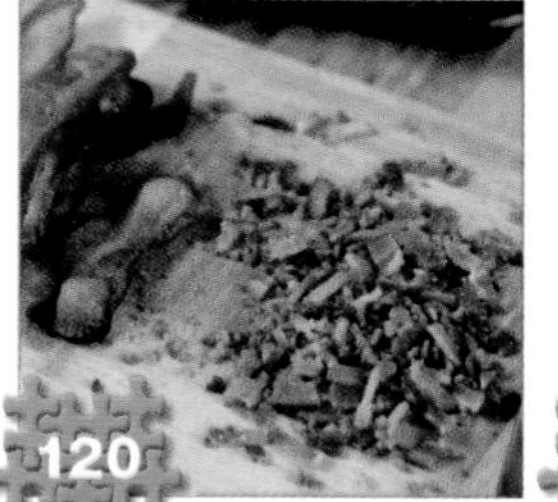
120 Crispy Bacon and Bacon Bits

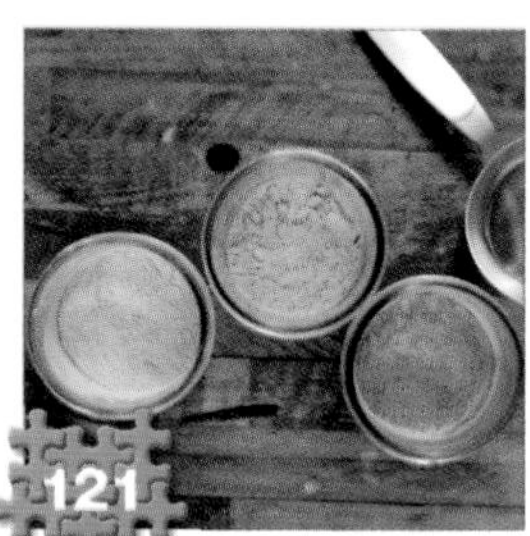
121 Homemade Fruit and Vegetable Flours

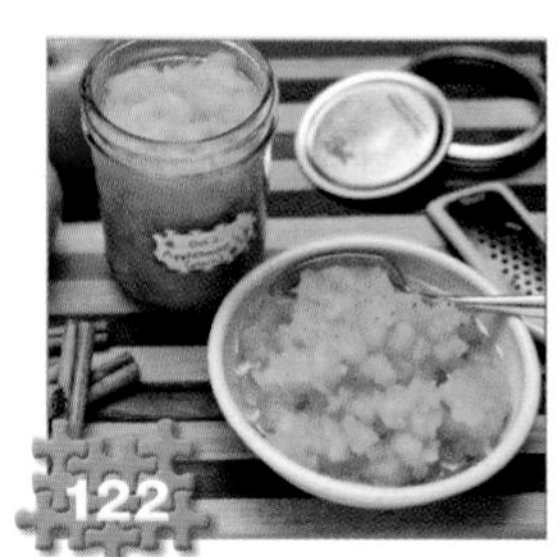
122 Applesauce

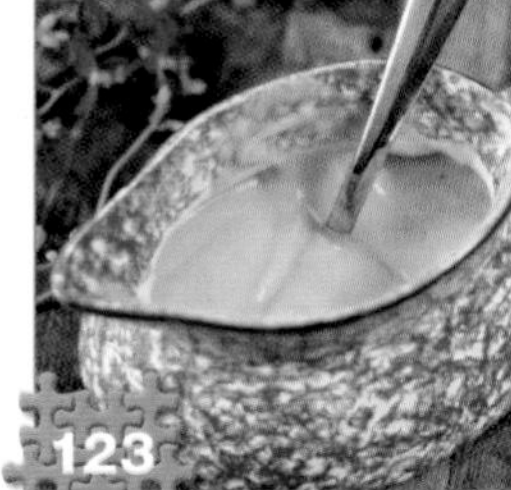
123 Cauliflower Gravy

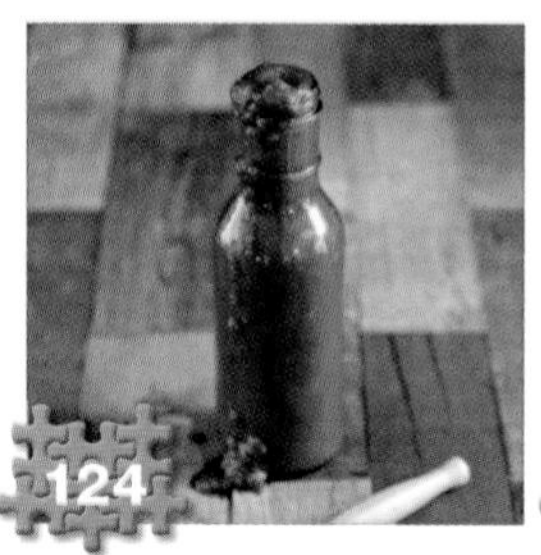
124 Barbecue Sauce

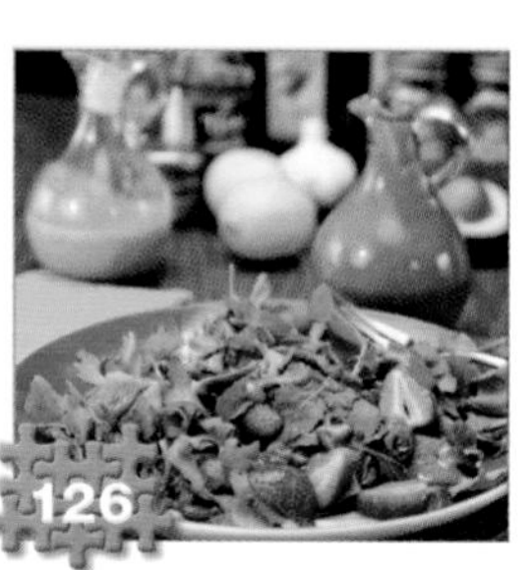
126 Salad Dressing

Breakfast Foods

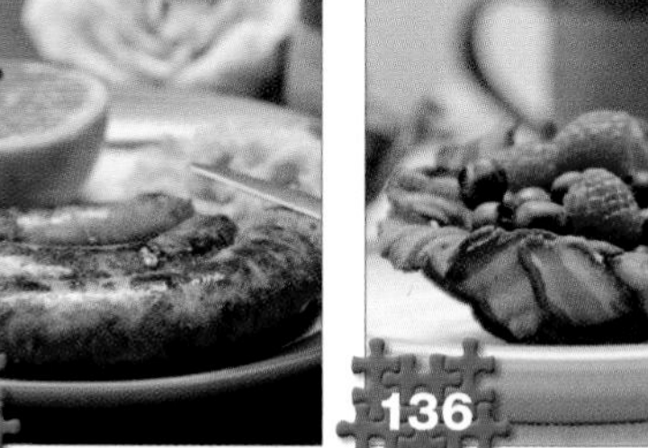
131 Homemade Sausage (9 Variations)

136 Bacon Fruit Cups

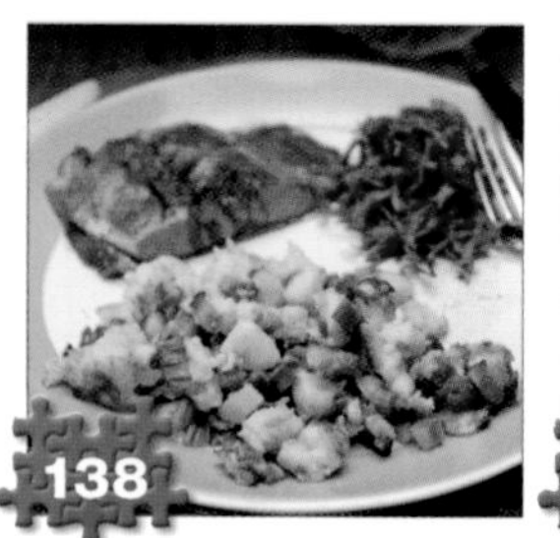
138 Taro Hash

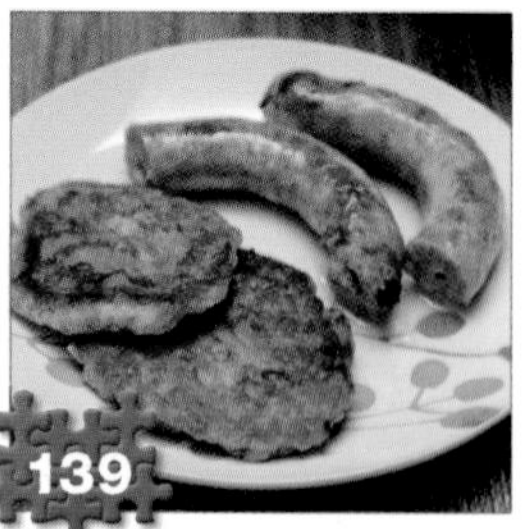
139 Plantain and Apple Fritters

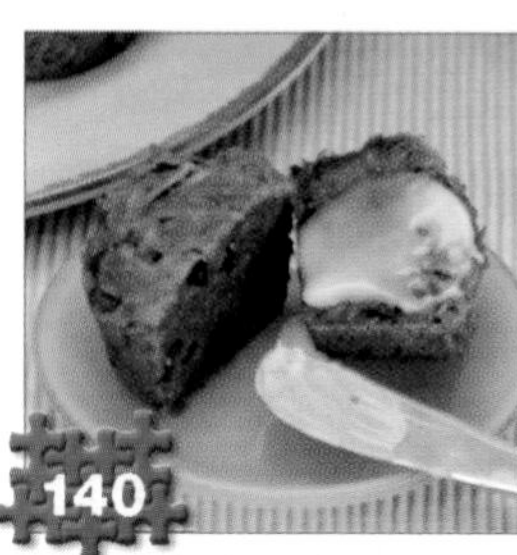
140 Carrot-Raisin Muffins

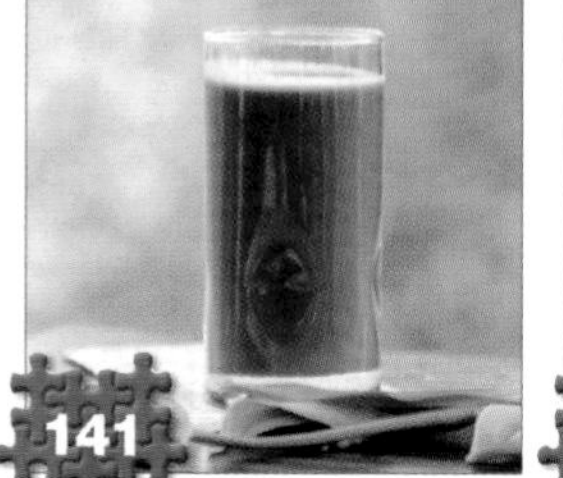
141 Superfood Smoothie

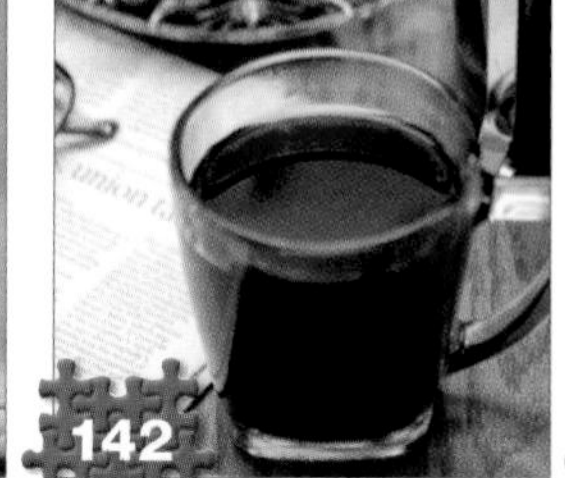
142 Breakfast Brew

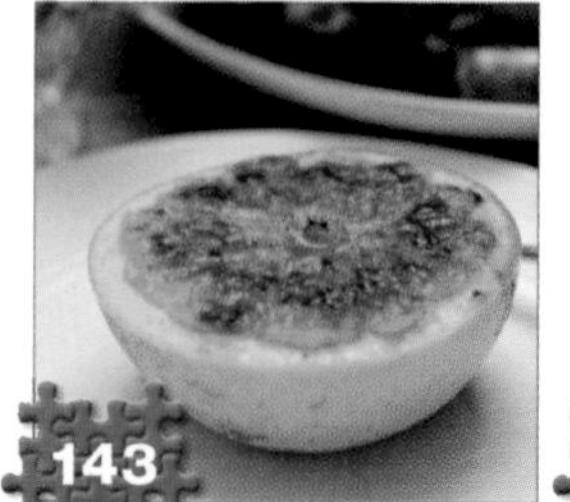
143 Cinnamon Broiled Grapefruit

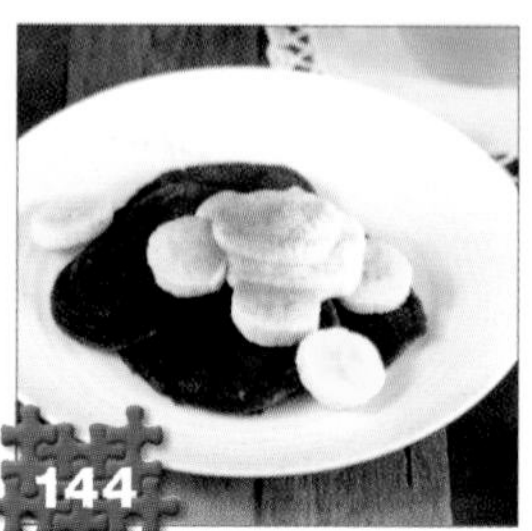
144 Banana "Nut" Pancakes

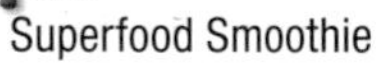

Appetizers, Salads, and Snacks

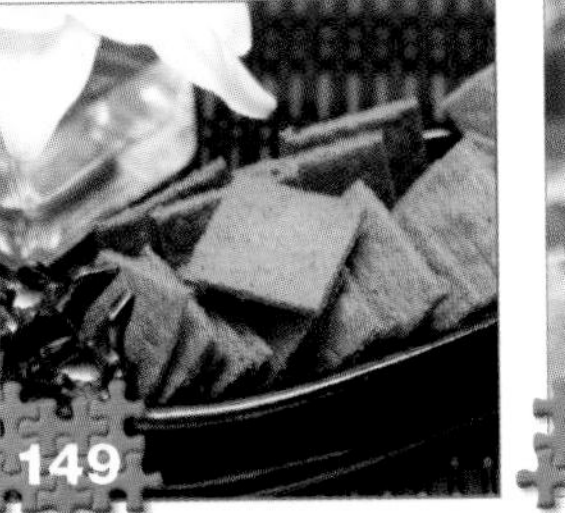

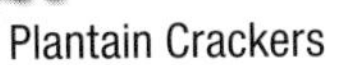
Plantain Crackers

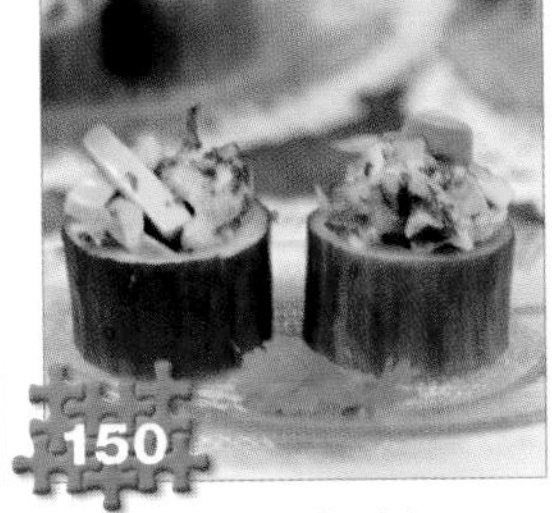

Ahi Tuna Ceviche

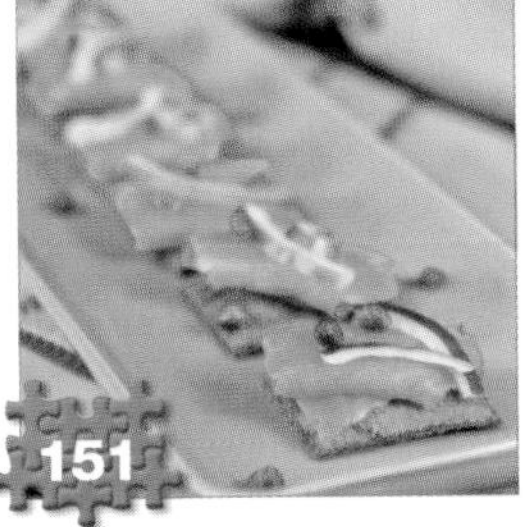

Lox Canapé

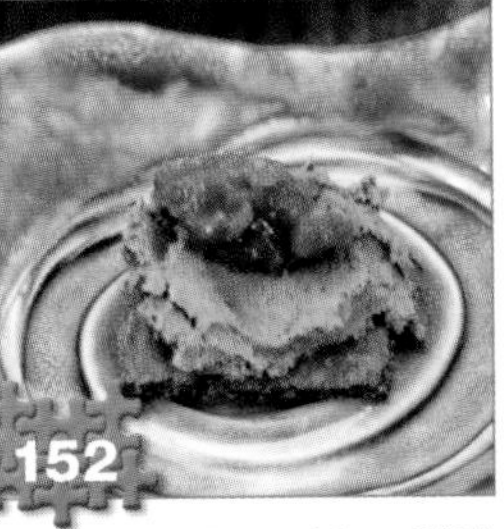

Bacon and Bison Liver Pâté with Fresh Fig Jam

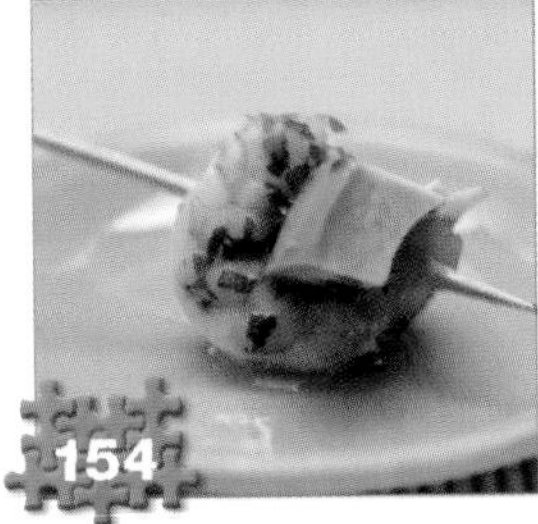

Shrimp and Avocado Skewers

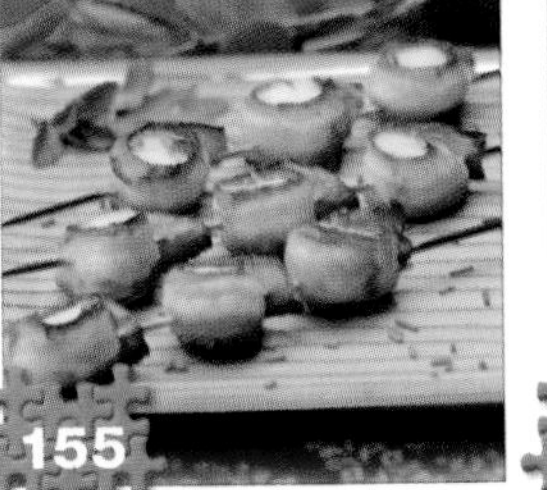

Bacon-Wrapped Scallops

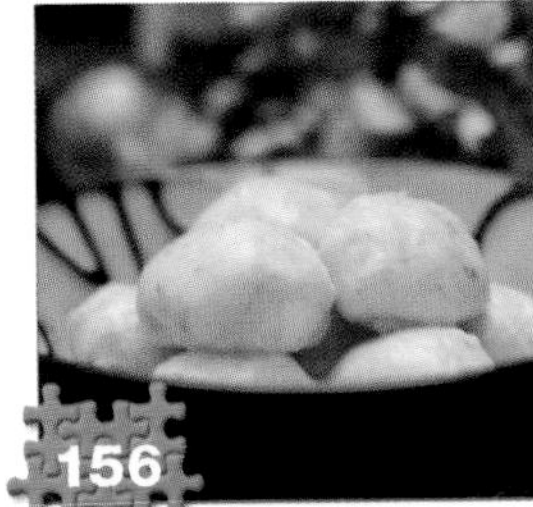

Har Gow–Inspired Shrimp Balls

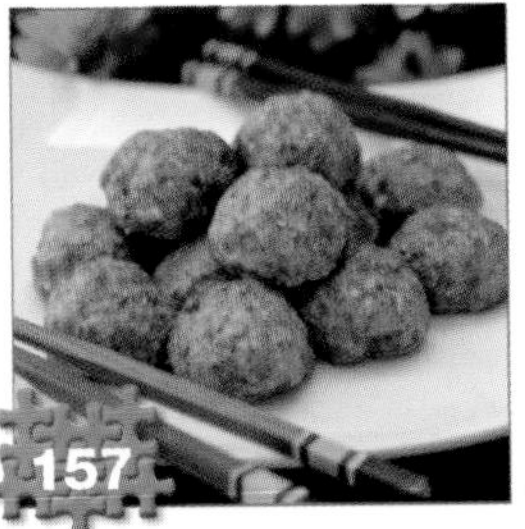

Pot Sticker Meatballs

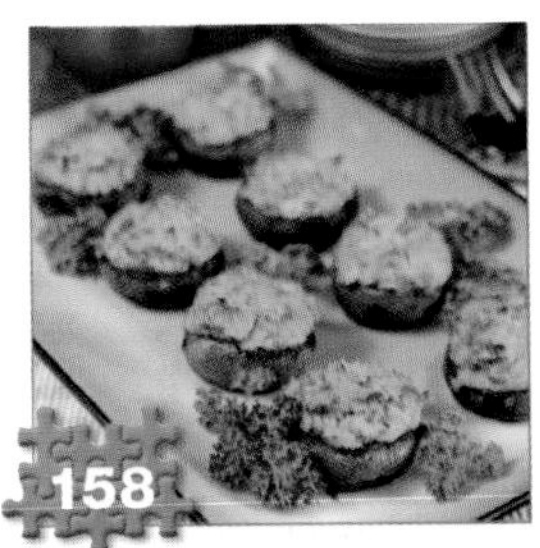

Crab-Stuffed Mushroom Caps

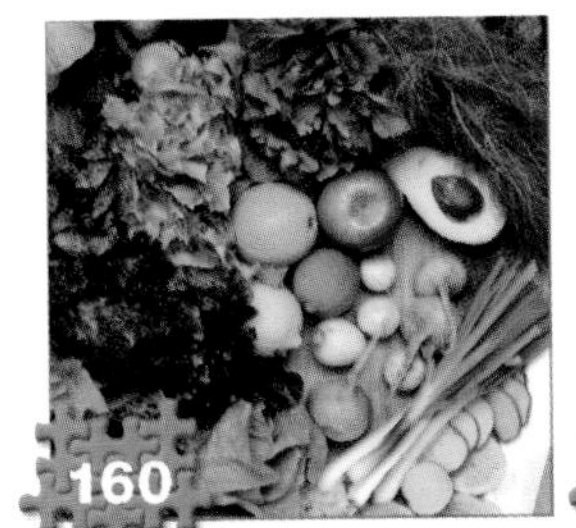

Garden Salad

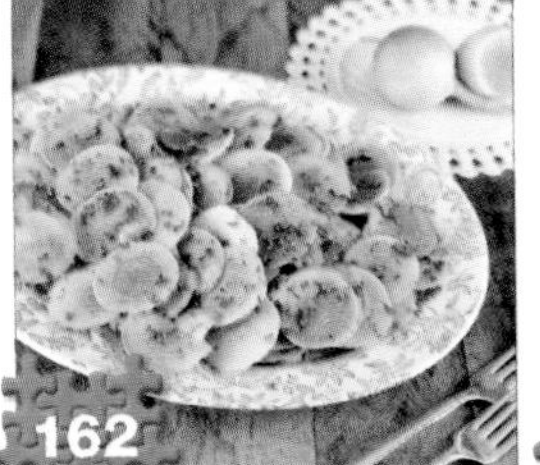

Radish Salad

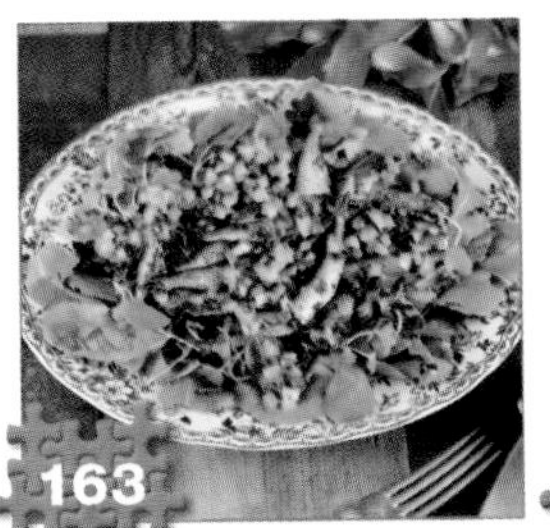

Sardine Salad

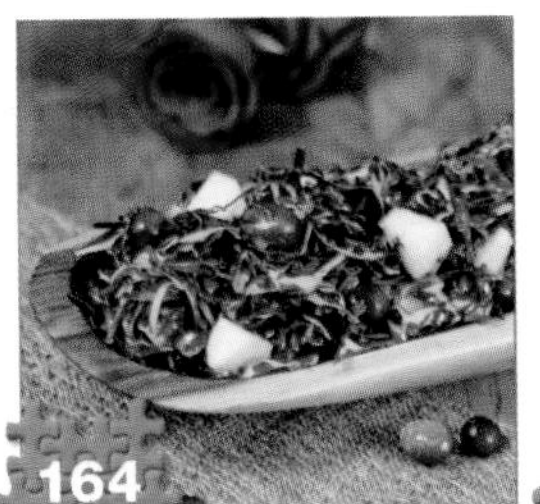

Cran-Apple Coleslaw

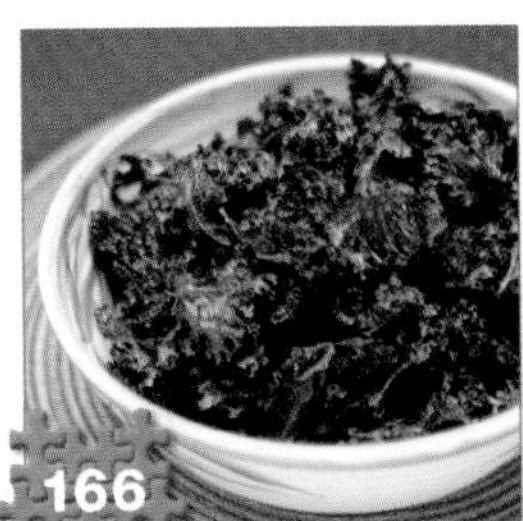

Kale Chips

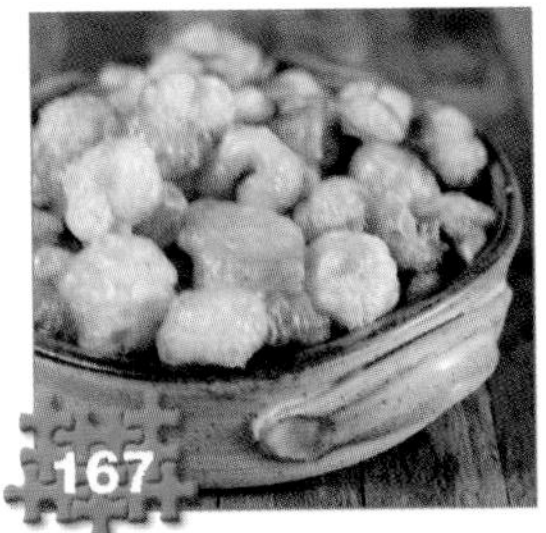

Pork Rinds

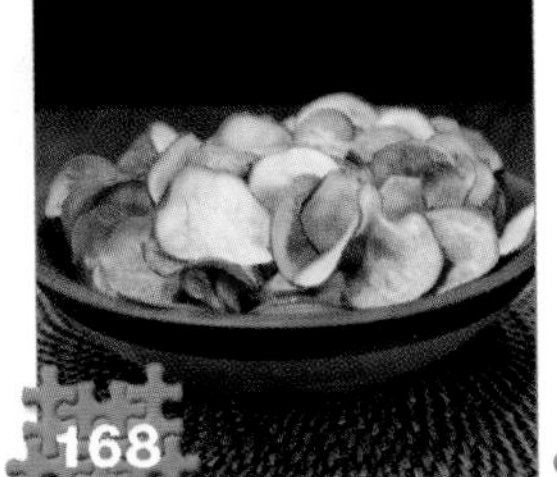

Sweet Potato Chips

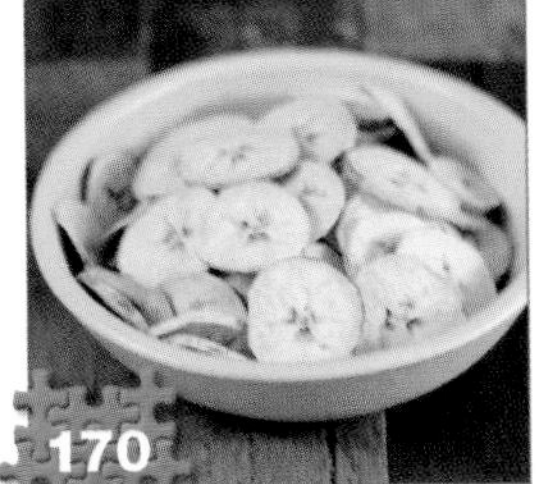

Dehydrator Plantain Chips

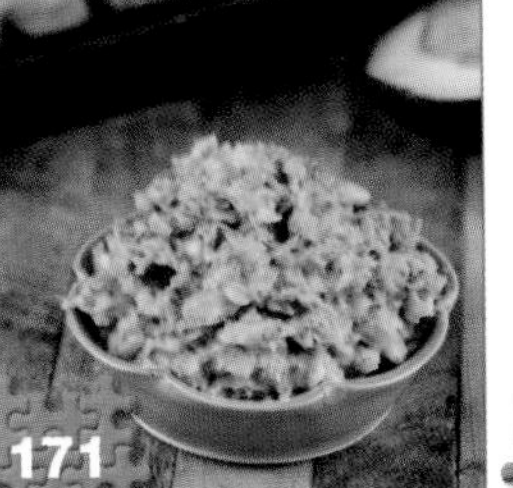

Guacamole

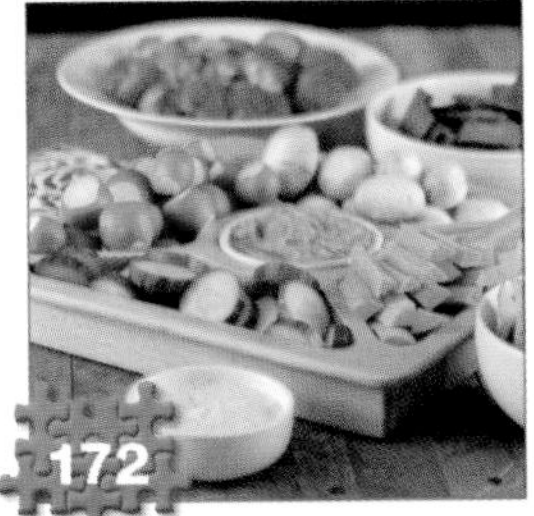

Veggies and Dip

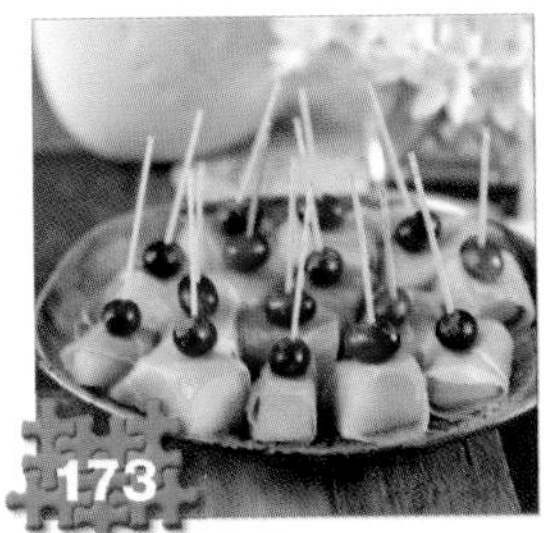

Prosciutto-Wrapped Melon

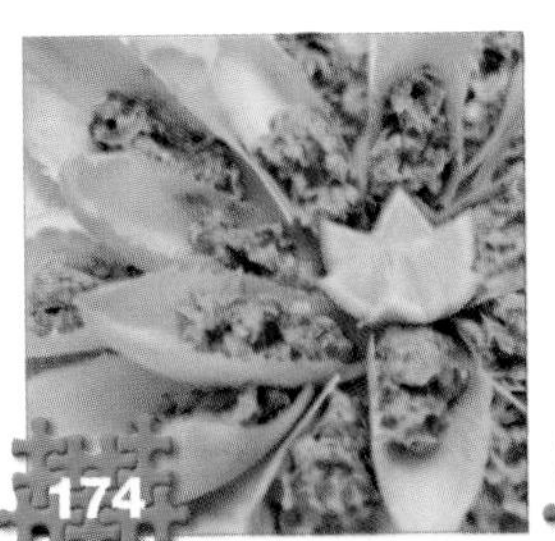

Smoked Salmon and Roe Endive Boats

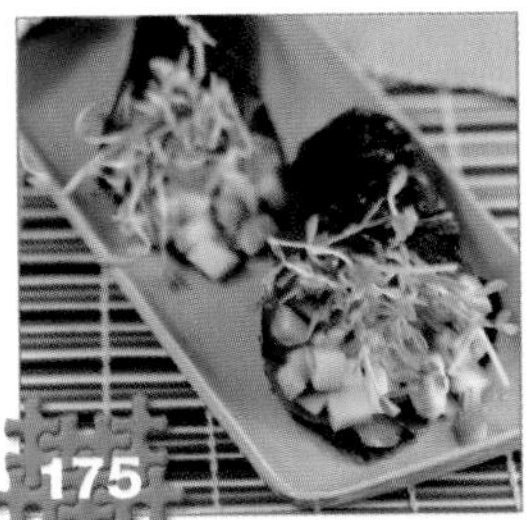

Smoked Salmon and Mango Salsa Nori Wraps

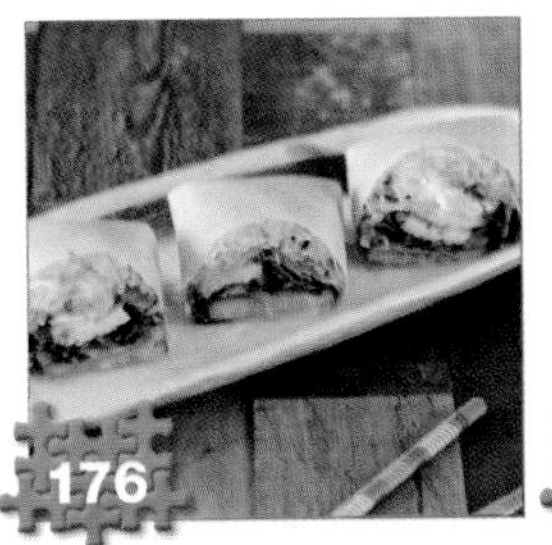

Vietnamese-Style Fresh "Spring Rolls"

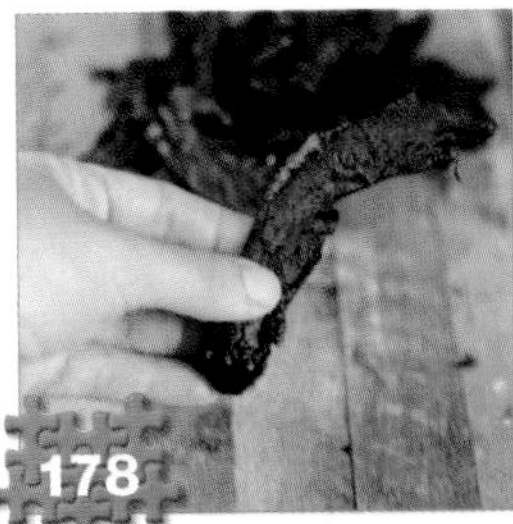

Sweet-and-Sour Beef Heart Jerky

Soups and Stews

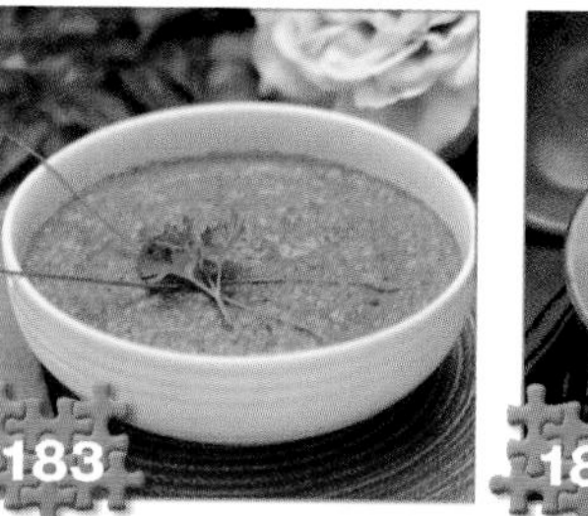
183 “Cream” of Broccoli Soup

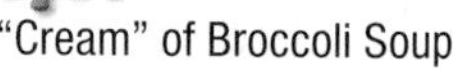

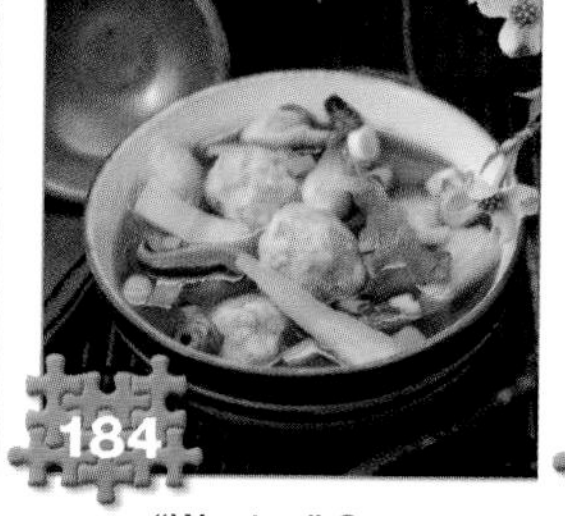
184 “Wonton” Soup

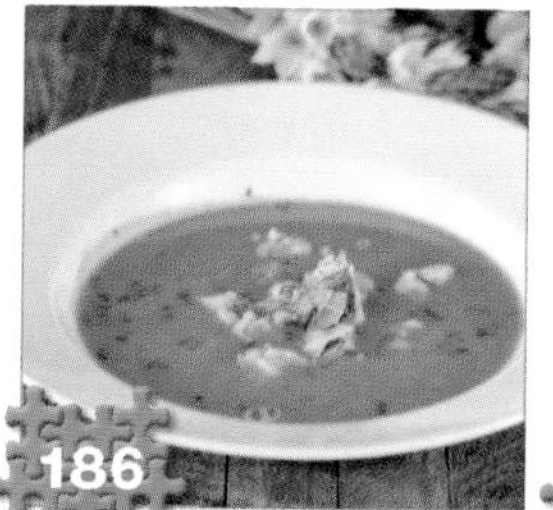
186 Lobster Bisque

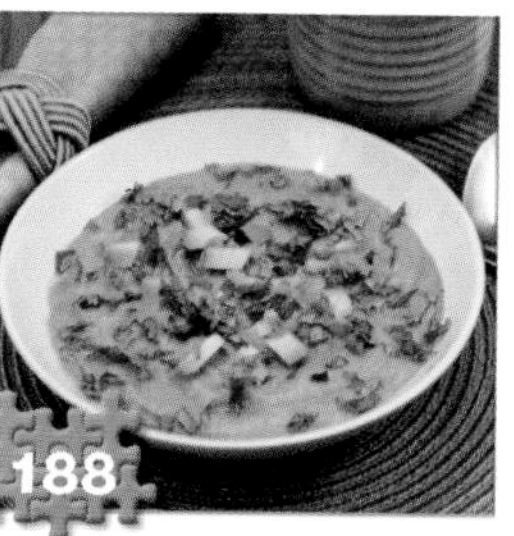
188 Garden Green Vichyssoise

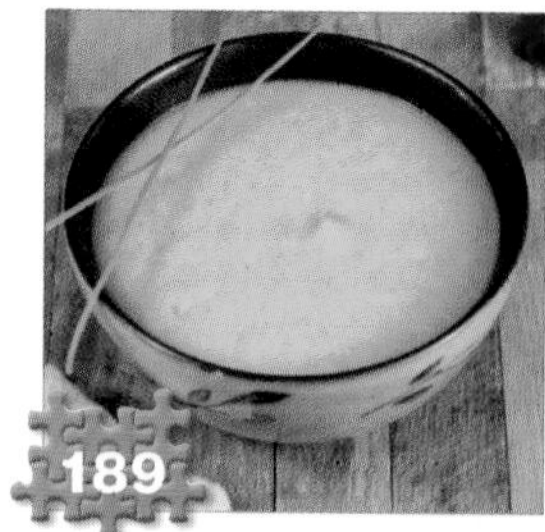
189 Carrot-Ginger Soup

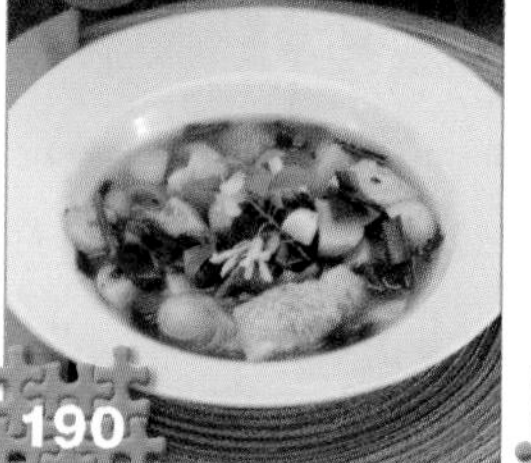
190 Seafood and Leek Soup

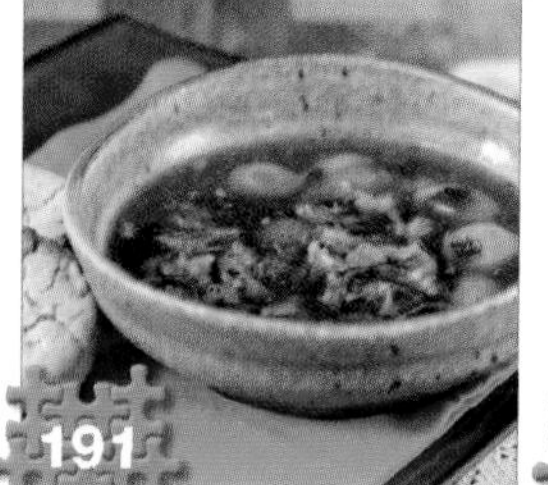
191 Oxtail and Pearl Onion Soup

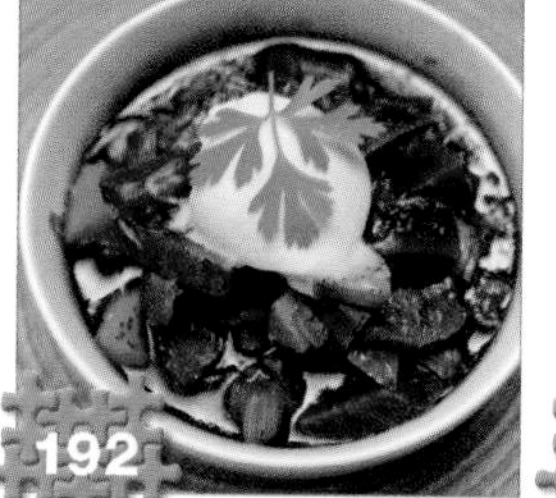
192 Beef Heart Borscht

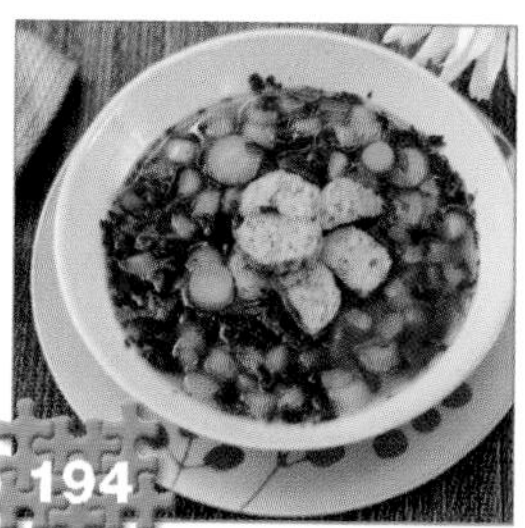
194 Vegetable Soup with Chicken Sausage

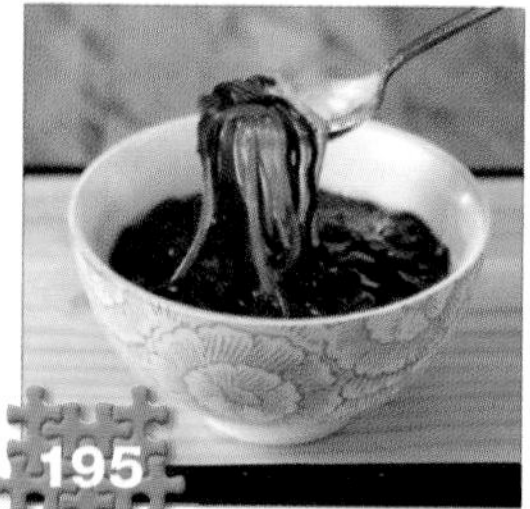
195 Asian-Inspired Noodle Soup

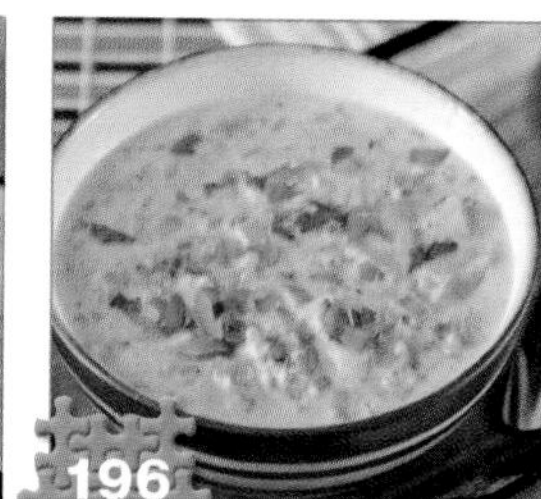
196 New England Clam Chowder

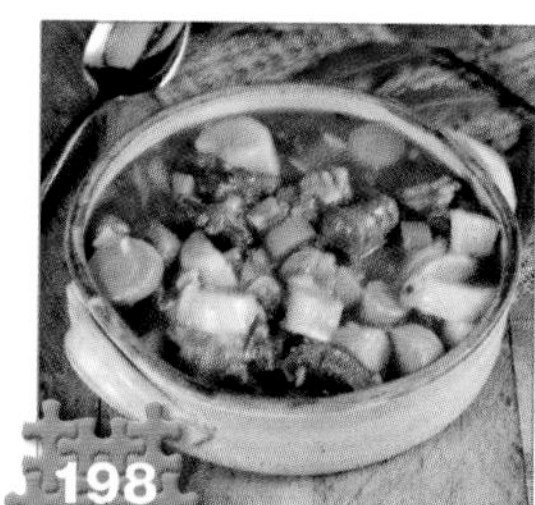
198 Beef Cheek and Daikon Radish Stew

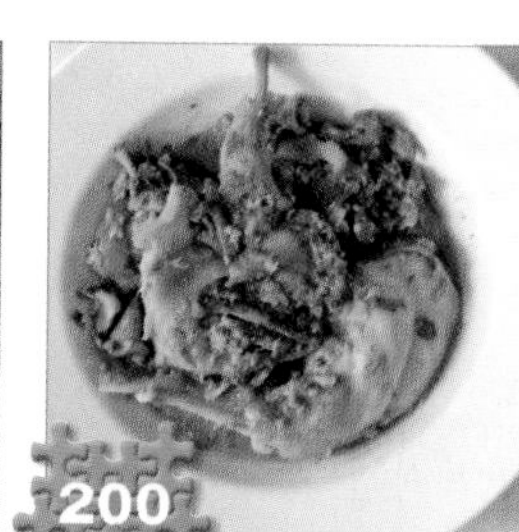
200 Rabbit and Wild Mushroom Stew

Meat and Poultry

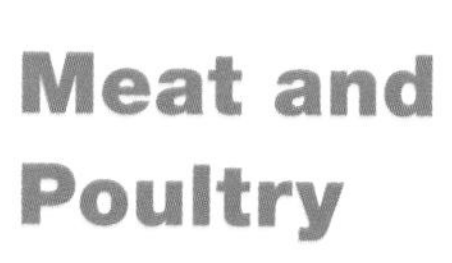

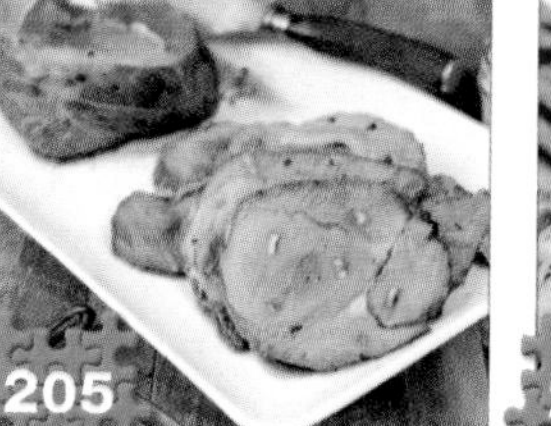
205 Garlic and Rosemary Roast Beef

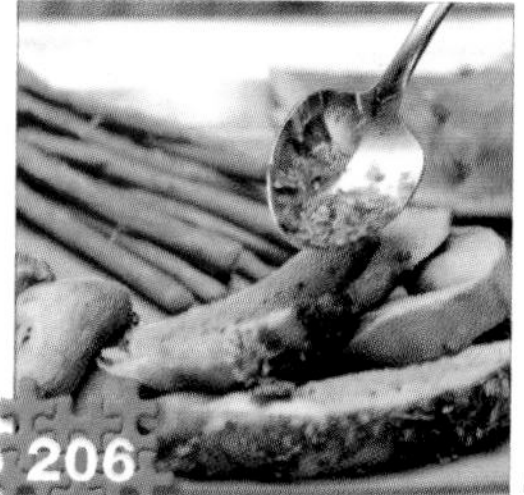
206 Leg of Lamb with Mint Vinegar

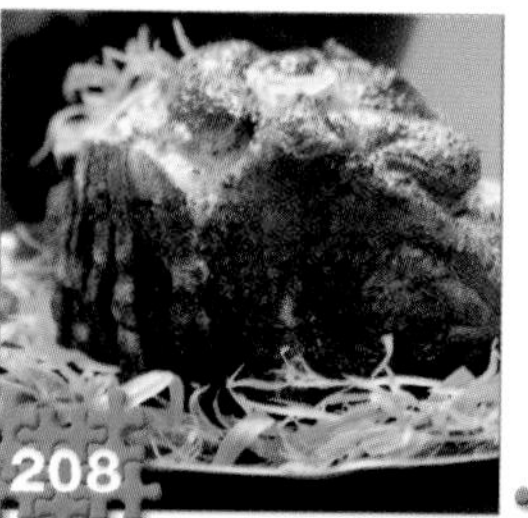
208 Tarragon Roasted Pork

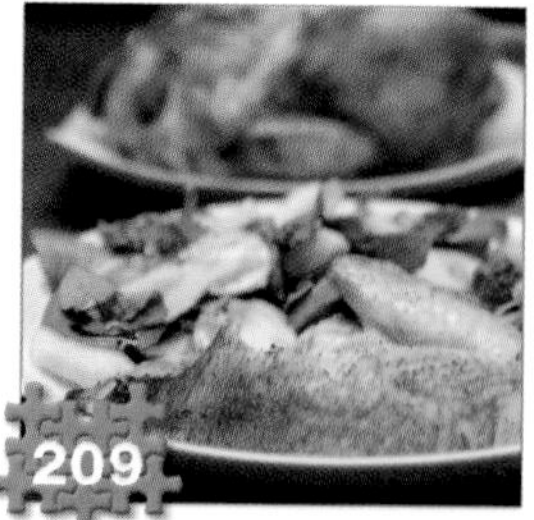
209 Roasted Chicken

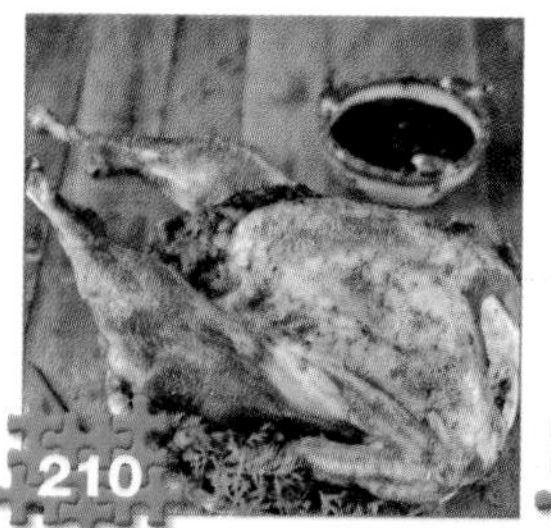
210 Whole Turkey with Mofongo Stuffing

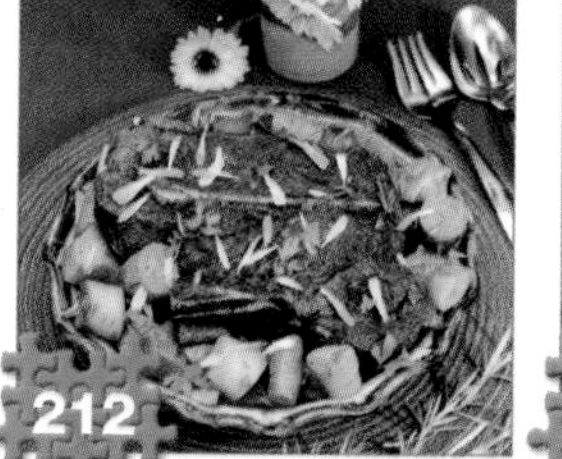
212 Rustic Bison Pot Roast

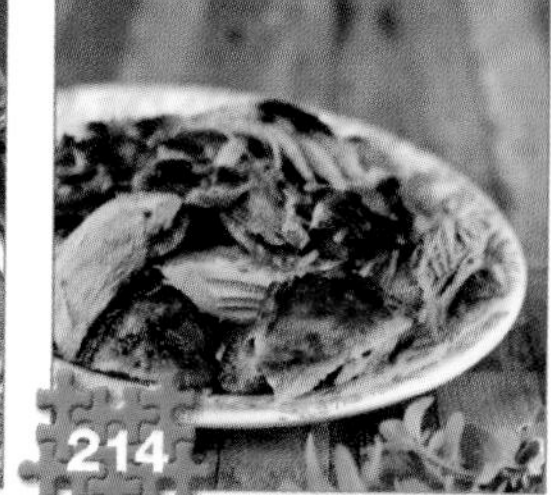
214 Garlic-Roasted Pork Shoulder

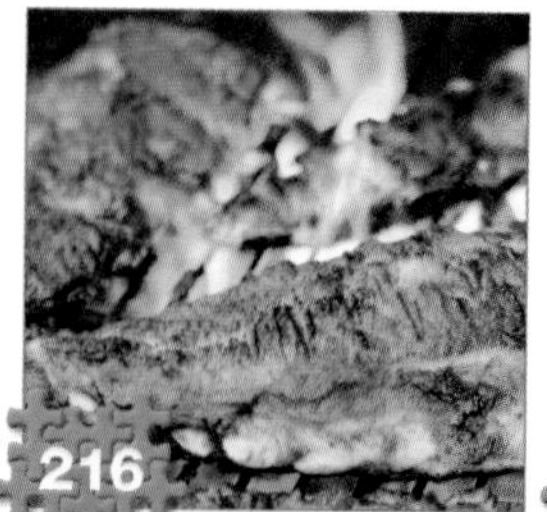
216 BBQ Pork Ribs

217 Greek-Inspired Lamb Chops

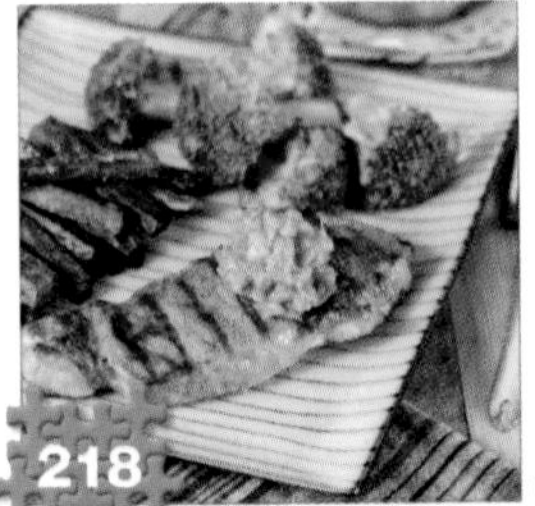
218 Simple Grilled Steak with Rhubarb Chutney

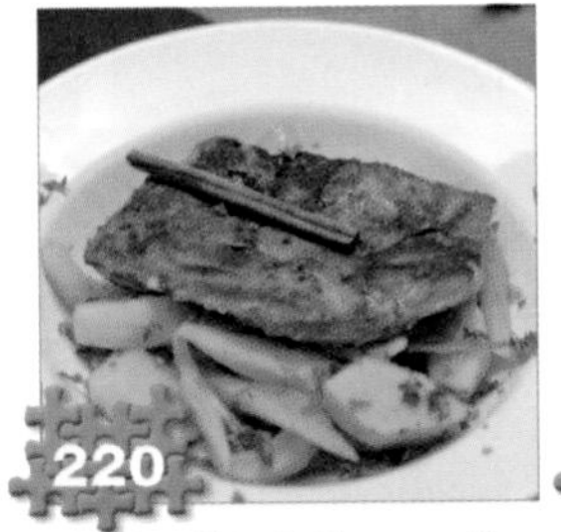
220 Braised Pork Chops with Apple and Fennel

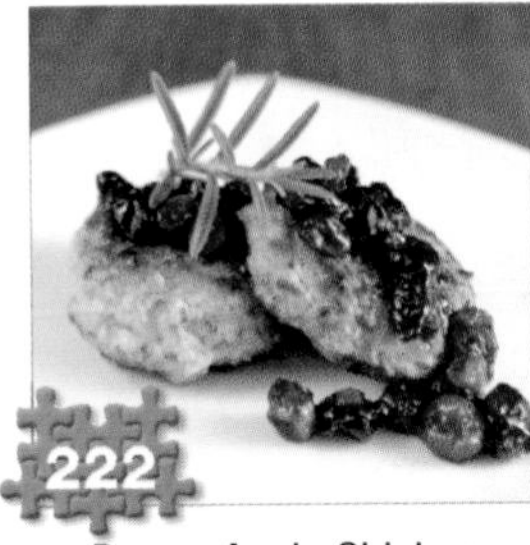
222 Bacon-Apple Chicken Burgers with Maple-Cranberry Sauce

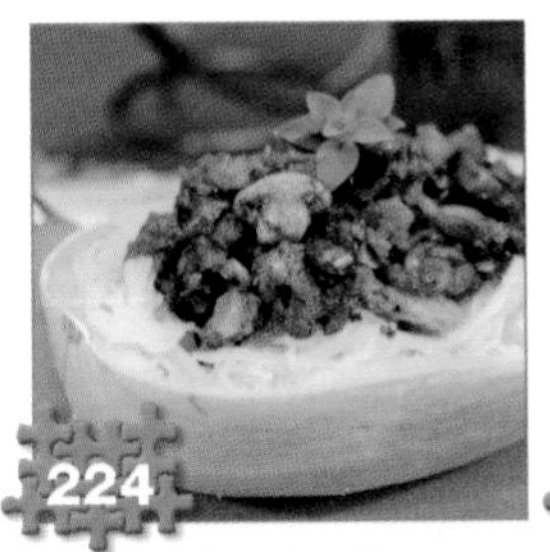
224 "Spaghetti"

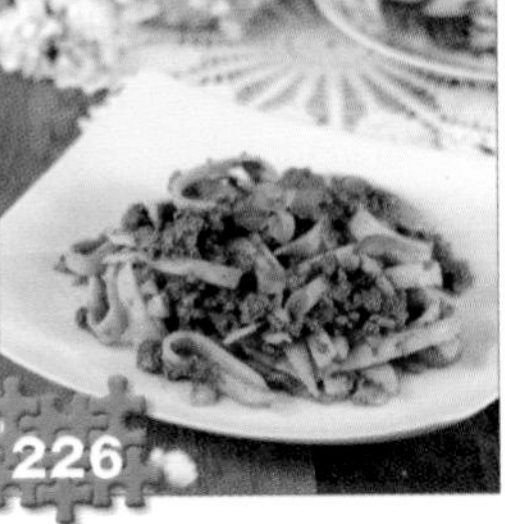
226 Sweet Potato Linguine with Bolognese Sauce

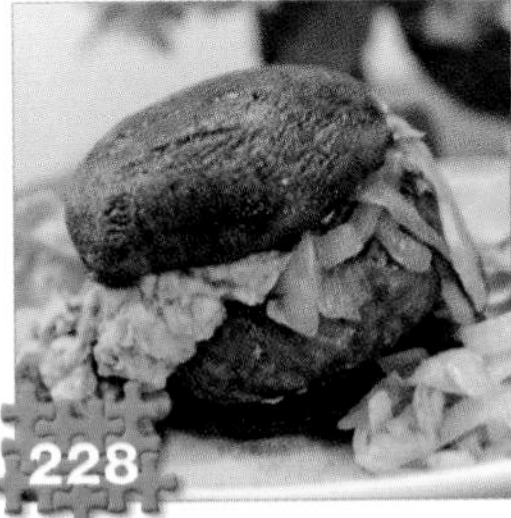
228 Burgers with Caramelized Onions and Portobello "Buns"

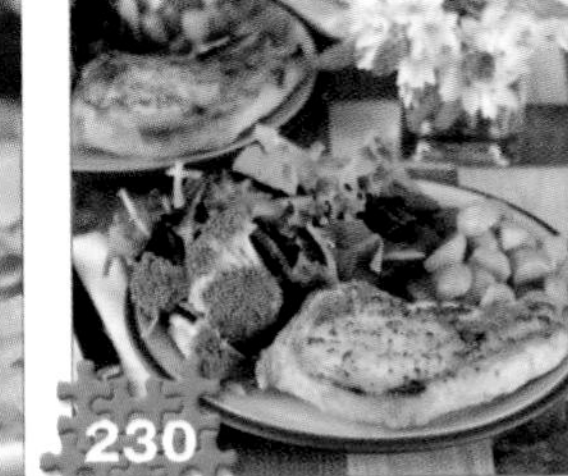
230 Lemon and Thyme Broiled Pork Chops

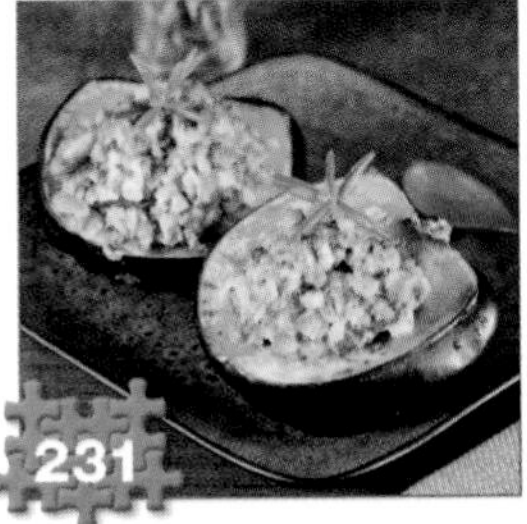
231 Pork Pie–Stuffed Acorn Squash

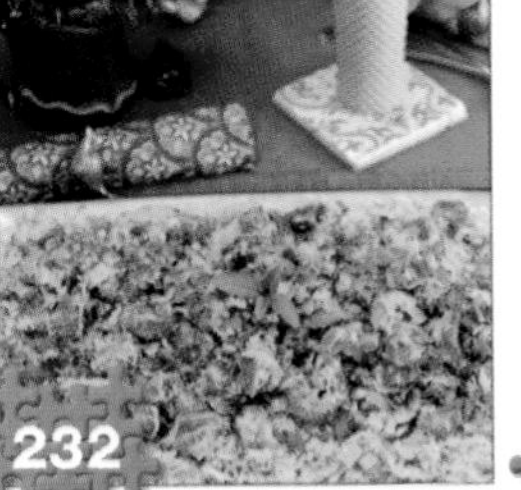
232 Lamb "Biryani"

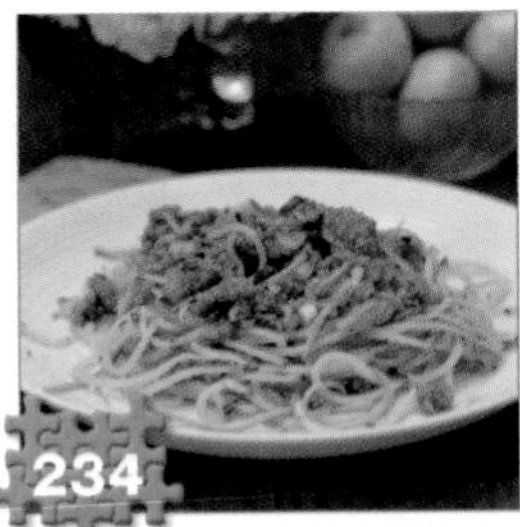
234 Pork Pad Thai

Fish and Shellfish

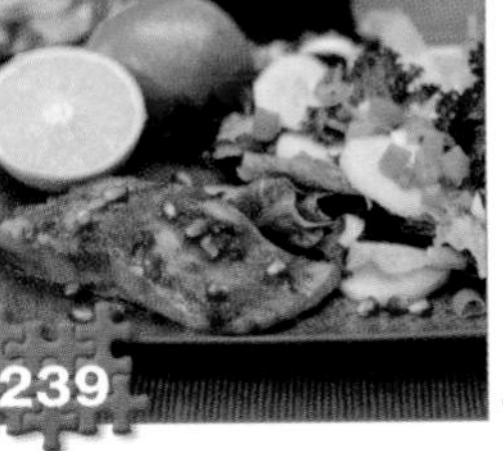
239 Pomegranate Molasses–Glazed Salmon

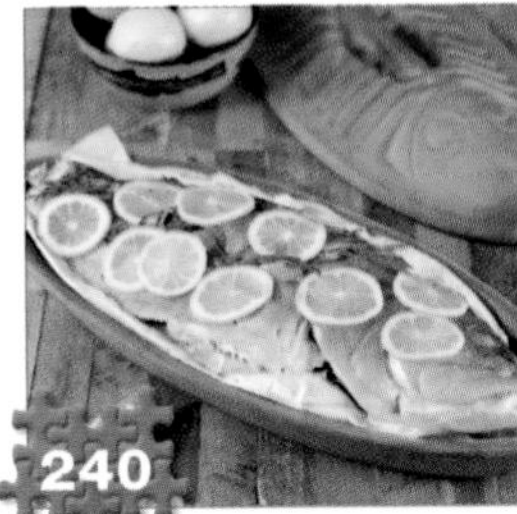
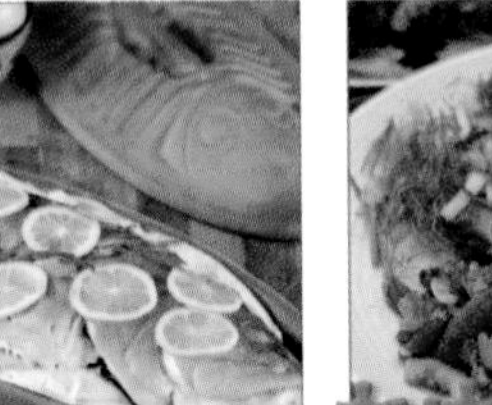
240 Baked Whole Fish

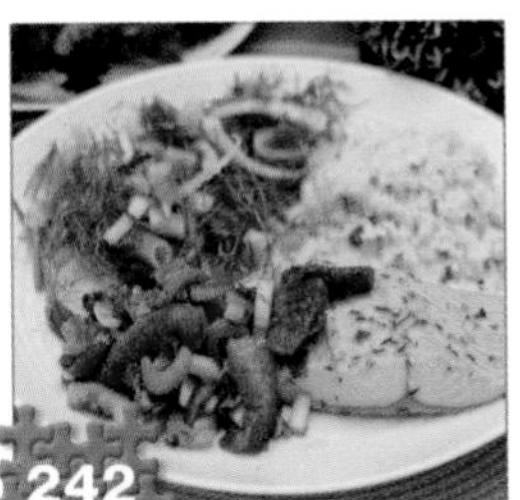
242 Lemon and Thyme Broiled Salmon with Blood Orange Salsa

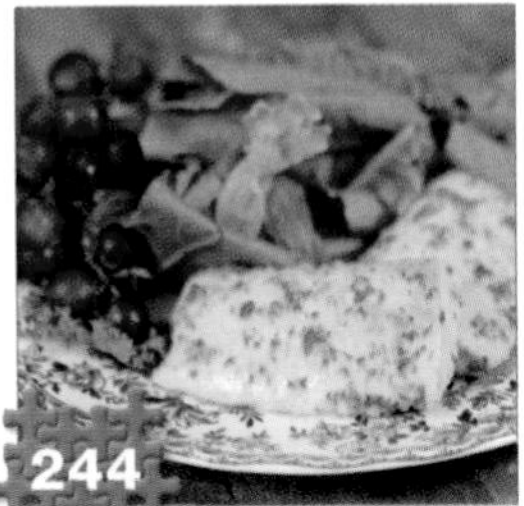
244 Simple Baked Whitefish

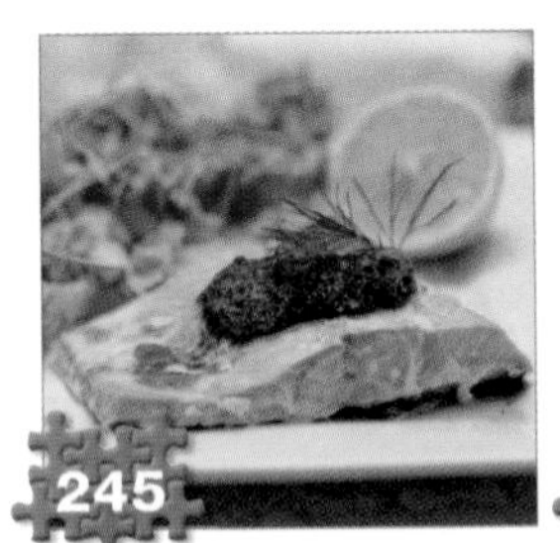
245 Salmon with Maître D' "Butter"

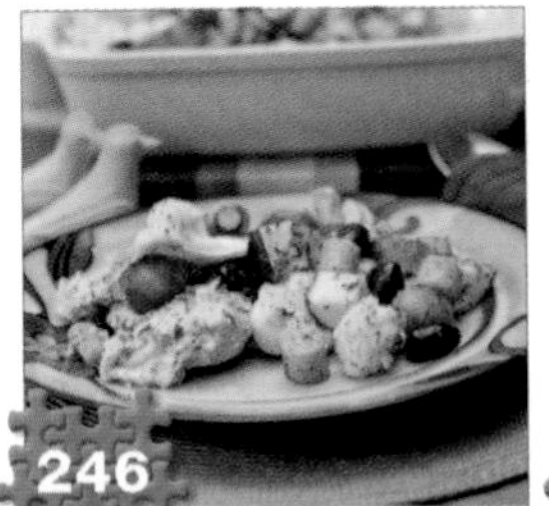
246 Mediterranean Mahi Mahi

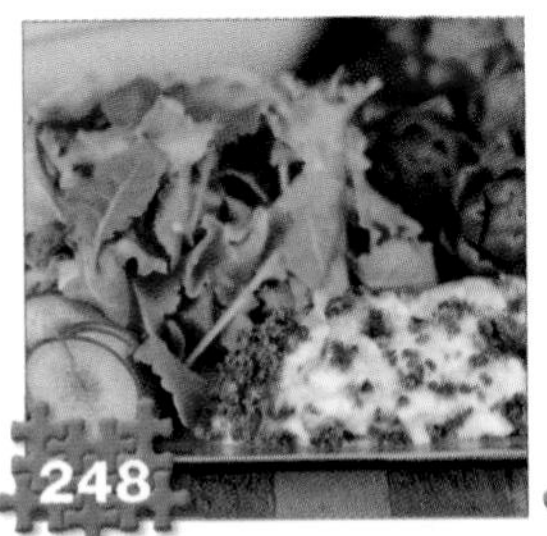
248 Scalloped Hake and Oysters

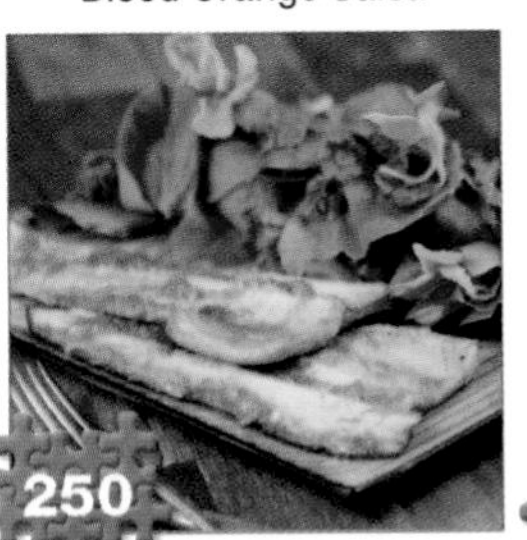
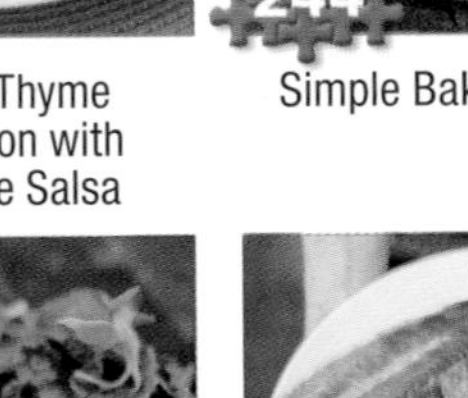
250 Teriyaki-Poached Trout

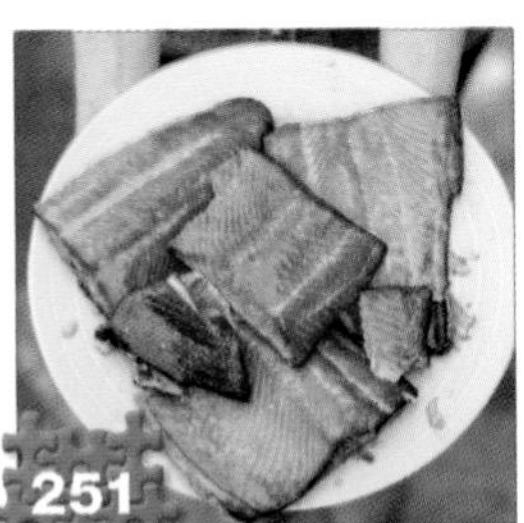
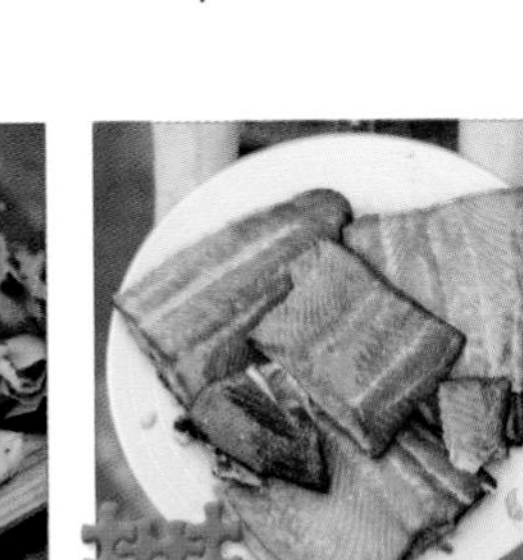
251 Smoked Salmon

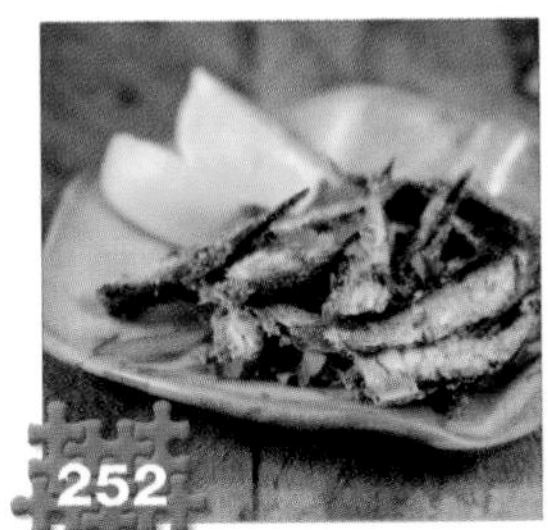
252 Pan-Fried Sardines

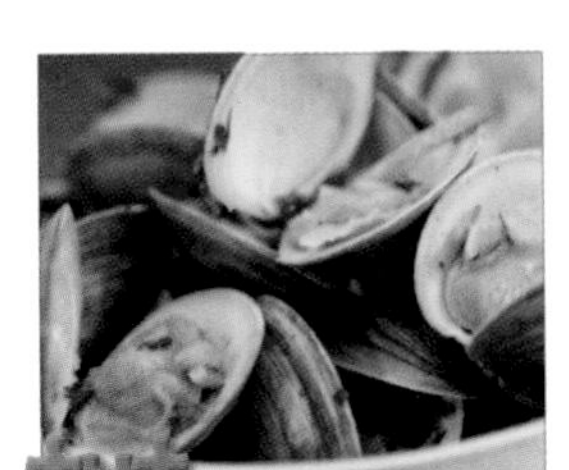
253 Steamed Clams

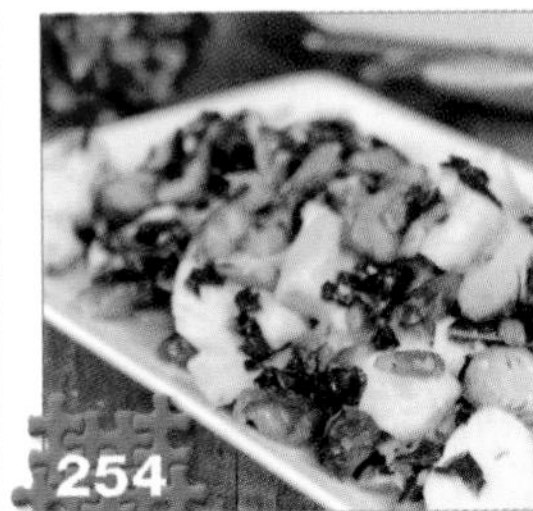
254 Bacon-Braised Whitefish and Brussels

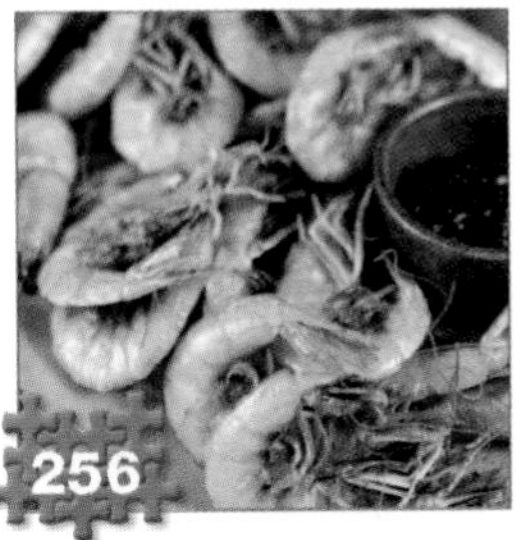
256 Deep-Fried Whole Shrimp with Cocktail Sauce

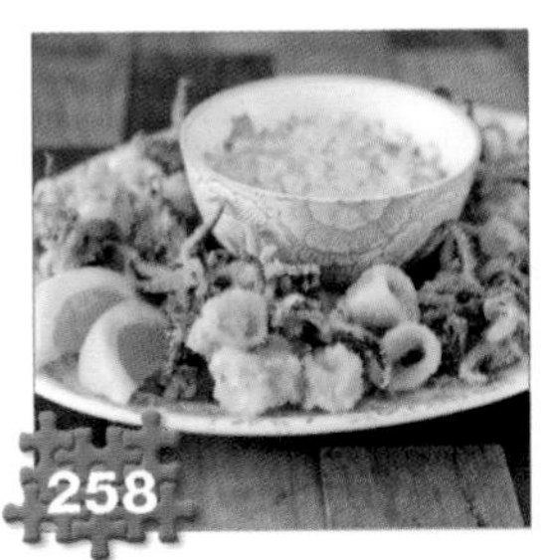
258 Calamari with Tzatziki Sauce

Offal

Side Dishes

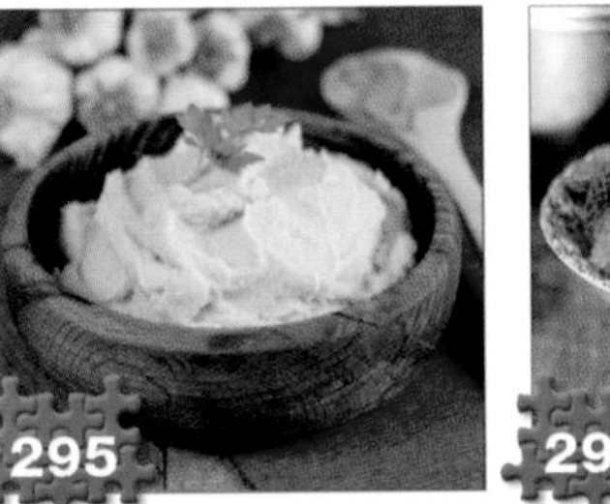
295 Cauliflower Mash

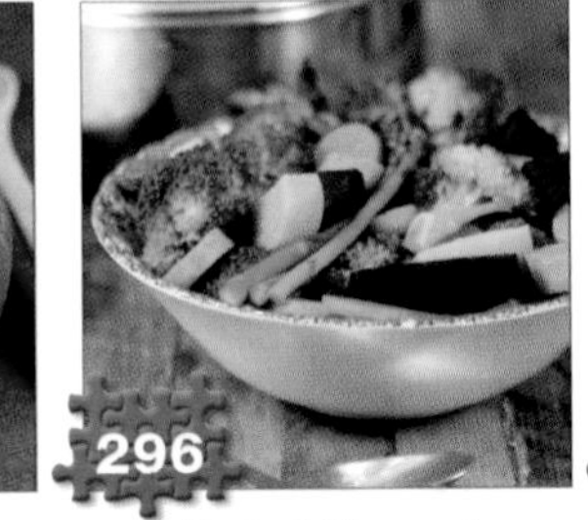
296 Perfect Steamed Vegetables

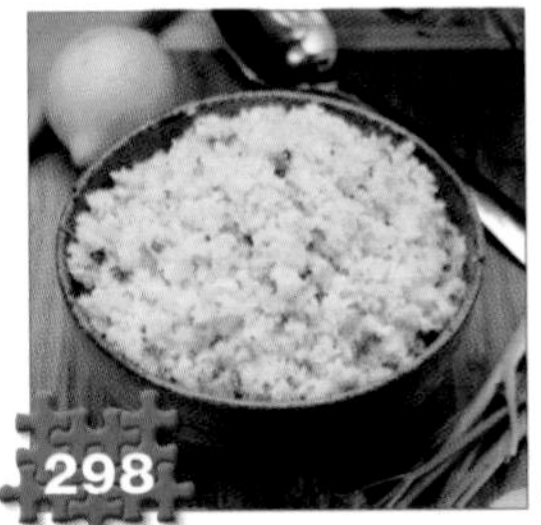
298 Cauliflower Rice—Three Ways

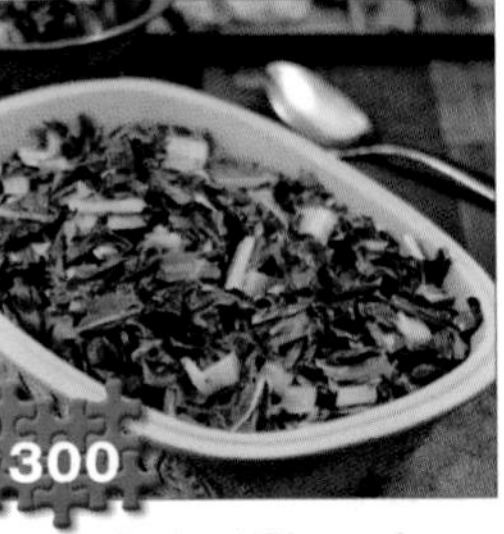
300 Braised Greens

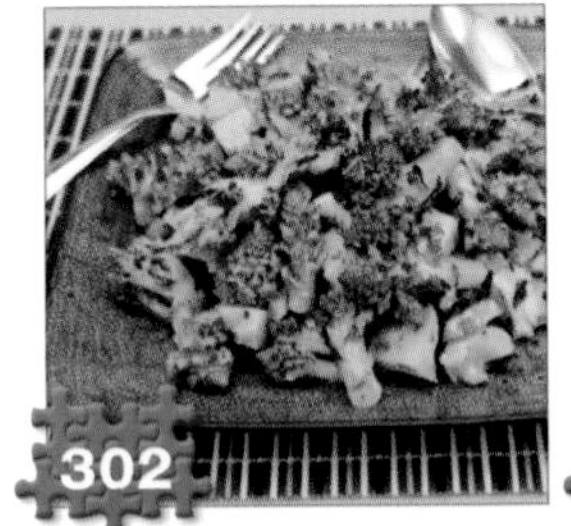
302 Roasted Broccoflower

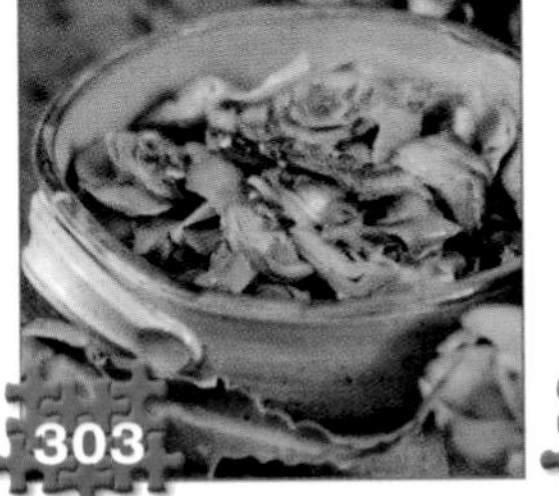
303 Garlicky Artichoke Hearts

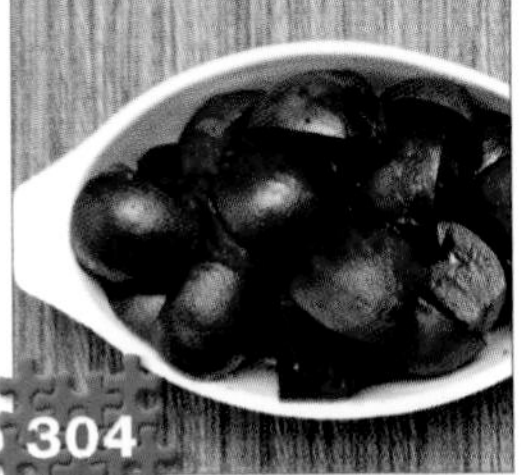
304 Balsamic-Roasted Beets

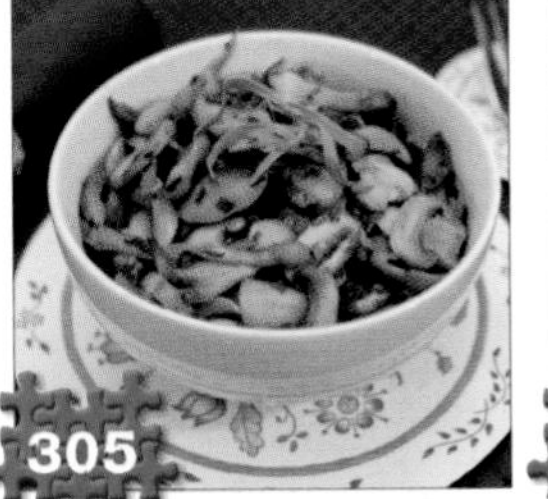
305 Wild Mushrooms and Tarragon

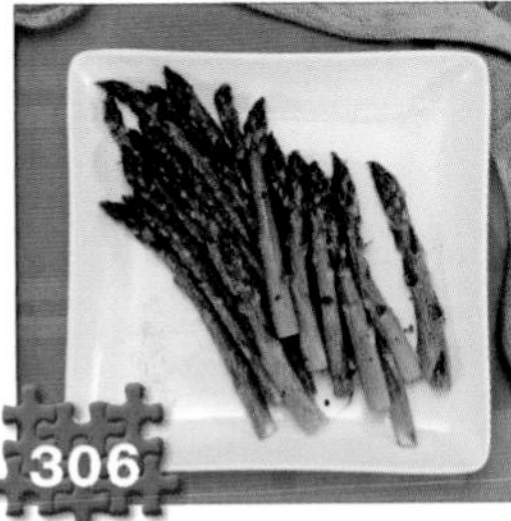
306 Easy Broiled Asparagus

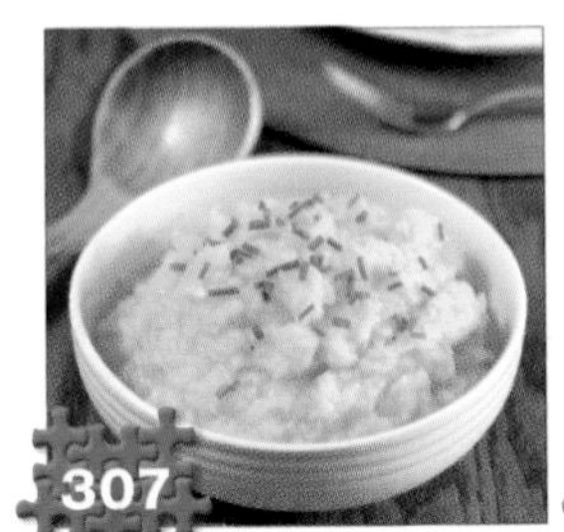
307 Mashed Acorn Squash with Forty Cloves of Garlic

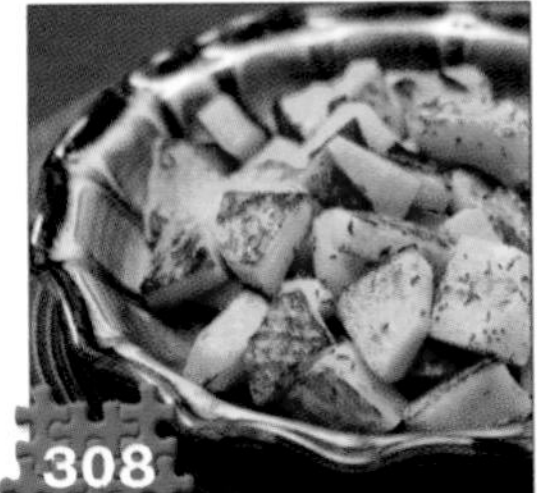
308 Roasted Butternut Squash

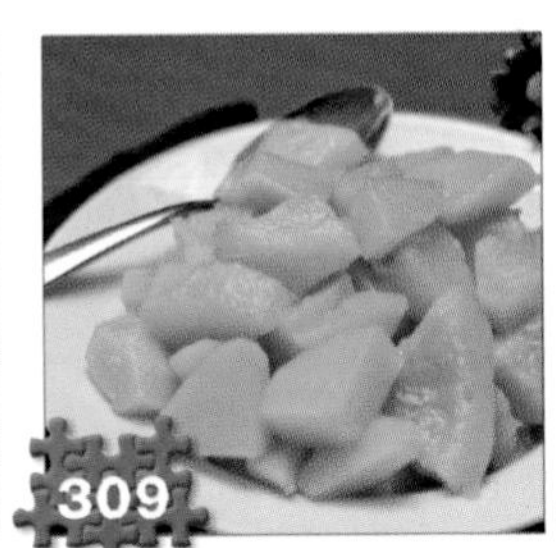
309 Maple-Braised Butternut Squash

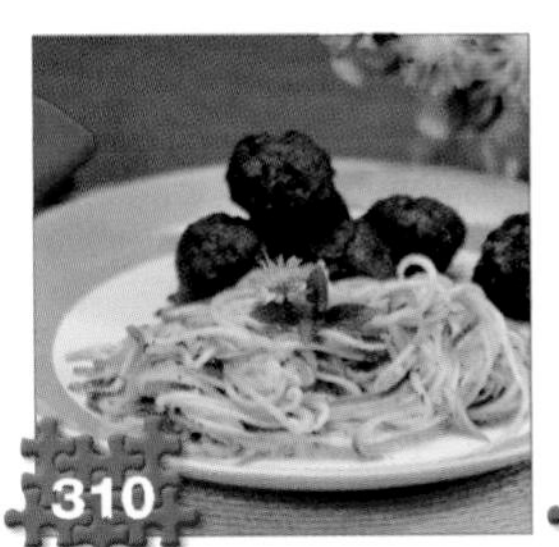
310 Mint Pesto Zucchini "Pasta"

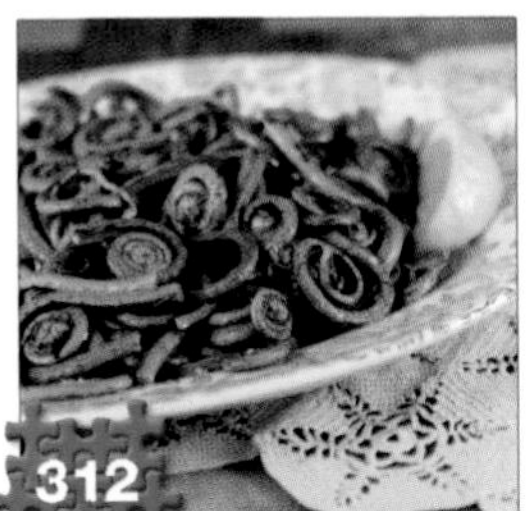
312 Fiddleheads

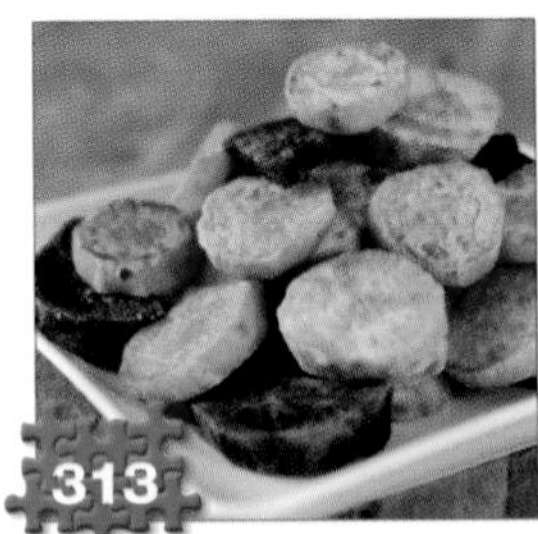
313 Roasted Sweet Potato

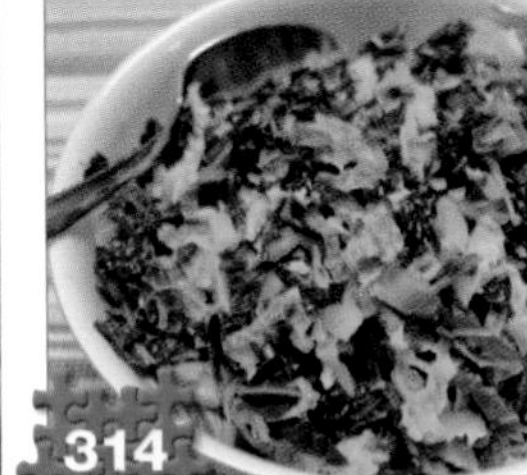
314 Bacon-Braised Savoy Cabbage and Apple

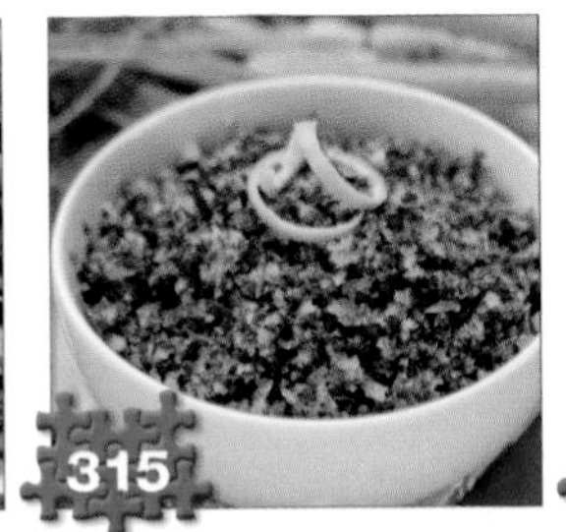
315 Whole Carrot "Tabouleh"

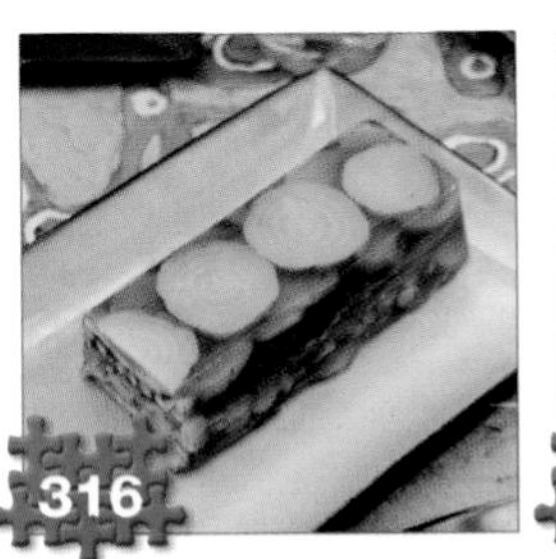
316 Vegetable Terrine

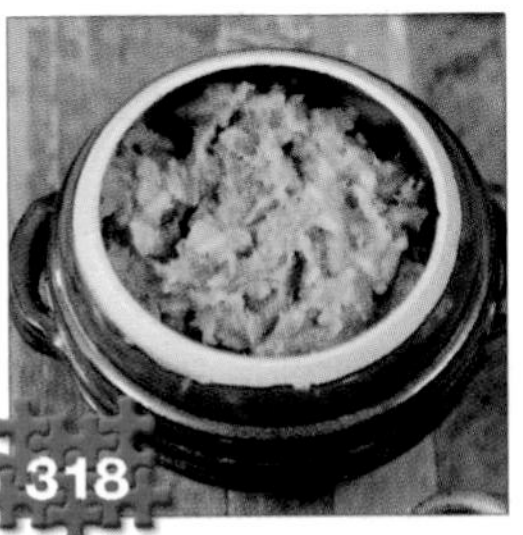
318 Kufu

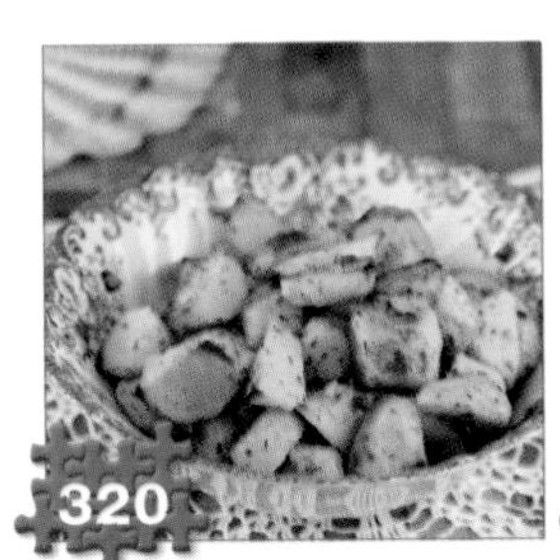
320 Savory Roasted Taro

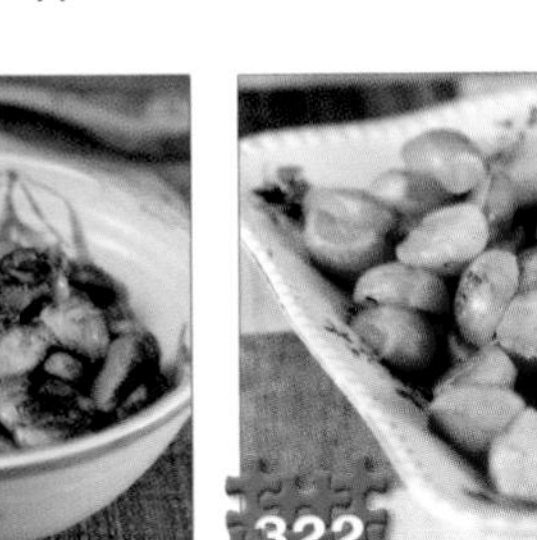
321 Bacon-Braised Brussels Sprouts

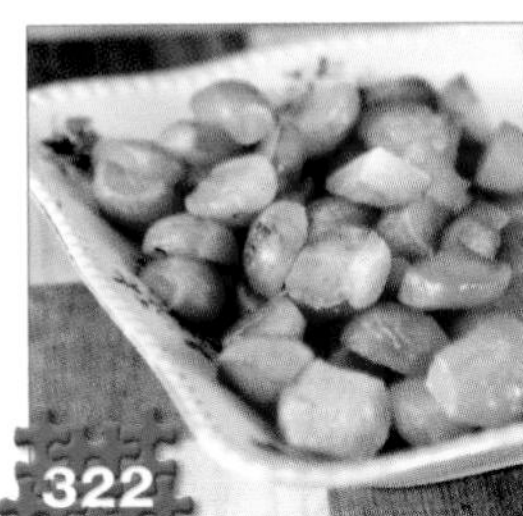
322 Roasted Radishes

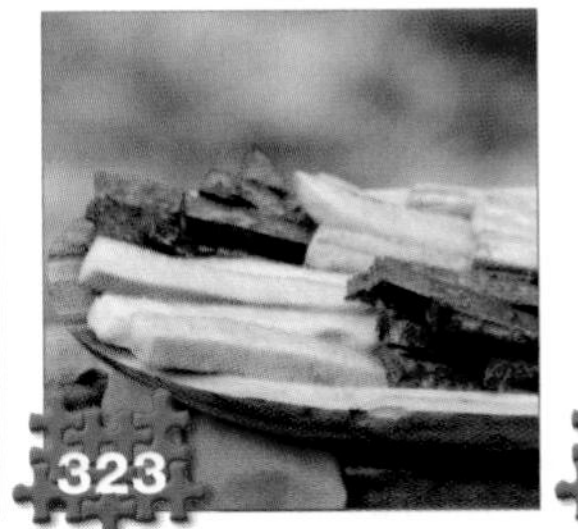
323 French Fries

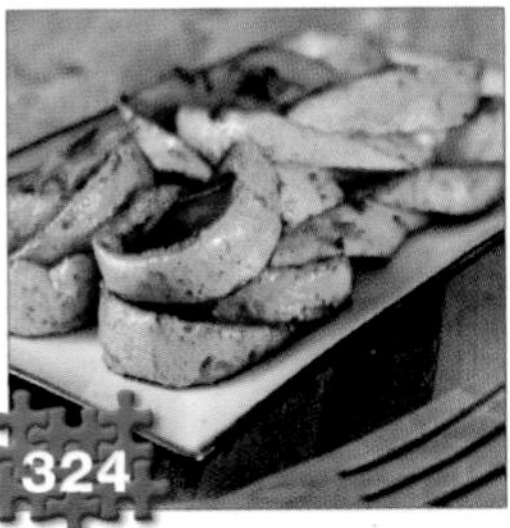
324 Spiced Kabocha Squash

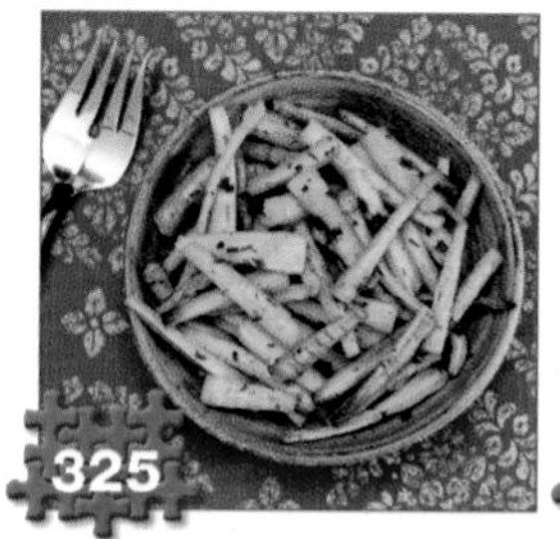

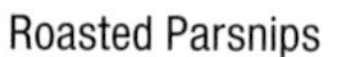

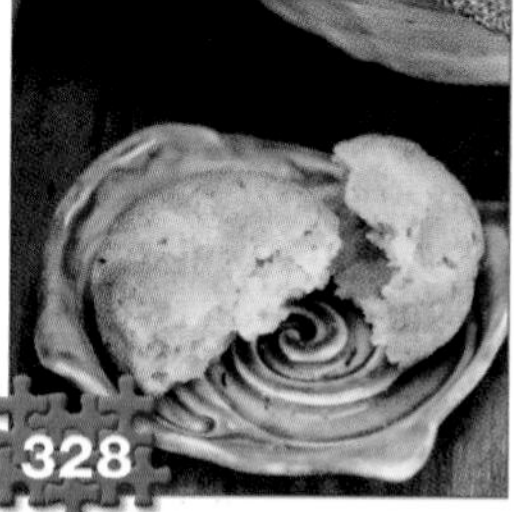

Sweet Treats and Beverages

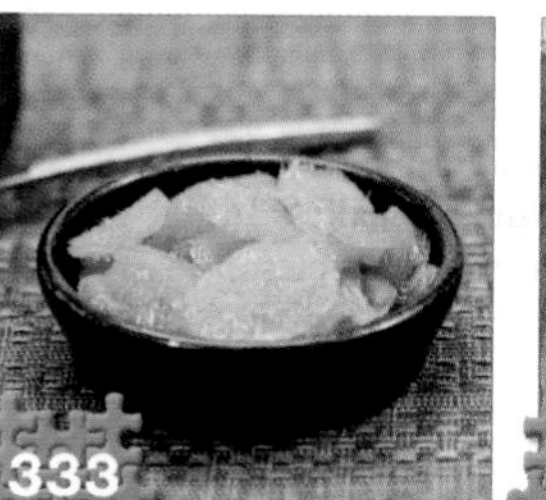

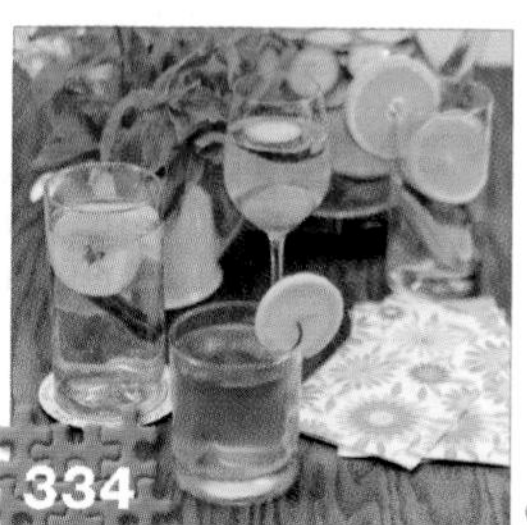

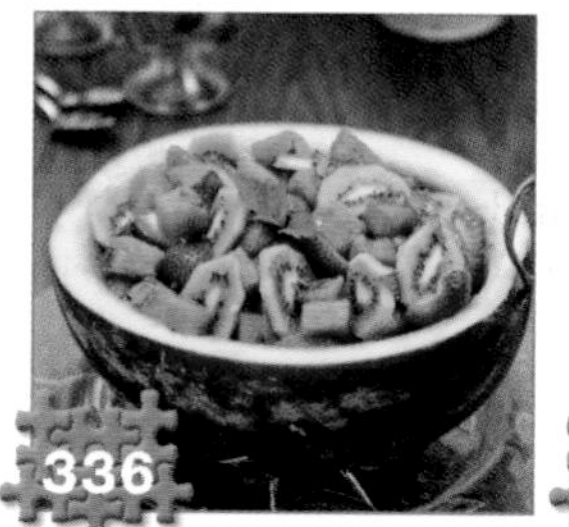

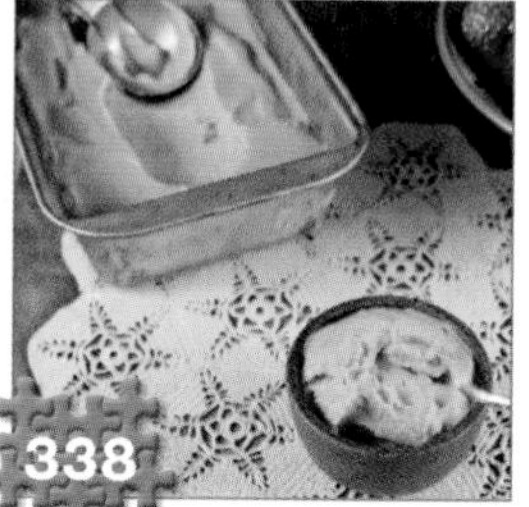

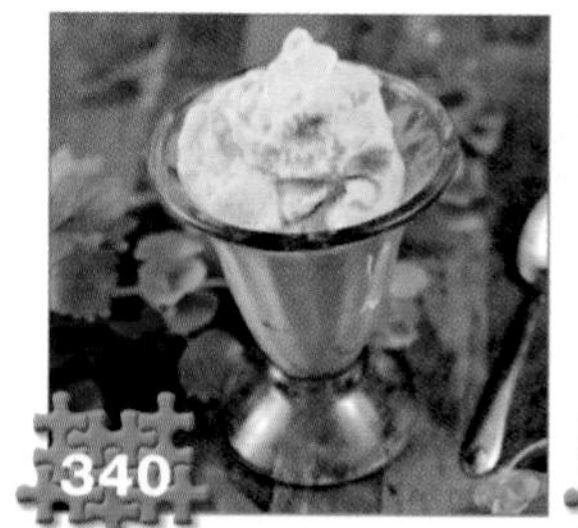

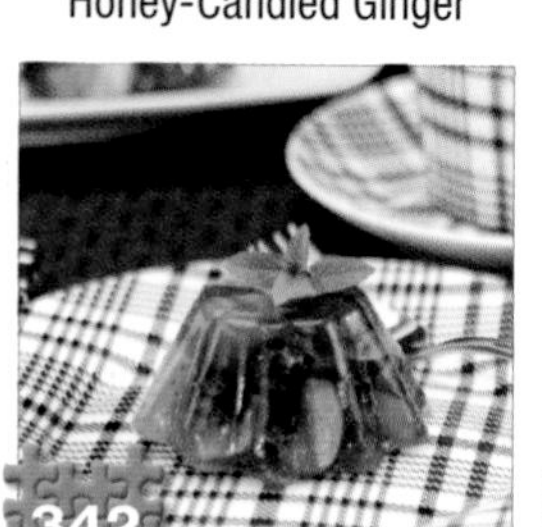

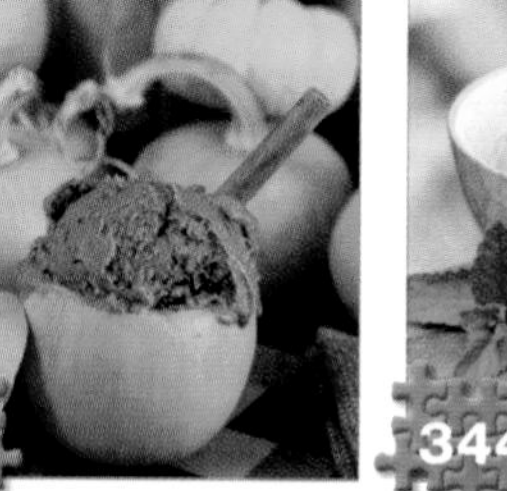

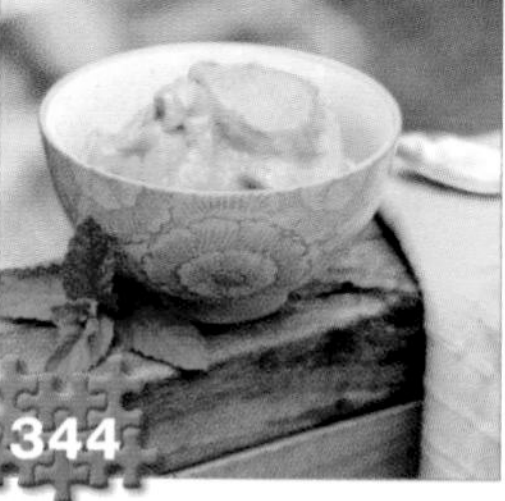

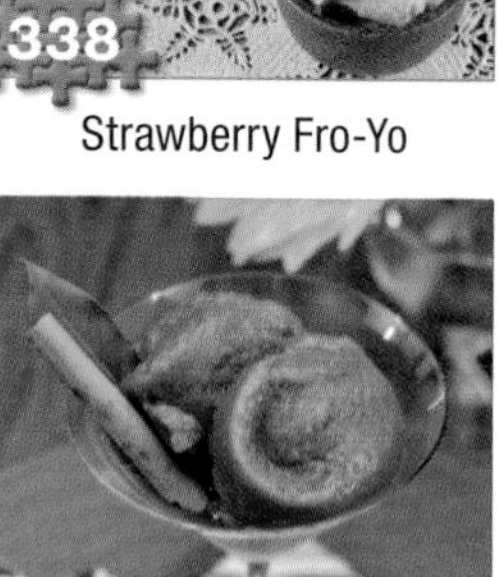

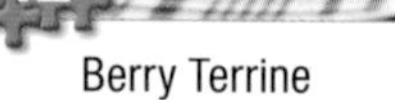
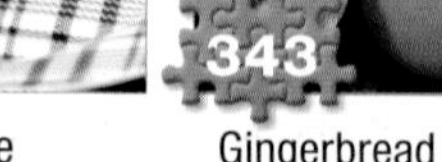
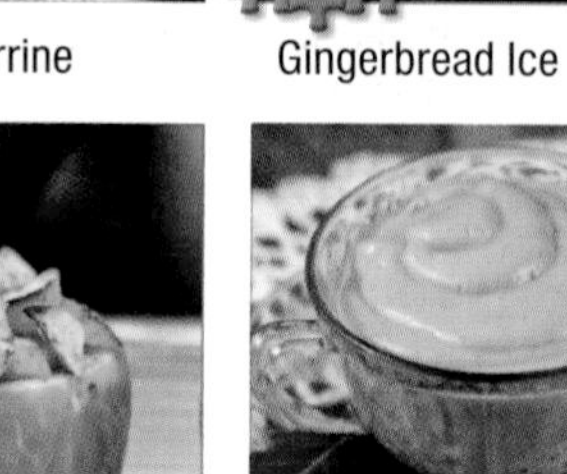
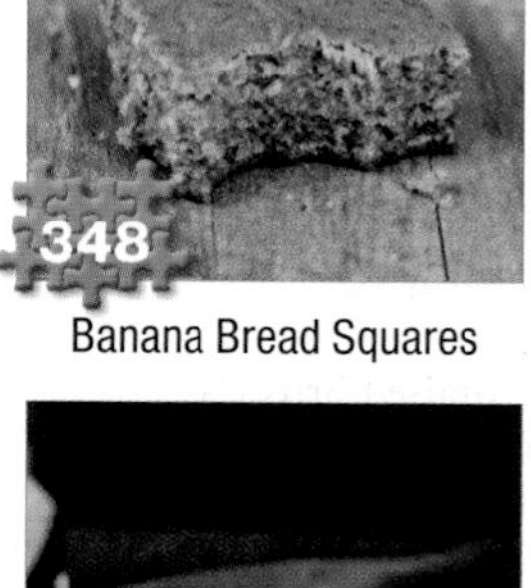

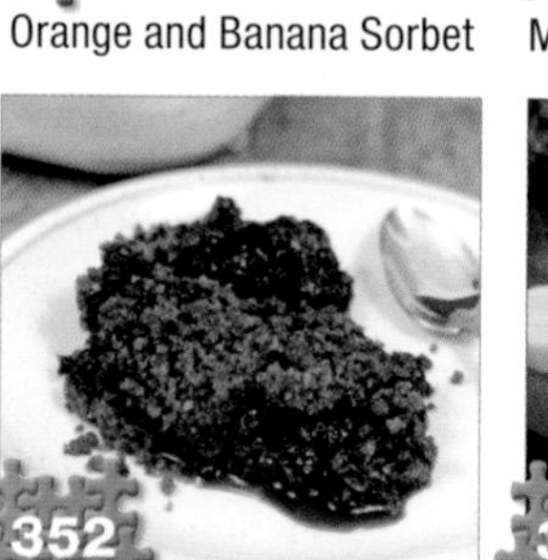
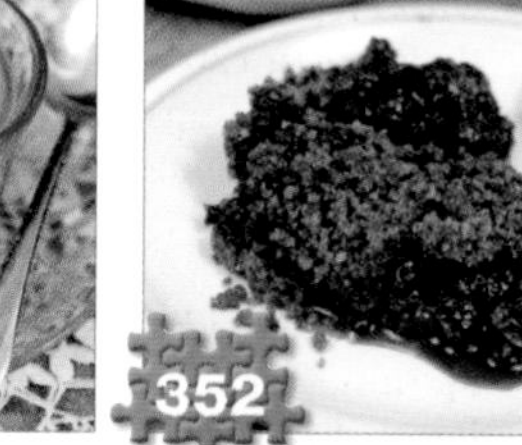
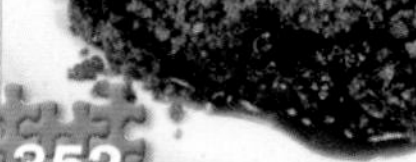
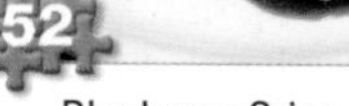

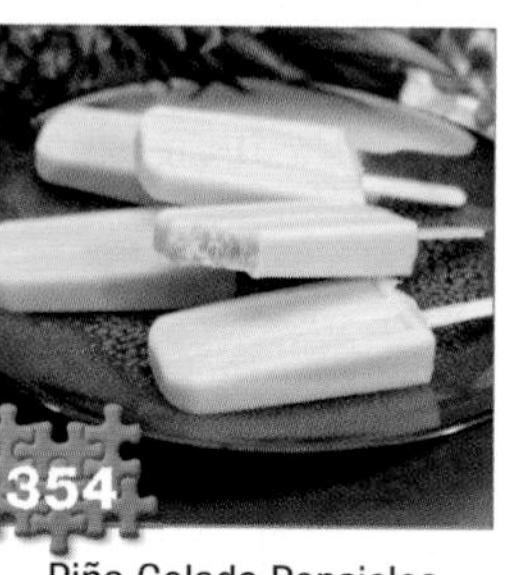
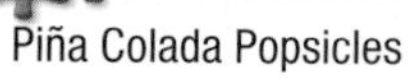

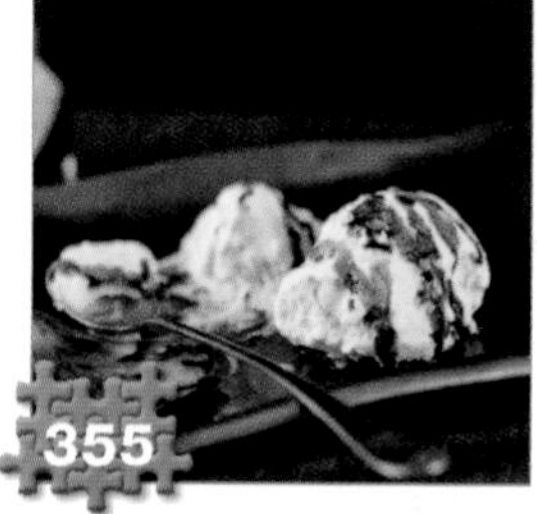

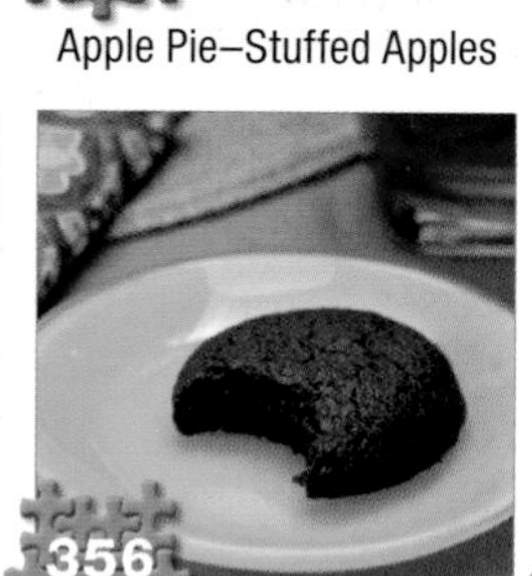

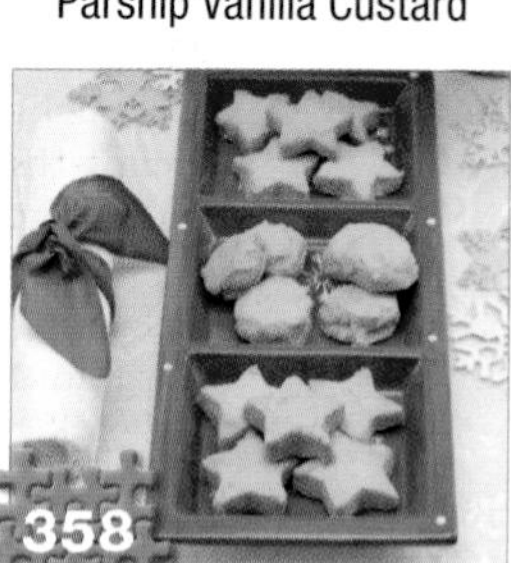
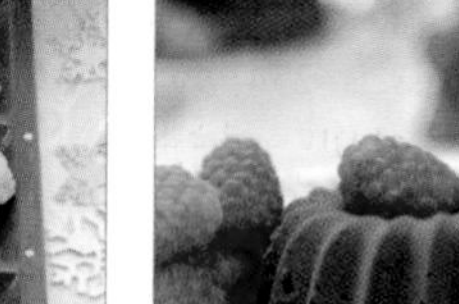

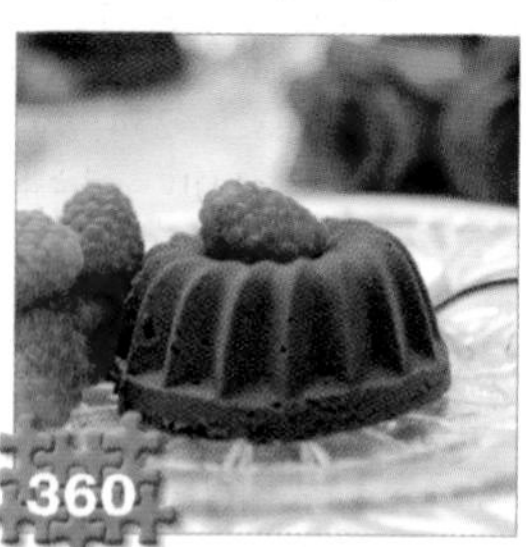
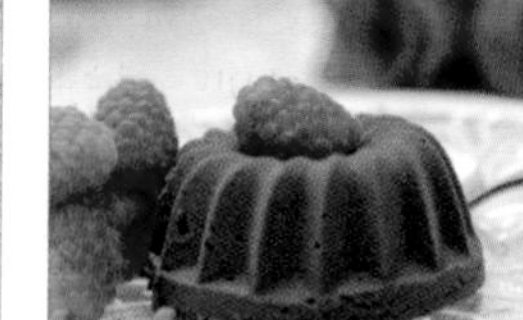
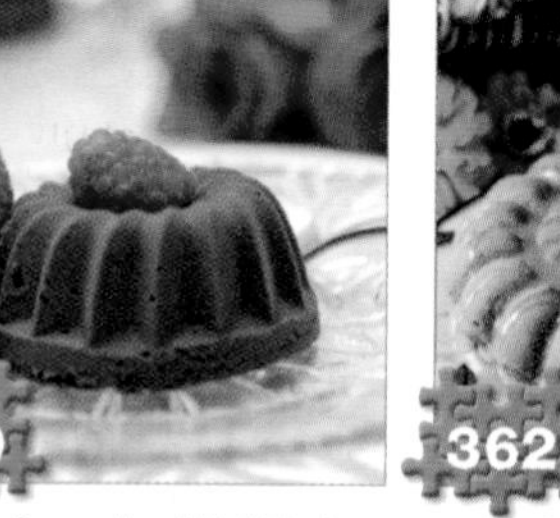

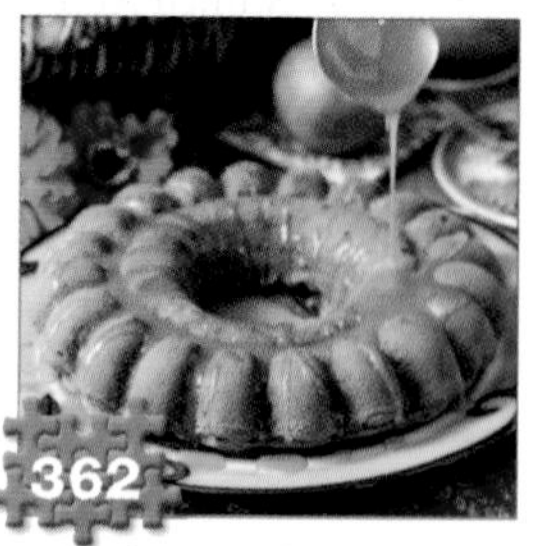
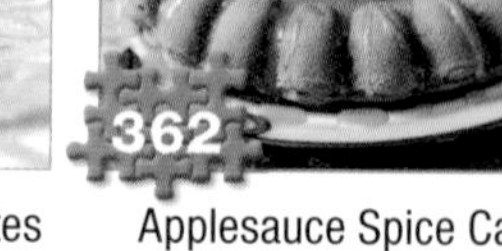

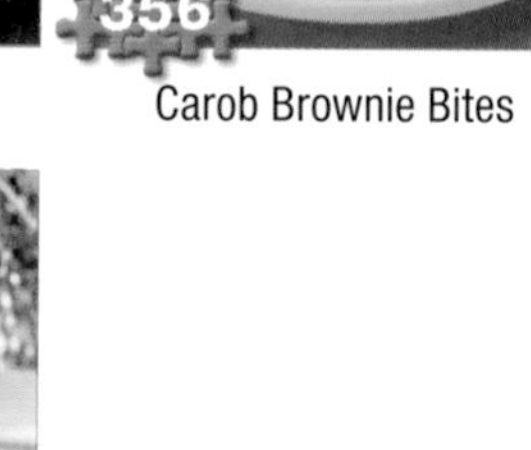
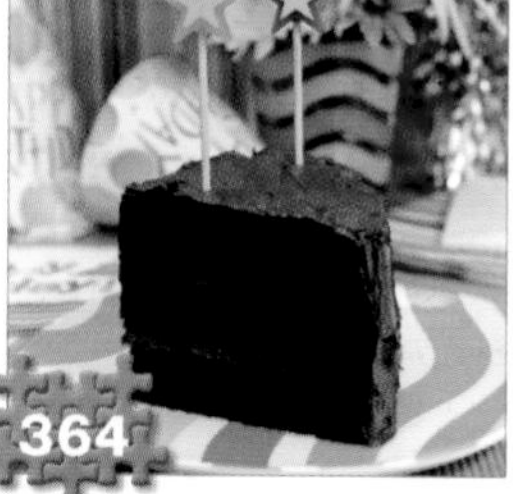

Index

Week 1

Shopping List

Meat
bacon (10–16 oz.)
beef tongue (2½–3 lbs.)
ground beef (1 lb.)
ground pork (5 lbs.)
top sirloin or rib roast (3–4 lbs.)

Seafood
hake (2½ lbs. of fillets)
oysters (2 lbs., shucked)
salmon (4–6 [6–8 oz.] fillets)
whole fish, gutted and scaled (such as red snapper, 3–5 lbs.)

Fruits
avocados (3)
banana (1)
berries, melon, or other fruit (1 cup for Bacon Fruit Cups)
blood oranges (2 lbs.)
grapefruit (1–2)
lemons (3–4)
lime (1)

Nonperishables
albacore tuna (5 oz. can)
capers
raisins (½ cup)
ingredients for your favorite salad dressing (oil, vinegar, herbs, etc.)

Vegetables
asparagus (2 lbs.)
broccoflower (4–5 heads, enough for 8 cups of florets and stems)
broccoli (2 lbs.)
butternut squash (2 lbs.)
cabbage or other vegetable for fermenting (3 lbs.)
carrots (1½ lbs.)
cauliflower (2½ heads)
celery root (1 large)
celery (1 head or heart)
cilantro (fresh)
dill (fresh)
fennel (2 small bulbs)
garlic (2–3 heads)
ginger root
golden beets (2–3 medium)
green plantains (6–8 medium)
mushrooms (wild, 1½ lbs.)
onions (2 large)
parsley (fresh)
portobello mushroom caps (4–6)
red onion (1)
rosemary (fresh)
shallot (1 large)
sweet potatoes (2 lbs.)
tarragon (fresh)
thyme (fresh)
zucchini (1 medium)
greens for braising (for 7 meals)
leafy greens plus add-ons for salads (for 5 meals)
leafy greens and superfood add-ons for Superfood Smoothie (for 1 meal)
large lettuce leaves (such as romaine or butterleaf) for Tuna Salad Wraps
seasonings for Cauliflower Rice (garlic, herbs, lemon, etc.)
veggies for steaming (for 3 meals)

Pantry Items
apple cider vinegar
avocado oil
baking soda
balsamic vinegar
bay leaf powder, or make your own using dried bay leaves
bay leaves
Bone Broth (9¼ cups, or ingredients to make 1 batch—page 110)
cinnamon (ground)
cinnamon stick
cloves (whole)
coconut oil (extra-virgin)
gelatin
lard
lemon juice (or additional fresh lemons to make your own)
mace
maple syrup (grade B)
marjoram (dried)
muscovado sugar or evaporated cane juice
olive oil (extra-virgin)
protein powder for Superfood Smoothie
pumpkin powder (½ cup, or 2 cups puréed pumpkin to make your own)
saffron
sage (dried)
salt (pink or gray)
tallow, bacon fat, and/or duck fat
thyme (dried)
truffle salt (optional)
turmeric (dried)
white wine (1¾ cups) or more broth

Other
casings for sausage (optional)
pickles (raw fermented, or ingredients to make your own—page 114)
sauerkraut (raw fermented, if not making your own)
vegetable juice (8–16 oz., or veggies to make your own)

Plan Ahead

- Bacon Bits: ¼ cup for Scalloped Hake and Oysters—make some extra bacon on Saturday morning
- Broth
- Carrot-Raisin Muffins
- Coconut Milk Yogurt
- English Bangers: Either precook sausage patties or stuff sausage into casings and then parboil; let cool and then freeze
- Green Tea and Garlic Pickles for Tuna Salad Wraps—or you can buy pickles if you prefer
- Plantain Crackers (double batch)
- Pumpkin powder for Carrot-Raisin Muffins (or buy online)
- Salad Dressing
- Sauerkraut: Note that this needs to ferment, typically for a week

Tip: If you bake a big enough whole fish on Saturday, you can use it for making the Scalloped Hake and Oysters on Sunday and for leftovers on Monday.

Meal Plan

	Breakfast	Lunch	Dinner
SATURDAY	Bacon Fruit Cups (page 136)	Baked Whole Fish (page 240)	Garlic and Rosemary Roast Beef (page 205)
	Braised Greens (page 300)	Maple-Braised Butternut Squash (page 309)	Perfect Steamed Vegetables (page 296)
	Sauerkraut (page 112)	Garden Salad (page 160)	Cauliflower Mash (page 295)
		Easy Broiled Asparagus (double batch; page 306)	
SUNDAY	English Bangers (page 132)	Beef Tongue with Celery Root and Fennel Slaw (page 270)	Scalloped Hake and Oysters (page 248)
	Braised Greens (page 300)	Plantain Crackers (double batch; page 149)	Braised Greens (page 300)
	Cinnamon Broiled Grapefruit (page 143)	Vegetable Terrine (page 316)	Roasted Broccoflower (page 302)
MONDAY	English Bangers (leftover)	Scalloped Hake and Oysters (leftover)	Baked Whole Fish (leftover)
	Maple-Braised Butternut Squash (leftover)	Braised Greens (page 300)	Roasted Sweet Potato (page 313)
	Roasted Broccoflower (leftover)	Cauliflower Mash (leftover)	Garden Salad (page 160)
	Sauerkraut (leftover)		Vegetable Terrine (leftover)
TUESDAY	Garlic and Rosemary Roast Beef (leftover)	Beef Tongue with Celery Root and Fennel Slaw (leftover)	Scalloped Hake and Oysters (leftover)
	Roasted Sweet Potato (leftover)	Plantain Crackers (leftover)	Easy Broiled Asparagus (leftover)
	Perfect Steamed Vegetables (page 296)	Garden Salad (page 160)	Wild Mushrooms and Tarragon (page 305)
	Cinnamon Broiled Grapefruit (page 143)	Roasted Broccoflower (leftover)	
WEDNESDAY	English Bangers (leftover)	Garlic and Rosemary Roast Beef (leftover)	Beef Tongue with Celery Root and Fennel Slaw (leftover)
	Carrot-Raisin Muffins (page 140)	Plantain Crackers (leftover)	Roasted Sweet Potato (leftover)
	Vegetable Terrine (leftover)	Braised Greens (page 300)	Garden Salad (page 160)
	Sauerkraut (leftover)	Wild Mushrooms and Tarragon (leftover)	"Cream" of Broccoli Soup (page 183)
THURSDAY	Superfood Smoothie (page 141)	Tuna Salad Wrap (page 260)	Lemon and Thyme Broiled Salmon with Blood Orange Salsa (page 242)
		"Cream" of Broccoli Soup (leftover)	Plantain Crackers (leftover)
			Braised Greens (page 300)
			Cauliflower Rice (page 298)
FRIDAY	English Bangers (leftover)	Lemon and Thyme Broiled Salmon with Blood Orange Salsa (leftover)	Burgers with Caramelized Onions and Portobello "Buns" (page 228)
	Carrot-Raisin Muffins (leftover)	Garden Salad (page 160)	Roasted Sweet Potato (leftover)
	Braised Greens (page 300)	Cauliflower Rice (leftover)	Perfect Steamed Vegetables (page 296)
	Sauerkraut (leftover)		

Week 2

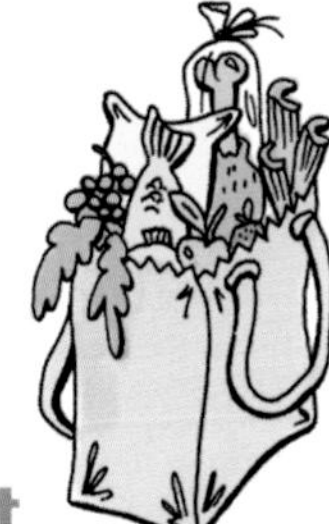

Shopping List

Meat

- bacon (16–20 oz.)
- ground beef (1 lb.)
- ground lamb (4 lbs.)
- ground pork (1 lb.)
- liver (1 lb., ground preferred)
- pork ribs (7–8 lbs.)

Seafood

- mahi mahi (4–6 [6 oz.] fillets)
- whitefish (3–4 [6–8 oz.] fillets)
- lox (2–3 oz.)

Fruits

- apples (4)
- avocado (1)
- banana (1)
- berries (½–1 cup for Coconut Milk Yogurt)
- cranberries (½ cups fresh or frozen)
- ingredients for your favorite fruit salad (for 3 meals)
- lemons (3)
- mango (1)

Nonperishables

- capers
- clams (3 [5–6 oz.] cans)
- coconut milk yogurt (1⅔ cups, or ingredients to make your own—page 118)
- ingredients for your favorite dip (avocado or coconut milk yogurt plus herbs—page 172)
- ingredients for your favorite salad dressing (oil, vinegar, herbs, etc.)
- nori sheets (2)
- olives (whole green or black, ¾ cup)
- sardines (2 [4 oz.] cans)

Vegetables

- artichoke hearts (12 oz.)
- arugula or mustard greens (6–10 cups)
- basil (fresh)
- beets (6–8)
- Brussels sprouts (1 lb.)
- butternut squash (2 lbs.)
- carrots (2 lbs.)
- cauliflower (1½ heads)
- celery (1 head or heart)
- chives (fresh)
- cucumber (1)
- garlic (1½–2 heads)
- ginger root
- green onion (1)
- onions (4)
- oregano (fresh)
- parsley (fresh)
- parsnips (2 lbs.)
- plantains (1 green and 2 ripe)
- radishes (8 oz.)
- red cabbage (1 lb.)
- red onion (1)
- rosemary (fresh)
- sage (fresh)
- savoy cabbage (1 head)
- sunflower sprouts (½ cup)
- taro root (1 lb.)
- tarragon (fresh)
- thyme (fresh)
- turmeric root
- turnip (1 large)
- zucchini (1 medium)
- greens for braising (for 3 meals)
- leafy greens plus add-ons for salads (for 3 meals)
- leafy greens and superfood add-ons for Superfood Smoothie (for 2 meals)
- starchy root vegetable for French Fries (1 lb.)
- veggies for steaming (for 4 meals)
- your favorite veggies to dip (for 2 meals)

Pantry Items

- apple cider vinegar
- avocado oil
- balsamic vinegar
- bay leaves (dried)
- Bone Broth (12–12½ cups, or ingredients to make 1½ batches—page 110)
- cinnamon (ground)
- coconut aminos
- coconut oil (extra-virgin)
- coconut water vinegar
- fish sauce
- gelatin
- honey
- lard
- lemon juice (or additional fresh lemons to make your own)
- mace
- marjoram (dried)
- molasses (blackstrap)
- olive oil (extra-virgin)
- oregano (dried)
- pomegranate molasses
- protein powder for Superfood Smoothie
- red palm oil
- rosemary (dried)
- sage (dried)
- salt (pink or gray)
- savory (dried)
- tallow, bacon fat, and/or duck fat
- tarragon (dried)
- thyme (dried)
- truffle salt (optional)
- turmeric (ground)

Other

- casings for sausage (optional)
- coconut cream (2 cups, or ingredients to make your own—page 116)
- lactobacillus-based probiotic supplement (if making homemade Coconut Milk Yogurt)
- vegetable juice (16–24 oz., or veggies to make your own)

Plan Ahead

- Barbecue Sauce for Pork Ribs
- Broth
- Coconut Cream (if making your own)
- Coconut Milk Yogurt
- Herbes de Provence for mahi mahi
- Hidden Liver Meatloaf
- Lamb Sausage: Either precook sausage patties or stuff sausage into casings and then parboil; let cool and then freeze
- Salad Dressing

Meal Plan

	Breakfast	Lunch	Dinner
SATURDAY	Lamb Sausage (page 132)	New England Clam Chowder (page 196)	Hidden Liver Meatloaf (page 272)
	Taro Hash (page 138)	Garden Salad (page 160)	French Fries (page 323)
	Perfect Steamed Vegetables (page 296)		Bacon-Braised Brussels Sprouts (page 321)
			Cauliflower Mash (page 295)
SUNDAY	Lamb Sausage (leftover)	New England Clam Chowder (leftover)	Simple Baked Whitefish (page 244)
	Taro Hash (leftover)	Garden Salad (page 160)	Balsamic-Roasted Beets (page 304)
	Bacon-Braised Savoy Cabbage and Apple (page 314)		Perfect Steamed Vegetables (page 296)
	Coconut Milk Yogurt (page 118) and fresh berries		Cauliflower Mash (leftover)
MONDAY	Superfood Smoothie (page 141)	Sardine Salad (page 163)	New England Clam Chowder (leftover)
		French Fries (leftover)	Garden Salad (page 160)
TUESDAY	Hidden Liver Meatloaf (leftover)	Simple Baked Whitefish (leftover)	BBQ Pork Ribs (page 216)
	Plantain and Apple Fritter (page 139)	Fruit Salad (page 336)	Balsamic-Roasted Beets (leftover)
	Braised Greens (page 300)	Veggies and Dip (page 172)	Cran-Apple Coleslaw (page 164)
	Cauliflower Mash (leftover)		Bacon-Braised Brussels Sprouts (leftover)
WEDNESDAY	Lamb Sausage (leftover)	BBQ Pork Ribs (leftover)	Mediterranean Mahi Mahi (page 246)
	Plantain and Apple Fritter (leftover)	Fruit Salad (leftover)	Roasted Butternut Squash (page 308)
	Perfect Steamed Vegetables (page 296)	Cran-Apple Coleslaw (leftover)	Braised Greens (page 300)
	Coconut Milk Yogurt (leftover)	Veggies and Dip (leftover)	Garlicky Artichoke Hearts (page 303)
THURSDAY	Crispy Bacon (page 120)	Mediterranean Mahi Mahi (leftover)	BBQ Pork Ribs (leftover)
	Plantain and Apple Fritter (leftover)	Fruit Salad (leftover)	Roasted Parsnips (page 325)
	Bacon-Braised Savoy Cabbage and Apple (leftover)	Perfect Steamed Vegetables (page 296)	Cran-Apple Coleslaw (leftover)
		Garlicky Artichoke Hearts (leftover)	Carrot-Ginger Soup (page 189) with bacon
FRIDAY	Superfood Smoothie (page 141)	Smoked Salmon and Mango Salsa Nori Wraps (page 175)	Mediterranean Mahi Mahi (leftover)
		Roasted Butternut Squash (leftover)	Roasted Parsnips (leftover)
		Cran-Apple Coleslaw (leftover)	Braised Greens (page 300)
			Carrot-Ginger Soup with bacon (leftover)

Week 3

Shopping List

Meat

- bacon (8 oz.)
- beef heart (3 lbs., ground preferred)
- ground beef (1 lb.)
- ground chicken or turkey (4 lbs.)
- ground lamb (1 lb.)
- ground pork (2 lbs.; or 1 lb. each ground pork and pork fat))
- lamb chops (2 lbs.)
- whole chickens (2, 4–6 lbs. each)

Seafood

- littleneck clams (4–5 lbs.)
- salmon (3–4 [6–8 oz.] fillets)
- whitefish (1½–2 lbs.)

Fruits

- apples (4–5)
- avocados (4–5)
- banana (1)
- Granny Smith apples (2)
- grapefruit (1)
- ingredients for your favorite fruit salad (for 3 meals)
- lemons (4)

Nonperishables

- black olives (4 oz.)
- ingredients for your favorite salad dressing (oil, vinegar, herbs, etc.)
- raisins (2 tablespoons)

Vegetables

- acorn squash (2 large)
- asparagus (1 lb.)
- basil (fresh)
- Brussels sprouts (1 lb.)
- cabbage or other veggies for fermenting (3 lbs.)
- carrots with greens (2 lbs.)
- cauliflower (2 heads)
- cilantro (fresh)
- dill (fresh)
- garlic (6–8 heads)
- kale (2 bunches)
- kohlrabi (½ cup)
- leeks (4)
- mint (fresh)
- mushrooms (any type, ½ lb.)
- mushrooms (wild, 1½ lbs.)
- onions (2)
- oregano (fresh)
- parsley (fresh)
- radishes (1 lb.)
- spaghetti squash (1 large or 2 small)
- spinach (2 cups)
- sweet potatoes (1 or 2)
- taro root (2 lbs.)
- tarragon (fresh)
- turnip (½ cup)
- zucchini (2 lbs.)
- greens for braising (for 4 meals)
- leafy greens plus add-ons for salads (for 4 meals)
- leafy greens and superfood add-ons for Superfood Smoothie (for 1 meal)
- seasonings for Cauliflower Rice (garlic, herbs, lemon, etc.)
- veggies for steaming (for 4 meals)

Pantry Items

- avocado oil
- Bone Broth (9 cups, or ingredients to make 1 batch—page 110)
- cinnamon (ground)
- coconut oil (extra-virgin)
- fish sauce
- garlic powder
- kuzu starch
- lard
- lemon juice (or additional fresh lemons to make your own)
- marjoram (dried)
- olive oil (extra-virgin)
- onion powder
- protein powder for Superfood Smoothie
- red wine (1 cup) or substitute (see page 85)
- rosemary (dried)
- sage (dried)
- salt (pink or gray)
- savory (dried)
- tallow, bacon fat, and/or duck fat
- thyme (dried)
- truffle salt (optional)
- white wine (½ cup, or additional broth and lemon juice)

Other

- casings for sausage (optional)
- sauerkraut (raw fermented, if not making your own)
- vegetable juice (8–16 oz., or veggies to make your own)

Plan Ahead

- Apple-Chicken Sausage for Vegetable Soup: Either precook sausage patties or stuff sausage into casings and then parboil; let cool and then freeze
- Applesauce
- Beef Heart Sausage: Either precook sausage patties or stuff sausage into casings and then parboil; let cool and then freeze
- Broth
- Kale Chips
- Maître D' "Butter"
- Poultry Seasoning for Roasted Chicken
- Salad Dressing
- Sauerkraut: Note that this needs to ferment, typically for a week
- Sweet Potato Chips

Meal Plan

	Breakfast	Lunch	Dinner
SATURDAY	Beef Heart Sausage (page 132)	Vegetable Soup with Chicken Sausage (page 194)	Greek-Inspired Lamb Chops (page 217)
	Applesauce (page 122)	Garden Salad (page 160)	Mashed Acorn Squash with Forty Cloves of Garlic (page 307)
	Perfect Steamed Vegetables (page 296)		Braised Greens (page 300)
	Sauerkraut (page 112)		Cauliflower Rice (page 298)
SUNDAY	Vegetable Soup with Chicken Sausage (leftover)	Greek-Inspired Lamb Chops (leftover)	Roasted Chicken (page 209)
	Garden Salad (page 160)	Mashed Acorn Squash with Forty Cloves of Garlic (leftover)	Whole Carrot "Tabouleh" (page 315)
		Braised Greens (page 300)	Mint Pesto Zucchini "Pasta" (page 310)
		Cauliflower Rice (leftover)	Roasted Radishes (page 322)
MONDAY	Beef Heart Sausage (leftover)	Steamed Clams (page 253)	Bacon-Braised Whitefish and Brussels (page 254)
	Cinnamon Broiled Grapefruit (page 143)	Mashed Acorn Squash with Forty Cloves of Garlic (leftover)	Garden Green Vichyssoise (page 188)
	Perfect Steamed Vegetables (page 296)	Mint Pesto Zucchini "Pasta" (leftover)	
	Sauerkraut (leftover)	Roasted Radishes (leftover)	
TUESDAY	Roasted Chicken (leftover)	Steamed Clams (leftover)	"Spaghetti" (page 224)
	Applesauce (leftover)	Sweet Potato Chips (page 168)	Fruit Salad (page 336)
	Perfect Steamed Vegetables (page 296)	Garden Green Vichyssoise (leftover)	Garden Salad (page 160)
	Sauerkraut (leftover)		
WEDNESDAY	Beef Heart Sausage (leftover) or Apple Chicken Sausage (leftover)	Roasted Chicken (leftover)	Salmon with Maître D' "Butter" (page 245)
	Garden Green Vichyssoise (leftover)	Fruit Salad (leftover)	Savory Roasted Taro (page 320)
		Kale Chips (page 166)	Braised Greens (page 300)
		Whole Carrot "Tabouleh" (leftover)	Wild Mushrooms and Tarragon (page 305)
THURSDAY	Superfood Smoothie (page 141)	Salmon with Maître D' "Butter" (leftover)	Bacon-Braised Whitefish and Brussels (leftover)
		Fruit Salad (leftover)	Wild Mushrooms and Tarragon (leftover)
		Kale Chips (leftover)	
		Easy Broiled Asparagus (page 306)	
FRIDAY	Beef Heart Sausage (leftover)	"Spaghetti" (leftover)	Roasted Chicken (leftover)
	Applesauce (leftover)	Sweet Potato Chips (leftover)	Savory Roasted Taro (leftover)
	Perfect Steamed Vegetables (page 296)	Garden Salad (page 160)	Braised Greens (page 300)
	Sauerkraut (leftover)		Easy Broiled Asparagus (leftover)

Week 4

Shopping List

Meat

- bacon (2½ lbs.)
- bison liver (1 lb.)
- ground beef (1 lb.)
- ground chicken or turkey (2–2½ lbs.)
- lamb chops (2 lbs.)
- pork roast (4–5 lbs.)
- steaks (2 [4–8 oz.])

Seafood

- salmon (4–6 [6–8 oz.] fillets)
- trout (3–4 [6–8 oz.] fillets)

Fruits

- apples (3)
- avocados (7)
- banana (1)
- berries, melon, or other fruit (1 cup for Bacon Fruit Cups)
- blood oranges (2 lbs.)
- cranberries (2 cups, fresh or frozen)
- lemons (3–4)
- limes (2–3)
- orange (1)

Nonperishables

- albacore tuna (1 [5 oz.] can)
- sardines (2 [4 oz.] cans)
- capers
- ingredients for your favorite salad dressing (oil, vinegar, herbs, etc.)

Vegetables

- arugula or mustard greens (6–10 cups)
- broccoflower (4 or 5 heads, enough for 8 cups of florets and stems)
- broccoli (2 lbs.)
- butternut squash (2 lbs.)
- cabbage or other veggies for fermenting (3 lbs.)
- cauliflower (2 heads)
- celery (1 head or heart)
- cilantro (fresh)
- garlic (3 heads)
- ginger root
- green onion (1)
- mint (fresh)
- onions (2)
- oregano (fresh)
- parsley (fresh)
- plantains (2–4 green)
- portobello mushroom caps (4–6)
- red onion (1)
- rhubarb (8 oz.)
- rosemary (fresh)
- sweet potatoes (2 lbs.)
- taro root (1 lb.)
- tarragon (fresh)
- thyme (fresh)
- zucchini (2 lbs.)
- greens for braising (for 1 meal)
- large lettuce leaves (such as romaine or butterleaf) for Tuna Salad Wraps
- leafy greens plus add-ons for salads (for 4 meals)
- leafy greens and superfood add-ons for Superfood Smoothie (for 2 meals)
- raw vegetables for dipping (2 meals)
- seasonings for Cauliflower Rice (garlic, herbs, lemon, etc.)
- starchy root vegetable for French Fries (1 lb.)
- veggies for steaming (for 4 meals)

Pantry Items

- avocado oil
- balsamic vinegar
- Bone Broth (4 cups, or ingredients to make ½ batch—page 110)
- cinnamon (ground)
- coconut aminos
- coconut oil (extra-virgin)
- coconut water vinegar
- cloves (ground)
- garlic powder
- lard
- lemon juice (or additional fresh lemons to make your own)
- lime juice (or additional fresh limes to make your own)
- mace
- maple syrup (grade B)
- olive oil (extra-virgin)
- onion powder
- oregano (dried)
- protein powder for Superfood Smoothie
- salt (pink or gray)
- tallow, bacon fat, and/or duck fat
- tarragon (dried)
- truffle salt (optional)
- turmeric (ground)
- white wine (½ cup) or more broth

Other

- casings for sausage (optional)
- pickles (raw fermented, or ingredients to make your own, page 114)
- sauerkraut (raw fermented, if not making your own)
- vegetable juice (16–32 oz., or veggies to make your own)

Plan Ahead

- Broth
- Green Tea and Garlic Pickles for Tuna Salad Wraps—or you can buy pickles if you prefer
- Plantain Chips or Crackers
- Rhubarb Chutney
- Salad Dressing
- Sauerkraut: Note that this needs to ferment, typically for a week
- Steak Spice

Meal Plan

	Breakfast	Lunch	Dinner
SATURDAY	Bacon Fruit Cups (page 136)	Bacon-Apple Chicken Burgers with Maple-Cranberry Sauce (page 222)	Teriyaki-Poached Trout (page 250)
	Garden Salad (page 160)	Roasted Butternut Squash (page 308)	Cauliflower Rice (page 298)
		Roasted Broccoflower (page 302)	Perfect Steamed Vegetables (page 296)
SUNDAY	Bacon-Apple Chicken Burgers with Maple Cranberry Sauce (leftover)	Tuna Salad Wrap (page 260)	Tarragon Roasted Pork (page 208)
	Roasted Broccoflower (leftover)	Plantain Chips (page 170) or Crackers (page 149)	Roasted Butternut Squash (leftover)
	Sauerkraut (page 112)	"Cream" of Broccoli Soup (page 183)	Braised Greens (page 300)
MONDAY	Superfood Smoothie (page 141)	Teriyaki-Poached Trout (leftover)	50/50/50 Burgers (page 289) with Portobello "Buns" (page 228)
		Cauliflower Rice (leftover)	French Fries (page 323)
		Garden Salad (page 160)	Guacamole (page 171)
			Raw Veggies
TUESDAY	Bacon-Apple Chicken Burgers with Maple Cranberry Sauce (leftover)	Tarragon Roasted Pork (leftover)	Simple Grilled Steak with Rhubarb Chutney (page 218)
	Roasted Butternut Squash (leftover)	Plantain Chips or Crackers (leftover)	Roasted Sweet Potato (page 313)
	Perfect Steamed Vegetables (page 296)	Garden Salad (page 160)	Perfect Steamed Vegetables (page 296)
WEDNESDAY	50/50/50 Burgers (leftover)	Tarragon Roasted Pork (leftover)	Lemon and Thyme Broiled Salmon with Blood Orange Salsa (page 242)
	Taro Hash (page 138)	French Fries (leftover)	Garden Salad (page 160)
	Sauerkraut (leftover)	Guacamole (leftover)	"Cream" of Broccoli Soup (leftover)
		Raw Veggies	
THURSDAY	Superfood Smoothie (page 141)	Sardine Salad (page 163)	Greek-Inspired Lamb Chops (page 217)
		Plantain Chips or Crackers (leftover)	Mint Pesto Zucchini "Pasta" (page 310)
			Roasted Sweet Potato (leftover)
FRIDAY	50/50/50 Burgers (leftover)	Greek-Inspired Lamb Chops (leftover)	Lemon and Thyme Broiled Salmon with Blood Orange Salsa (leftover)
	Taro Hash (leftover)	Mint Pesto Zucchini "Pasta" (leftover)	"Cream" of Broccoli Soup (leftover)
	Sauerkraut (leftover)	Roasted Sweet Potato (leftover)	Perfect Steamed Vegetables (page 296)

Week 5 (Low FODMAP)

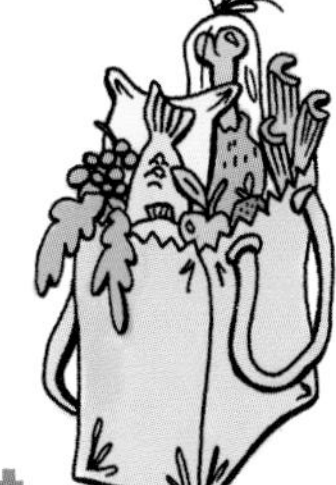

Shopping List

Meat
bacon (1 lb.)
beef heart (2 lbs.)
bison chuck roast (3–4 lbs.)
ground beef (4 lbs.)
ground pork (4 lbs.)
leg of lamb (4–6 lbs.)
liver (½ lb.)

Seafood
salmon (2–3 [6–8 oz.] fillets)
sea scallops (1 lb. frozen, or buy fresh midweek)
shrimp (1 lb.)
squid (1 lb.)

Nonperishables
bamboo shoots (2 [5 oz.] cans)
sardines (2 [4 oz.] cans)
water chestnuts (2 [5 oz.] cans)
ingredients for your favorite salad dressing (oil, vinegar, herbs, etc.)
kelp noodles (1 lb.)

Vegetables
arugula or mustard greens (6–10 cups)
baby bok choy (6–8 oz.)
bok choy (1 bunch)
butternut squash (2 lbs.)
cabbage or other veggies for fermenting (3 lbs.)
carrots (1½ lbs.)
celery (2 stalks)
cucumber (1 or 2, if making Tzatziki)
dill (fresh, if making Tzatziki)
ginger root
green garlic (2–3 stalks)
green onions (12–15)
kale (1 bunch)
leeks (2–3)
mint (fresh)
oyster mushrooms (4 oz.)
parsley (fresh)
parsnips (3 lbs.)
plantains (2–4 green)
rosemary (fresh)
sage (fresh)
shiitake mushrooms (3 fresh or dried)
spaghetti squash (3–4 lbs.)
tarragon (fresh)
thyme (fresh)
zucchini (2 lbs.)
greens for braising (for 5 meals)
leafy greens and superfood add-ons for Superfood Smoothie (for 1 meal)
leafy greens plus add-ons for salads (for 5 meals)
starchy root vegetable for French Fries (1 lb.)
veggies for steaming (for 6 meals)

Fruits
banana (1 green)
ingredients for your favorite fruit salad (for 2 meals)
lemons (2)

Pantry Items
arrowroot powder
bay leaves (dried)
Bone Broth (10½–12½ cups, or ingredients to make 1½ batches—page 110)
cloves (ground)
coconut oil (extra-virgin)
coconut water vinegar or white wine vinegar
fish sauce
lard
lemon juice (or fresh lemons to make your own)
mace (ground)
marjoram (dried)
olive oil (extra-virgin)
oregano (dried)
protein powder for Superfood Smoothie
red wine (½ cup) or more broth
rosemary (dried)
sage (dried)
salt (pink or gray)
savory (dried)
tallow, bacon fat, and/or duck fat
tapioca starch
thyme (dried)

Other
casings for sausage (optional)
coconut milk yogurt (½ cup, or ingredients to make your own—page 118; if making Tzatziki)
sauerkraut or other fermented veggies (raw fermented, if not making your own)
vegetable juice (8–16 oz., or veggies to make your own)

⚠ When following a low-FODMAP meal plan, remember to check recipes for FODMAP ALERT modifications.

Plan Ahead

- Broth
- Farmer's Sausage: Either precook sausage patties or stuff sausage into casings and then parboil; let cool and then freeze
- Kale Chips
- Plantain Crackers or Chips
- Salad Dressing
- Sauerkraut or other fermented veggies

Meal Plan

	Breakfast	Lunch	Dinner
SATURDAY	Farmer's Sausage (page 132)	Calamari with Tzatziki Sauce (page 258)	Rustic Bison Pot Roast (page 212)
	Braised Greens (page 300)	French Fries (page 323)	Perfect Steamed Vegetables (page 296)
	Sauerkraut or other fermented veggies (page 112)	Garden Salad (page 160)	
SUNDAY	Rustic Bison Pot Roast (leftover)	"Wonton" Soup (page 184)	Hidden Offal Swedish Meatballs (page 282)
	Perfect Steamed Vegetables (leftover)	Plantain Chips (page 170) or Crackers (page 149)	Zucchini Noodles (page 310)
		Kale Chips (page 166)	Garden Salad (page 160)
MONDAY	Hidden Offal Swedish Meatballs (leftover)	"Wonton" Soup (leftover)	Leg of Lamb with Mint Vinegar (page 206)
	Zucchini Noodles (leftover)	Garden Salad (page 160)	Roasted Butternut Squash (page 308)
	Kale Chips (leftover)		Braised Greens (page 300)
TUESDAY	Rustic Bison Pot Roast (leftover)	Calamari with Tzatziki Sauce (leftover)	Beef Heart "Chow Mein" (page 278)
	Roasted Butternut Squash (leftover)	French Fries (leftover)	Perfect Steamed Vegetables (page 296)
	Braised Greens (leftover)	Garden Salad (page 160)	
WEDNESDAY	Farmer's Sausage (leftover)	Hidden Offal Swedish Meatballs (leftover)	Leg of Lamb with Mint Vinegar (leftover)
	Roasted Butternut Squash (leftover)	Zucchini Noodles (leftover)	Roasted Parsnips (page 325)
	Perfect Steamed Vegetables (leftover)	Fruit Salad (page 336)	Braised Greens (page 300)
	Sauerkraut or other fermented veggies (leftover)		
THURSDAY	Farmer's Sausage (leftover)	Sardine Salad (page 163)	Asian-Inspired Salmon en Papillote (page 262)
	Roasted Parsnips (leftover)	Plantain Chips or Crackers (leftover)	Spaghetti Squash Noodles (page 224)
	Braised Greens (leftover)	Fruit Salad (leftover)	Perfect Steamed Vegetables (page 296)
	Sauerkraut or other fermented veggies (leftover)		
FRIDAY	Superfood Smoothie (page 141)	Bacon-Wrapped Scallops (page 155)	Leg of Lamb with Mint Vinegar (leftover)
		Plantain Chips or Crackers (leftover)	Spaghetti Squash Noodles (leftover)
		Perfect Steamed Vegetables (leftover)	Garden Salad (page 160)
		Kale Chips (leftover)	

Week 6 (Low FODMAP)

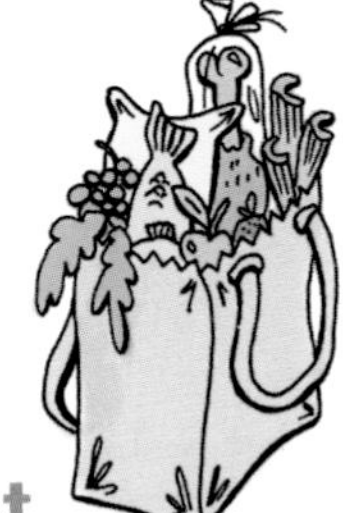

Shopping List

Meat
bacon (4 slices)
ground pork (6 lbs.)
oxtail (2 lbs.)
pork chops (2 lbs.)
steaks (3–4, 4–8 oz. each)

Seafood
mahi mahi (4–6 [6 oz.] fillets)
mixed shellfish (1 lb.)
salmon (5–6 [6–8 oz.] fillets)
whitefish (3–4 [6–8 oz.] fillets)

Fruits
banana (1 green)
ingredients for your favorite fruit salad (for 4 meals)
lemons (5)
limes (2–3)
orange (1) or orange juice (¼ cup)

⚠ When following a low-FODMAP meal plan, remember to check recipes for FODMAP ALERT modifications.

Vegetables
arugula or mustard greens (6–10 cups)
butternut squash (1 lb.)
cabbage or other veggies for fermenting (3 lbs.)
carrots (1 lb.)
celery (2 stalks)
cilantro (fresh)
fiddlehead ferns (3 cups)
ginger root
green garlic (1–2 stalks)
green onions (5–6)
kabocha squash (1 large)
kale (1 bunch)
kohlrabi (2 lbs.)
leeks (3 lbs.)
mixed greens (12 cups collards, mustard greens, turnip greens, etc.)
oregano (fresh)
parsley (fresh)
parsnips (2 lbs.)
plantains (2–4 green)
radishes (8 oz.)
rosemary (fresh)
sage (fresh)
taro root (3 lbs.)
tarragon (fresh)
thyme (fresh)
turmeric root
turnips (2 lbs.)
zucchini (1 medium)
greens for braising (for 6 meals)
leafy greens and superfood add-ons for Superfood Smoothie (for 1 meal)
leafy greens plus add-ons for salads (for 6 meals)
veggies for steaming (for 5 meals)

Nonperishables
capers
ingredients for your favorite salad dressing (oil, vinegar, herbs, etc.)
olives (whole green or black, ¾ cup)
sardines (2 [4 oz.] cans)

Pantry Items
avocado oil
Bone Broth (10 cups and 6 cups fish, or ingredients to make 1 batch of each—page 110)
cloves (whole)
cinnamon (ground)
coconut aminos
coconut oil (extra-virgin)
coconut water vinegar
fish sauce
ginger (ground)
lard
lemon juice (or additional fresh lemons to make your own)
mace
marjoram (dried)
olive oil (extra-virgin)
oregano (dried)
pomegranate molasses
protein powder for Superfood Smoothie
red palm oil
red wine (1 cup) or more broth
rosemary (dried)
sage (dried)
salt (pink or gray)
savory (dried)
tallow, bacon fat, and/or duck fat
tarragon (dried)
thyme (dried)
truffle salt
turmeric (ground)

Other
casings for sausage (optional)
sauerkraut or other fermented veggies (raw fermented, if not making your own)
vegetable juice (8–16 oz., or veggies to make your own)

Plan Ahead

- Broth
- Breakfast Sausage: Either precook sausage patties or stuff sausage into casings and then parboil; let cool and then freeze
- Herbes de Provence for mahi mahi
- Kale Chips
- Plantain Chips or Crackers
- Salad Dressing
- Sauerkraut or other fermented veggies

Meal Plan

	Breakfast	Lunch	Dinner
SATURDAY	Breakfast Sausage (page 132)	Pork Pad Thai (page 234)	Simple Baked Whitefish (page 244)
	Braised Greens (page 300)	Perfect Steamed Vegetables (page 296)	Savory Roasted Taro (page 320)
	Sauerkraut or other fermented veggies (page 112)		Garden Salad (page 160)
	Fruit Salad (page 336)		Fiddleheads (page 312)
SUNDAY	Pork Pad Thai (leftover)	Pomegranate Molasses–Glazed Salmon (page 239)	Mediterranean Mahi Mahi (page 246)
	Braised Greens (page 300)	Carrot-Ginger Soup, butternut squash variation (page 189)	Perfect Steamed Vegetables (page 296)
	Sauerkraut or other fermented veggies (leftover)	Garden Salad (page 160)	Kale Chips (page 166)
		Fiddleheads (leftover)	
MONDAY	Breakfast Sausage (leftover)	Sardine Salad (page 163)	Seafood and Leek Soup (page 190)
	Braised Greens (page 300)	Savory Roasted Taro (leftover)	Plantain Chips (page 170) or Crackers (page 149)
	Sauerkraut or other fermented veggies (leftover)	Perfect Steamed Vegetables (page 296)	Garden Salad (page 160)
TUESDAY	Superfood Smoothie (page 141)	Simple Baked Whitefish (leftover)	Lemon and Thyme Broiled Pork Chops (page 230)
		Carrot-Ginger Soup, butternut squash variation (leftover)	Oxtail-Braised Greens (page 284)
		Braised Greens (page 300)	Roasted Parsnips (page 325)
WEDNESDAY	Breakfast Sausage (leftover)	Pomegranate Molasses–Glazed Salmon (leftover)	Simple Grilled Steak (page 218)
	Roasted Parsnips (leftover)	Fruit Salad (leftover)	Spiced Kabocha Squash (page 324)
	Braised Greens (page 300)	Perfect Steamed Vegetables (page 296)	Garden Salad (page 160)
	Kale Chips (page 166)		
THURSDAY	Lemon and Thyme Broiled Pork Chops (leftover)	Seafood and Leek Soup (leftover)	Mediterranean Mahi Mahi (leftover)
	Oxtail-Braised Greens (leftover)	Plantain Chips or Crackers (leftover)	Perfect Steamed Vegetables (page 296)
	Fruit Salad (leftover)	Garden Salad (page 160)	Kale Chips (leftover)
FRIDAY	Breakfast Sausage (leftover)	Simple Grilled Steak (leftover)	Lemon and Thyme Broiled Pork Chops (leftover)
	Plantain Chips or Crackers (leftover)	Fruit Salad (leftover)	Oxtail-Braised Greens (leftover)
	Roasted Parsnips (leftover)	Garden Salad (page 160)	Spiced Kabocha Squash (leftover)
	Braised Greens (page 300)		Sauerkraut or other fermented veggies (leftover)

Reading Labels

Trying to figure out whether a product is Paleo Approach friendly? It helps to know the many aliases that some pervasive foods go by.

☒ Gluten in Foods

Avoiding gluten can take some effort. Ingredients derived from wheat and other gluten-containing grains are found in a vast array of packaged and manufactured foods, but also in some ingredients not normally considered to be processed foods. The following list includes some of these hidden—and not-so-hidden—sources of gluten.

- Asian rice paper
- atta flour
- bacon (check ingredients)
- barley
- barley grass
- barley malt
- beer (unless gluten-free)
- bleached or unbleached flour
- bran
- bread flour
- breading
- brewer's yeast
- bulgur
- coating mixes
- communion wafers
- condiments
- couscous
- croutons
- dinkle (spelt)
- durum
- einkorn
- emmer (durum wheat)
- farina
- farro (called emmer wheat except in Italy)
- food starch
- French fries
- fu (a dried form of gluten)
- gliadin
- glue used on some envelopes, stamps, and labels
- gluten peptides
- glutenin
- graham
- gravies
- hydrolyzed wheat gluten
- hydrolyzed wheat protein
- ice cream (may contain flour as an anticrystallizing agent)
- imitation fish
- kamut
- lunch meats
- maida (Indian wheat flour)
- malt
- malt vinegar
- marinades
- matzah (aka matso)
- medications (prescription or over the counter)
- mir (a wheat and rye cross)
- nutritional and herbal supplements
- oats
- panko (bread crumbs)
- pilafs (containing orzo)
- prepared foods
- processed cereals (often contain barley malt)
- rye
- salad dressings
- sauces
- seitan
- self-basting poultry
- semolina
- soup bases and bouillon
- soy or rice drinks (barley malt or malt enzymes may be used during manufacturing)
- soy sauce (unless wheat-free)
- spelt
- spice mixes (often contain wheat as an anticaking agent, filler, or thickening agent)
- starch
- stuffings
- syrups
- thickeners
- triticale
- wheat
- wheat bran
- wheat germ
- wheat grass
- wheat starch

Common Sources of Gluten/Wheat Contamination:

- art supplies: paint, clay, glue, and play dough (can be transferred to the mouth if hands aren't washed)
- flour dust
- foods sold in bulk (often contaminated by scoops used in other bins and by flour dust)
- grills, pans, cutting boards, utensils, toasters and other appliances, and oils that have been used for preparing foods containing gluten
- household products (may be transferred to the lips and ingested)
- knives (double-dipping knives into food spreads after spreading on bread can leave gluten-containing crumbs)
- millet, white rice flour, buckwheat flour, sorghum flour, and soy flour (commonly contaminated)
- personal care products, especially shampoos (may be transferred to the lips and ingested)
- powder coating inside rubber gloves (may be derived from wheat)
- waxes or resins on fruits and vegetables

☒ Gluten Cross-Reactors

Some foods have a higher likelihood of cross-reacting with gluten, meaning that the antibodies your body makes against gluten recognize similar proteins in these foods, so your body sees these foods and gluten as being one and the same. While gluten sensitivity doesn't automatically mean that you are sensitive to all or any of these foods, it's prudent to be cautious of them:

- brewer's/baker's/nutritional yeast
- corn
- dairy proteins (casein, casomorphin, butyrophilin, whey)
- instant coffee
- millet
- oats
- potatoes
- rice
- sorghum

☒ Corn in Foods

Ingredients derived from corn can be found in the vast majority of packaged and manufactured foods. If you are very sensitive to corn-derived products, avoiding these pervasive ingredients can be overwhelming. However, avoiding processed foods in general will make a huge difference. You may or may not need to go to the extent of avoiding all traces of corn-derived ingredients (in medications, for example); however, being aware of where corn exposure may be sneaking into your life will help you identify whether it is a problem. The following list includes some hidden—and not-so-hidden—sources of corn.

Ingredients Derived from Corn

- acetic acid
- alcohol
- alpha tocopherol
- artificial flavorings
- artificial sweeteners
- ascorbates
- ascorbic acid
- aspartame
- astaxanthin
- baking powder
- barley malt
- bleached flour
- blended sugar
- brown sugar
- calcium citrate
- calcium fumarate
- calcium gluconate
- calcium lactate
- calcium magnesium acetate (CMA)
- calcium stearate
- calcium stearoyl lactylate
- caramel and caramel color
- carboxymethylcellulose sodium
- cellulose, microcrystalline
- cellulose, powdered
- cetearyl glucoside
- choline chloride
- citric acid
- citrus cloud emulsion (CCS)
- cocoglycerides
- confectioners' sugar
- corn oil
- corn sweetener
- corn sugar
- corn syrup
- corn syrup solids
- cornmeal
- cornstarch
- crosscarmellose sodium
- crystalline dextrose
- crystalline fructose
- cyclodextrin
- datum (dough conditioner)
- decyl glucoside
- decyl polyglucose
- dextrin
- dextrose (also found in IV solutions)
- dextrose anything (such as monohydrate or anhydrous)
- d-Gluconic acid
- distilled white vinegar
- drying agent
- erythorbic acid
- erythritol
- ethanol
- Ethocel 20
- ethylcellulose
- ethyl acetate
- ethyl alcohol
- ethyl lactate
- ethyl maltol
- ethylene
- Fibersol-2
- flavorings
- food starch
- fructose
- fruit juice concentrate
- fumaric acid
- germ/germ meal
- gluconate
- gluconic acid
- glucono delta-lactone
- gluconolactone
- glucosamine
- glucose
- glucose syrup (also found in IV solutions)
- glutamate
- gluten
- gluten feed/meal
- glycerides
- glycerin
- glycerol
- golden syrup
- grits
- hominy
- honey
- hydrolyzed corn
- hydrolyzed corn protein
- hydrolyzed vegetable protein
- hydroxypropyl methylcellulose
- hydroxypropyl methylcellulose phthalate (HPMCP)
- inositol
- invert syrup or sugar
- lactate
- lactic acid
- lauryl glucoside
- lecithin
- linoleic acid
- lysine
- magnesium fumarate
- maize
- malic acid
- malonic acid
- malt syrup from corn
- malt, malt extract
- maltitol
- maltodextrin
- maltol
- maltose
- mannitol
- margarine
- methyl gluceth
- methyl glucose
- methyl glucoside
- methylcellulose
- modified cellulose gum
- modified cornstarch
- modified food starch
- molasses (corn syrup may be present; check label)
- mono- and diglycerides
- monosodium glutamate (MSG)
- monostearate
- natural flavorings
- olestra/Olean
- polenta
- polydextrose
- polylactic acid (PLA)
- polysorbates (e.g., Polysorbate 80)
- polyvinyl acetate
- potassium citrate
- potassium fumarate
- potassium gluconate
- powdered sugar
- pregelatinized starch
- propionic acid
- propylene glycol
- saccharin
- salt (iodized)
- semolina (unless from wheat)
- simethicone
- sodium carboxymethylcellulose
- sodium citrate
- sodium erythorbate
- sodium fumarate
- sodium lactate
- sodium starch glycolate
- sodium stearoyl fumarate
- sorbate
- sorbic acid
- sorbitan
- sorbitan monooleate
- sorbitan trioleate
- sorbitol
- sorghum (syrup and/or grain may be mixed with corn)
- Splenda (artificial sweetener)
- starch
- stearic acid
- stearoyls
- sucralose (artificial sweetener)
- sucrose
- sugar
- talc
- threonine
- tocopherol (vitamin E)
- treacle
- triethyl citrate
- unmodified starch
- vanilla, natural flavoring
- vanilla, pure or extract
- vanillin
- vinegar, distilled white
- vinyl acetate
- vitamin C
- vitamin E
- vitamin supplements
- xanthan gum
- xylitol
- yeast
- zea mays
- zein

☒ Soy in Foods

Soy is another ingredient that has permeated the food supply. Soy lecithin and soy protein are especially common ingredients to find in packaged goods. The following list includes foods that are derived from soy:

- bean curd
- bean sprouts
- chocolate (soy lecithin may be used in manufacturing)
- edamame (fresh soybeans)
- hydrolyzed soy protein (HSP)
- kinako
- miso (fermented soybean paste)
- mono- and diglycerides
- monosodium glutamate (MSG)
- natto
- nimame
- okara
- shoyu
- soy albumin
- soy cheese
- soy fiber
- soy flour
- soy grits
- soy ice cream
- soy lecithin
- soy meal
- soy nuts
- soy pasta
- soy protein (concentrate, hydrolyzed, isolate)
- soy sauce
- soy sprouts
- soy yogurt
- soya
- soybean (curds, granules)
- soybean oil
- soymilk
- tamari
- tempeh
- teriyaki sauce
- textured vegetable protein (TVP)
- tofu (dofu, kori-dofu)
- yuba

Potentially Cross-Contaminated Foods Must Be Labeled:

- "may contain soy"
- "produced on shared equipment with soy"
- "produced in a facility that also processes soy"

Products That Commonly Contain Soy

- Asian cuisine (Chinese, Korean, Japanese, Thai)
- baked goods
- baking mixes
- bouillon cubes
- candy
- cereal
- chicken (raw or cooked) processed with chicken broth
- chicken broth
- deli meats
- energy bars
- imitation dairy foods, such as soymilk, vegan cheese, and vegan ice cream
- infant formula
- margarine
- mayonnaise
- meat products with fillers; for example, burgers and sausages
- nutrition bars
- nutrition supplements (vitamins)
- peanut butter and peanut butter substitutes
- protein powders
- sauces, gravies, and soups
- smoothies
- vegetable broth
- vegetarian meat substitutes (veggie burgers, imitation chicken patties, imitation lunch meats, imitation bacon bits)
- waxes or horticultural oils on fruits

☒ Sugar in Foods

When you are reading food labels, it is helpful to know how to decipher which ingredients are sugar. While most of them are refined, some are unrefined (which typically means that the sugar retains some minerals). It is also common for manufactured products to contain more than one form of sugar. The following ingredients are all forms of sugar:

- agave
- agave nectar
- barley malt
- barley malt syrup
- beet sugar
- brown rice syrup
- brown sugar
- cane crystals
- cane juice
- cane sugar
- caramel
- coconut sugar
- corn sweetener
- corn syrup
- corn syrup solids
- crystalline fructose
- date sugar
- dehydrated cane juice
- demerara sugar
- dextrin
- dextrose
- diastatic malt
- evaporated cane juice
- fructose
- fruit juice
- fruit juice concentrate
- galactose
- glucose
- glucose solids
- golden syrup
- high-fructose corn syrup
- honey
- inulin
- invert sugar
- jaggery
- lactose
- malt syrup
- maltodextrin
- maltose
- maple syrup
- molasses
- monk fruit (luo han guo)
- muscovado sugar
- palm sugar
- panela
- panocha
- rapadura
- raw cane sugar
- raw sugar
- refined sugar
- rice bran syrup
- rice syrup
- saccharose
- sorghum
- sorghum syrup
- sucanat
- sucrose
- syrup
- treacle
- turbinado sugar
- yacon syrup

☒ Dairy in Foods

Dairy ingredients are more and more commonly used in manufactured and prepackaged foods. The following ingredients found on a label indicate the presence of milk protein.

- milk — acidophilus milk, buttermilk, buttermilk blend, buttermilk solids, cultured milk, condensed milk, dried milk, dry milk solids (DMS), evaporated milk, fat-free milk, fully cream milk powder, goat's milk, Lactaid milk, lactose-free milk, low-fat milk, malted milk, milk derivative, milk powder, milk protein, milk solids, milk solid pastes, nonfat dry milk, nonfat milk, nonfat milk solids, pasteurized milk, powdered milk, sheep's milk, skim milk, skim milk powder, sour milk, sour milk solids, sweet cream buttermilk powder, sweetened condensed milk, sweetened condensed skim milk, whole milk, 1% milk, 2% milk
- butter — artificial butter, artificial butter flavor, butter extract, butter fat, butter flavored oil, butter solids, dairy butter, natural butter, natural butter flavor, whipped butter
- casein & caseinates — ammonium caseinate, calcium caseinate, hydrolyzed casein, iron caseinate magnesium caseinate, potassium caseinate, sodium caseinate, zinc caseinate
- cheese — cheese flavor (artificial and natural), cheese food, cottage cheese, cream cheese, imitation cheese, vegetarian cheeses with casein
- cream, whipped cream
- curds
- custard
- dairy product solids
- galactose
- ghee (cultured ghee may be OK)
- half & half
- hydrolysates — casein hydrolysate, milk protein hydrolysate, protein hydrolysate, whey hydrolysate, whey protein hydrolysate
- ice cream, ice milk, sherbet
- lactalbumin, lactalbumin phosphate
- lactate solids
- lactic yeast
- lactitol monohydrate
- lactoglobulin
- lactose
- lactulose
- milk fat, anhydrous milk fat
- nisin preparation
- nougat
- pudding
- quark
- recaldent
- rennet, rennet casein
- Simplesse (fat replacer)
- sour cream, sour cream solids, imitation sour cream
- whey — acid whey, cured whey, delactosed whey, demineralized whey, hydrolyzed whey, powdered whey, reduced mineral whey, sweet dairy whey, whey powder, whey protein, whey protein concentrate, whey solids
- yogurt (regular or frozen), yogurt powder

May contain milk:

- caramel flavoring
- flavoring
- high-protein flour
- lactic acid
- lactic acid starter culture
- natural flavoring

"Nondairy" products may contain casein. Foods covered by the FDA labeling laws that contain milk must be labeled "contains milk"; however, prescription and over-the-counter medications are exempt.